Lippincott's Illustrated 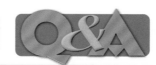 Review of

Histology

Illustrated Interactive Q & A

Guiyun Zhang, MD, PhD

Assistant Professor
Department of Pathology, Anatomy and Cell Biology
Jefferson Medical College
Thomas Jefferson University
Philadelphia, Pennsylvania

Bruce A. Fenderson, PhD

Professor
Department of Pathology, Anatomy and Cell Biology
Jefferson Medical College
Thomas Jefferson University
Philadelphia, Pennsylvania

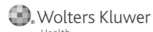 Wolters Kluwer
Health

Philadelphia • Baltimore • New York • London
Buenos Aires • Hong Kong • Sydney • Tokyo

Acquisitions Editor: Crystal Taylor
Product Manager: Amy Weintraub
Production Project Manager: Marian A. Bellus
Manufacturing Manager: Margie Orzech
Designer: Doug Smock
Compositor: SPi Global

Two Commerce Square
2001 Market Street
Philadelphia, PA 19103 USA
LWW.com

Printed in China

Library of Congress Cataloging-in-Publication Data
Zhang, Guiyun, author.
  Lippincott's illustrated Q & A review of histology / Guiyun Zhang, Bruce A. Fenderson.
     p. ; cm.
  Illustrated Q & A review of histology
  Includes index.
  ISBN 978-1-4511-8830-1
 I. Fenderson, Bruce A., author. II. Title. III. Title: Illustrated Q & A review of histology.
  [DNLM: 1. Histology—Examination Questions. QS 518.2]
  QM32
  611.0076—dc23

                                                                                      2013051149

To purchase additional copies of this book, call our customer service department at (800) 638-3030 or fax orders to (301) 223-2320. International customers should call (301) 223-2300.

Visit Lippincott Williams & Wilkins on the Internet: http://www.LWW.com. Lippincott Williams & Wilkins customer service representatives are available from 8:30 am to 6:00 pm, EST.

To my husband, Biao Zuo, and my son, Ran Zuo,
whose love, humor, and unconditional support have accompanied me
on my academic path and made this project most enjoyable;

To all of my students,
whose excitement and passion for learning provided
great initial stimulation for this project.

—Guiyun—

To my parents, Douglas and Joyce,
who shared their time and love, showed me the joy of learning,
encouraged me to read books and practice my violin,
clarified the difference between playing notes and making music,
emphasized the virtues of honesty and hard work,
taught me by example, and set me on a good path in life.

—Bruce—

Reviewers

Thomas Erickson
University of North Dakota School of Medicine
and Health Sciences
Grand Forks, ND

Adam Burch
College of Osteopathic Medicine of the
Pacific-Northwest
Western University of Health Sciences
Lebanon, OR

Marielle Kulling
Michigan State University College of
Osteopathic Medicine
Lansing, MI

Tyler Barnes
Mercer University School of Medicine
Savannah, GA

Preface

Lippincott's Illustrated Q&A Review of Histology presents the key concepts of modern tissue structure and function in the form of clinical vignette-style questions. Using the format of the National Board of Medical Examiners (NBME), the questions address the major topics in histology and cell biology presented in primary textbooks and atlases such as (1) Ross & Pawlina: *Histology: A Text and Atlas*; (2) Mescher: *Junqueira's Basic Histology*; (3) Gartner & Hiatt: *Color Atlas of Histology*; (4) Cui: *Atlas of Histology with Functional and Clinical Correlations*; and (5) Eroschenko: *diFiore's Atlas of Histology*. In addition to being a learning companion to these excellent textbooks, our illustrated questions and answers will serve as a stand-alone resource for self-assessment and board review.

The questions are prepared at a level appropriate for all preclinical basic science students. They provide a roadmap for students learning histology and pathology and preparing for the United States Medical Licensing Examination (USMLE). Students in the allied health sciences (e.g., nursing and physician assistant programs) will also find considerable didactic value in clinical vignette-style questions. Clinical vignette-style questions strengthen problem-solving skills and simulate the practice of medicine.

This book is also intended for undergraduate students of cellular and developmental biology. Histology is the science of biological design at the cellular and tissue level of complexity. Mastery of this body of knowledge enables students to evaluate normal tissue differentiation and provides a foundation for basic research in cell biology. The questions and answers in this book address core concepts of form and function. They are suitable for all students of biology and do not assume prior training in pathology or medicine. From this perspective, the clinical vignettes provide a human context for basic science.

Key features of this illustrated histology text include

- Multiple choice questions that follow the USMLE template. Each vignette is followed by a question stem that addresses a key concept in cell biology/histology.
- Answer choices appear homogeneous and are listed alphabetically to avoid unintended cueing.
- Explanations are linked to the clinical vignettes and address key concepts. Incorrect answers are explained in context.
- Over 480 full-color images illustrate important histologic features and highlight the complexity of life.
- Tissues with similar histological features are compared, providing a challenging comprehensive review.
- Side-by-side comparisons of normal tissue and histopathology provide a bridge to clinical problem solving and diagnostic pathology.

We hope that this illustrated review of histology will help students appreciate the complexity and beauty of human form and function. We also hope that our selection of images and questions will help future generations of health professionals think critically and make informed decisions. One way that students can practice critical thinking is to formulate their own questions concerning tissue organization and mechanisms of disease. We are mindful of the words of James Thurber, who penned, "It is better to know some of the questions than all of the answers." We wish our students success in their life-long learning adventure. *Have fun with your basic science training and never stop learning.*

Guiyun Zhang
Bruce A. Fenderson

Acknowledgments

We gratefully acknowledge the staff at Lippincott Williams & Wilkins. We are particularly indebted to Catherine Noonan, Stephanie Roulias, and Amy Weintraub for expert help with manuscript preparation. The contributions of the editors and authors of *Lippincott's Illustrated Q&A Review of Rubin's Pathology*, 2nd edition; *Rubin's Pathology: Clinicopathologic Foundations of Medicine*, 6th edition; *Atlas of Histology with Functional and Clinical Correlations*; and *Color Atlas of Histology with Functional and Clinical Correlations* were invaluable in the preparation of this text.

We are deeply indebted to the authors of the University of Iowa Virtual Slide Box and the Jefferson Medical College Virtual Slide Box for their permission to create static images of digital slides. We are indebted to our many colleagues: William Kocher (Cooper Medical School of Rowan University) for sharing his concept of presenting side-by-side comparisons of normal tissue and histopathology that are featured in Chapter 21; Gyorgy Hajnoczky and David Weaver (Thomas Jefferson University, Department of Pathology, Anatomy and Cell Biology) for providing beautiful fluorescent images of intracellular organelles that appear on the book cover and in Chapter 1; Fred Dee (University of Iowa, Department of Pathology), David Birk (University of South Florida, Department of Molecular Pharmacology & Physiology), and Robert Ogilvie (Medical University of South Carolina) for permission to create digital snapshots of histology slides; Emanuel Rubin (Thomas Jefferson University, Department of Pathology) for permission to create digital snapshots of pathology slides; Stephen Peiper (Chair, Department of Pathology, Anatomy and Cell Biology, Thomas Jefferson University) for providing an excellent environment for pursuing scholarship in medical education; Fred Gorstein and Richard Schmidt (Thomas Jefferson University, Department of Pathology, Anatomy and Cell Biology) and Jennifer Fisher (Rowan University, School of Osteopathic Medicine) for critical comments on the manuscript; Mitch Eddy (National Institute of Environmental Health Sciences, Laboratory of Reproductive and Developmental Toxicology) for help with images of developing mouse embryos; Ashlie Burkart and Alina Dulau Floria (Thomas Jefferson University, Department of Pathology, Anatomy and Cell Biology) for providing examples of histopathology; and MBF Bioscience for permission to use Biolucida, their digital slide-viewing software.

Contents

Chapter 1

Cell Biology

QUESTIONS

Select the single best answer.

1 You are investigating maternal factors that regulate the cell cycle during early development. A mouse embryo is flushed from the uterine tube, treated with acid Tyrode solution to remove its zona pellucida, and examined by phase microscopy (shown in the image). The embryo exhibits a cleavage furrow and appears to be undergoing cytokinesis. These events take place during what phase of mitosis?

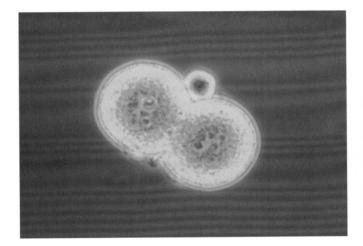

(A) Anaphase
(B) Interphase
(C) Metaphase
(D) Prophase
(E) Telophase

2 What intracellular protein complex links microtubules of the spindle apparatus to sister chromatids during mitosis and meiosis?

(A) Astral fibers
(B) Centrioles
(C) Centromere
(D) Centrosome
(E) Kinetochore

3 As part of your research, you examine integral membrane proteins in cleavage-stage mouse embryos using fluorescence microscopy (shown in the image). A pulse of high-intensity UV light is directed at a small patch on the surface of one blastomere, thereby causing an immediate loss of fluorescence emission (photobleaching). Over the next 10 minutes, fluorescence emission from this patch of membrane recovers. Which of the following cellular properties/processes best explains these experimental findings?

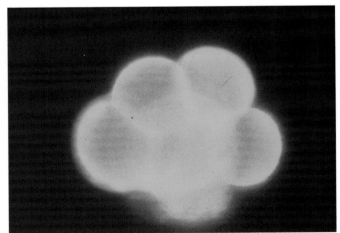

(A) Lipid raft assembly
(B) Membrane fluidity
(C) Patching and capping
(D) Protein trafficking
(E) Receptor-mediated endocytosis

1

4 You are studying cell migration during embryonic development. Neural tubes are harvested from post-implantation mouse embryos and placed in culture on plastic dishes coated with fibronectin. Time-lapse imaging reveals neural crest cells migrating away from the explanted tissue. The cells are observed to undergo continuous changes in cell shape, including the formation and retraction of lamellipodia. What protein is the principal mediator of membrane ruffling and locomotion in these cultured cells?

(A) Actin
(B) Desmin
(C) Lamin
(D) Tubulin
(E) Vimentin

5 A skin biopsy is examined at a double-headed microscope. The surgical pathologist directs your attention to waxy/lipid material filling the cytoplasm of secretory cells forming a sebaceous gland (shown in the image). Secretion of this waxy material to the pilosebaceous canal involves programmed cell death (apoptosis). Which of the following cytologic features provides evidence of apoptosis in this gland?

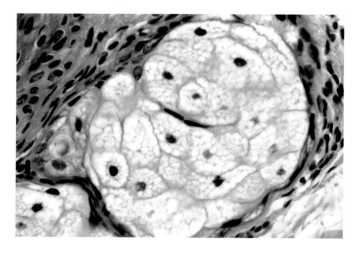

(A) Aggregation of intermediate filaments
(B) Disaggregation of polyribosomes
(C) Membrane blebs
(D) Mitochondrial swelling
(E) Nuclear pyknosis

6 A sample of adrenal cortex obtained at autopsy is fixed with formalin, embedded in paraffin, sectioned at 6 μm, stained with H&E, and examined by light microscopy (shown in the image). Cells of the zona fasciculata appear washed out and "spongy" due to an accumulation of cholesterol and other precursors for steroid hormone biosynthesis. Electron microscopic examination of these "steroid factory" cells would be expected to show an abundance of which of the following organelles?

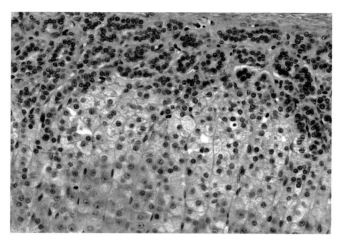

(A) Autophagic vacuoles
(B) Dense-core secretory granules
(C) Golgi apparatus
(D) Rough endoplasmic reticulum
(E) Smooth endoplasmic reticulum

7 A portion of the small intestine is collected at autopsy, and sections are stained with periodic acid–Schiff (PAS) and counterstained with hematoxylin. The mucosa of the intestine is examined by light microscopy (shown in the image). PAS is particularly useful for identifying which of the following biological materials?

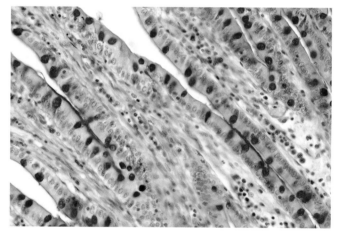

(A) Collagens
(B) Lipids
(C) Nucleic acids
(D) Proteins
(E) Sugars

8 You are asked to lead a seminar on intracellular protein trafficking. What organelle provides a microenvironment for the posttranslational modification and sorting of membrane and secretory proteins?

(A) Golgi apparatus
(B) Lysosome
(C) Peroxisome
(D) Plasma membrane
(E) Smooth endoplasmic reticulum

9 Hematopoietic stem cells are cultured in vitro at 37°C in the presence of recombinant erythropoietin. A photomicrograph of a typical "burst-forming unit" committed to the erythrocyte pathway of differentiation is shown in the image. Which of the following histochemical stains can be used as a "vital dye" to distinguish viable from nonviable cells in your cell culture?

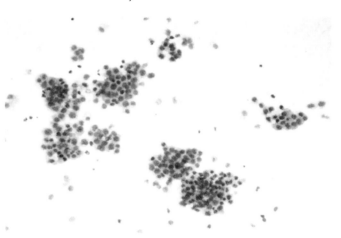

(A) Aldehyde fuchsin
(B) Hematoxylin and eosin
(C) Luxol fast blue/cresyl violet
(D) Periodic acid–Schiff
(E) Trypan blue

10 Hepatocytes in a liver biopsy are examined by electron microscopy. The parallel lines with knob-like features (arrows, shown in the image) represent which of the following intracellular organelles?

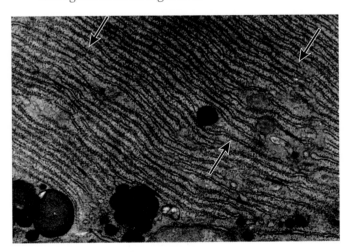

(A) Endoplasmic reticulum
(B) Golgi apparatus
(C) Mitochondria
(D) Nucleus
(E) Peroxisomes

11 A small muscular artery is examined in the pathology department. Smooth muscle fibers in the tunica media appear red, whereas collagen bundles in the tunica adventitia appear blue (shown in the image). This slide was most likely colored using which of the following histochemical stains?

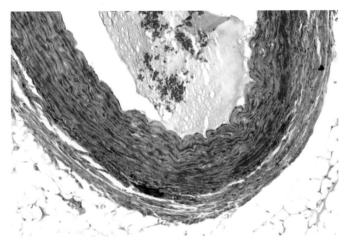

(A) Aldehyde fuchsin
(B) Hematoxylin and eosin
(C) Luxol fast blue/cresyl violet
(D) Masson trichrome
(E) Periodic acid–Schiff

12 A digital slide of a sympathetic chain ganglion is examined in the histology laboratory. Large multipolar neurons are surrounded by nerve fibers and connective tissue (shown in the image). Identify the dark basophilic region within the nucleus of these ganglion cells.

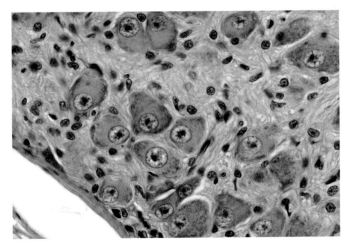

(A) Basal body
(B) Centrosome
(C) Golgi apparatus
(D) Nucleolus
(E) Peroxisome

13 A spinal cord smear preparation is obtained at autopsy and stained with Luxol fast blue/cresyl violet. The large octopus-like cells on this slide are multipolar motor neurons (shown in the image). What protein forms intracellular tracts that deliver organelles and vesicles to distant nerve terminals via anterograde axonal transport?

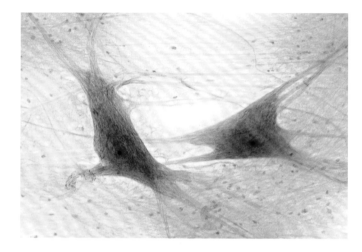

(A) Actin
(B) Clathrin
(C) Lamin
(D) Tubulin
(E) Ubiquitin

14 The motor neurons described in Question 13 are labeled by immunocytochemistry using antibodies directed against a neuron-specific protein that helps maintain the shape of dendrites and axons. This structural protein forms which of the following intracellular organelles?
(A) Endoplasmic reticulum
(B) Intermediate filaments
(C) Microfilaments
(D) Microtubules
(E) Plasma membrane

15 A soft tissue biopsy is examined in the pathology department. Normal adipocytes are examined at high magnification (shown in the image). The clear space that has pushed the cytoplasm and nucleus to the periphery of these cells is best described by which of the following terms?

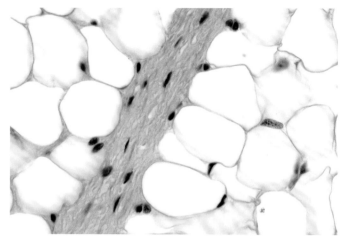

(A) Endosome
(B) Granule
(C) Inclusion
(D) Vacuole
(E) Vesicle

16 You are studying the role of mitochondrial dysfunction in alcoholic liver disease. Genes for an inner mitochondrial membrane protein and a red fluorescent protein are spliced, and the fusion protein is expressed in mouse embryo fibroblasts. The distribution of mitochondria in the transfected cells is visualized by confocal fluorescence microscopy (shown in the image). Inhibition of the electron transport chain in this organelle leads to which of the following reversible changes in cell behavior?

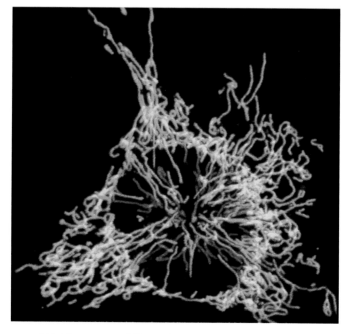

(A) Extension of filopodia
(B) Hydropic swelling
(C) Intracellular lipid storage
(D) Membrane ruffling
(E) Protooncogene activation

17 Release of cytochrome c from the organelle described in Question 16 activates which of the following cellular processes?
(A) Apoptosis
(B) Autophagy
(C) Cell division
(D) Cell motility
(E) Exocytosis

18 Fluorescent fusion proteins are used to monitor the distribution of organelles in a myoblast cell line. The distribution of mitochondria and microfilaments is examined by confocal fluorescence microscopy (shown in the image). In this composite image, DNA is colored blue, microfilaments are colored green, and mitochondria are colored red. Which of the following cell adhesion proteins forms anchoring junctions that link actin microfilaments to adhesive glycoproteins on the surface of the culture dish?

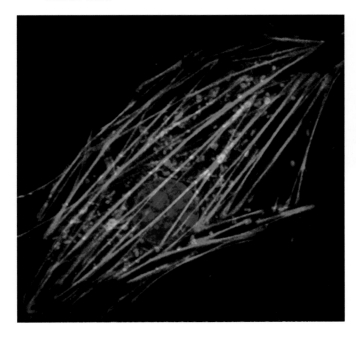

(A) Cadherins
(B) Cloudins
(C) Connexins
(D) Integrins
(E) Selectins

19 Which of the following cellular processes describes the uptake of extracellular fluids and small particles by the cell described in Question 18?
(A) Autophagy
(B) Exocytosis
(C) Involution
(D) Phagocytosis
(E) Pinocytosis

20 The genes for green fluorescent protein and tubulin are spliced, and the fusion protein is expressed in a myoblast cell line. The distribution of microtubules is monitored by confocal fluorescence microscopy (shown in the image). During mitosis, these cytoskeletal proteins are reorganized to coordinate chromosome separation. Which of the following organelles is the principal microtubule-organizing center in these myoblasts?

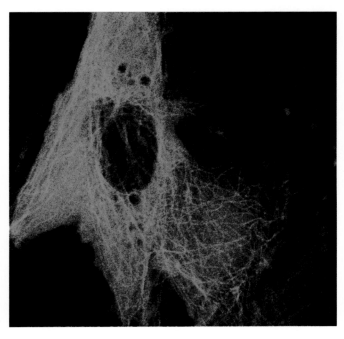

(A) Astral fibers
(B) Basal body
(C) Centromeres
(D) Centrosomes
(E) Kinetochores

21 You attend a national meeting on regenerative medicine. One of the talks focuses on cellular senescence and cancer. Reactivation of the gene for which of the following nuclear proteins may enable some cancer cells to escape cellular senescence, continue to proliferate, and maintain genomic stability?
(A) DNA helicase
(B) Lamin A
(C) Oct 4 transcription factor
(D) Rb tumor suppressor protein
(E) Telomerase

22 The gene for green fluorescent protein is modified by the addition of a signal sequence that targets the translation product to the lumen of the endoplasmic reticulum (ER). The distribution of the rough ER in a transfected myoblast cell line is monitored by confocal fluorescence microscopy (shown in the image). Which of the following families of proteins facilitates proper protein folding in the ER, cytoplasm, and nucleus of this muscle stem cell?

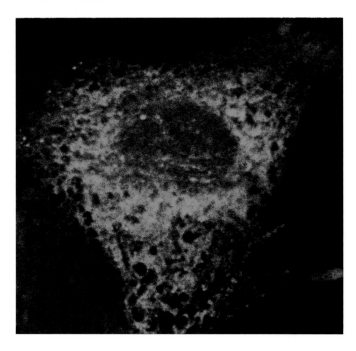

(A) Chaperones
(B) Clathrins
(C) Cyclins
(D) Lamins
(E) Ubiquitin ligases

23 Hepatocytes from a liver biopsy are examined by electron microscopy. Identify the elongated organelles shown in the image.

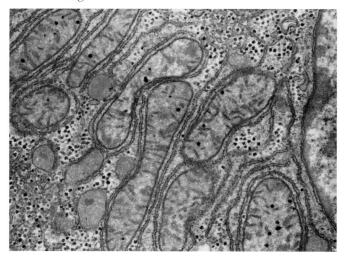

(A) Endoplasmic reticulum
(B) Golgi apparatus
(C) Lysosomes
(D) Mitochondria
(E) Peroxisomes

24 A 23-year-old man presents with a 6-month history of yellow skin and sclerae. Physical examination shows mild jaundice and peritoneal ascites. The patient is subsequently diagnosed with α-1-antitrypsin deficiency. A liver biopsy stained with PAS reveals globular inclusions of misfolded α-1-antitrypsin (shown in the image). The abundance of these abnormal glycoproteins has apparently overwhelmed normal degradation pathways. Which of the following cellular processes describes the normal mechanism for specifically targeting and degrading misfolded proteins within cells?

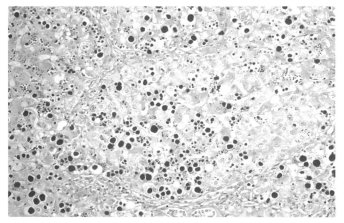

(A) Activation of the caspase enzyme cascade
(B) Activation of the ubiquitin–proteasome pathway
(C) Delivery of acid hydrolases to lysosomes
(D) Fusion of secretory vesicles with the plasma membrane
(E) Generation of reactive oxygen species

25 A 42-year-old woman presents with increasing abdominal girth and yellow discoloration of her skin and sclera. Physical examination reveals hepatomegaly and evidence of liver failure (jaundice). A Prussian blue stain of a liver biopsy is shown in the image. This stain identifies which of the following elements?

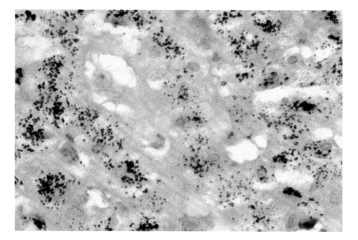

(A) Calcium
(B) Cobalt
(C) Copper
(D) Iron
(E) Potassium

26 A kidney biopsy from a 44-year-old man is examined by electron microscopy. The nucleus of an endothelial cell exhibits a peripheral ring of dark-stained chromatin (arrow, shown in the image). Which of the following best describes the functional significance of the dark-stained ring of marginal chromatin observed in this electron micrograph?

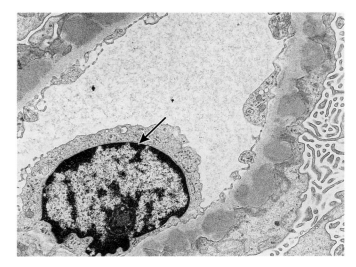

(A) DNA replication center
(B) Kinetochore complex assembly
(C) Nucleosome assembly
(D) Organization of inactive chromatin
(E) Ribosomal RNA biosynthesis

27 Which of the following proteins contributes to the structural matrix that anchors chromatin to the nuclear membrane during interphase of the cell cycle?
(A) Desmin
(B) Keratin
(C) Lamin
(D) Perlecan
(E) Vimentin

28 An 85-year-old woman with Alzheimer disease dies in her sleep. At autopsy, hepatocytes are noted to contain golden cytoplasmic granules that do not stain with Prussian blue (shown in the image). This "wear-and-tear" pigment of aging (lipofuscin) accumulates primarily within which of the following cellular organelles?

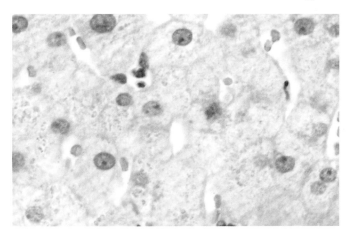

(A) Endosomes
(B) Golgi apparatus
(C) Lysosomes
(D) Peroxisomes
(E) Vacuoles

29 You are involved in a translational research project to develop small-molecule inhibitors of pepsin secretion by chief cells in the stomach mucosa. Chief cells store precursor enzymes within zymogen granules. By electron microscopy, these "protein factory" cells would most likely show an abundance of which of the following intracellular organelles?
(A) Centrosomes
(B) Endosomes
(C) Phagolysosomes
(D) Rough endoplasmic reticulum
(E) Smooth endoplasmic reticulum

30 A 55-year-old woman learns that she has high levels of serum cholesterol (greater than 280 mg/dL; normal less than 200 mg/dL) and is at increased risk for development of ischemic heart disease. The patient asks you to explain the normal pathway for serum cholesterol uptake and clearance. You explain to her that low-density lipoprotein (LDL) receptors present in her liver bind LDL cholesterol and internalize it by forming coated vesicles (endosomes). Which of the following structural proteins mediates LDL receptor internalization by organizing small buds of plasma membrane into endosomes?
(A) Actin
(B) Clathrin
(C) Desmin
(D) Laminin
(E) Vimentin

31 A 23-year-old woman complains of recurrent bone pain and increasing abdominal girth. Physical examination reveals enlargement of the patient's liver and spleen (hepatosplenomegaly). A spleen biopsy reveals large macrophages, with a fibrillar appearance reminiscent of "wrinkled tissue paper" (shown in the image). The patient is subsequently diagnosed with Gaucher disease. She carries mutations in the genes for glucocerebrosidase. Without this hydrolytic enzyme, glucocerebroside accumulates within which of the following cellular organelles?

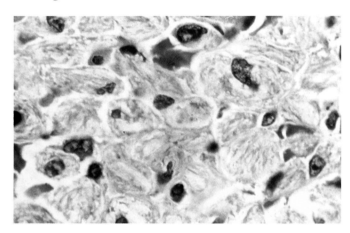

(A) Autophagic vacuoles
(B) Endoplasmic reticulum
(C) Lysosomes
(D) Mitochondria
(E) Peroxisomes

32 You are studying the differentiation of epithelial cells lining the intestinal mucosa and identify a common stem cell for the secretory lineage that gives rise to Paneth cells, enterocytes, and goblet cells. Which of the following terms describes the developmental potential of these gastrointestinal stem cells?
(A) Embryonic
(B) Metaplastic
(C) Multipotent
(D) Nullipotent
(E) Pluripotent

33 A cervical biopsy is obtained from a 42-year-old woman with a history of abnormal Pap smears. The tissue is tested for human papillomavirus (HPV) by in situ hybridization using cDNA probes. Evidence of HPV viral genome is detected in cells in the cervical biopsy (dark blue spots, shown in the image). The patient is told that she is at increased risk for the development of cervical cancer. She asks you to elaborate. You explain that HPV encodes an early gene (*E6*) that activates a cellular protein that, in turn, accelerates the degradation of the p53 tumor suppressor protein. Name the protein that is activated by HPV E6.

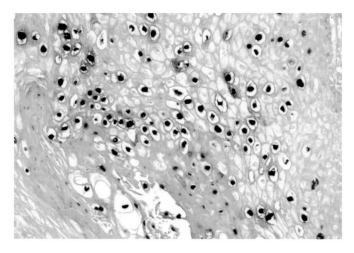

(A) β-Catenin
(B) Cathepsin
(C) Glucuronyl transferase
(D) GTP-activating protein
(E) Ubiquitin ligase

34 You join a research laboratory to investigate the growth and differentiation of human embryonic stem (ES) cells. These remarkable cells have been shown to differentiate into a wide variety of somatic cell types including (1) dopamine-producing neurons, (2) cardiac myocytes, and (3) insulin-producing pancreatic islet cells. ES cells are similar or equivalent to which of the following populations of cells/tissues in the early embryo?
(A) Amnion
(B) Chorion
(C) Epiblast
(D) Hypoblast
(E) Trophoblast

35 As part of your research, you investigate the role of cyclins and cyclin-dependent kinases in regulating ES cell growth in vitro. These rapidly dividing cells spend most of their time in which phase of the mitotic cell cycle?
(A) G0
(B) G1
(C) G2
(D) M
(E) S

36 You are invited to give a seminar on the molecular mechanisms of lineage formation and cell differentiation. During the seminar, you are asked to list the primary germ layers of the embryo and discuss their derivatives. Blood vessels and hematopoietic stem cells originate from which of the following tissues/structures during embryogenesis?

(A) Ectoderm
(B) Endoderm
(C) Mesoderm
(D) Neural crest
(E) Notochord

37 The principal investigator of your laboratory asks you whether pluripotent ES cells can differentiate into neural crest cells or primordial germ cells. You suggest that cellular and molecular markers would help you answer that question. Markers for which of the following cells could be used to monitor neural crest cell differentiation in vitro?

(A) Cardiac myocytes
(B) Hepatocytes
(C) Keratinocytes
(D) Melanocytes
(E) Enterocytes

ANSWERS

1 **The answer is E: Telophase.** After fertilization, the male and female pronuclei join to form the nucleus of the zygote. Maternal enzymes and transcription factors regulate nuclear reprogramming and activate zygotic gene transcription. The first cleavage division takes place about 24 hours after fertilization. During this mitotic cell division, sister chromatids are partitioned to genetically identical daughter cells (blastomeres). Mitosis consists of four phases: prophase, metaphase, anaphase, and telophase. Chromosome condensation occurs during prophase (choice D). The mitotic spindle organizes sister chromatids during metaphase (choice C). Chromosomes are pulled apart during anaphase (choice A). Cytokinesis, nuclear membrane formation, and DNA unwinding occur during telophase. A contractile ring of actin and nonmuscle myosin forms the cleavage furrow. After telophase, the daughter cells enter interphase of the cell cycle (choice B). The blastomeres at this stage are totipotent. They become smaller in size with each subsequent cell division. Totipotency of the blastomeres is lost after the third cleavage division (eight-cell stage) as the embryo undergoes compaction to form the blastocyst.
Keywords: Cell cycle, mitosis, cleavage division

2 **The answer is E: Kinetochore.** The spindle apparatus organizes and separates chromosomes during mitosis and meiosis. Microtubules of the spindle apparatus link chromosomes to microtubule organizing centers and mediate the movement of paired chromosomes to opposite poles of the cell during anaphase. Centromeres (choice C) are repetitive DNA sequences that provide a point of attachment between the sister chromatid and a nucleation site for the assembly of the kinetochore protein complex. Kinetochores are attachment sites for microtubules of the spindle apparatus. Each kinetochore binds 15 to 20 microtubules. Bundles of microtubules (spindle fibers) originate from microtubule-organizing centers (centrosomes, choice D). Centrosomes are composed of two centrioles (choice B) and a zone of pericentriolar proteins that regulate microtubule nucleation. Centrosomes are associated with the nuclear membrane during interphase and replicated during S phase of the cell cycle. They move to opposite poles of the cell during mitotic prophase as the nuclear envelope disintegrates. Astral fibers (choice A) are microtubules that anchor centrosomes to the plasma membrane. Dyneins are molecular motor proteins that move chromosomes along the spindle apparatus. Failure of sister chromatids to separate during anaphase is referred to as nondisjunction. The resulting embryos are said to exhibit genetic mosaicism.
Keywords: Kinetochore, mitosis, cell cycle

3 **The answer is B: Membrane fluidity.** The plasma membrane separates the cytoplasm and intracellular organelles from the external environment. Loss of plasma membrane integrity results in cell death (necrosis). The plasma membrane is a fluid mosaic of lipids and proteins. Integral proteins pass through the lipid bilayer, whereas peripheral proteins do not. Membrane proteins are essential for cell viability and differentiated cell functions. For examples, membrane proteins serve as pumps, enzymes, channels, receptors, structural molecules, and attachment sites. Oligosaccharides and polysaccharides conjugated to membrane proteins and sphingolipids form a cell surface coat (glycocalyx). In polarized epithelial cells, the plasma membrane exhibits distinct apical, basal, and lateral domains. Fluorescence recovery after photobleaching (FRAP) is an experimental technique that can be used to measure the rate at which lipids and proteins move by lateral diffusion within the plane of the membrane. The viscosity of the plasma membrane has been compared to that of thick molasses. Tight junctions provide a barrier to the lateral diffusion of membrane proteins and lipids. In some cells, the plasma membrane forms microdomains (lipid rafts, choice A) that regulate cell signaling. Patching and capping (choice C) describe the clustering of cell surface molecules by specific cross-linking agents, such as antibodies or pollen. Protein trafficking and endocytosis (choices D and E) do not regulate the lateral diffusion of lipids and proteins in the plasma membrane.
Keywords: Membrane fluidity, fluid mosaic model

4 **The answer is A: Actin.** Motility is a remarkable property of cells that is essential for embryonic development, wound healing, and lymphocyte trafficking. Cell locomotion involves the coordinated assembly and disassembly of actin microfilaments. Actin filaments are helical structures, with a growing end that adds globular (G-actin) to filamentous F-actin. Assembly of microfilaments can generate membrane protrusions, such as filopodia and lamellipodia. Changes in the shape of lamellipodia over time are referred to as "membrane ruffling." During cell locomotion, the leading edge of the plasma membrane displays cell–substrate adhesion proteins that bind glycoproteins in the extracellular matrix. Desmin and vimentin (choices B and E) are intermediate filament proteins found in mesenchymal cells. Lamins (choice C) are nuclear matrix proteins that stabilize the nuclear membrane and organize chromatin. Tubulins (choice D) form the spindle apparatus, regulate intracellular transport, and control the movement of cilia and flagella.
Keywords: Neural crest cells, actin microfilaments

5 **The answer is E: Nuclear pyknosis.** Apoptosis is a programmed pathway of cell death that is activated by a variety of extracellular and intracellular signals. It is often a self-defense mechanism, destroying cells that harbor viruses or have acquired genetic alterations. In this example, secretory cells of the sebaceous gland initiate programmed cell death in order to release their intracellular stores of lipid and wax. This process of exocytosis is referred to as holocrine secretion. Cytologic features of cells undergoing apoptosis include nuclear condensation (pyknosis) and chromatin fragmentation (karyorrhexis and karyolysis). Pyknotic nuclei are small, shrunken, and deeply basophilic (shown in the image). The other cytologic findings are features of acute reversible cell injury.

Keywords: Pyknosis, programmed cell death

6 **The answer is E: Smooth endoplasmic reticulum.** Intracellular membranes establish compartment boundaries and organelles that serve different cellular functions. Examples of membrane-bound intracellular organelles include the nucleus, endoplasmic reticulum, Golgi apparatus, mitochondria, peroxisomes, lysosomes, endosomes, and secretory vesicles. The endoplasmic reticulum (ER) is composed of parallel membrane sheets and sacs that are specialized for protein and lipid biosynthesis. Smooth ER lacks ribosomes, and its surface appears smooth when examined by electron microscopy. Smooth ER is particularly abundant in cells that synthesize lipids (e.g., fatty acids, phospholipids, cholesterol, and steroid hormones). In skeletal and cardiac muscle, smooth ER sequesters calcium and regulates muscle contraction. In the liver, smooth ER provides a large surface area for oxidative enzymes (e.g., cytochromes) that degrade toxins and carcinogens. The other organelles may be present in steroid-producing cells, but they would not be abundant.

Keywords: Adrenal cortex, smooth endoplasmic reticulum

7 **The answer is E: Sugars.** Periodic acid–Schiff (PAS) reagent is a histochemical stain that is useful for identifying carbohydrates (oligosaccharides and polysaccharides). In this section of the small intestine, PAS stains mucus-producing goblet cells. Mucins are heavily glycosylated glycoproteins that protect the intestinal mucosa and lubricate the luminal contents. Hematoxylin is a basic dye that is commonly used to identify cell nuclei (nucleic acids) in paraffin sections. Cellular structures that retain hematoxylin are said to be basophilic. Cellular structures that retain eosin are said to be eosinophilic. PAS does not stain collagens, lipids, nucleic acids, or proteins (choices A to D).

Keywords: Goblet cells, periodic acid–Schiff reagent

8 **The answer is A: Golgi apparatus.** The Golgi apparatus is an intracellular organelle that regulates posttranslational modification and sorting of membrane and secretory proteins. Like the ER, the Golgi apparatus is composed of flat membrane sacs (vesicles). Newly synthesized proteins leave the ER in small transport vesicles that fuse with the Golgi membrane network. Here, a variety of glycosyltransferase enzymes attach linear and branched oligosaccharide chains to the asparagine residues (N-linked

glycans) and serine/threonine residues (O-linked glycans) of membrane and secretory proteins. The ultimate destination of each protein is determined by intrinsic signal peptides and patterns of protein glycosylation. Mature vesicles leave trans-Golgi membranes as secretory vesicles that may be stored in apical cytoplasm or as transport vesicles that deliver proteins/glycoproteins to various organelles or membrane domains (e.g., apical, basal, or lateral membranes). Lysosomes (choice B) are vesicles filled with acid hydrolases that degrade cellular debris. Peroxisomes (choice C) are small vesicles filled with catalase and other enzymes that remove reactive oxygen species (e.g., hydrogen peroxide). None of the other organelles are involved in the posttranslational modification of membrane and secretory proteins.

Keywords: Golgi apparatus

9 **The answer is E: Trypan blue.** Trypan blue is a nontoxic (vital) dye that is retained by dead cells but excluded by viable nonphagocytic cells. When trypan blue is added to an aliquot of cells in suspension, the percentage of viable cells in the sample can be determined rapidly using a benchtop hemocytometer. One simply divides the number of viable cells in an aliquot by the total number of cells examined. Hematoxylin and eosin (H&E, choice B) are the most commonly used dyes in histology and histopathology. Aldehyde fuchsin (choice A) can be used to identify elastic fibers and mast cell secretory granules. Luxol fast blue/cresyl violet (choice C) is commonly used to stain nervous tissue. As mentioned above, PAS (choice D) is commonly used to identify carbohydrate-rich cellular components and secretions (e.g., mucus). Erythropoietin is a kidney hormone that promotes the survival and growth of hematopoietic cells that are committed to the erythrocyte pathway of differentiation.

Keywords: Hyperplasia, erythropoietin, hematopoiesis

10 **The answer is A: Endoplasmic reticulum.** This electron micrograph demonstrates ultrastructural features of rough endoplasmic reticulum (ER). These flat membrane vesicles provide a large surface area for protein synthesis (translation). The small knob-like features are ribosomes that are actively synthesizing membrane and secretory proteins. Signal peptides mediate the attachment of ribosomes to the rough ER. Signal recognition particles, docking proteins, and translocator proteins collaborate to shepherd these proteins through the lipid bilayer. Cytosolic proteins are synthesized by "free ribosomes." None of the other organelles exhibit the ultrastructural features of rough ER.

Keywords: Rough endoplasmic reticulum

11 **The answer is D: Masson trichrome.** This slide specimen reveals key histologic features of a muscular artery. Erythrocytes in the vascular lumen and smooth muscle cells in the tunica media appear red. Collagen fibers in the tunica media appear blue. This striking pattern of tissue staining was obtained using Masson trichrome. Trichrome reagents use two or more acid dyes to stain tissues with contrasting colors (e.g., red and blue). Trichrome staining methods are widely used for differentiating smooth muscle fibers from collagen connective tissue. This is helpful, because these tissues look similar in slides that are stained using H&E.

Keywords: Arteries, trichrome stain

12 The answer is D: Nucleolus. In eukaryotic cells, the nucleus maintains the integrity of the genome and regulates complex patterns of gene expression. The nucleus provides a microenvironment for the myriad structural proteins and enzymes that control DNA replication, DNA repair, chromatin assembly, and RNA synthesis. The nucleoplasm contains many different types of RNAs, including messenger (mRNA), ribosomal (rRNA), transfer (tRNA), and small nuclear (snRNA). Genes that encode the rRNAs are clustered in a nonmembranous region of the nucleus, termed the nucleolus. The nucleolus stains intensely with basic dyes and is visible within the nucleus of these ganglion cells. The outer margin of the double-membrane nuclear envelope is visible in this H&E slide preparation. Basal bodies (choice A) are modified centrioles located at the base of cilia and flagella. Centrosomes (choice B) and Golgi apparatus (choice C) are perinuclear, but these organelles cannot be identified by light microscopy. Peroxisomes (choice E) are located in the cytosol.

Keywords: Nucleolus, motor neurons

13 The answer is D: Tubulin. Axons are cellular processes that convey electrochemical signals away from neuronal cell bodies. These elongated structures are largely dependent on the neuronal cell body for the delivery of organelles and vesicles and for the removal of cellular waste (e.g., abnormal proteins). Axonal transport is an intracellular shuttle/delivery system that uses microtubules and motor proteins (e.g., kinesin and dynein) to transport vesicles to and from the synaptic membrane. Microtubules are rigid hollow tubes composed of repeating units of αβ-tubulin dimers. These polymeric structures grow from nucleation sites within centrosomes. Tubulins comprise a family of proteins that regulate diverse cellular activities, including: (1) chromosome separation during mitosis and meiosis, (2) intracellular vesicle transport, and (3) the whip-like movement of cilia and flagella. Clathrin (choice B) forms coated membrane vesicles during receptor-mediated endocytosis. Ubiquitin (choice E) is a protein that tags other proteins for degradation by proteasomes. None of the other proteins mediate axonal (axoplasmic) transport.

Keywords: Axonal transport, motor neurons

14 The answer is B: Intermediate filaments. The cytoskeleton is an intracellular network of filamentous proteins that provides structural support, transports organelles, regulates cell motility, and controls cell division. It includes microtubules composed of tubulin, microfilaments composed of actin, and intermediate filaments composed of tissue-specific fibrous proteins. Unlike microtubules and microfilaments, intermediate filaments are nonpolar structures composed of protein building blocks that vary from one tissue to another. Intermediate filament protein families include keratins, lamins, vimentins, desmins, and neurofilament proteins. Keratins protect the external surface of the skin. Lamins stabilize the inner nuclear membrane, organize chromatin, and regulate gene expression. Neurons express neurofilament proteins that provide flexible, structural support to help maintain complex patterns of axons and dendrites within the central and peripheral nervous system. Microtubules and microfilaments are present in nerve axons and dendrites and contribute to cell structure, but they are not composed of neuron-specific fibrous proteins. None of the other organelles provide structural support to neurons or glial cells.

Keywords: Cytoskeleton, intermediate filaments

15 The answer is C: Inclusion. Differentiated cells synthesize a wide variety of proteins, lipids, and carbohydrates that are stored, transported, or secreted. Adipocytes synthesize and store large quantities of triglycerides. Lipid droplets in the cytoplasm coalesce to form a large inclusion that pushes the cytoplasm and nucleus to the periphery of the cell (shown in the image). Glycogen, hemosiderin (denatured ferritin), and lipofuscin (cross-linked lipids and proteins) are also stored as cytoplasmic inclusions. Other metabolic products are packaged within membrane-bound organelles, termed vesicles (choice E). The cytoplasm of most cells is filled with innumerable small vesicles. With the help of microtubules and motor proteins, vesicles transport proteins, lipids, and carbohydrates from one organelle to another (e.g., from ER to Golgi or plasma membrane to lysosome). Large membrane-bound organelles are referred to as vacuoles (choice D). Examples of vacuoles include phagolysosomes and autophagic vacuoles. Endosomes (choice A) are vesicles that internalize ligands and cell surface receptors and transport them to lysosomes for degradation or for recycling back to the plasma membrane. Granules (choice B) are secretory vesicles that are commonly stored in apical cytoplasm. During exocytosis, secretory granules fuse with the plasma membrane, releasing their contents to the extracellular space.

Keywords: Adipocytes, inclusions

16 The answer is B: Hydropic swelling. Fusion proteins containing fluorescent protein markers can be used to examine the distribution of organelles in living cells. In this experiment, mitochondria are identified as long, coiled, rope-like structures. These ATP energy-producing organelles are derived from the oocyte at the time of fertilization. They carry their own DNA, synthesize many of their own proteins, and replicate autonomously during interphase. Mitochondria can assume different sizes and shapes, and they often localize to sites within the cell where energy is most needed. When cellular levels of ATP are depleted (e.g., by exposure to toxins or lack of oxygen), cells undergo acute hydropic swelling. This increase in cell volume is caused by an inability of the plasma membrane Na/K ATPase to pump sodium out of the cell. Without adequate levels of ATP to fuel the membrane pump, sodium and water are retained within the cell, and the cell swells. Inhibition of the mitochondrial electron transport chain over an extended period of time will lead to cellular atrophy. ATP depletion does not lead to the other listed changes in cell morphology or behavior.

Keywords: Mitochondria, hydropic swelling

17 **The answer is A: Apoptosis.** Apoptosis is a programmed pathway of cell death that is triggered by a variety of extracellular and intracellular signals. It is often a self-defense mechanism, destroying cells that have been infected with pathogens or those in which genomic alterations have occurred. Mitochondria play a key role in regulating apoptosis. In response to cellular stress, mitochondria open an outer membrane "permeability transition pore" that permits the release of cytochrome c from the inner mitochondrial membrane to the cytoplasm. Within the cytoplasm, cytochrome c triggers an apoptotic cascade that leads to the activation of effector enzymes (caspases) that degrade chromatin and destabilize the cytoskeleton. During development, apoptosis deletes unwanted cells in limb buds to form the digits. None of the other cellular processes are activated by the release of cytochrome c from mitochondria.

Keywords: Apoptosis, mitochondrial permeability transition pore

18 **The answer is D: Integrins.** This beautiful fluorescent image provided by David Weaver and Gyorgy Hajnoczky at Thomas Jefferson University shows the subcellular location of microfilaments, mitochondria, and chromatin in a cultured myoblast. The actin bundles (colored green) are aligned along an axis of cell polarity and migration. These microfilaments make connections with the plasma membrane at sites of cell–substrate adhesion. Microfilaments attach to proteins along the inner leaflet of the plasma membrane. These attachment proteins include α-actinin, vinculin, paxillin, talin, and integrin. Integrins are transmembrane receptors that mediate cell signaling and cell–substrate adhesion. They link microfilaments of the cytoskeleton to various proteins in the extracellular matrix, including laminin, vitronectin, fibronectin, and collagen. Integrins help regulate cell shape, motility, and differentiation. Cadherins (choice A), cloudins (choice B), and selectins (choice E) mediate cell–cell adhesion. Connexins (choice C) form intercellular pores that permit gap junction communication.

Keywords: Integrins, microfilaments, cell adhesion

19 **The answer is E: Pinocytosis.** Uptake of fluid and macromolecules at the cell surface is referred to as endocytosis. This energy-dependent cellular activity provides cells with essential fluids, nutrients, and proteins. It also enables specialized cells to internalize large particles (e.g., cellular debris and bacteria) for degradation within phagolysosomes. Endocytosis involves the formation of vesicles at the plasma membrane by a process of vesicle budding. Three general mechanisms of endocytosis are described: (1) pinocytosis (constitutive uptake of fluid and small particles), (2) phagocytosis (uptake of large particles by macrophages and other phagocytic cells; choice D), and (3) receptor-mediated endocytosis (clathrin-dependent uptake of specific ligands). Pinocytotic vesicles can be identified by electron microscopy. They are particularly abundant in the cytoplasm of vascular endothelial cells. Autophagy (choice A) enables cells to degrade and eliminate unwanted or damaged organelles. Exocytosis (choice B) is an energy-dependent process of secretion that involves fusion of secretory vesicles with the plasma membrane.

Keywords: Pinocytosis

20 **The answer is D: Centrosomes.** As mentioned above, microtubules are rigid hollow tubes composed of repeating units of αβ-tubulin dimers. They regulate diverse cellular activities, including chromosome separation during mitosis and meiosis, intracellular vesicle transport, and the movement of cilia and flagella. These polymeric structures grow from nucleation sites within centrosomes. Centrosomes are composed of two centrioles positioned at right angles and a zone of pericentriolar proteins that regulate microtubule nucleation. Centrosomes are associated with the nuclear membrane during interphase and replicated during S-phase of the cell cycle. Basal bodies (choice B) are modified centrioles located at the base of cilia and flagella. Kinetochores (choice E) are protein complexes on chromosomes that provide attachment sites for the spindle apparatus during cell division. None of the other organelles is a primary microtubule-organizing center in nonciliated, muscle stem cells.

Keywords: Centrosome, cell cycle

21 **The answer is E: Telomerase.** Telomerase is a nuclear enzyme that adds repetitive DNA sequences to maintain the length of chromosome telomeres. Somatic cells that are undergoing cellular senescence (i.e., loss of proliferative capacity) do not normally express telomerase. With each round of somatic cell replication, the telomere shortens. The length of telomeres may act as a "molecular clock" that governs the life span of replicating cells, providing a mechanism for cellular senescence. Because cancer cells and embryonic cells express high levels of telomerase, reactivation of this enzyme is thought to enable these cells to escape senescence, proliferate, and maintain genomic stability. Mutations affecting

DNA helicase and lamin A (choices A and B) are associated with accelerated aging syndromes (progeria). Oct 4 (choice C) is a transcription factor that is essential for pluripotency and self-renewal in embryonic stem cells. Tumor suppressor proteins (choice D) *restrain* the cell cycle. The genes for Rb and p53 tumor suppressor proteins are among the most commonly mutated genes in human cancers.

Keywords: Telomerase, neoplasia

22 **The answer is A: Chaperones.** For many proteins, polypeptide folding is prone to error and requires the assistance of molecular chaperones. Chaperones are a family of proteins found in the nucleus, cytoplasm, and ER that assist other proteins in assuming their correct three-dimensional conformation. They also prevent protein aggregation and target abnormally folded proteins for proteolytic degradation. Chaperones that are up-regulated in response to cellular stress are referred to as "heat shock proteins." Mutations in chaperone genes have been linked to a number of chronic diseases, termed chaperonopathies. None of the other proteins regulates protein folding.

Keywords: Chaperones, protein folding

23 **The answer is D: Mitochondria.** This transmission electron micrograph reveals elongated, tubular mitochondria in the cytoplasm of hepatocytes. Mitochondria have inner and outer membranes that provide compartments for the enzymes and cytochromes that mediate glycolysis and oxidative phosphorylation. Folds of the inner mitochondrial membrane (cristae) provide additional surface area for energy production (shown in the image). Electron transport proteins and ATP synthase are associated with the inner membrane. Enzymes that carry out the citric acid (Krebs) cycle are present within the mitochondrial matrix that is surrounded by the inner membrane. When cells are deprived of oxygen, mitochondria swell and their cristae become less prominent. None of the other organelles exhibit the ultrastructural features of mitochondria.

Keywords: Mitochondria, hepatocytes

24 **The answer is B: Activation of the ubiquitin–proteasome pathway.** Abnormal or unwanted proteins are degraded within lysosomes or targeted for degradation by proteasomes. Proteasomes are protein complexes that bind and degrade proteins that have been "tagged" with ubiquitin, a 76-amino-acid protein. Protein ubiquitination is a complex process that requires a variety of enzymes, including activators, conjugating enzymes, and ubiquitin ligases. α-1-Antitrypsin deficiency is a heritable disorder in which mutations in the gene for α-1-antitrypsin yield an insoluble protein. These globules stain red with PAS. The mutant protein is not easily exported from the cells. It accumulates causing cell injury and cirrhosis. α-1-Antitrypsin deficiency is the most common genetic cause of liver disease in infants and children and the most frequent genetic disease for which liver transplantation

is indicated. Caspases (choice A) mediate apoptotic cell death. Reactive oxygen species (choice E) contribute to the lysis of bacteria and necrotic debris in the phagolysosomes of inflammatory cells.

Keywords: α-1-Antitrypsin deficiency, proteasomes

25 **The answer is D: Iron.** Prussian blue is a common histochemical stain for iron. In this liver biopsy, Prussian blue identifies iron deposits within the cytoplasm of hepatocytes (dark blue inclusions, shown in the image). Iron is carried in the serum by transferrin, picked up by cell surface transferrin receptors, and internalized via receptor-mediated endocytosis. Within cells, iron is bound by ferritin. Hemosiderin is a partially denatured form of ferritin that aggregates easily. It is recognized microscopically as yellow-brown granules in the cytoplasm, which turn blue with the Prussian blue reaction. The patient described in this clinical vignette suffers from hereditary hemochromatosis, a genetic abnormality of iron absorption in the small intestine. Excess iron is stored mostly in the form of hemosiderin, primarily in the liver. Clinical symptoms of hereditary hemochromatosis include cirrhosis, diabetes, skin pigmentation, and heart disease. Patients are at increased risk for the development of hepatocellular carcinoma. None of the other elements forms molecular complexes with Prussian blue.

Keywords: Hereditary hemochromatosis

26 **The answer is D: Organization of inactive chromatin.** Chromatin is composed of DNA, RNA, and protein. In routine H&E slide preparations, nuclear chromatin binds hematoxylin and is said to be basophilic. Patterns of gene expression are regulated, in part, by global changes in chromatin packing. Inactive chromatin, heterochromatin, is highly condensed and deeply basophilic. Much of the heterochromatin in this endothelial cell is found along the periphery of the nucleus. This is referred to as marginal chromatin. By contrast, active chromatin, euchromatin, is dispersed within the nucleoplasm and lightly stained. Chromatin is supported and organized by structural proteins that provide points of attachment between chromatin and the inner nuclear membrane. None of the other cell processes describe the function of heterochromatin.

Keywords: Chromatin, heterochromatin

27 **The answer is C: Lamin.** A network of intermediate filament proteins is associated with the inner nuclear membrane. This nuclear (fibrous) lamina stabilizes the nuclear membrane, organizes chromatin, and regulates gene expression. It is composed largely of lamin A and lamin C proteins that form intermediate filaments. Lamin receptors bind these filamentous proteins to the nuclear membrane. During cell division, the nuclear lamina and nuclear membrane disintegrate to facilitate chromosome segregation and separation. Lamin gene mutations are associated with a variety of diseases (laminopathies) including Hutchinson-Gilford progeria. Patients with

progeria undergo accelerated aging. Perlecan (choice D) is a basement membrane protein. None of the other intermediate filament proteins (choices A, B, and E) anchors chromatin to the nuclear membrane.
Keywords: Nucleus, nuclear lamins

28 The answer is C: Lysosomes. Lysosomes are acidic vesicles that degrade proteins, lipids, and carbohydrates. They are filled with a variety of acid hydrolases that degrade macromolecules to their constituent parts (e.g., amino acids and simple sugars). In some situations, lysosomes are unable to degrade cellular debris. Examples include (1) endogenous substrates that are not catabolized because a key enzyme is missing (lysosomal storage diseases), (2) insoluble endogenous pigments (lipofuscin and melanin), and (3) exogenous particulates (silica and carbon). Examination of this patient's liver at autopsy reveals insoluble "wear-and-tear" pigment of aging. These pigments are composed of cross-linked lipids and proteins (peroxidation products) that accumulate over time. Lipofuscin is stored within the lysosomes of long-lived cells in the brain, heart, and liver. None of the other organelles store lipofuscin.
Keywords: Aging, lipofuscin, lysosomes

29 The answer is D: Rough endoplasmic reticulum. As mentioned above, the endoplasmic reticulum (ER) is composed of parallel membrane sheets and sacs that are specialized for protein and lipid biosynthesis. Smooth ER lacks ribosomes, and its surface appears smooth when examined by electron microscopy. Smooth ER is particularly abundant in cells that synthesize lipids. By contrast, cells that are actively synthesizing proteins feature an abundance of rough ER. Rough ER features bound ribosomes, and its surface appears rough when examined by electron microscopy. Signal sequences, recognition particles, docking proteins, and translocator proteins collaborate to guide proteins destined for secretion through the lipid bilayer. Chief cells store precursor proteins (e.g., pepsinogen) in membrane-bound dense-core granules.
Keywords: Stomach, chief cells, endoplasmic reticulum

30 The answer is B: Clathrin. The LDL receptor is a transmembrane glycoprotein that regulates plasma cholesterol by mediating endocytosis and recycling of apolipoprotein (apo) E. Lacking LDL receptor function, high levels of LDL circulate, are taken up by tissue macrophages, and accumulate to form arterial plaques (atheromas). Receptor-mediated endocytosis is a mechanism for uptake of specific ligands and receptors that is regulated by clathrin. Clathrin stabilizes small invaginations of the plasma membrane, forming coated vesicles (endosomes). Coated vesicles are transported to lysosomes, where ligands and receptors are separated, and receptors are recycled to the plasma membrane. None of the other proteins regulates receptor-mediated endocytosis.
Keywords: Receptor-mediated endocytosis, clathrin

31 The answer is C: Lysosomes. Gaucher disease is characterized by the accumulation of glucosylceramide in the lysosomes of macrophages. The underlying abnormality in Gaucher disease is a deficiency in glucocerebrosidase—a lysosomal acid hydrolase. The hallmark of this disorder is the presence of lipid-laden macrophages (Gaucher cells) in the spleen, liver sinusoids, lymph nodes, lungs, and bone marrow. Gaucher cells are derived from resident macrophages in the respective organs (e.g., Kupffer cells in the liver and alveolar macrophages in the lung). None of the other organelles stores glucosylceramide in patients with Gaucher disease.
Keywords: Gaucher disease, lysosomes

32 The answer is C: Multipotent. Development proceeds from clusters of self-renewing stem cells to beautiful networks of highly differentiated cells. How stem cells acquire instructions for differentiation remains a mystery. When these instructions are revealed, stem cell–based therapies may transform medicine, providing a source of replacement cells and tissues for patients with chronic diseases. The zygote and early cleavage stage blastomeres are totipotent cells, meaning that they have the ability to form all embryonic and extraembryonic tissues. The inner cell mass of the blastocyst is composed of pluripotent embryonic stem cells (choices A and E) that give rise to all embryonic cells and tissues. Pluripotent embryonic stem (ES) cells can be isolated from human blastocysts and cultured in vitro. ES cells that lose the ability to undergo differentiation are said to be nullipotent (choice D). Metaplastic cells (choice B) have undergone a change in differentiation from one pathway to another. Examples of metaplasia include squamous metaplasia in the lungs of smokers and glandular metaplasia in the esophagus of patients with acid reflux. The correct answer for this question is multipotent (choice C). Gastrointestinal stem cells that have the ability to differentiate into a limited number of derivatives are best described as multipotent, adult stem cells.
Keywords: Stem cells

33 The answer is E: Ubiquitin ligase. Epithelial cells in this cervical biopsy exhibit distinct perinuclear vacuoles (shown in the image). These sharply demarcated, clear zones surround the nuclei of HPV-infected cells. The vacuoles are filled with actively replicating virus particles (virions). The gene products of oncogenic DNA viruses, like HPV, are known to inactivate tumor suppressor proteins. Recent studies indicate that they do so, by accelerating the degradation of p53 via the ubiquitin–proteasome pathway (see Question 24). Loss of p53 permits cells to escape cellular senescence and proliferate. Mutations in GTP-activating protein (choice D) are associated with neurofibromatosis. None of the other proteins accelerates the degradation of p53 in cervical epithelial cells.
Keywords: Cervical cancer, proteasomes, HPV

34 **The answer is C: Epiblast.** As mentioned above, pluripotent ES cells can be isolated from the inner cell mass of the blastocyst. When provided with a feeder layer and appropriate growth factors, they can propagate indefinitely. The ability of these remarkable cells to differentiate into derivatives of all three primary germ layers is shared by epiblast cells of the bilaminar embryo. Pluripotent ES cells have been shown to form primordial germ cells that give rise to meiotic cells and gametes. Pluripotency of the epiblast is lost after gastrulation. The other embryonic tissues (choices A, B, D, and E) may be multipotent, but they are not pluripotent.

Keywords: Embryonic stem cells

35 **The answer is B: G1.** The cell cycle can be divided into discrete phases that are referred to as G1, S, G2, and M. Cells that have exited the cell cycle are said to reside in G0. Together, G1, S, and G2 constitute interphase. DNA is replicated for cell division during S-phase. Progression of cells through G1 and G2 are regulated by cyclins and cyclin-dependent kinases. These gap phases provide critical checkpoints for cell division. In most rapidly proliferating cells, G1 is the longest and most variable phase of the cell cycle (*not* choices A, C, D, and E). During G1, cells "evaluate" the integrity of their genome. DNA damage that cannot be repaired typically leads to programmed cell death. M phase is divided into prophase, metaphase, anaphase, and telophase (see Question 1).

Keywords: Cell cycle, mitosis, cyclins

36 **The answer is C: Mesoderm.** During development, cells activate sets of genes to generate intricate patterns of tissues and organs that make up the human body. The engine that drives this incredible diversity of cells and tissues is gastrulation. At the beginning of the 3rd week of development, epiblast cells undergo an epithelial–mesenchymal transition. They invaginate and migrate to form the three primary germ layers: ectoderm, mesoderm, and endoderm. Derivatives of ectoderm include epidermis of the skin, neural retina, and central nervous system. Derivatives of mesoderm include muscle, cartilage, bone, blood vessels, and hematopoietic cells. Derivatives of endoderm include liver, pancreas, and urinary bladder. In addition to forming different types of cells, the embryo organizes cells into tissues and organs. This amazing process of shaping the embryo is referred to as morphogenesis. None of the other embryonic tissues give rise to blood vessels and hematopoietic stem cells.

Keywords: Mesoderm, gastrulation

37 **The answer is D: Melanocytes.** Cellular and molecular markers provide important tools for studying cell differentiation. Some markers characterize stem cells, whereas other markers identify features of terminally differentiated cells. Markers commonly used to identify pluripotent human ES cells include alkaline phosphatase, SSEA-4, and transcription factors (Oct-3/4 and Nanog). Markers of mesoderm include intermediate filament proteins (desmin and nestin), bone morphogenetic protein (BMP4), and fibroblast growth factor (FGF2). Markers of early endoderm include α-fetoprotein, β-catenin, and transcription factors of the *sox* gene family. Neural crest cells give rise to a wide range of differentiated cells, including melanocytes, Schwann cells, and dorsal root sensory ganglion cells. Antibodies to melanin granules could be used for following the differentiation of neural crest cells in vitro. Neural crest cells do not give rise to the other differentiated cells listed.

Keywords: Stem cells, neural crest cells

Chapter 2

Epithelial Tissue

QUESTIONS

Select the single best answer.

1 Epithelial cells line the gastrointestinal tract, respiratory tree, cardiovascular system, and genitourinary system and cover the skin. Which of the following cellular properties best distinguishes lining/coating epithelial cells from other cells/tissues in the body?

(A) Apical and basal membrane domains
(B) Cell–cell anchoring junctions
(C) Cell–extracellular matrix anchoring junctions
(D) Communicating (gap) junctions
(E) Pericellular lamina externa

2 Digital slides illustrating various tissues are examined in the histology laboratory. Your instructor asks you to discuss the epithelium that lines the collecting ducts in the renal medulla (arrows, shown in the image). Identify the type of epithelium.

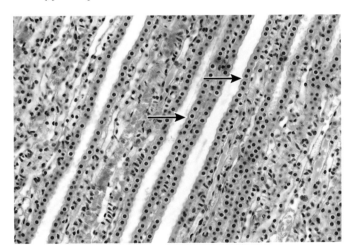

(A) Pseudostratified cuboidal
(B) Simple columnar
(C) Simple cuboidal
(D) Simple squamous
(E) Stratified columnar

3 You continue to examine the digital slide described in Question 2 and identify a new visual field located near the tip of a renal papilla. The epithelium that lines these ducts (arrows, shown in the image) exhibits which of the following patterns of morphology?

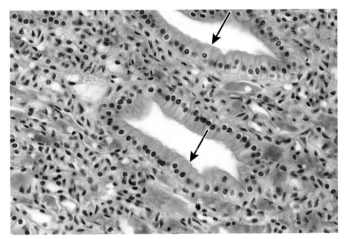

(A) Pseudostratified cuboidal
(B) Simple columnar
(C) Simple cuboidal
(D) Simple squamous
(E) Stratified columnar

4 Your instructor reminds you that epithelial cells have membrane channels that permit ions and small signaling molecules to pass between adjacent cells. Which of the following proteins forms these intercellular (gap) junctions?

(A) Cadherins
(B) Connexins
(C) Netrins
(D) Perforins
(E) Porins

5 A 50-year-old woman complains about a red papule on her right arm. Biopsy of the skin lesion reveals numerous, benign vascular channels filled with erythrocytes.

The endothelial cells that line these vascular channels (arrows, shown in the image) exhibit which of the following patterns of epithelial tissue morphology?

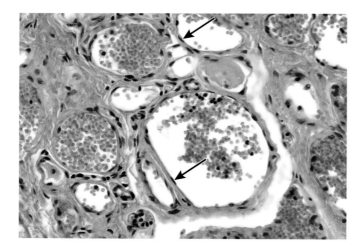

(A) Pseudostratified cuboidal
(B) Simple columnar
(C) Simple cuboidal
(D) Simple squamous
(E) Stratified columnar

6 A portion of the upper esophagus, collected at autopsy, is fixed with formalin, embedded in paraffin, sectioned at 6 μm, stained with H&E, and examined by light microscopy (shown in the image). Identify the type of epithelium.

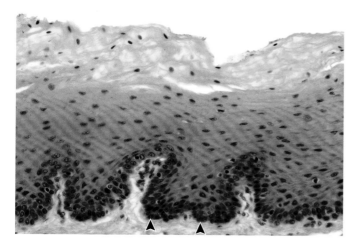

(A) Keratinized stratified squamous
(B) Nonkeratinized stratified squamous
(C) Pseudostratified columnar
(D) Stratified cuboidal
(E) Transitional

7 You are investigating the role of cell adhesion molecules in embryonic development. Sections of a gastrula-stage mouse embryo are stained with periodic acid–Schiff reagent and counterstained with methylene blue. Which of the following families of proteins forms anchoring junctions between adjacent epithelial cells in the neural ectoderm of this embryo (arrow, shown in the image)?

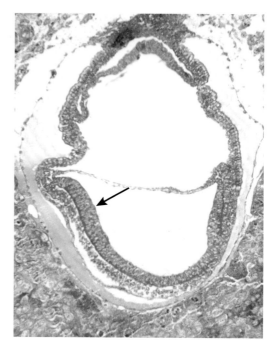

(A) Cadherins
(B) Cloudins
(C) Integrins
(D) Occludins
(E) Selectins

8 Further examination of the embryo described in Question 7 reveals fluid-filled cavities above and below the amnion (shown in the image). Which of the following proteins plays an important role in regulating fluid transport and cavity formation in this embryo?
(A) Catalase
(B) Cytochrome p450
(C) Na/K ATPase
(D) Perforin
(E) Superoxide dismutase

9 A 58-year-old man presents with a pigmented skin lesion on the lateral aspect of his right leg. A punch biopsy of the skin lesion is examined by light microscopy. Which of the following types of epithelium describes the patient's epidermis (indicated by the double arrow, shown in the image)?

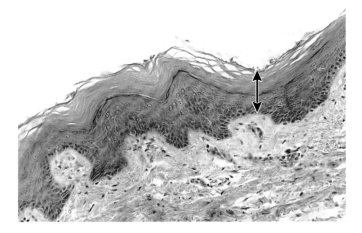

(A) Keratinized stratified squamous
(B) Nonkeratinized stratified squamous
(C) Pseudostratified columnar
(D) Stratified cuboidal
(E) Transitional

10 Further examination of the skin biopsy described in Question 9 reveals the ducts of sweat glands (arrows, shown in the image). Which of the following types of epithelium lines these excretory channels?

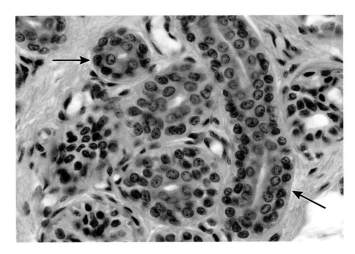

(A) Pseudostratified columnar
(B) Stratified columnar
(C) Stratified cuboidal
(D) Stratified squamous
(E) Transitional

11 A 25-year-old woman spends an afternoon raking leaves. Later that evening, she discovers fluid-filled blisters on the palms of her hands. Leakage of fluid from dermal capillaries at sites of minor injury in the hands of this patient is regulated by changes in which of the following intercellular junctions?

(A) Gap junctions
(B) Hemidesmosomes
(C) Macula adherens (desmosomes)
(D) Zonula adherens
(E) Zonula occludens

12 A 64-year-old man presents with a small mass on the inner surface of his lower lip. Biopsy of the mass reveals chronic inflammatory cells. As you examine the biopsy, you observe a large sweat duct surrounded by loose connective tissue (shown in the image). Identify the type of epithelium.

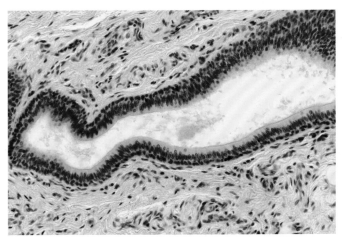

(A) Pseudostratified columnar
(B) Stratified columnar
(C) Stratified cuboidal
(D) Stratified squamous
(E) Transitional

13 A 10-year-old girl scrapes her elbow on the sidewalk while skateboarding. Physical examination reveals a 5-cm superficial skin abrasion. Which of the following cellular processes regulates regeneration of the epidermis in this patient's superficial abrasion?

(A) Differentiation of myoepithelial cells and wound contraction
(B) Loss of cell contact inhibition of growth and motility
(C) Platelet activation and intravascular coagulation
(D) Proliferation of capillary endothelial cells (angiogenesis)
(E) Stimulation of fibroblasts to deposit a provisional extracellular matrix

14 A 58-year-old woman presents with painless hematuria (blood in her urine). Urine cultures are negative for *E. coli*. A biopsy of the urinary bladder is examined in the pathology department (shown in the image). Identify the type of epithelium.

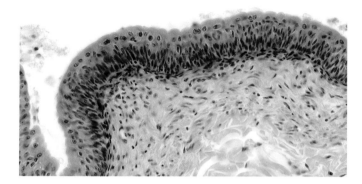

(A) Pseudostratified columnar
(B) Stratified columnar
(C) Stratified cuboidal
(D) Stratified squamous
(E) Transitional

15 A section of trachea obtained at autopsy is stained with H&E and examined at high magnification (shown in the image). Identify the type of the lining epithelium.

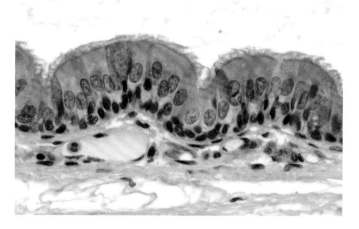

(A) Ciliated pseudostratified columnar with goblet cells
(B) Glandular epithelium
(C) Keratinized stratified squamous
(D) Nonkeratinized stratified squamous
(E) Simple columnar with goblet cells

16 Which of the following membrane junctions anchors the epithelial cells described in Question 15 to extracellular matrix molecules in the underlying basal lamina?
(A) Gap junctions
(B) Hemidesmosomes
(C) Macula adherens
(D) Zonula adherens
(E) Zonula occludens

17 Which of the following proteins regulates the motility of cilia found along the apical membrane domain of the columnar epithelial cells described in Questions 15 and 16?
(A) Actin
(B) Desmin
(C) Keratin
(D) Tubulin
(E) Vimentin

18 A biopsy of small intestine is examined at high magnification in the pathology department. Identify the apical membrane feature indicated by the arrows (shown in the image).

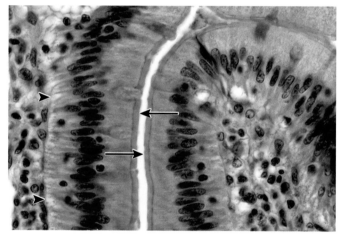

(A) Basal lamina
(B) Glycocalyx
(C) Lamina propria
(D) Striated brush border
(E) Terminal web

19 Electron microscopic examination of the epithelial cells described in Question 18 reveals basolateral membrane infoldings (interdigitations). What is the most likely function of this membrane specialization?
(A) Endocytosis
(B) Enzyme secretion
(C) Exocytosis
(D) Fluid transport
(E) Immune surveillance

20 A section of the intestinal biopsy described in Questions 18 and 19 is stained with periodic acid–Schiff (PAS) and examined at high magnification (shown in the image). Identify the type of epithelium.

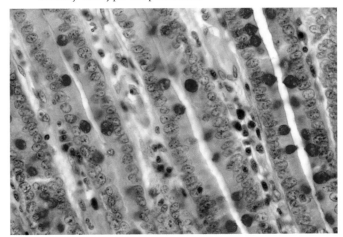

(A) Pseudostratified cuboidal
(B) Simple columnar
(C) Simple cuboidal
(D) Simple squamous
(E) Stratified columnar

21 Which of the following terms best describes the PAS-positive goblet cells identified in the image for Question 20?
(A) Multicellular endocrine glands
(B) Multicellular exocrine mucous glands
(C) Multicellular exocrine serous glands
(D) Unicellular enteroendocrine glands
(E) Unicellular exocrine mucous glands

22 Organs of the anterior neck are examined by a double-headed microscope. The pathology resident asks you to describe the small, tightly packed cells with central nuclei (shown in the image). These cells exhibit which of the following patterns of epithelial cell differentiation?

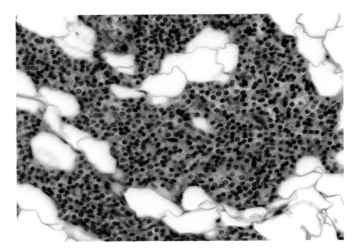

(A) Complex stratified
(B) Glandular
(C) Pseudostratified
(D) Simple squamous
(E) Stratified cuboidal

23 A sample of the epididymis, collected at autopsy, is examined by light microscopy in the pathology department. The nuclei of sperm are visible within the lumen of the duct. Epithelial cells lining the epididymis exhibit long stereocilia (shown in the image). Which of the following proteins determines the shape and size of these specialized apical membrane structures?

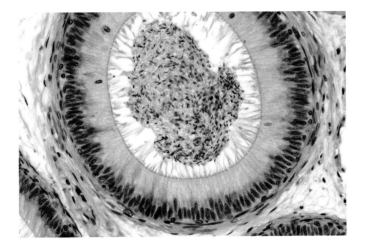

(A) Actin
(B) Desmin
(C) Keratin
(D) Tubulin
(E) Vimentin

24 You attend a lecture on the physiology of lactation and breast-feeding. Under the influence of pregnancy-associated hormones, epithelial cells of the mammary gland secrete lipids, carbohydrates, and proteins. The lipid components of breast milk are released from the apical surface of the glandular epithelial cells as a lipid droplet within an envelope of the plasma membrane. Which of the following terms best describes this mechanism of secretion?
(A) Apocrine
(B) Eccrine
(C) Endocrine
(D) Holocrine
(E) Merocrine

25 A section of the submandibular gland is stained with H&E and examined in the histology laboratory (shown in the image). The secretory units indicated by the arrows are composed primarily of which of the following types of epithelial cells?

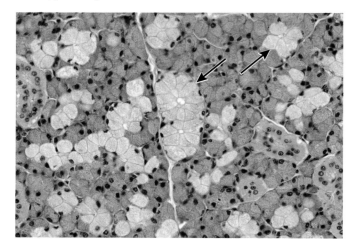

(A) Endocrine
(B) Goblet
(C) Mucous
(D) Paracrine
(E) Serous

26 In addition to collagen and proteoglycan, the basal lamina of the epithelial cells identified in Question 25 consists of which of the following structural proteins?
(A) Desmoplakin
(B) Laminin
(C) Talin
(D) Vimentin
(E) Vinculin

27 The distribution of organelles in cultured endothelial cells is examined using immunocytochemical techniques. A peripheral web of filamentous proteins is identified by confocal fluorescence microscopy (arrowhead, shown in the image). This web consists primarily of which of the following filamentous proteins?

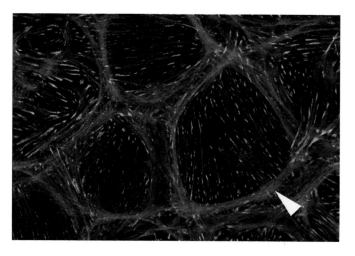

(A) Actin
(B) Desmin
(C) Lamin
(D) Nestin
(E) Tubulin

28 A 68-year-old woman presents with a breast lump that she discovered 5 days ago. A biopsy reveals ductal carcinoma. Immunohistochemical assays are performed to investigate the role of cell adhesion molecules in malignancy. In contrast to normal ductal epithelial cells, this patient's cancer cells exhibit decreased expression of a cell adhesion protein (absence of brown stain indicated by the asterisk, shown in the image). Which of the following cell adhesion proteins was most likely down-regulated in this patient's ductal carcinoma?

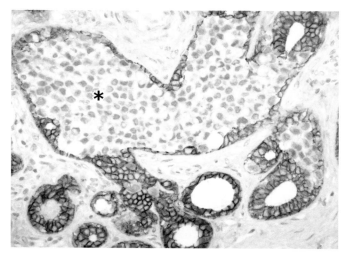

(A) Cadherin
(B) Fibronectin
(C) Integrin
(D) Laminin
(E) Selectin

29 A 58-year-old woman with a history of diabetes complains of swelling of her ankles. Physical examination reveals edema of the lower extremities. A kidney biopsy is obtained. Which of the following histochemical stains can be used to highlight the patient's glomerular basement membrane when examined by light microscopy?
(A) Aldehyde fuchsin
(B) Hematoxylin and eosin
(C) Luxol fast blue/cresyl violet
(D) Periodic acid–Schiff
(E) Trypan blue

30 A neurula-stage mouse embryo is stained by immuno-histochemistry with monoclonal antibodies directed to stage-specific embryonic antigens. A marker for embryonic ectoderm is colored brown, and a marker for early mesoderm is colored red. Which of the following terms best describes the region of the embryo indicated by the asterisk (shown in the image)?

(A) Ectoderm
(B) Endoderm
(C) Intermediate mesoderm
(D) Mesenchyme
(E) Somitic mesoderm

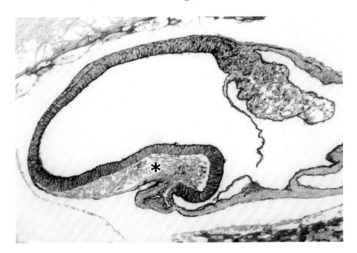

ANSWERS

1 **The answer is A: Apical and basal membrane domains.** The body is woven together with aggregates of cells (tissues) that collaborate to serve a common function. These tissue functions include (1) protection, transport, and secretion (epithelial tissue); (2) contraction and movement (muscle tissue); (3) reception and transmission of information (neural tissue); and (4) support (connective tissue). Epithelial tissue is divided into two general types based on function, namely lining/coating and glandular. Lining or coating epithelium is further classified on the basis of morphology (e.g., simple or stratified). In addition to absorption, secretion, and protection, epithelial cells provide receptors for the special sense organs. Lining/coating epithelial cells exhibit polarity. They have distinct apical and basal membrane domains; they feature close apposition of lateral membrane borders; and they synthesize a basal lamina that provides attachment and structural support. None of the other cellular features is unique to epithelial cells. Most cells/tissues feature anchoring and communicating cell junctions. Adipocytes, nerves, and muscle cells secrete a pericellular matrix that is referred to as lamina externa (choice E).
Keywords: Epithelial tissue, cell polarity

2 **The answer is C: Simple cuboidal.** This image shows parallel rows of cuboidal epithelial cells lining collecting ducts in the medulla of the kidney. The cells are more or less square (cuboidal) with central basophilic nuclei. The epithelial cells exhibit distinct polarity. Their apical membrane lines the lumen of the duct, whereas their basal membrane makes contact with a basal lamina of various adhesive glycoproteins. The basal lamina is not visible by light microscopy. The epithelium is said to be simple, because it is composed of a single layer (monolayer) of cells. Straight capillaries (vasa vecta) are observed to travel in parallel with the ducts. None of the other types of epithelium describes the morphology of these urinary collecting ducts.
Keywords: Kidney, collecting ducts

3 **The answer is B: Simple columnar.** This image shows a single layer of columnar epithelial cells lining a collecting duct. The cells are taller than they are wide. The nuclei are located near the base of the cells. Compared to cuboidal cells, columnar cells are generally believed to be more metabolically active. The apical cytoplasm of these columnar cells may be filled with organelles involved in fluid transport and/or secretion. In this H&E slide preparation, the cell nuclei are basophilic, whereas the cytoplasm is acidophilic. The red patches/smudges shown in the image represent clumps of hemolyzed red blood cells. None of the other types of epithelium describes the morphology of these urinary collecting ducts.
Keywords: Kidney, collecting ducts

4 **The answer is B: Connexins.** The lateral membrane borders of epithelial cells contain a variety of integral and peripheral membrane proteins that mediate cell adhesion and cell communication. Communicating (gap) junctions are formed by the assembly of subunits of the connexin family of integral membrane proteins. Together, 12 connexin proteins join to form a pore (connexon) that provide ionic coupling between adjacent cells. Gap junctions permit the rapid exchange of ions, metabolites, and small signaling molecules between cells and throughout the epithelium. Gap junctions are present in most tissues of the body (from nerve to muscle). They help tissues share resources and coordinate functions. Cadherins (choice A) are calcium-dependent cell adhesion molecules. Netrins (choice C) are secreted proteins involved in axon guidance during development. Perforins (choice D) are cytolytic proteins produced by killer T lymphocytes. Porins (choice E) are channel proteins found in the outer membrane of gram-negative bacteria.
Keywords: Gap junctions, cell communication

5 **The answer is D: Simple squamous.** This skin biopsy demonstrates vascular channels lined by thin cells with minimal cytoplasm and elongated nuclei. These flat scalelike cells form a simple squamous epithelium. Epithelial cells that line the heart, blood vessels, and lymphatic channels are referred to as endothelial cells. They have tight junctions that provide a permeability barrier between blood and extravascular tissues. In response to local injury, vascular endothelial cells initiate coagulation and inflammation. Mesothelium refers to the simple squamous epithelium that lines the pericardium, pleural cavities, and peritoneum. Hemangiomas are benign neoplasms of capillary endothelial cells. Erythrocytes within blood vessels can be used as a "histologic rulers," because they measure about 8 μm in diameter and their size is generally invariant. None of the other types of epithelium describes histologic features of vascular endothelial cells.
Keywords: Hemangiomas, endothelial cells

6 **The answer is B: Nonkeratinized stratified squamous.** This section of the esophagus reveals a stratified epithelium composed of multiple cell layers. Basal stem cells (arrowheads, shown in the image) undergo sequential changes in cell size, shape, nuclear morphology, and gene expression as they are pushed up toward the surface. The upper layer of this stratified epithelium is composed of squamous cells. This tissue is referred to as a nonkeratinized stratified squamous epithelium, because it lacks an external coating of insoluble keratin protein. Evidence of nuclear pyknosis (chromatin condensation) in the superficial region of this epithelium indicates that the keratinocytes are undergoing cellular senescence. None of the other types of epithelium describes histologic features of the esophageal mucosa.
Keywords: Esophagus, stem cells

7 **The answer is A: Cadherins.** During gastrulation, epiblast cells invaginate along the primitive streak to form mesodermal cells that migrate between the epiblast and the hypoblast. Cells that remain in the epiblast layer form the presumptive neural plate. This epithelial tissue is characterized by the presence of anchoring junctions that bind cells together and organize cytoskeletal proteins. Anchoring junctions include (1) zonula adherens junctions (cadherins linked to actin microfilaments) and (2) macula adherens junctions (cadherins linked to intermediate filaments). Cadherins are a family of calcium-dependent proteins that mediate cell adhesion, cell migration, and transmembrane signaling. Cadherins mediate epithelial cell–cell adhesion by forming "zipper-like" molecular interactions at the cell surface. Cloudins and occludins (choices B and D) form tight junctions (zonula occludens). Integrins (choice C) mediate cell–substrate adhesion at sites of focal adhesions and hemidesmosomes. Selectins (choice E) mediate leukocyte margination and extravasation during inflammation.

Keywords: Cadherins, gastrulation

8 **The answer is C: Na/K ATPase.** The amnion is a thin membrane sac that surrounds the embryo and fetus. It provides a protective, fluid-filled environment that permits the embryo to fold properly and develop normal limb appendages. Epithelial cells in the embryo and adult express a variety of transport proteins and pumps that move fluid and electrolytes from one compartment to another. For example, Na/K ATPase is a membrane pump that regulates water transport (uptake) in the gastrointestinal tract and kidney. This integral membrane protein uses ATP to transport sodium across the plasma membrane. If the pump is restricted to the lateral/basal membrane of a polarized epithelial cell, then transport of sodium toward the underlying basal lamina will cause water to flow across the epithelium to maintain isosmotic balance. Water can also move in the opposite direction across an epithelium to form a fluid-filled cavity. None of the other proteins regulates fluid or electrolyte transport.

Keywords: Na/K ATPase, amnion, chorion

9 **The answer is A: Keratinized stratified squamous.** This patient's skin biopsy shows a stratified epithelium composed of multiple cell layers. The superficial layer of this stratified epithelium features squamous cells that have undergone programmed cell death. As they undergo apoptosis, the keratinocytes leave behind an insoluble layer of keratin intermediate filament proteins (eosinophilic layer, visible in the image). None of the other types of epithelium describes histologic features of the epidermis.

Keywords: Skin, keratins

10 **The answer is C: Stratified cuboidal.** This image shows sweat ducts that are lined by a double layer of cuboidal epithelial cells. The cell nuclei are aligned in discrete rows. Tight (occluding) junctions between the ductal epithelial cells form an impermeable barrier. As a result of these zonula occludens junctions, the lateral membrane borders between adjacent ductal cells are not visible by light microscopy (shown in the image). Stratified cuboidal epithelium is rarely encountered in histopathology. It may reflect the need for greater support, or it may represent a transition zone for epithelial tissues that are switching from simple to stratified. None of the other types of epithelium describe histologic features of these sweat ducts in the dermis of the skin.

Keywords: Skin, eccrine sweat glands

11 **The answer is E: Zonula occludens.** As mentioned above, capillary endothelial cells are characterized by the presence of tight junctions that establish a permeability barrier between blood and extravascular interstitial tissue. These occluding junctions (zonula occludens) bring the lipid bilayers of adjacent cells into close proximity. Zonula occludens are composed principally of three proteins: occludin, claudin, and junctional adhesion molecule. The extracellular portions of these transmembrane proteins form a zipper-like structure that seals the intercellular space and limits *paracellular* fluid transport. Parenthetically, *transcellular* transport occurs when biomolecules move across the plasma membrane. In response to injury (e.g., mechanical friction raking leaves), inflammatory cells release cytokines and signaling molecules (e.g., histamine) that trigger capillary endothelial cells to disassemble tight junctions and form intercellular gaps. These cellular changes lead to the leakage of fluid from the blood into the surrounding extravascular space (referred to as edema fluid). In some organs, capillary endothelial cells exhibit small windows (fenestrae) that facilitate the transport of biomolecules across the endothelium. None of the other intercellular junctions regulates vascular permeability.

Keywords: Tight junctions, zonula occludens

12 **The answer is B: Stratified columnar.** This image shows stratified columnar epithelium lining an excretory duct in the lip. The cell nuclei are aligned in two distinct rows. The cells facing the lumen are taller than they are wide, hence the classification of this epithelium as stratified columnar. The duct is supported by loose connective tissue. Stratified columnar epithelium is rarely encountered in histopathology. None of the other types of epithelial tissue describes the histologic features of this large excretory duct.

Keywords: Excretory duct

13 The answer is B: Loss of cell contact inhibition of growth and motility. Superficial abrasions of the skin heal by a process of regeneration. Regeneration involves epithelial cell proliferation and migration. In brief, maturation of the epidermis requires an intact layer of basal stem cells that are in direct contact with one another. If this contact is disrupted, basal cells at the margin of the wound become activated. They proliferate and close the wound through cell migration. When epithelial continuity is reestablished, cell migration and cell division cease, and normal epidermal maturation resumes. This mechanism of epithelial growth regulation is referred to as "contact inhibition of growth and motility." The epidermal basement membrane provides a crucial "road map" that guides basal stem cells during regeneration of the epithelium. The other choices describe responses to deep wounds that involve the formation of granulation tissue.
Keywords: Skin abrasion, epithelial regeneration

14 The answer is E: Transitional. The renal calyces, ureters, urinary bladder, and proximal urethra are lined by a transitional epithelium. This "urothelium" is specialized to accommodate distention. Urothelium is stratified and appears to consist of five or six cell layers when the bladder is empty (shown in the image). Upon distention, however, the same epithelium would appear to consist of only three layers. The superficial cells are typically described as being cuboidal and dome shaped, because they appear to bulge into the lumen. Hematuria may be a symptom of an ascending urinary tract infection or (less commonly) bladder cancer. None of the other types of epithelium describes histologic features of the bladder mucosa.
Keywords: Urinary bladder, urothelium

15 The answer is A: Ciliated pseudostratified columnar with goblet cells. This image illustrates histologic features of the "respiratory epithelium" that lines the conducting airways of the lungs. Careful examination of this section of the trachea reveals (1) ciliated columnar epithelial cells, (2) distinct sizes/shapes of cell nuclei within the epithelium, and (3) numerous large secretory cells (goblet cells). Cilia are specialized apical membrane organelles that beat in a whiplike fashion to remove mucus and inhaled particles from the lungs. They function as a "mucociliary ladder." The distinct populations of cell nuclei shown in the image suggest that there are distinct populations of cells within the epithelium. If these cells are layered, then the epithelium is stratified. On the other hand, if these cells make contact with the underlying basement membrane, then the epithelium is said to be "pseudostratified." Although it is difficult to demonstrate by light microscopy, respiratory epithelium is pseudostratified. The basal membrane domains of all cells

in the epithelium are attached to the common basement membrane. Goblet cells secrete a protective mucus. None of the other types of epithelium describes the distinct histologic features of respiratory epithelium.
Keywords: Respiratory epithelium, mucociliary ladder

16 The answer is B: Hemidesmosomes. Membrane junctions that anchor cells to the extracellular matrix include focal adhesions and hemidesmosomes. Focal adhesions link the extracellular matrix to intracellular actin bundles through integrin membrane receptors. Focal adhesions are dynamic structures that regulate changes in cell motility and differentiation. By contrast, hemidesmosomes provide stable connections between polarized epithelial cells and the underlying basal lamina. Hemidesmosomes link the extracellular matrix to intermediate filament proteins through integrin membrane receptors. The distinction between the basal lamina and basement membrane is often a point of confusion. Basal laminae are pericellular deposits of glycoproteins and proteoglycans that are secreted by epithelial cells. This layer is very thin and cannot be visualized by light microscopy. By contrast, basement membranes are thicker and may be visualized by light microscopy, particularly in sections that are stained for carbohydrate using periodic acid–Schiff (PAS). Basement membranes consist of two layers of extracellular matrix: (1) glycoproteins and proteoglycans of the basal lamina and (2) type III collagen (reticular) fibers secreted by connective tissue fibroblasts. None of the other membrane junctions anchors epithelial cells to the basal lamina.
Keywords: Hemidesmosomes, basal lamina

17 The answer is D: Tubulin. Cilia are amazing apical membrane extensions that serve a variety of functions including whiplike movement and signal transduction. Motile cilia generate a mucociliary ladder that removes inhaled particles from the lungs, whereas immotile cilia provide mechanoreceptors that monitor gravity and acceleration in the ear. Recently, cilia have been shown to generate tiny currents that regulate the development of left/right asymmetry in the embryo. Without these "nodal cilia," the internal organs may be randomly placed. Cilia arise from membrane-associated microtubule-organizing centers, termed basal bodies. These organelles regulate the polymerization of $\alpha\beta$-tubulin dimers to form a core of microtubules that are referred to as the axoneme. In motile cilia, the axoneme is composed of a central pair of microtubules surrounded by nine microtubule doublets (9 + 2 configuration). Molecular motor proteins (e.g., dynein) hydrolyze ATP to initiate sliding movements of microtubules within the axoneme. Actin (choice A) polymerizes to form microfilaments. Desmin, keratin, and vimentin (choices B, C, and E) are intermediate filament proteins.
Keywords: Cilia, tubulin

18 The answer is D: Striated brush border. This high magnification photomicrograph of the small intestine reveals epithelial cells that are specialized for absorption. The apical membranes of these enterocytes are packed with delicate, fingerlike projections (microvilli) that provide increased surface area for enzymes and transport proteins. These nonmotile organelles are lined by actin microfilaments. In H&E-stained slide preparations, microvilli appear as a striated (brush-like) border along the external surface of the lining epithelium. Basal laminae (choice A) are extracellular matrix deposits along the basal membrane. Glycocalyx (choice B) is a molecular coat of oligosaccharides along the external surface of the apical membrane. Lamina propria (choice C) is connective tissue that fills the core of the intestinal villi. The faint, eosinophilic line that runs parallel to the striated brush border is a terminal web of actin microfilaments (choice E).
Keywords: Microvilli, striated brush border

19 The answer is D: Fluid transport. Epithelial cells that line the gastrointestinal (GI) tract transport fluid from the lumen of the gut to the underlying connective tissue. This transcellular transport mechanism is facilitated by basolateral membrane infoldings that provide increased surface area for proteins that pump sodium outside the cell. Water from the lumen of the GI tract follows the sodium gradient that is established by these pumps. After leaving the cell, water and electrolytes are drained by postcapillary venules and lymphatic channels. Careful examination of the image provided for Question 18 reveals spaces between the basolateral membranes of the epithelial cells (arrowheads, shown in the image). These open spaces provide indirect evidence for fluid transport in this tissue. Basolateral membrane folds do not regulate the other cellular processes listed.
Keywords: Na/K ATPase

20 The answer is B: Simple columnar. This beautiful photomicrograph shows a linear array of cell nuclei in the simple columnar epithelium that lines the mucosa of the small intestine. The nuclei are monomorphic and located near the basal region of these epithelial cells. The nuclei contain primarily euchromatin, suggesting an active pattern of gene expression. This slide preparation also illustrates the delicate nature of the lamina propria (connective tissue) that supports the avascular epithelium. Oxygen and nutrients move by passive diffusion into the overlying epithelium from capillaries in the lamina propria. None of the other types of epithelium describes histologic features of the intestinal mucosa.
Keywords: Intestinal villi

21 The answer is E: Unicellular exocrine mucous glands. Epithelial cells form glands that are specialized for the secretion of various molecules, including mucus,

enzymes, saline solution, hormones, and other signaling molecules. These glands may be unicellular (e.g., goblet cells in the gastrointestinal tract) or multicellular (e.g., pancreas). Glands that secrete products onto a surface, either directly or indirectly via a communicating duct, are referred to as *exocrine* glands. By contrast, glands that lack a communicating duct system are referred to as *endocrine* glands. This image reveals scattered PAS-positive goblet cells in the jejunum of the small intestine. These secretory epithelial cells are best described as unicellular exocrine mucous glands. None of the other terms describes histologic features of intestinal goblet cells.
Keywords: Goblet cells, unicellular glands

22 The answer is B: Glandular. As mentioned previously, epithelial tissue can be broadly classified as lining/coating or glandular. This autopsy specimen reveals glandular tissue in the parathyroid gland. The epithelial cells are small, monomorphic, and tightly packed with indistinct cell boarders. They secrete parathyroid hormone, which is taken up by capillaries to enter the systemic circulation. In contrast to lining/coating epithelial cells, these glandular epithelial cells appear to lack polarity. However, closer inspection reveals that these epithelial cells are organized into anastomosing cords and clusters. The endocrine cells are surrounded by adipocytes. The large clear spaces in these connective tissue cells are remnants of lipid inclusions that were extracted during tissue preparation. None of the other types of epithelium describes histologic features of the parathyroid gland.
Keywords: Parathyroid glands

23 The answer is A: Actin. Stereocilia are found only in the epididymis and on certain sensory cells of the inner ear. Despite their name, these apical membrane structures are really long, immotile microvilli. Like microvilli, stereocilia are filled with organized bundles of actin filaments. In the epididymis, stereocilia provide increased surface area for absorption of fluid. In the inner ear, these delicate structures serve as exquisitely sensitive mechanoreceptors. Tubulin (choice D) organizes cilia. Desmin, keratin, and vimentin (choices B, C, and E) are intermediate filament proteins.
Keywords: Epididymis, stereocilia

24 The answer is A: Apocrine. Exocrine glands use different mechanisms for secreting their products. These mechanisms are described as (1) apocrine (budding of apical cytoplasm); (2) merocrine (choice E, fusion of membrane-bound secretory vesicles with the plasma membrane); and (3) holocrine (choice D, release of a cellular inclusion following programmed cell death). Eccrine (choice B) refers to the secretion of water and salt by dermal sweat glands. Endocrine secretion (choice C) also involves the fusion of secretory vesicles with the plasma membrane (merocrine secretion). However, endocrine glands are ductless glands that release hormones directly into the circulatory system.

Keywords: Lactation, secretion, apocrine secretion

25 **The answer is C: Mucous.** The submandibular gland is a mixed exocrine gland that features both serous and mucous secretory units (referred to as acini). Serous secretions are protein rich and watery, whereas mucous secretions are carbohydrate rich and viscous. The arrows shown on this image identify pale cells with compressed peripheral nuclei. The cells are clustered around a narrow central lumen. These epithelial cells secrete heavily glycosylated proteins (mucins) that do not take up H&E. They would, however, stain with periodic acid–Schiff. Goblet cells (choice B) are unicellular mucous glands found in the gastrointestinal tract. Paracrine cells (choice D) secrete signaling molecules (paracrine factors) that influence cells in close proximity. None of the other types of differentiated cells exhibit cytologic features of mucous cells in the submandibular gland.

Keywords: Submandibular glands

26 **The answer is B: Laminin.** Epithelial cells secrete an adhesive matrix of glycoproteins and proteoglycans along their basal membrane. This pericellular basal lamina provides support and links epithelial cells to the underlying connective tissue. Basal laminae and connective tissue collagen fibers (joined together) form basement membranes that are visible in some tissues. Molecular components of the basal lamina include laminin, entactin, nidogen, type IV collagen, and proteoglycans (e.g., heparan sulfate). Assembly of the basal lamina is initiated by the attachment of integrin membrane receptors to laminin in the pericellular matrix. Entactin and nidogen form connections between laminin and type IV collagen. In addition to providing structural support, basal laminae sequester signaling molecules that regulate epithelial cell growth and differentiation. Desmoplakin, talin, and vinculin (choices A, C, and E) are attachment proteins that interact with cadherin and/or integrin receptors to form cell–cell anchoring junctions. Vimentin (choice D) is an intermediate filament protein.

Keywords: Basal lamina, laminin

27 **The answer is A: Actin.** Cytoskeletal proteins include microtubules (composed of tubulin), microfilaments (composed of actin), and intermediate filaments (composed of tissue-specific filamentous proteins). Actin filaments are found in most cells. In epithelial cells and tissues, actin filaments organize microvilli and regulate changes in cell shape and cell locomotion. In many lining

epithelial cells, actin filaments form a dense terminal web that stabilizes the apical membrane domain (including microvilli). Lamins (choice C) are intermediate filament proteins that organize nuclear chromatin. Tubulins (choice E) form microtubules that regulate vesicle transport and cell division. Desmin and nestin (choices B and D) are intermediate filament proteins expressed by muscle cells and neural stem cells, respectively.

Keywords: Terminal web, microfilaments

28 **The answer is A: Cadherin.** Cadherins are a family of calcium-dependent cell adhesion proteins. They form "zipper-like" anchoring junctions at the cell surface that mediate cell adhesion and transmembrane signaling. A variety of studies have shown that E-cadherin gene expression is reduced in most epithelial cancers (carcinomas). Without E-cadherin, neoplastic cells undergo an epithelial–mesenchymal transition, penetrate basement membranes, and invade capillary/lymphatic channels. Up-regulation of cadherin gene expression has been shown to suppress the invasion and metastasis of malignant cells. Fibronectin and laminin (choices B and D) are extracellular matrix glycoproteins. Integrins (choice C) mediate cell–substrate adhesion. P-selectin mediates the attachment of neutrophils to activated endothelial cells during acute inflammation.

Keywords: Breast cancer, cadherins

29 **The answer is D: Periodic acid–Schiff.** Basement membranes can be visualized in tissues that are stained with periodic acid–Schiff. This histochemical reagent binds sugars that are abundant in basement membranes at the junction between epithelial cells and the underlying connective tissue. The glomerular basement membrane has been shown to contain an abundance of heparan sulfate proteoglycan. Diabetes mellitus, a complex metabolic disease associated with glucosuria and polyuria, is the leading cause of end-stage renal disease in the United States, accounting for a third of all patients with chronic renal failure. In this condition, the glomeruli show diffuse mesangial matrix expansion and thickening of the glomerular basement membrane. Diabetic glomerulosclerosis results in progressive renal failure. None of the other histochemical stains are particularly useful for visualizing basement membranes by light microscopy.

Keywords: Basement membranes, diabetes mellitus

30 **The answer is D: Mesenchyme.** This embryo has completed gastrulation and is forming the neural tube and heart. The asterisk (shown in the image) identifies loosely arranged spindle cells that are floating in a noncollagenous extracellular matrix. This loose connective tissue is referred to as embryonic mesenchyme. Mesenchyme in the head region will contribute to the development of musculoskeletal structures in the head and neck. Ectoderm (choice A) will form the skin and central nervous system. Endoderm (choice B) will form the gastrointestinal tract and extramural gut derivatives (e.g., lungs and liver). Intermediate mesoderm (choice C) will give rise to the genitourinary system. Somitic mesoderm will form the dermis, skeletal muscle, and axial skeleton. Reciprocal inductive interactions between mesenchyme and epithelium will regulate organogenesis, providing the embryo with form and function.

Keywords: Mesenchyme, neurulation

Chapter 3

Connective Tissue

QUESTIONS

Select the single best answer.

1 A 60-year-old woman presents with several small, pearly nodules on the back of her neck. A biopsy of one lesion reveals a basal cell carcinoma and adjacent areas of normal skin (shown in the image). The area indicated by the asterisk is typically composed of which of the following tissue types?

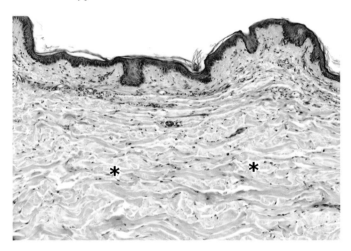

(A) Dense, irregular connective tissue
(B) Dense, regular connective tissue
(C) Glandular epithelium
(D) Skeletal muscle
(E) Smooth muscle

2 For the biopsy described in Question 1, which of the following types of connective tissue is found directly beneath the basophilic surface epithelium? This tissue is highly cellular and contains capillary loops that provide nutrients and oxygen to the overlying epithelium.
(A) Adipose tissue
(B) Dense irregular connective tissue
(C) Elastic connective tissue
(D) Loose connective tissue
(E) Reticular connective tissue

3 A 43-year-old woman presents with a mass in her right breast that she first detected 4 months ago. A firm 4-cm mass is palpated on breast examination. An excisional biopsy is obtained (shown in the image). The area indicated by arrows is primarily composed of which of the following types of connective tissue?

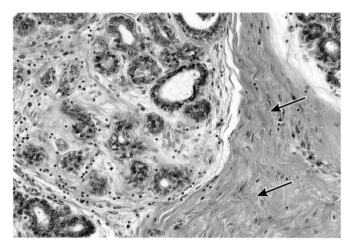

(A) Dense irregular
(B) Dense regular
(C) Elastic
(D) Loose
(E) Reticular

4 Which of the following cells are responsible for the synthesis and deposition of collagens and other extracellular matrix proteins in the area of the breast biopsy specified in Question 3?
(A) Adipocytes
(B) Fibroblasts
(C) Glandular epithelial cells
(D) Macrophages
(E) Plasma cells

5 A biopsy of an axillary lymph node from the patient described in Question 3 is examined by light microscopy. In this silver-stained section (shown in the image), the irregular black lines indicated by the arrows

30

represent which of the following stromal connective tissue components?

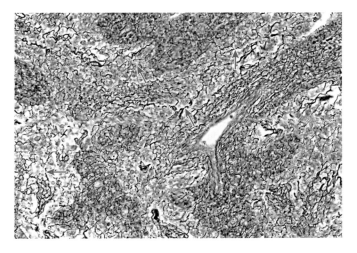

(A) Elastic fibers
(B) Fibrillin microfibrils
(C) Fibronectin glycoproteins
(D) Heparin sulfate proteoglycans
(E) Reticular fibers

6 The delicate stromal fibers described in Question 5 are composed primarily of which of the following structural proteins?
(A) Collagen type I
(B) Collagen type II
(C) Collagen type III
(D) Elastin
(E) Fibrillin

7 Which of the following bone marrow–derived cells is typically found within open spaces formed by the extracellular matrix fibers described in Question 5? These cells are believed to play an important role in anticancer immune surveillance.
(A) Lymphocytes
(B) Mast cells
(C) Macrophages
(D) Neutrophils
(E) Plasma cells

8 A 3-year-old girl is found to have extremely pliable skin. Her parents note that she bruises easily and that her joints can be hyperextended. Biochemical and genetic studies establish a diagnosis of Ehlers-Danlos syndrome. This patient's genetic disease is caused by an abnormality or deficiency of which of the following proteins?
(A) Actin
(B) Collagen
(C) Elastin
(D) Fibrillin
(E) Myosin

9 A 68-year-old man presents with a 2-week history of abdominal discomfort. A CT scan reveals a dilated and calcified segment of the abdominal aorta proximal to the bifurcation. Prior to surgery, the patient suffers a massive heart attack and expires. The abdominal aorta is examined at autopsy (shown in the image). Loss of which of the following cellular/biochemical components of the aortic media contributed the most to the development of this patient's abdominal aneurysm?

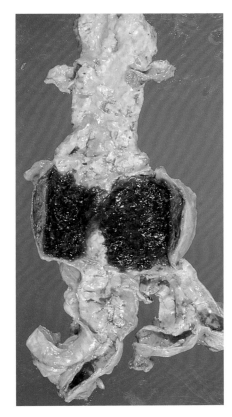

(A) Collagen type I fibers
(B) Elastic fibers/lamellae
(C) Heparin sulfate proteoglycans
(D) Reticular (type III collagen) fibers
(E) Smooth muscle bundles

10 A 12-month-old boy is brought to the emergency room for examination of his right arm following a tumble at school. Radiologic examination of the limb reveals a recent fracture of the right ulna and evidence of several additional healing fractures. Further testing demonstrates that this child has osteogenesis imperfecta, an autosomal dominant genetic disease caused by mutations in the gene for which of the following structural proteins?
(A) Collagen type I
(B) Collagen type II
(C) Elastin
(D) Fibrillin-1
(E) Laminin

11 Type I collagen described in Question 10 belongs to which subfamily of collagens?
(A) Anchoring fibril–forming collagens
(B) Fibril-associated collagens
(C) Fibril-forming collagens
(D) Network-forming collagens
(E) Transmembrane collagens

12 In patients with osteogenesis imperfecta, gene mutations that change which of the following amino acids can block the formation of collagen triple helices?
(A) Glycine
(B) Histidine
(C) Leucine
(D) Lysine
(E) Proline

13 During fibrillogenesis of type I collagen, the triple helix of the procollagen molecule is formed at which of the following locations?
(A) Extracellular space
(B) Golgi apparatus
(C) Nucleus
(D) Rough endoplasmic reticulum
(E) Secretory vesicles

14 A 28-year-old marine complains of gingivitis, skin hemorrhages, multiple infections, and poor wound healing. Laboratory studies suggest vitamin C deficiency (scurvy). Lack of vitamin C in this patient primarily affects which of the following essential steps in collagen fibrillogenesis?
(A) Cleavage of uncoiled collagen propeptides
(B) Formation of tropocollagen fibrils
(C) Galactosylation of hydroxylysine residues
(D) Hydroxylation of proline and lysine residues
(E) Secretion of procollagen into extracellular space

15 A 2-year-old girl with itchy skin and respiratory distress is brought to the emergency room by her parents 30 minutes after eating peanut butter cookies. On physical examination, the patient shows flushing and swelling of her lips and eyelids. Hives are present over her face and arms. Vital signs are blood pressure 90/40 mm Hg and pulse 100 per minute. Which of the following inflammatory cells is primarily responsible for the development of increased vascular permeability in this patient with a severe peanut allergy?
(A) Eosinophils
(B) Macrophages
(C) Mast cells
(D) Neutrophils
(E) Plasma cells

16 A 17-year-old boy presents with yellow and red-crusted lesions over his face of 5-day duration. He is a member of the high school wrestling team and has a recent history of intermittent low-grade fever. Skin cultures are positive for *Streptococcus pyogenes*. Spread of this bacterial infection within the patient's dermis may occur if the intrinsic viscosity of dermal connective tissue is altered by infection. Which of the following connective tissue components determines the viscosity of connective tissue and provides a protective barrier that limits the spread of deep-seeded bacterial infections in the skin?
(A) Collagen type I fibers
(B) Elastic fibers
(C) Fibroblast
(D) Ground substance
(E) Reticular (type III collagen) fibers

17 Which of the following connective tissue components binds the most water and regulates the crucial biological functions of the viscous and highly hydrated ground substance described in Question 16?
(A) Elastic fibers
(B) Fibroblasts
(C) Glycoproteins
(D) Glycosaminoglycans
(E) Proteoglycan core proteins

18 The parents of a 3-year-old boy are concerned that their son shows signs of physical and mental retardation. After a series of physical and laboratory examinations, the child is diagnosed with Hurler syndrome. This rare genetic disease is caused by disordered degradation and abnormal accumulation of which of the following connective tissue structural components?
(A) Collagen fibers
(B) Elastic fibers
(C) Glycoproteins
(D) Glycosaminoglycans
(E) Proteoglycan core proteins

19 Which of the following components of connective tissue links cells to the extracellular matrix to help maintain tissue integrity and regulate cell behavior?
(A) Proteoglycans
(B) Glycoproteins
(C) Collagen fibers
(D) Elastic fibers
(E) Glycosaminoglycans

20 A 12-year-old girl has a 1.5-cm birthmark (benign congenital nevus) removed from her left upper thigh under local anesthesia. Which of the following families of cell adhesion molecules is the principal component of the "provisional matrix" that mediates cell-to-matrix interactions during wound healing in this patient?
(A) Cadherins
(B) Fibronectins
(C) Integrins
(D) Laminins
(E) Selectins

21 The right lower limb of a 6-year-old boy becomes swollen and enlarged following a visit to South Africa. He is diagnosed with lymphatic filariasis. The patient's soft tissue swelling (edema) is caused by an accumulation of which of the following connective tissue components?

(A) Collagen fibers
(B) Glycoproteins
(C) Glycosaminoglycans
(D) Proteoglycans
(E) Tissue fluid

22 A 65-year-old woman jogger with a history of tendonitis affecting the pes anserinus at the knee suffers a massive stroke and expires. A section of her left sartorius tendon is examined at autopsy (shown in the image). This collagen-rich connective tissue is important in transmitting force from muscle to bone. Which of the following best describes this type of connective tissue?

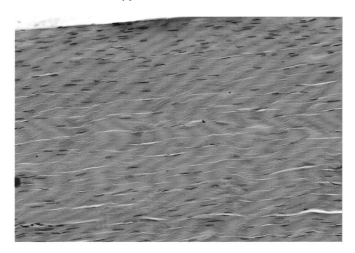

(A) Dense irregular
(B) Dense regular
(C) Elastic
(D) Loose
(E) Reticular

23 A 48-year-old man is admitted to the hospital with a fever of 38°C (103°F), night sweats, persistent cough, and prolonged diarrhea. Stool culture reveals the presence of acid-fast bacilli that are identified as *Mycobacterium avium–intracellulare*. Immune responses to the pathogen are known to involve IgA antibodies that are secreted into the lumen of the small intestine. This immunoglobulin is produced and secreted by which of the following bone marrow–derived cells?

(A) Eosinophils
(B) Macrophages
(C) Mast cells
(D) Neutrophils
(E) Plasma cells

24 A biopsy of the small intestine is sectioned and stained with H&E (shown in the image). Identify the cell indicated by the arrow.

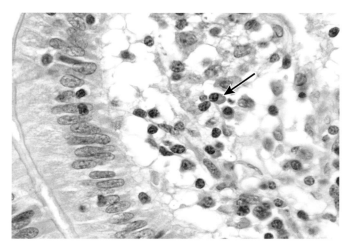

(A) Eosinophil
(B) Macrophage
(C) Mast cell
(D) Neutrophil
(E) Plasma cell

25 A 44-year-old woman presents with a 2-week history of fever and painful joints. Physical examination shows skin pigmentation, glossitis (inflammation of tongue), and generalized lymphadenopathy. The patient has lost 9 kg (20 lb) over the past 6 months. She reports that her stools are pale and foul smelling. Biopsy of the small intestine is shown in the image. Identify the cells indicated by the arrows.

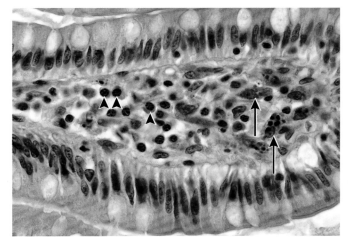

(A) Eosinophils
(B) Fibroblasts
(C) Macrophages
(D) Mast cells
(E) Plasma cells

26 In the image shown for Question 25, which of the following types of connective tissue best describes the cellular layer that lies below the simple columnar, lining epithelium?
(A) Adipose tissue
(B) Dense irregular connective tissue
(C) Elastic connective tissue
(D) Loose connective tissue
(E) Reticular connective tissue

27 A section of the aorta is examined at autopsy using a special stain (shown in the image). Identify the tissue type in the region indicated by the double arrow.

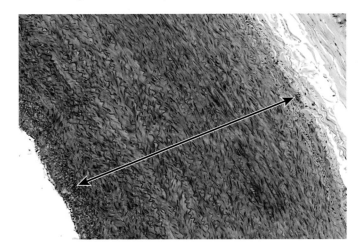

(A) Dense irregular connective tissue
(B) Dense regular connective tissue
(C) Elastic connective tissue
(D) Reticular connective tissue
(E) Smooth muscle tissue

28 A 38-year-old woman delivers a stillborn neonate with craniofacial abnormalities at 24 weeks gestation. A section of fetal skull is examined by light microscopy (shown in the image). Which of the following types of connective tissue best describes this autopsy specimen?

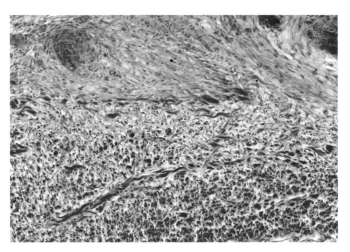

(A) Dense irregular connective tissue
(B) Hyaline cartilage
(C) Mesenchyme
(D) Nonmineralized bone
(E) Red bone marrow

29 An obese, 18-year-old man (BMI = 32 kg/m²) presents with questions regarding his weight. The patient admits to an unusually strong appetite and uncontrolled food intake. His behavior may be related to decreased serum concentration of which of the following hormones?
(A) Cholecystokinin
(B) Ghrelin
(C) Glucagon
(D) Leptin
(E) Melatonin

30 Thick Camper fascia from the abdomen of a 72-year-old man is examined at autopsy (shown in the image). Which of the following best describes histologic features of this tissue?

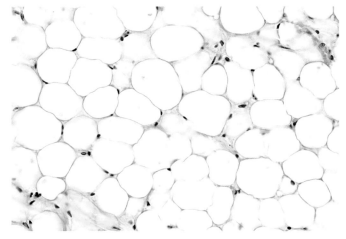

(A) Multilocular adipose tissue with cellular hyperplasia
(B) Multilocular adipose tissue with cellular hypertrophy
(C) Unilocular adipose tissue with cellular hyperplasia
(D) Unilocular adipose tissue with cellular hypertrophy
(E) Unilocular adipose tissue with cellular metaplasia

31 The adipocytes described in Question 30 are surrounded and supported by a network that is composed chiefly of which of the following fibers?
(A) Collagen
(B) Elastic
(C) Reticular
(D) Skeletal muscle
(E) Smooth muscle

32 In addition to providing body insulation and maintaining energy homeostasis, adipose tissue is considered to be an important organ for which of the following biological functions?

(A) Calcium storage

(B) Endocrine secretion

(C) Hematopoiesis

(D) Immune surveillance

(E) Wound healing

33 A 58-year-old obese man (BMI = 33 kg/m²) complains of headaches and blurry vision of 5-month duration. On physical examination, the blood pressure is 190/148 mm Hg. Malignant hypertension in this patient may be due, in part, to an increase in the serum concentration of which of the following adipocyte-produced hormones?

(A) Adiponectin

(B) Angiotensinogen

(C) Estrogens

(D) Leptin

(E) Resistin

34 A 15-year-old girl suffers from anorexia nervosa. During your physical examination of the patient, you understand that, despite inadequate nutrition, white adipose tissue will generally remain undiminished in mass in which of the following anatomic locations?

(A) Breast

(B) Greater omentum

(C) Mesentery of the small intestine

(D) Periorbital space

(E) Subcutaneous fascia

ANSWERS

1 **The answer is A: Dense, irregular connective tissue.** Basal cell carcinoma is the most common malignant tumor in persons with pale skin. It usually develops on the sun-damaged skin of people with fair skin and freckles. In this skin biopsy, dense irregular connective tissue in the dermis shows coarse, randomly oriented and eosinophilic collagen fibers and bundles with few cells. It can be found in the dermis, organ capsules, and between glandular tissues. Dense, regular connective tissue (choice B) is characterized by coarse collagen fiber/bundles that are regularly oriented and well organized. Glandular epithelia (choice C) are highly cellular and well organized. Skeletal muscle fibers (choice D) would show a uniform distribution with flattened peripheral nuclei. Smooth muscle fibers (choice E) would appear more cellular with abundant nuclei located in the center of each muscle fiber.
Keywords: Basal cell carcinoma, dense irregular connective tissue

2 **The answer is D: Loose connective tissue.** Loose connective tissue is the most common connective tissue type found throughout the body and provides support to other structures (e.g., epithelial tissues, blood vessels, muscles). In this skin biopsy, the tissue layer underlying the epithelium demonstrates characteristic features of loose connective tissue. It is highly cellular and vascular and contains loosely packed collagen fibers that are not identifiable by light microscopy. Elastic and reticular fibers are present in loose connective tissue, but the dominant fibers are collagenous. Therefore, choices C and E are incorrect. Since the collagenous fibers are loosely packed and there are no or few adipocytes, choices A and B are also incorrect.
Keywords: Basal cell carcinoma, loose connective tissue

3 **The answer is A: Dense irregular.** Breast cancer is the most common malignancy of women in the United States, and mortality from this disease among women is second only to that of lung cancer. In the normal portion of this breast biopsy, the indicated area surrounds lobules of the mammary gland. This area features densely packed collagen fibers oriented in different directions, with fewer cells than in the area immediately surrounding and cushioning the glandular epithelium (loose connective tissue). It may be confusing to students that collagen fibers in a localized area may appear "regular," particularly when viewed at high magnification; however, when examined over larger distance scales, the collagen fibers surrounding breast lobules are irregular. Therefore, choices B, C, D, and E are incorrect.
Keywords: Breast cancer, dense irregular connective tissue

4 **The answer is B: Fibroblasts.** For collagenous connective tissues present in skin and tendon, all of the components of the extracellular matrix (e.g., collagen fibers, elastic fibers, and ground substance) are produced by fibroblasts. Fibroblasts synthesize and secrete procollagen molecules of various types, as well as precursor molecules that form elastic fibers. Collagen and elastic fiber assembly and packing occur in the extracellular space. By contrast, elastic connective tissue components found in large arteries and veins are produced by smooth muscle cells. For the patient described in Question 3, invasion of stromal connective tissue by malignant cells usually incites a pronounced fibroblastic proliferation. This "desmoplasia" creates a palpable mass, which is the most common initial sign of ductal carcinoma of breast. Invasive ductal carcinoma usually manifests as a hard, fixed mass that is often referred to as scirrhous carcinoma. On gross examination, the tumor is typically firm and shows irregular margins. None of the other choices synthesizes large amounts of collagen.
Keywords: Fibroblasts, extracellular matrix

5 **The answer is E: Reticular fibers.** Reticular fibers are delicate, branching fibers that form a three-dimensional meshwork and supporting stroma. Reticular fibers are found in highly cellular organs, such as lymph nodes, spleen, liver, and pancreas. Routine H&E staining does not reveal the presence of reticular fibers. Reticular fibers appear black in slides treated with special silver stains. Elastic fibers (choice A) are composed of elastin and fibrillin microfibrils (choice B), and they are best visualized using special elastic stains. Fibronectin glycoproteins and heparin sulfate proteoglycans (choices C and D) are components of ground substance that do not show fibrous features when examined by light microscopy.
Keywords: Breast cancer, lymph nodes, reticular fibers

6 **The answer is C: Collagen type III.** Small-diameter, branching reticular fibers are composed mainly of type III collagen. Type I collagen (choice A) is the major component of collagenous fibers, whereas type II collagen (choice B) forms fibrils in the matrix of cartilage. Elastin and fibrillin (choices D and E) are major components of elastic fibers or lamellae.
Keywords: Reticular fibers

7 **The answer is C: Macrophages.** In lymph nodes and spleen, macrophages reside within the sinus-like spaces formed by reticular fibers. Here, they monitor material that passes through the organ. Pathogens and malignant cells are captured and phagocytosed by macrophages that reside in regional lymph nodes. Lymphocytes (choice A) form the parenchyma of lymph nodes. Plasma cells (choice E) and neutrophils (choice D) may be present in lymph nodes, but they are not specifically associated with reticular fibers. Mast cells (choice B) are typically found in loose connective tissue.
Keywords: Macrophage, lymph node

8 **The answer is B: Collagen.** Ehlers-Danlos syndrome (EDS) is a group of rare, autosomal dominant, inherited disorders of connective tissue that feature remarkable hyperelasticity and fragility of the skin and joint hypermobility. The common feature of most types of EDS is a generalized defect in collagen, including abnormalities in its molecular structure, synthesis, secretion, and degradation. Patients typically can stretch their skin many centimeters, and trivial injuries can lead to serious wounds. Because sutures do not hold well, dehiscence of surgical incisions is common. Hypermobility of the joints allows unusual extension and flexion. Abnormalities would not be expected in the other cell/tissue components listed.
Keywords: Ehlers-Danlos syndrome

9 **The answer is B: Elastic fibers/lamellae.** Aneurysms are localized dilations of blood vessels caused by a congenital or acquired weakness. An aneurysm is defined as an increase in the vessel's diameter by at least 50%. Forms of aneurysm include saccular, fusiform, and dissecting (tear in the media). The large majority of aneurysms of the abdominal aorta in elderly patients are related to atherosclerosis. The aneurysm in this patient was opened longitudinally to reveal a large mural thrombus within the lumen (see photograph). Loss of internal and external elastic fibers/lamina in the aortic wall is associated with aortic dilation and increased risk of rupture. Loss or deficiency of the other components is not believed to play a direct role in the pathogenesis of abdominal aortic aneurysm.
Keywords: Aneurysm, elastic lamellae/fibers

10 **The answer is A: Collagen type I.** Mutations in the type I collagen gene cause a deficiency in the synthesis of type I collagen and abnormal fibrillogenesis. Well-organized collagen fibers are the principal organic component of bone. They provide bone with flexibility. Brittle bones and frequent fractures are common complaints in patients with osteogenesis imperfecta. Mutations affecting type II collagen (choice B) are associated with Kniest dysplasia or type 2 achondrogenesis (cartilage abnormalities). Mutations affecting fibrillin-1 (choice D) cause Marfan syndrome (defective elastic fiber formation). Mutations affecting elastin (choice C) would cause vascular disorders. Laminins (choice E) are a family of adhesive glycoproteins in the extracellular matrix. Mutations in the laminin beta-2 gene are associated with Pierson syndrome, a congenital disease with neurological, renal, and ocular deficits.
Keywords: Osteogenesis imperfecta

11 **The answer is C: Fibril-forming collagens.** Collagen is a protein superfamily composed of at least 27 types. Based on their structural and amino acid similarities, collagens are divided into several subfamilies. Type I collagen, as well as collagen types II, III, V, and XI contain uninterrupted glycine–proline–hydroxyproline repeats, and their triple-helical molecules assemble into fibrils.

Therefore, these collagens comprise a fibril-forming subfamily (fibrillar collagens). Fibril-associated collagens (choice B), such as types XII and XIV, have interruptions in their triple helices; they associate with the surface of collagen fibrils and regulate fibril assemble. Some collagens, for example, type VII, form anchoring fibrils (choice A) that bind the basal lamina to the underlying connective tissue. Network-forming collagens (choice D) create complex networks, such as type IV collagen in basement membranes, type VI collagen forming a pericellular filamentous network in cartilage, and type VIII and X collagen networks in tissues. Transmembrane collagens (choice E), such as types XVII and XIII, link cells with extracellular matrix glycoproteins.
Keywords: Collagens

12 **The answer is A: Glycine.** To form a collagen triple helix, every third amino acid in each of the three procollagen α-chains must be glycine. Other amino acids can occur in the other two positions, but the most abundant amino acids in collagen are hydroxyproline and hydroxylysine. A gene mutation involving glycine at the third position will affect the formation of the triple helix and block the synthesis and deposition of collagen fibrils/fibers.
Keywords: Collagens, osteogenesis imperfecta

13 **The answer is D: Rough endoplasmic reticulum.** Formation of type I collagen fibers in connective tissue involves intracellular procollagen synthesis, as well as extracellular assembly of collagen molecules into fibrils and fibers. The procollagen α-chains are synthesized and further modified in the rough endoplasmic reticulum (rER) through a series of posttranslational modifications, including, but not limiting to (1) hydroxylation of proline and lysine residues, (2) cleavage of the signal peptide from the pro-α-chains, and (3) glycosylation of specific hydroxylysine residues. The modified pro-α-chains form triple helical procollagen molecules that are further stabilized by hydrogen and disulfide bonds in the rER. Procollagen molecules are then transported into the Golgi apparatus (choice B), where they are packed into secretory vesicles (choice E) and secreted into the extracellular space (choice A).
Keywords: Collagen, posttranslational modifications

14 **The answer is D: Hydroxylation of proline and lysine residues.** Intra- and interchain hydrogen bonds, disulfide bonds, and chaperone proteins are all essential for the formation of the triple-helical structure of procollagen. Hydroxyl groups added to proline and lysine residues during posttranslational processing provide the structural basis for hydrogen bonding. Vitamin C (ascorbic acid) is an essential cofactor for enzymes that regulate hydroxylation of proline and lysine. These enzymes are lysyl hydroxylase and prolyl hydroxylase. Vitamin C deficiency causes defects in the formation of triple helical procollagen, and this results in poor wound healing.

Skin hemorrhages arise from capillaries that have weak walls and are easily damaged by minor trauma. Impaired collagen synthesis also leads to gingivitis and alveolar bone resorption, which may lead eventually to loss of teeth. None of the other biochemical steps in collagen fibrillogenesis are affected by vitamin C deficiency.
Keywords: Scurvy, vitamin C deficiency

15 **The answer is C: Mast cells.** Antigens binding to receptors on the surface of mast cells trigger the release of inflammatory mediators such as histamine. Release of this vasoactive mediator from stored mast cell granules causes an immediate hypersensitivity reaction. The other cells are involved in inflammation, but they do not initiate immediate hypersensitivity. Eosinophils (choice A) are involved in the defense against parasitic infestations. Macrophages and neutrophils (choices B and D) respond to cell injury. They internalize debris and pathogens via phagocytosis. Macrophages also "present" foreign antigens to lymphocytes to initiate immune responses. Plasma cells (choice E) synthesize and secrete immunoglobulin (antibody).
Keywords: Peanut allergy, type 1 hypersensitivity reaction

16 **The answer is D: Ground substance.** Ground substance is a highly hydrated, transparent mixture of macromolecules occupying the extracellular space located between cells and fibrous components of the connective tissue. This complex mixture of macromolecules is viscous and serves to lubricate joints and internal organs. Due to its high viscosity, ground substance can also serve as a barrier to invading bacteria and other microorganisms and helps prevent them from spreading by lateral diffusion into adjacent tissues. However, some bacteria secrete hyaluronidase, an enzyme that degrades proteoglycans. This enzyme significantly reduces the viscosity of ground substance, enabling hyaluronidase-positive bacteria to be more invasive. Impetigo in this patient represents a localized, intraepidermal infection with *S. pyogenes*. It spreads by close contact and most commonly affects children. Minor trauma allows inoculation of bacteria. The intraepithelial pustule that forms will eventually rupture and leak a purulent inflammatory exudate.
Keywords: Impetigo, ground substance

17 **The answer is D: Glycosaminoglycans.** Proteoglycans, glycosaminoglycans, and glycoproteins are the three major groups of macromolecules found in the ground substance of connective tissue. Glycosaminoglycans (GAGs) are linear heteropolysaccharides formed by repeating disaccharide units. GAGs are categorized into seven distinct groups based on their specific sugar residues and degree of sulfation. These groups include hyaluronan, chondroitin-4-sulfate and chondroitin-6-sulfate, dermatan sulfate, keratan sulfate, heparan sulfate, and heparin. The largest and most ubiquitous GAG is hyaluronic acid. The carbohydrate chains of this polyanion typically contain thousands of monosaccharides. GAGs

are highly negatively charged, and they attract/retain a large volume of water. This hydrated gel lubricates tissues and absorbs shock. GAGs bound to core proteins form large macromolecular structures termed proteoglycans. Whereas GAG chains retain large amounts of water, the core proteins of proteoglycans (choice E) do not bind water. Glycoproteins (choice C) contain multivalent domains that interconnect and stabilize cells within the extracellular matrix. Fibrous components and cells (choices A and B) are not involved directly in regulating the viscosity of ground substance.
Keywords: Ground substance

18 **The answer is D: Glycosaminoglycans.** Hurler syndrome is a rare genetic disorder characterized by excess accumulation of glycosaminoglycans in tissue. Highly glycosylated proteoglycans are constantly synthesized and degraded within lysosomes. Deficiency of these crucial lysosomal enzymes blocks substrate degradation and leads to intracellular accumulation of glycosaminoglycans. Symptoms of these "mucopolysaccharidoses" depend on the particular enzyme that is deficient. In Hurler syndrome, deficiency of alpha-L-iduronidase causes heparan sulfate and dermatan sulfate to accumulate in various tissues and organs. Hurler syndrome presents in early childhood, and patients may die at young age.
Keywords: Hurler syndrome, glycosaminoglycans

19 **The answer is B: Glycoproteins.** Glycoproteins are secreted molecules that contain linear or branched N-linked and O-linked oligosaccharides. Adhesive glycoproteins of the extracellular matrix possess binding domains for collagen fibrils, proteoglycans, GAGs, and other glycoproteins. These glycoproteins also contain binding sites for cells and interact with cell surface receptors (e.g., integrins). These multiadhesive features enable glycoproteins to link cells and tissues to extracellular matrix to maintain tissue integrity. They also provide signals for cell proliferation and cell migration. None of the other components exhibit multiple binding domains that link cells to the matrix.
Keywords: Glycoproteins

20 **The answer is B: Fibronectins.** Fibronectins are perhaps the most abundant multiadhesive glycoproteins in the extracellular matrix of connective tissues. Plasma-derived fibronectin is also deposited at sites of tissue injury to facilitate wound healing. During the initial phase of healing, fibronectin in the extravasated plasma is cross-linked to fibrin, collagen, and other extracellular matrix components by the action of transglutaminases. This cross-linking provides a provisional stabilization of the wound during the first several hours and provides a substrate for cell adhesion and migration. Cadherins (choice A) and integrins (choice C) are cell–cell adhesion molecules. Like the selectin family of cell adhesion proteins, they are found at the cell surface and are not part of the extracellular matrix. Laminins (choice D) are present

in basement membranes. Selectins (choice E) are sugar-binding glycoproteins that mediate the initial attachment of leukocytes to endothelial cells at sites of inflammation.
Keywords: Nevus, wound healing

21 **The answer is E: Tissue fluid.**   A small amount of tissue fluid is normally retained in extracellular/interstitial space. This fluid is similar in ion composition to blood plasma. In certain pathologic conditions, fluid passes through the capillary wall and accumulates in the tissue resulting in soft tissue edema. Conditions associated with generalized edema include lymphatic obstruction secondary to filarial infestations of regional lymph nodes; decreased venous return to the heart due to congestive heart disease; increased capillary hydrostatic pressure; and loss of plasma protein (reduced oncotic pressure). Filariasis is caused by infestation of filarial nematodes that reside in lymphatic vessels and lymph nodes, thereby causing lymphatic obstruction and lymphedema. Severe and massive lymphedema is referred to as elephantiasis. Filariasis is common in Africa and South Asia.
Keywords: Filariasis, edema

22 **The answer is B: Dense regular.**   Dense regular connective tissue is found in tendons and ligaments, where coarse strong collagen fibers are organized into regularly oriented, parallel bundles. Elongated fibroblasts are located in spaces that are parallel to the collagen fibers. In longitudinal sections of tendon (shown in the image), fibroblast nuclei appear as linear dark lines interspersed with collagen bundles. The cytoplasm of fibroblasts cannot be distinguished from collagen in H&E slide preparations. The organization of collagen fibers in dense regular connective tissue serves to resist forces generated in the same direction, in response to stress. As a result, dense regular connective tissue is adapted to transmit force from muscle to bone in tendons or transmit force from bone to bone in ligaments. Dense regular connective tissue exhibits a small amount of ground substance and few cells or vessels. None of the other types of connective tissue exhibit histologic features of tendon.
Keywords: Tendons, dense regular connective tissue

23 **The answer is E: Plasma cells.**   *M. avium* and *M. intracellulare* are similar mycobacterial species that cause identical diseases and are, therefore, classified together as *M. avium–intracellulare* complex (MAC). MAC is a rare, granulomatous, pulmonary disease in immunocompetent persons, but it is a progressive systemic disorder in patients with AIDS. One-third of all AIDS patients develop overt MAC infections. The proliferation of organisms and the recruitment of macrophages produce expanding lesions, ranging from epithelioid granulomas containing few organisms to loose aggregates with foamy macrophages. Plasma cells are located in various locations throughout the body including the lamina propria of the gastrointestinal tract. Plasma cells (derived from B lymphocytes) produce soluble

antibodies that target invading pathogens for destruction. None of the other inflammatory cells secrete antibodies.
Keywords: Acquired immunodeficiency, plasma cells

24 **The answer is E: Plasma cell.**   Plasma cells are considered to be immigrant cells that migrate from the vascular space into connective tissues. In routine H&E-stained sections, the nuclei of mature plasma cells display a characteristic "clock-face" or "cartwheel" appearance with a prominent, centrally located nucleolus and clumps of heterochromatin along the periphery of the nucleus. Plasma cell cytoplasm is typically basophilic, owing to an abundance of rER that facilitates active protein synthesis. An extensive Golgi apparatus may also be seen as a pale-stained area in close proximity to the nucleus. None of the other cells exhibit cytologic features of plasma cells.
Keywords: Plasma cells

25 **The answer is C: Macrophages.**   Whipple disease is a rare infectious disorder of the small intestine in which malabsorption is the most prominent feature. The disorder typically features infiltration of the small bowel mucosa by macrophages that are packed with small, rod-shaped bacilli (*Tropheryma whippelii*). Infiltrates of macrophages containing bacilli may be found in other organs, including the lymph nodes and heart. Macrophages bind and internalize pathogens and necrotic tissue debris. As seen in the image, macrophages are large cells with eosinophilic cytoplasm containing phagocytosed material. Plasma cells are identified with arrowheads (shown in the image). None of the other cells are phagocytes.
Keywords: Whipple disease, macrophages

26 **The answer is D: Loose connective tissue.**   The lamina propria is a cellular layer of loose connective tissue that underlies the lining epithelium of the gastrointestinal (GI) tract. Loosely packed collagen fibers and some elastic fibers are present in the lamina propria, but they are not readily apparent in routine H&E-stained preparations. The lamina propria of the GI tract contains an abundance of cells, including numerous capillaries and lymphatic vessels (shown in the image). None of the other types of connective tissue describes histologic features of the lamina propria.
Keywords: Loose connective tissue, lamina propria

27 **The answer is C: Elastic connective tissue.**   Elastic connective tissue is found in large elastic arteries and some ligaments along the vertebral column (e.g., ligamentum flavum). In some tissues, elastic fibers (ligamentum flavum) or elastic lamellae (large arteries) comprise the predominant extracellular structural component. Collagen fibers/bundles are also present, but they are far less abundant than in collagenous connective tissue. In the tunica media (the middle layer of large arterial walls), layers of smooth muscle fibers (choice E) are found between elastic lamellae and collagen fibers. In most types of connective tissue, fibroblasts synthesize the extracellular components; however, smooth muscle cells synthesize the connective tissue found in large elastic arteries (elastic lamellae, collagen fibers, and ground substance). None of the other connective tissues listed feature elastic fibers/lamellae as a major structural component.

Keywords: Elastic connective tissue

28   The answer is C: Mesenchyme.   Mesenchyme is embryonic primitive connective tissue that gives rise to all the adult connective tissue types. Muscle tissues, vascular, and urogenital systems are also derived from embryonic mesenchyme. In a routine H&E preparation, mesenchymal cells appear small and spindle shaped. Fine, delicate, and sparse collagen fibers are scattered between the cells. Undifferentiated mesenchymal cells may be present in adult connective tissue, but they cannot be distinguished from fibroblasts on H&E staining. The other tissues are examples of adult connective tissue, and they do not describe histological features of embryonic mesenchyme.

Keywords: Mesenchyme

29   The answer is D: Leptin.   Leptin is a 16-kD polypeptide hormone produced by adipocytes in white adipose tissue. It acts on leptin receptors in the hypothalamus to regulate food intake and energy use. Unlike short-term weight control hormones, such as peptide YY, inhibition of appetite by leptin has a long-term effect on weight. Absence or decreased serum levels of leptin result in uncontrolled food intake and obesity. Cholecystokinin (choice A) is secreted by mucosal epithelial cells of the small intestine and regulates digestion in the small intestine by stimulating the release of digestive enzymes and bile. Glucagon (choice C) is secreted by the pancreas and raises blood glucose levels. Together with insulin, glucagon helps maintain stable levels of blood glucose. Melatonin (choice E), secreted by the pineal gland, regulates the rhythmic sleep–wake cycle. Ghrelin (choice B) is produced by the small intestine and functions as a "meal initiator" by stimulating the sense of hunger. Overproduction of ghrelin in patients with Prader-Willi syndrome can cause compulsive eating and obesity.

Keywords: Obesity

30   The answer is D: Unilocular adipose tissue with cellular hypertrophy.   In white adipose tissue, adipocytes are large, crowded, polyhedral cells. The cells are filled with one single droplet of lipid (i.e., unilobular cells). The cytoplasm and nucleus are pushed to the periphery of the cell. In routine histological preparations, lipid extraction during tissue processing causes adipocytes to assume a signet ring profile. Excessive energy intake with less energy expenditure results in obesity, with a significant accumulation of adipose tissue. In childhood, obesity results from increases in the size (hypertrophy) of adipocytes, as well as the formation of new adipocytes (hyperplasia). In adults, obesity principally involves accumulation of lipid within existing adipocytes (hypertrophy). Multilocular adipose tissue (choices A and B), termed brown adipose tissue, is mainly

found in newborns. Unilocular adipose tissue with cellular hyperplasia (choice C) occurs in early childhood but does not contribute to the pathogenesis of adult obesity.

Keywords: Obesity, adipose tissue

31   The answer is C: Reticular fibers.   Adipocytes synthesize and secrete reticular (type III collagen) fibers that form an interwoven network that provides support. These reticular networks are only visible using special stains. They are invisible by H&E staining. The meshwork of polygonal strands seen in the image shown in Question 30 consists of the cytoplasm of two adjacent adipocytes and the thin layer of the extracellular matrix that is located between them. Rich supply of blood vessels and nerves are found in the extracellular spaces between the crowded adipocytes. Elastic fibers and collagen fibers are also present in the extracellular matrix between adipocytes, but unlike reticular fibers, they do not form an interwoven network. Skeletal and smooth muscle fibers (choices D and E) are not found in white adipose tissue.

Keywords: Obesity, adipocytes

32   The answer is B: Endocrine secretion.   A variety of hormones, growth factors, and cytokines are produced in white adipose tissue. Leptin (discussed earlier in this chapter) is a polypeptide hormone secreted by adipocytes that helps regulate food intake and body weight control. Therefore, adipose tissue is not only an organ for energy storage; it also serves as an endocrine organ. Adipose tissue does not regulate the other biological functions listed.

Keywords: Adipose tissue

33   The answer is B: Angiotensinogen.   Adipocytes produce the polypeptide hormone, angiotensinogen (AGE). This hormone is also secreted by other tissues/organs (e.g., liver). Over production of AGE is associated with systemic hypertension. For this reason, obese individuals commonly suffer from systemic hypertension. None of the other adipocyte-produced hormones regulates systemic blood pressure.

Keywords: Obesity, systemic hypertension

34   The answer is D: Periorbital space.   White adipose tissue found throughout the body functions as an organ for energy storage, insulation, cushioning, and hormone secretion. When caloric intake is reduced, as in this case of anorexia nervosa (a disorder with irrational fear of gaining weight and extreme restriction of food), lipids within adipocytes are broken down and mobilized to provide energy. White adipose tissue in most regions of the body (choices A, B, C, and E) is depleted of lipid. However, white adipose tissue in certain parts of the body (e.g., beneath the epicardium, in the periorbital space, in the palms of the hands, and in soles of the feet) remain largely undiminished during long periods of starvation, so as to maintain cushioning functions in these critical areas.

Keywords: Anorexia nervosa

Chapter 4

Cartilage and Bone

QUESTIONS

Select the single best answer.

1 A 16-year-old track and field athlete asks for advice on protecting her knee joints from "wear-and-tear" injury. In this connection, articular cartilage acts as an excellent shock absorber and provides resilience against load. This critical biomechanical function is attributed chiefly to which of the following components of cartilage?
(A) Extracellular calcium phosphate
(B) Extracellular water
(C) Intracellular glycogen
(D) Intracellular water
(E) Membrane glycoproteins

2 For the patient described in Question 1, which of the following cartilage components plays the most important role in binding extracellular (interstitial) water?
(A) Collagen type II fibrils
(B) Glycosaminoglycans
(C) Membrane glycolipids
(D) Membrane glycoproteins
(E) Proteoglycan core proteins

3 A 59-year-old obese woman (BMI = 33 kg/m²) complains of sharp pain and stiffness of her knee joints. The pain is typically worse following exercise and prolonged use of her joints. She is diagnosed with degenerative osteoarthritis. Which of the following best describes the pathogenesis of joint pain in this patient?
(A) Acute inflammation of joint ligaments
(B) Chronic inflammation of the synovium with pannus formation
(C) Degeneration of articular cartilage
(D) Degeneration of cortical bone
(E) Reduced volume of synovial fluid

4 The knee joint of a 68-year-old woman is examined at autopsy. The articular cartilage shown in the image differs from hyaline cartilage in which of the following ways?

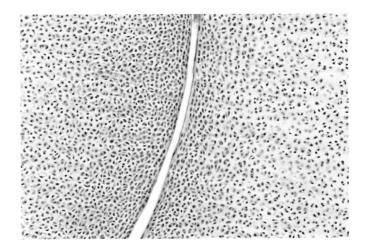

(A) Absence of blood vessels in the cartilage matrix
(B) Absence of perichondrium
(C) Amorphous cartilaginous matrix
(D) Chondrocytes organized in isogenous groups
(E) Chondrocytes located within lacunae

5 Which of the following types of collagen is the principal protein forming the intricate, three-dimensional meshwork found in hyaline cartilage throughout the body?
(A) Type I
(B) Type II
(C) Type III
(D) Type V
(E) Type VI

6 The collagen molecules of the type described in Question 5 self-aggregate to form which of the following structures in hyaline cartilage?
(A) Bundles
(B) Fibers
(C) Fibrils
(D) Filaments
(E) Procollagens

7 Which of the following proteins is the most abundant proteoglycan core protein found in hyaline cartilage?
(A) Aggrecan
(B) Biglycan
(C) Decorin
(D) Lumican
(E) Versican

8 Which of the following components of hyaline cartilage links the chondrocyte cell surface with the surrounding extracellular matrix and thereby helps regulate the turnover, degeneration, and repair of hyaline cartilage?
(A) Collage type II fibrils
(B) Collagen type IV fibrils
(C) Glycoproteins
(D) Glycosaminoglycans
(E) Proteoglycans

9 A 64-year-old man with a history of smoking presents with chest pain and hemoptysis. Chest x-ray demonstrates a bronchial mass, and a CT-guided needle biopsy reveals squamous cell carcinoma. The tumor and tissue margin containing bronchial cartilage are resected, and the specimen is examined by light microscopy (shown in the image). The matrix of the hyaline cartilage appears heterogeneous in color. Which of the following best describes the region indicated by the arrows?

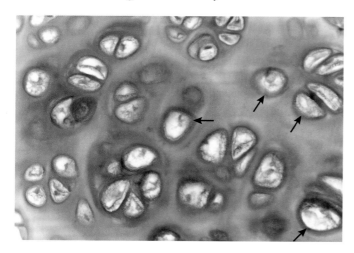

(A) Inner layer of the perichondrium
(B) Interterritorial matrix
(C) Outer layer of the perichondrium
(D) Pericellular matrix
(E) Territorial matrix

10 For the patient described in Question 9, what is the principal collagen type found within the region indicated by the arrows?
(A) Type II
(B) Type VI
(C) Type IX
(D) Type X
(E) Type XI

11 For the surgical specimen described in Question 9, which of the lettered arrows on the photomicrograph identifies the interterritorial matrix?

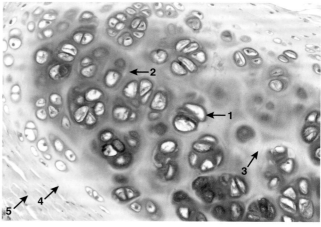

(A) Arrow 1
(B) Arrow 2
(C) Arrow 3
(D) Arrow 4
(E) Arrow 5

12 For the surgical specimen described in Question 9, which of the following patterns of cartilage growth is demonstrated (evidenced) by the heterogeneous distribution of proteoglycans, glycoproteins, and collagens within the hyaline cartilage matrix?
(A) Appositional growth from chondroblasts
(B) Appositional growth from chondrocytes
(C) Interstitial growth from chondroblasts
(D) Interstitial growth from chondrocytes

13 A surgical specimen containing normal cartilage is examined by light microscopy (shown in the image). The tissue/substance present within the rectangular box is best described as which of the following?

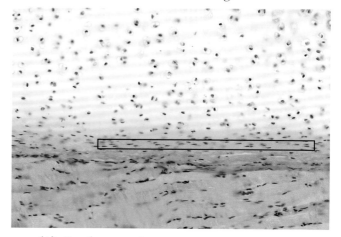

(A) Cartilage matrix
(B) Inner layer of the perichondrium
(C) Interstitial matrix
(D) Outer layer of the perichondrium
(E) Pericellular matrix

14 A 70-year-old woman with a mediastinal mass is diagnosed with primary lung cancer. The surgical specimen includes normal bronchial cartilage tissue and malignant cells. Slides are examined in the department of pathology (shown in the image). Identify the cells/structures indicated by the circles?

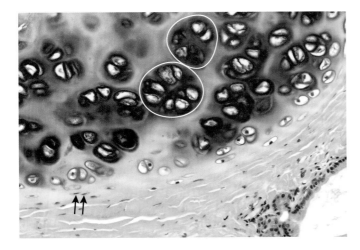

(A) Chondroblasts
(B) Ground substance
(C) Interterritorial matrix
(D) Isogenous groups
(E) Lacunae

15 For the surgical specimen described in Question 14, the nuclei indicated by the arrows shown in the image belong to which of the following types of connective tissue cells?
(A) Chondroblasts
(B) Chondrocytes
(C) Endothelial cells
(D) Fibroblasts
(E) Myofibroblasts

16 Which of the following cells is responsible for appositional growth of hyaline cartilage during growth and development?
(A) Chondroblasts in the perichondrium
(B) Chondrocytes in matrix lacunae
(C) Chondrocytes in isogenous groups
(D) Fibroblasts in the perichondrium
(E) Mesenchymal stem cells in the perichondrium

17 The parents of a 3-year-old boy complain that their child has a high fever, sore throat, and hoarse voice. On physical examination, the child's epiglottis appears swollen and erythematous. The boy is diagnosed with acute bacterial epiglottitis. In considering this case, you recall that the epiglottis at the entrance to the larynx is composed primarily of which of the following types of connective tissue?
(A) Dense, irregular connective tissue
(B) Dense, regular connective tissue
(C) Elastic cartilage
(D) Fibrocartilage
(E) Hyaline cartilage

18 Cartilage obtained at autopsy of a 50-year-old woman is examined by light microscopy (shown in the image). Which of the following histologic features in this photomicrograph is most useful for determining the specific type of cartilage?

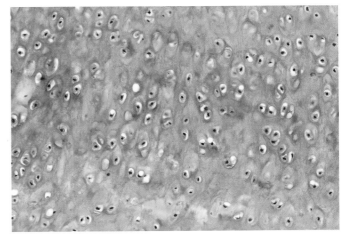

(A) Density of proteoglycans in the matrix
(B) Elastic fibers in the matrix
(C) Orientation of type II collagen fibers in the matrix
(D) Thickness of the surrounding perichondrium
(E) Type I collagen fibers in the matrix

19 A herniated intervertebral disc was removed surgically from the lumbar region of a 48-year-old man. Which of the following types of connective tissue is located within the peripheral annulus of this patient's intervertebral disc?
(A) Dense, irregular connective tissue
(B) Dense, regular connective tissue
(C) Elastic cartilage
(D) Fibrocartilage
(E) Hyaline cartilage

20 Fibrocartilage is a type of connective tissue characterized by resistance to tearing and compression. It combines which of the following basic histologic features?
(A) Elastic cartilage and dense, irregular connective tissue
(B) Elastic cartilage and dense, regular connective tissue
(C) Hyaline cartilage and dense, irregular connective tissue
(D) Hyaline cartilage and dense, regular connective tissue
(E) Hyaline cartilage and elastic cartilage

21 Which of the following types of cartilage or bone is found in the epiphyseal growth plates of children and adolescents?
(A) Articular cartilage
(B) Elastic cartilage
(C) Fibrocartilage
(D) Hyaline cartilage
(E) Immature bone

22 A 58-year-old man with a history of ischemic heart disease is scheduled for coronary artery bypass graft surgery. Before cutting the costal cartilage to open the chest cavity, the surgeon is mindful that healing of cartilage is problematic. She understands that hyaline cartilage has a limited capacity to undergo repair and regeneration due to which of the following intrinsic attributes?
(A) Avascularity of the cartilage matrix
(B) Cell cycle arrest of differentiated chondrocytes
(C) Deficiency of chondroblasts in the perichondrium
(D) Overgrowth of fibroblasts at the wound site
(E) Presence of growth inhibitory cytokines released by neutrophils

23 A 55-year-old man complains of bone pain affecting his right femur. X-ray of the leg reveals a thickened bone shaft and a mass with poorly defined borders. Biopsy of the mass is examined by light microscopy (shown in the image). Based on morphology, which of the following is the most likely diagnosis for this malignant neoplasm?

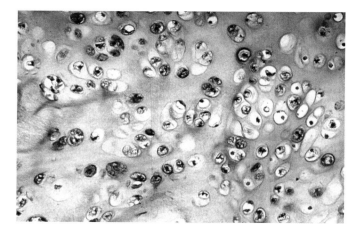

(A) Chondroma
(B) Chondrosarcoma
(C) Fibroma
(D) Osteoma
(E) Osteosarcoma

24 Which of the following osteocyte-derived biomolecules is the major structural component present in bone matrix?
(A) Aggrecan
(B) Collagen type I
(C) Collagen type II
(D) Fibronectin
(E) Glycosaminoglycan

25 Which of the following connective tissue cells initiates the mineralization of the bone matrix during growth and bone remodeling throughout life?
(A) Bone-lining cells
(B) Osteoblasts
(C) Osteocytes
(D) Osteoclasts
(E) Osteoprogenitor cells

26 A 57-year-old woman undergoes spine fusion surgery. Following the procedure, the surgeon prescribes osteogenic protein-1 (OP-1) to promote bone growth and healing. OP-1 (also referred as bone morphogenic protein-7) has been shown to stimulate the differentiation of mesenchymal stem cells to yield which of the following cell types?
(A) Chondroblasts
(B) Fibroblasts
(C) Myoblasts
(D) Osteoblasts
(E) Osteoclasts

27 Bone obtained at the autopsy of a 68-year-old man is examined by light microscopy (shown in the image). Identify the structures indicated by the circles.

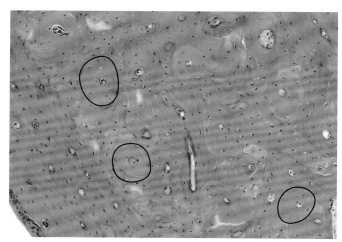

(A) Bone spicules
(B) Haversian canals
(C) Haversian systems
(D) Interstitial lamellae
(E) Volkmann canals

28 A ground (polished) section of bone from the patient described in Question 27 is examined under high magnification (shown in the image). Identify the features indicated by the arrows.

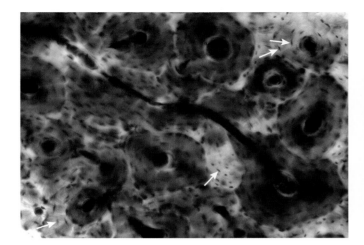

(A) Canaliculi
(B) Haversian canals
(C) Lacunae
(D) Lamellae
(E) Volkmann canals

29 A higher magnification figure is obtained from the bone specimen described in Question 28 (shown in the image). Identify the thin lines indicated by the arrows and the structures that occupy this space.

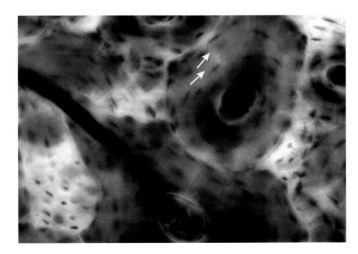

(A) Canaliculi and cytoplasmic processes of osteocytes
(B) Haversian canal and neurovascular structures
(C) Lacunae and osteoclasts
(D) Lacunae and osteocytes
(E) Volkmann canal and neurovascular structures

30 A 21-year-old man is brought to the emergency room in a coma 1 hour after hitting his head against a metal pole while skate boarding. CT scan of the head reveals a skull fracture and epidural hemorrhage (shown in the image, note arrow). The epidural hematoma developing in this patient forms between which of the following two anatomic structures?

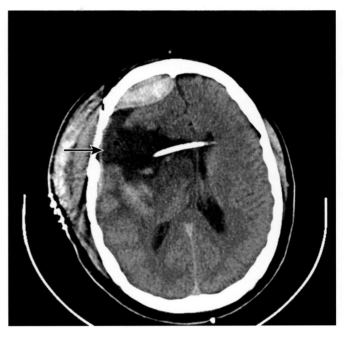

(A) Arachnoid and pia mater
(B) Dura and arachnoid mater
(C) Periosteal and meningeal layers of dura mater
(D) Periosteum and skull
(E) Pia mater and brain

31 The function of the periosteum in supporting new bone growth is determined fundamentally by paracrine/endocrine signals that regulate the differentiation of which of the following connective tissue cells?
(A) Fibroblasts
(B) Osteoblasts
(C) Osteoclasts
(D) Osteocytes
(E) Osteoprogenitor cells

32 Spongy bone is examined by light microscopy (shown in the image). Which of the following best describes the epithelium (indicated by arrows) that lines the surface of bone spicules in spongy bone and the internal surface of compact bone?

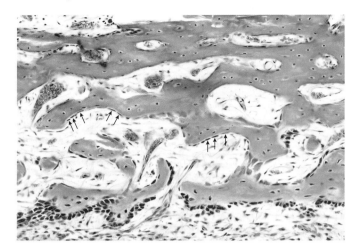

(A) Articular cartilage
(B) Endosteum
(C) Perichondrium
(D) Periosteum
(E) Sharpy fibers

33 A portion of the skull was obtained at the autopsy of a fetus with trisomy 21 (Down syndrome). A developing bone spicule is shown in the image. The light-stained line indicated by the arrows represents which of the following bone structures?

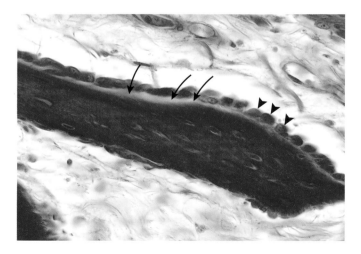

(A) Endosteum
(B) Lacuna
(C) Lamella
(D) Osteoid
(E) Periosteum

34 For the autopsy specimen described in Question 33, the arrowheads shown in the image identify which of the following types of connective tissue cells?
(A) Bone-lining cells
(B) Osteoblasts
(C) Osteoclasts
(D) Osteocytes
(E) Osteoprogenitor cells

35 A bone biopsy taken from a 12-year-old girl was examined by light microscopy (shown in the image). Identify the cells indicated by the arrows.

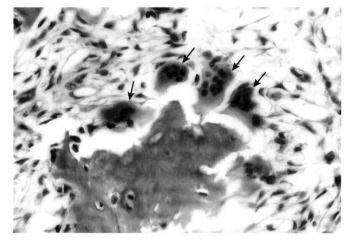

(A) Macrophages
(B) Megakaryocytes
(C) Osteoblasts
(D) Osteoclasts
(E) Osteocytes

36 Osteoclasts are derived from which of the following types of cells?
(A) Bone-lining cells
(B) Mononuclear hematopoietic progenitor cells
(C) Mesenchymal stem cells
(D) Osteoblasts
(E) Osteoprogenitor cells

37 A 6-year-old boy with mild hydrocephalus suffers chronic infections and dies of intractable chronic anemia. At autopsy, his bones are dense and misshapen. The femur in particular shows obliteration of the marrow space. Hematopoietic bone marrow cells are sparse. The diagnosis is osteopetrosis, a rare genetic disorder caused by dysfunction of which of the following cell types?
(A) Chondroblasts
(B) Fibroblasts
(C) Osteoblasts
(D) Osteoclasts
(E) Osteocytes

38 A 58-year-old woman fractures her hip after slipping on an icy sidewalk. An x-ray reveals generalized osteopenia (reduced bone density). A femoral head obtained from another patient with this condition reveals attenuated bony trabeculae (shown in the image on the right). Normal bone is shown in the image on the left. Which of the following best explains the pathogenesis of osteopenia in this postmenopausal woman?

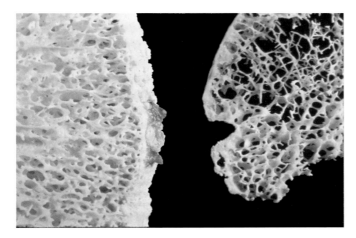

(A) Decreased osteoclast activity
(B) Increased mineralization of bone
(C) Increased osteoblast activity
(D) Increased osteoclast activity
(E) Increased osteocyte activity

39 A 42-year-old woman presents to the emergency room with a spontaneous fracture of her humeral head. She has suffered from malabsorption secondary to Crohn disease for 20 years. Histologically, the humeral head shows bony trabeculae that are covered by a thicker than normal layer of osteoid (shown in the image). In this section, the osteoid is stained red, and mineralized bone is stained black. Which of the following best describes the pathogenesis of osteomalacia in this patient?

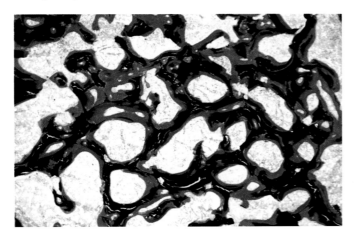

(A) Decreased new bone formation by osteoblasts
(B) Enhanced bone resorption by activated osteoclasts
(C) Impaired mineralization of new bone matrix
(D) Impaired osteocyte activity
(E) Increased calcification of bone matrix

40 For the patient described in Question 39, impaired mineralization of the new bone matrix was most likely caused by a chronic deficiency of which of the following vitamins?
(A) Vitamin A
(B) Vitamin B
(C) Vitamin C
(D) Vitamin D
(E) Vitamin E

41 Which of the following bones forms via the intramembranous ossification pathway during embryonic and fetal development?
(A) Femur
(B) Mandible
(C) Pubis
(D) Scapulae
(E) Vertebrae

42 A 16-year-old girl is seen for her annual health checkup. Measurements taken in the office indicate that the patient has grown 15 cm over the past year. Which of the following cells in epiphyseal growth plates was chiefly responsible for the longitudinal growth of long bones in this patient?
(A) Chondrocytes in the hypertrophy zone of the growth plate
(B) Chondrocytes in the proliferation zone of the growth plate
(C) Chondrocytes in the resting zone of the growth plate
(D) Osteoblasts in the ossification zone
(E) Osteocytes in the ossification zone

43 A 28-year-old man with achondroplasia is admitted to the hospital for hip replacement due to severe osteoarthritis. He has short arms and legs and a relatively large head. Which of the following pathogenetic mechanisms is most likely responsible for this patient's inherited condition?
(A) Accelerated calcification of the bone matrix
(B) Arrest of the epiphyseal growth plate
(C) Enhanced bone resorption by activated osteoclasts
(D) Impaired mineralization of the new bone matrix
(E) Lack of secondary ossification centers

44 For the patient described in Question 43, which of the following mechanisms best explains the fact that the patient's head appears unusually large?
(A) Compensatory increase in head mesenchyme during development
(B) Disruption of compact bone formation in the skull
(C) Enhanced fusion of bone spicules in the skull
(D) Increased osteoblast activity in the skull
(E) Lack of defect in intramembranous bone formation

45 The distal end of the femur is examined at the autopsy of a 3-month-old child with Edward syndrome (trisomy 18). Longitudinal sections of the epiphyseal growth plate reveal evidence of zonation (shown in the image). Which of the labeled areas represents the zone of hypertrophy?

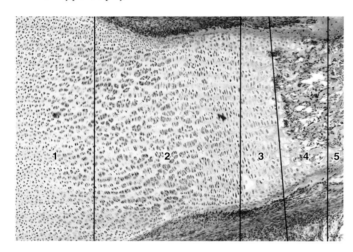

(A) Area 1
(B) Area 2
(C) Area 3
(D) Area 4
(E) Area 5

46 For the bone specimen described in Question 45, cells in which area are most active in producing the new cartilage matrix?
(A) Area 1
(B) Area 2
(C) Area 3
(D) Area 4
(E) Area 5

47 A 15-year-old girl complains of uneven shoulders that she first noticed 3 months ago while trying on a new dress. Physical examination reveals uneven back musculature and a prominent left scapula caused by rotation of the thoracic ribcage. Radiologic studies confirm mild scoliosis. This developmental abnormality is most likely caused by asymmetric growth of which of the following musculoskeletal structures?
(A) Cartilage growth plates
(B) Cement lines
(C) Intervertebral discs
(D) Intrinsic back muscles
(E) Ligaments and tendons

48 For the patient described in Question 47, which of the following zones within the affected end plates was primarily responsible for initiating asymmetric growth, thereby resulting in the development of mild scoliosis in this adolescent patient?
(A) Calcification
(B) Hypertrophy
(C) Ossification
(D) Proliferation
(E) Resting

49 A 14-year-old girl fractures her right fibula playing soccer. The leg is immobilized in a cast. During healing, a soft callus forms at the site of bone fracture. Which of the following represents the primary tissue composition of the patient's soft callus?
(A) Cartilage and dense connective tissue
(B) Immature and mature bone spicules
(C) Loose connective tissue, fibroblasts, and vascular endothelial cells
(D) Macrophages and plasma cells in a proteoglycan-rich ground substance
(E) Necrotic debris and extravasated blood

50 During bone fracture repair described in Question 49, the patient's soft callus is replaced by a bony callus. Which of the following best describes the primary tissue mass in the newly formed bony callus at the site of fracture?
(A) Cancellous
(B) Compact
(C) Lamellar
(D) Spongy
(E) Woven

ANSWERS

1 **The answer is B: Extracellular water.** Extracellular (interstitial) water accounts for 60% to 80% of the wet weight of cartilage and provides resilience to pressure loads applied to the cartilage matrix. None of the other choices contributes significantly to the resiliency of cartilage against pressure.
Keywords: Articular cartilage, interstitial water

2 **The answer is B: Glycosaminoglycans.** Glycosaminoglycans (GAGs) are linear polysaccharide chains with repeating disaccharide units that "decorate" core proteins forming proteoglycan monomers. The carboxyl and sulfate groups present on GAGs are highly negatively charged and therefore help bind a large amount of water via intermolecular hydrogen bonds. Collagen type II fibrils (choice A) provide tensile strength to cartilage and organize proteoglycan core proteins (choice E). None of the other components plays a significant role in binding extracellular water in cartilage.
Keywords: Articular cartilage, glycosaminoglycans, proteoglycans

3 **The answer is C: Degeneration of articular cartilage.** Articular cartilage covers the articular surface of bones and helps reduce friction during joint movement. With advancing age, articular cartilage may undergo progressive degeneration and be worn away, resulting in chronic osteoarthritis. Degenerative osteoarthritis is the single most common form of joint disease. Inflammation of synovium with pannus formation (choice B) occurs in patients with rheumatoid arthritis. None of the other choices are involved in the pathogenesis of degenerative osteoarthritis.
Keywords: Degenerative osteoarthritis

4 **The answer is B: Absence of perichondrium.** Unlike hyaline cartilage, articular cartilage does not have a superficial perichondrium. This feature provides a smooth surface for joint movement. Aside from this difference, the histologic features of articular and hyaline cartilage are the same and include absence of blood vessels in cartilage matrix (choice A), presence of an amorphous matrix (choice C), and arrangement of differentiated chondrocytes in isogenous groups and lacunae (choices D and E).
Keywords: Articular cartilage, perichondrium

5 **The answer is B: Type II.** Numerous collagen types have been identified in cartilage matrix; however, type II collagen is the most abundant. Collagen types II, VI, IX, X, and XI are referred as "cartilage-specific" collagens since they are only found in significant quantities in cartilaginous connective tissue.
Keywords: Hyaline cartilage, type II collagen

6 **The answer is C: Fibrils.** Unlike type I collagen, which organizes into fibers and fiber bundles, type II collagen can only aggregate into fibrils—the smallest fibrous collagen units. Collagen fibrils have a refractive index similar to matrix ground substance and are therefore not identifiable in routine histochemical preparations. For this reason, hyaline cartilage typically appears amorphous by light microscopy. Filaments (choice D) are cytoplasmic structural macromolecules (e.g., keratin and vimentin intermediate filaments).
Keywords: Hyaline cartilage, type II collagen

7 **The answer is A: Aggrecan.** Aggrecan is the most abundant proteoglycan core protein found in hyaline cartilage. This protein carries a large number of chondroitin sulfate GAG side chains. Aggrecan–GAG monomers associate with hyaluronan polysaccharide chains via a link protein to form vast proteoglycan aggregates. Hydrophilic proteoglycan aggregates bind interstitial (extracellular) water to the matrix, which accounts for the ability of cartilage to resist compressive forces associated with wear and tear. Lumican (choice D) carries keratan sulfate side chains. Biglycan (choice B), decorin (choice C) and versican (choice E) may have chondroitin sulfate side chains, but these proteins are commonly associated with blood vessels and skin.
Keywords: Hyaline cartilage, aggrecan

8 **The answer is C: Glycoproteins.** Many glycoproteins function as multivalent cell adhesion molecules. These glycoproteins have multiple binding domains that anchor cartilage matrix molecules to receptors on the chondrocyte cell surface; they help anchor cells to the matrix, maintain tissue integrity, and may mediate transmembrane signaling. Examples of glycoproteins that serve as important markers of cartilage turnover and degeneration include anchorin, tenascin, and fibronectin.
Keywords: Hyaline cartilage, glycoproteins

9 **The answer is D: Pericellular matrix.** The amorphous matrix of hyaline cartilage is not homogenous in color when viewed following H&E staining. The darkly blue-stained zone immediately surrounding chondrocytes is referred to as pericellular or capsular matrix. Pericellular matrix is newly secreted and deposited matrix. It contains a high concentration of basophilic proteoglycans, hence the darker blue color.
Keywords: Hyaline cartilage, pericellular matrix

10 **The answer is B: Type VI.** Collagen type VI is the principal collagen present in the pericellular cartilage matrix. Type VI collagen molecules form a network that helps anchor the chondrocyte to the surrounding matrix. Collagen type VI as well as types II, IX, X, and XI are collectively referred as cartilage-specific collagens since they are found in significant amounts only in cartilage

matrix thus far. Collagen type IX (choice C) and XI (choice E) primarily interact with type II collagen and regulate fibrillogenesis of type II fibrils. Collagen type X (choice D) is important in organizing collagen fibrils into a three-dimensional meshwork and is highly expressed by hypertrophic chondrocytes located in the hypertrophy zone of the growth plate. Researches have shown that type X collagen is involved in the apoptosis of chondrocytes in the growth plate. The other four cartilage-specific collagens are primarily found in interterritorial matrix.
Keywords: Pericellular matrix, type VI collagen

11 **The answer is C: Arrow 3.** Interterritorial matrix fills the space between isogenous groups of chondrocytes. It is more mature than the pericellular matrix (arrow 1). The territorial matrix (arrow 2) surrounds isogenous groups of chondrocytes. The interterritorial matrix contains eosinophilic type II collagen fibrils and, compared to the territorial matrix, exhibits a relative paucity of proteoglycan ground substance.
Keywords: Hyaline cartilage, interterritorial matrix

12 **The answer is D: Interstitial growth from chondrocytes.** Interstitial growth occurs as chondrocytes located in lacunae continuously deposit new matrix. The newly deposited pericellular matrix contains high concentrations of ground substance and appears darker blue when stained with H&E or methylene blue. Over time, this matrix is pushed away from chondrocytes and undergoes a maturation process characterized by increasing amounts of type II collagen fibrils and decreasing amounts of matrix proteoglycans.
Keywords: Cartilage, interstitial growth

13 **The answer is B: Inner layer of the perichondrium.** Hyaline and elastic cartilage connective tissues are surrounded by a perichondrium—a dense connective tissue capsule layer. When cartilage growth is active, an inner cellular and an outer fibrous layer can be observed within this perichondrium. Most of the cells along the inner layer of perichondrium are mesenchymal stem cells that may differentiate into chondroblasts that begin to secrete new cartilage matrix components. None of the other choices show this histologic appearance in this location.
Keywords: Cartilage, perichondrium

14 **The answer is D: Isogenous groups.** Singular chondrocytes grow within spherical spaces referred to as lacunae (lakes). In this protected microenvironment, they proliferate yielding daughter cells that reside in close proximity to one another. These coherent clusters of daughter cells represent isogenous groups. Following each mitotic division, daughter chondrocytes synthesize and deposit the new territorial matrix. None of the other choices show this distinctive morphology.
Keywords: Lung cancer, cartilage, isogenous group

15 **The answer is A: Chondroblasts.** Chondroblasts are found at the interface of cartilage proper and the perichondrium. They arise from mesenchymal stem cells found within the inner layer of the perichondrium (see Question 13). They actively synthesize and deposit matrix on the surface of an existing cartilage template. Once chondroblasts become enveloped within matrix lacunae, they are referred to as differentiated chondrocytes (choice B). Myofibroblasts (choice E) contribute to the healing of granulation tissue by "primary intention." Fibroblasts (choice D) are located in the outer perichondrium and surrounding connective tissue. Endothelial cells (choice C) are not found in this histologic location.
Keywords: Hyaline cartilage, chondroblasts

16 **The answer is A: Chondroblasts in the perichondrium.** Cartilage can grow via two different biological processes: appositional and interstitial growth. During appositional growth, new cartilage matrix is added on the surface of an existing cartilage template by chondroblasts in the perichondrium. These cells are themselves derived from pluripotent mesenchymal stem cells located in the inner layer of the perichondrium. Once chondroblasts become surrounded with the cartilage matrix in visible lacunae, they are referred to as chondrocytes. Chondrocytes undergo mitosis to form clusters (isogenous groups) that deposit new matrix within cartilage, a process referred to as interstitial growth (choice C). Fibroblasts (choice D) do not synthesize cartilage matrix.
Keywords: Cartilage, appositional growth

17 **The answer is C: Elastic cartilage.** The epiglottis is composed primarily of elastic cartilage. Elastic and hyaline cartilage are both surrounded by a dense connective tissue capsule (perichondrium). *Haemophilus influenzae* is the leading cause of epiglottitis in children worldwide; however, *Streptococcus pyogenes*, *S. pneumoniae*, and *Staphylococcus aureus* now represent a larger proportion of pediatric cases of epiglottitis in the United States.
Keywords: Epiglottitis, elastic cartilage

18 **The answer is B: Elastic fibers in the matrix.** Elastic cartilage is similar to hyaline cartilage, except for the presence of thick bundles of elastic fibers in the matrix. Shrunken chondrocytes located in "empty" lacunae is the characteristic feature of cartilage. Elastic fiber bundles in the matrix are the specific feature to distinguish elastic cartilage from amorphous hyaline cartilage. Type I collagen fibers in the cartilage matrix (choice E) is a defining characteristic of fibrocartilage. None of the other choices is a distinguishing feature of elastic cartilage.
Keywords: Elastic cartilage

19 The answer is D: Fibrocartilage. Intervertebral discs consist of a centrally located nucleus pulposus and a peripheral annulus fibrosus. The nucleus pulposus is composed largely of a gel-like matrix and functions as a cushion or shock absorber. The peripheral annulus fibrosus is composed of fibrocartilage and provides resilience against compression. Fibrocartilage does not possess a perichondrium. None of the other choices are found within the annulus fibrosus of intervertebral discs.
Keywords: Herniated intervertebral disc, fibrocartilage

20 The answer is D: Hyaline cartilage and dense, regular connective tissue. Fibrocartilage is commonly found in anatomic locations where pressure and shearing forces are frequently encountered. These anatomic locations include intervertebral discs, pubic symphysis, and insertion points of tendons and ligaments. The combination of hyaline cartilage with bundles of type I collagen makes fibrocartilage particularly resistant to compression, as well as tearing and shearing forces. Because fibrocartilage lacks a perichondrium layer, its development and repair depend on interstitial growth.
Keywords: Herniated disk, fibrocartilage

21 The answer is D: Hyaline cartilage. Epiphyseal plate refers to the cartilage disc that is present between the primary and secondary ossification centers during bone formation. It is the remnant of the hyaline cartilage model of the developing bone. At the ossification zone of the epiphyseal plate, newly formed immature bone spicules may be present, but they are not the major tissue type composing the epiphyseal plate.
Keywords: Epiphyseal plate, hyaline cartilage

22 The answer is A: Avascularity of the cartilage matrix. Hyaline cartilage has a limited capacity for repair and regeneration owing to poor vascular supply and the relative immobility of resident chondrocytes. Granulation tissue that forms at the wound surface is replaced over time by fibrous (collagen-rich) scar tissue, or in some cases, by bone arising from activated mesenchymal stem cells. If an injury to cartilage involves the perichondrium, mesenchymal stem cells can differentiate into fibroblasts and/or osteoblasts instead of chondroblasts. The mechanisms that regulate cartilage repair and regeneration are poorly understood.
Keywords: Hyaline cartilage

23 The answer is B: Chondrosarcoma. Chondrosarcomas are malignant tumors of bone that secrete cartilage matrix. The photomicrograph in this case shows malignant chondrocytes embedded in a cartilaginous matrix. Chondroma (choice A) is a benign tumor of cartilage (i.e., not malignant by definition). None of the other choices show this cartilaginous tissue morphology.
Keywords: Chondrosarcoma

24 The answer is B: Collagen type I. Type I collagen, organized into parallel and/or concentric lamellae, is the major structural component of bone matrix. Type I collagen together with traces of other collagens accounts for 90% of the total protein present in bone matrix. Ground substance including glycoproteins and proteoglycans are minor components, comprising 10% of total bone matrix protein. These organic components are mineralized by the deposition of calcium phosphate, mainly in the form of hydroxyapatite crystals $Ca_{10}(PO_4)_6(OH)_2$. Hydroxyapatite comprises about 50% of the dry weight of normal-density bone. Aggrecan (choice A) and glycosaminoglycans (choice E) comprise proteoglycans found in cartilage.
Keywords: Bone matrix, type I collagen

25 The answer is B: Osteoblasts. Osteoblasts are responsible for the secretion of a new bone matrix, as well as bone matrix calcification and mineralization. Osteoblasts are derived from resting osteoprogenitor cells (choice E). They can be found where active bone formation is occurring. Osteoblasts not only actively secrete organic components of the bone matrix, but also initiate the calcification process. When bone formation is not occurring, osteoblasts become quiescent and line the surfaces of the existing bone; hence they are referred to as bone lining cells (choice A). Osteocytes (choice C) are mature bone cells trapped within lacunae. They are derived from osteoblasts. Osteocytes can still synthesize a new matrix and also are involved in bone resorption, therefore maintaining the bone matrix. Osteoclasts (choice D) are bone resorption cells and actively involved in bone remodeling.
Keywords: Bone, osteoblasts

26 The answer is D: Osteoblasts. Bone morphogenic proteins (BMPs) are growth factors that appear to be specific to bone tissue. They have been shown to induce the differentiation of mesenchymal stem cells into osteoblasts that actively produce new bone matrix. Recombinant BMP-7 (also referred to as OP-1) is used clinically to promote bone formation and growth following orthopedic surgery. Osteoblasts deposit bone matrix and undergo differentiation to become osteocytes. The differentiation of mesenchymal stem cells into chondroblasts (choice A) is regulated by SOX-9. BMPs do not stimulate the differentiation of fibroblasts (choice B) or osteoclasts (choice E).
Keywords: Spinal fusion surgery, bone morphogenetic proteins

27 The answer is C: Haversian systems. In mature bone, collagen fibers are organized into lamellae. In compact bone, lamellae can be further organized into different patterns. In the center of a compact bone, lamellae are arranged into concentric sheets around a central canal that contains blood vessels and nerves, forming a cylindrical unit referred to as the haversian system or osteon. Because bone undergoes constant remodeling, new osteons develop and older osteons become incomplete, forming interstitial lamellae (choice D). Circumferential lamellae are found along the outer and inner circumferences of the bone, parallel to the surface of the bone. Volkmann canals (choice E) can be seen on the figure connecting the haversian canals (choice B). Bone spicules (choice A), also referred as trabeculae, form a three-dimensional meshwork in the marrow of spongy bone. Ultrastructural studies have shown that collagen fibers in bone spicules are organized into parallel lamellae lacking vascular cores.

Keywords: Compact bone, haversian system, osteon

28 **The answer is C: Lacunae.** Lacunae are spaces within the bone matrix that contain osteocytes in living tissue. In a ground section, where cells and other organic components are removed, lacunae appear as empty spaces. Canaliculi (choice A) are barely visible at this magnification; they are small channels within mineralized bone matrix that form a network connecting lacunae. The cytoplasmic processes of osteocytes are located within canaliculi and contact each other via gap junctions, thus allowing communication between adjacent osteocytes. Lamellae (choice D) are formed by collagen fibers organized into parallel and concentric sheets. Haversian canals (choice B) are the central canals of osteons that carry blood vessels and nerves into haversian systems. A Volkmann canal in longitudinal section is prominent in this photomicrograph. Volkmann canals run perpendicular to and thereby connect haversian canals and vessels in the periosteum and endosteum.

Keywords: Bone, lacunae

29 **The answer is A: Canaliculi and cytoplasmic processes of osteocytes.** Canaliculi are thin tunnels penetrating the bone matrix and connecting neighboring lacunae. Canaliculi and lacunae form a continuous network within the bone matrix. While lacunae host the cell bodies of osteocytes, canaliculi are occupied by the cytoplasmic processes of osteocytes, allowing communication between adjacent cells. A haversian canal (choice B) is visible in the image. It is a cylindrical canal in the center of a haversian system containing capillaries or small blood vessels and nerves. The Volkmann canal (choice E) is not present in this small field. It is typically oriented perpendicular to the haversian canal and hosts neurovascular structures. Multiple lacunae are present in the image, and they host the cell bodies of osteocytes.

Keywords: Compact bone, canaliculi

30 **The answer is D: Periosteum and skull.** Periosteum is a layer of dense connective tissue surrounding and attaching to the surface of the bone. It is richly innervated by pain sensory fibers. The middle meningeal artery, the major artery supplying the skull and dura mater, travels between the skull and the periosteum (periosteal layer of the dura mater). A fracture of the skull may tear this artery, and blood may accumulate between and separate the skull from the periosteum, resulting in a potentially lethal epidural hematoma. A hemorrhage between dura and arachnoid mater (choice B) is typically referred to as a subdural hematoma. Subarachnoid hemorrhage is bleeding into the subarachnoid space between the arachnoid and pia mater (choice A). Dural venous sinuses are located between the periosteal and the meningeal layers of dura mater (choice C). Pia is tightly adherent to the surface of the brain (choice E).

Keywords: Epidural hematoma, periosteum

31 **The answer is E: Osteoprogenitor cells.** Periosteum is a connective tissue capsule that covers the external surface of bone. In growing bone, the periosteum contains an outer fibrous layer and an inner cellular layer that is composed of osteoprogenitor cells. These multipotential stem cells are themselves derived from pluripotential mesenchymal stem cells. Upon activation, osteoprogenitor cells differentiate into osteoblasts to produce new bone matrix. The outer layer of periosteum is dense connective tissue with collagen type I fibers and scattered fibroblasts (choice A). Osteoblasts (choice B) are present at the interface between the bone surface and the periosteum. Osteocytes (choice D) are not present in the periosteum.

Keywords: Periosteum, osteoprogenitor cells

32 **The answer is B: Endosteum.** The single cell layer that lines the surface of bone facing the marrow cavity is referred as endosteum. This simple epithelium is composed of osteoprogenitor stem cells as well as activated osteoblasts (if bone growth is active), quiescent osteoblasts (if bone growth has ceased), or osteoclasts (if bone remodeling is ongoing). Articular cartilage (choice A) covers the articular surface of bones that are exposed to a joint cavity. Perichondrium (choice C) covers the surface of cartilage. Periosteum (choice D) surrounds the external surface of compact bone. Sharpy fibers (choice E) attach fibers in the periosteum to the bone matrix.

Keywords: Bone, endosteum

33 **The answer is D: Osteoid.** Osteoid represents a newly deposited, unmineralized bone matrix that is found on the surface of existing bone. Osteoid appears lighter stained than calcified bone matrix in routine preparations stained with H&E. Approximately 50% of fetuses with trisomy 21 (Down syndrome) are aborted spontaneously. Fetal karyotyping may be recommended for women who become pregnant over the age of 40. None of the other choices show this distinctive morphology.

Keywords: Intramembranous bone formation, osteoid

34 **The answer is B: Osteoblasts.** Osteoblasts differentiate from osteoprogenitor stem cells. They actively secrete and deposit new bone matrix. Osteoblasts are typically cuboidal in shape and line the surface of growing bone

spicules. Cells located within the lacunae of bone matrix are osteocytes (choice D). Bone-lining cells and osteo-progenitor cells (choices A and E) cannot be readily discerned by light microscopy.
Keywords: Intramembranous bone formation

35 **The answer is D: Osteoclasts.**   The distinguishing features of osteoclasts include large size and multiple nuclei (multinucleated giant cells). These distinctive cells contain a variety of hydrolytic enzymes, such as alkaline phosphatase, that facilitate bone resorption. Osteoclasts are found wherever bone formation and resorption are active. Macrophages (choice A) form multinucleated giant cells under certain pathologic conditions (e.g., foreign body reactions); however, these "granulomas" would not be expected in normal bone. Megakaryocytes (choice B) are platelet-forming cells present in red bone marrow. None of the other choices appear as multinucleated giant cells.
Keywords: Bone, osteoclasts

36 **The answer is B: Mononuclear hematopoietic progenitor cells.** Osteoclasts are bone marrow–derived cells. They are not related to the osteoprogenitor cell lineage (choice E). Rather, they represent the fusion of precursor cells derived from mononuclear progenitor cells in the bone marrow. This lineage also gives rise to tissue macrophages.
Keywords: Bone, osteoclasts

37 **The answer is D: Osteoclasts.**   Osteopetrosis, also known as "marble bone" disease or Albers-Schönberg disease, is a group of rare inherited disorders. It can be severe, sometimes fatal, affecting infants and children. The sclerotic skeleton in patients with osteopetrosis is the result of failed osteoclast function (i.e., failed bone resorption and remodeling). Because osteoclast function is arrested, osteopetrosis is characterized by block like radiodense bones, hence the term marble bone disease. Chondroblasts (choice A) and fibroblasts (choice B) do not regulate bone growth and development. Increased osteoblast and osteocyte activities (choices C and E) have not been demonstrated in patients with osteopetrosis.
Keywords: Osteopetrosis, Albers-Schönberg disease, osteoclasts

38 **The answer is D: Increased osteoclast activity.**   Osteoporosis is the most common bone disease characterized by progressive loss of bone mass. It commonly affects elderly postmenopausal women. Porous bone tissue can no longer provide adequate mechanical support and eventually results in bone fracture. Bone loss is the result of aggressive bone resorption by increased osteoclast activity and decreased bone deposition by osteoblasts (therefore, not choices A, C, and E). There is no evidence that the mineralization process is affected in patients with osteoporosis (choice B).
Keywords: Osteoporosis, osteopenia

39 **The answer is C: Impaired mineralization of new bone matrix.** Osteomalacia (soft bones) is a disorder of adults characterized by inadequate mineralization of newly formed bone matrix (thus choice E is incorrect). Broad (exaggerated) layers of osteoid rim the bony trabeculae in patients with osteomalacia. Decreased bone formation by osteoblasts (choice A) and enhanced bone resorption by activated osteoclasts (choice B) are typically observed in patients with osteoporosis.
Keywords: Osteomalacia

40 **The answer is D: Vitamin D.**   Abnormal metabolism of vitamin D and/or insufficient calcium in the diet is the primary cause of osteomalacia in adults and rickets in children. In these cases, the newly formed bone matrix cannot calcify normally. Malabsorption of vitamin D and calcium complicates a number of small intestinal diseases including celiac sprue, Crohn disease, and scleroderma. Vitamin A deficiency (choice A) affects endochondral bone growth. Insufficient amount of vitamin C (choice C) causes scurvy, in which collagen assembly is disrupted. There is no evidence that deficiencies of vitamins B and E (choices B and E) are associated with bone disease.
Keywords: Osteomalacia, vitamin D deficiency

41 **The answer is B: Mandible.**   The upper and lower limb bones of the appendicular skeleton develop through the process of endochondral ossification. Neural crest–derived flat bones of the skull, face, and clavicle are formed through a different process referred to as intramembranous ossification. Intramembranous ossification is a mechanism whereby bone is directly developed on the embryonic mesenchymal tissue, the membrane. Osteoblasts derived from mesenchymal cells deposit bone matrix at multiple locations and form multiple bone spicules. These bone spicules undergo remodeling and eventually form compact bone at both the external surfaces and remain as spongy bone within the bone cavity.
Keywords: Intramembranous bone formation

42 **The answer is B: Chondrocytes in the proliferation zone of the growth plate.**   Chondrocytes in the proliferation zone of the growth plate undergo mitosis and form longitudinal columns of stacked cells, a specialized form of isogenous groups. The stacked cells produce and deposit new cartilage matrix to increase the length of long bones during development. Chondrocytes in the hypertrophy zone (choice A) undergo apoptosis and no longer produce matrix. Chondrocytes in the resting zone (choice C) provide reserve cells for proliferation. Osteoblasts and osteocytes in the ossification zone (choices D and E) deposit bone matrix on calcified cartilage spicules and are not responsible for growth of the length of long bones.
Keywords: Endochondral bone formation, growth plate

43 **The answer is B: Arrest of the epiphyseal growth plate.** Achondroplasia refers to a syndrome of short-limbed dwarfism and macrocephaly and represents a failure of normal epiphyseal cartilage formation. It is the most common genetic form of dwarfism and is inherited as an autosomal dominant trait. Achondroplasia is caused by an activating mutation in the fibroblast growth factor-3 (FGF-3) receptor. This mutation negatively regulates chondrocyte proliferation and differentiation and arrests the development of the growth plate. The other steps of endochondral bone formation (choices A, C, D, and E) appear to be normal in patients with achondroplasia.
Keywords: Achondroplasia, endochondral bone formation, growth plate

44 **The answer is E: Lack of defect in intramembranous bone formation.** Epiphyseal growth plates in patients with achondroplasia exhibit attenuated proliferation zones and reduced zones of proliferating cartilage. Thus, endochondral bone formation is impaired, while intramembranous bone formation proceeds normally (i.e., lack of defect). For this reason, bones that develop via the intramembranous ossification pathway, such as flat bones of the neurocranium, appear relatively large. The thickness of long bones is normal, but their length is shortened. As a result, patients with achondroplasia appear to have short and thick limb bones.
Keywords: Achondroplasia, intramembranous ossification

45 **The answer is C: Area 3.** Epiphyseal plates are cartilaginous discs that lay between the diaphysis and the epiphysis of long bones. These growth plates control bone length and ultimately determine adult height. Five zones are visible in the growth plate shown in the photomicrograph. From epiphysis to diaphysis, they include zones of resting cartilage (choice A), proliferation (choice B), hypertrophy (choice C), calcification (choice D), and ossification (choice E). Chondrocytes in the zone of hypertrophy (area 3) are greatly enlarged, and the matrix located between columns of hypertrophic chondrocytes is compressed into thin septae.
Keywords: Epiphyseal growth plate, endochondral bone formation

46 **The answer is B: Area 2.** Chondrocytes in the zone of proliferation undergo several rounds of mitotic division. Cells within the same isogenous group are organized into longitudinal columns, and they actively deposit a new cartilage matrix. Owing to the longitudinal proliferation of chondrocytes in the proliferation zone, the structure of the growth plate remains essentially unchanged from early fetal life to skeletal maturity. The rate of mitosis and production of new cartilage matrix matches the speed of ossification from the diaphysis. This balance results in controlled longitudinal growth of long bones.
Keywords: Epiphyseal growth plate, endochondral bone formation

47 **The answer is A: Cartilage growth plates.** Cartilage growth plates in the vertebrae are referred as "end plates." In scoliosis, for unknown reasons, one side of these end plates grows faster than the other, resulting in lateral curvature of the vertebral column. The growth of the width of the vertebrae is from appositional growth of periosteum, a form of intramembranous ossification. This process is not affected in patients with scoliosis. The other choices are not related to the pathogenesis of scoliosis.
Keywords: Scoliosis, growth plates

48 **The answer is D: Proliferation.** Columns of chondrocytes in longitudinal isogenous groups actively deposit new bone matrix and result in longitudinal growth of vertebrae. Asymmetric growth of the cartilage growth plates appears to be caused primarily by an underlying asymmetry in the rate of cell cycle progression in affected chondrocytes. Asymmetry of hypertrophy, calcification, and ossification then ensue with time.
Keywords: Scoliosis, growth plates

49 **The answer is A: Cartilage and dense connective tissue.** During the healing process of a bone fracture, necrotic debris and extravasated blood are removed by neutrophils and macrophages. Blood vessels and fibroblasts then proliferate at the site of injury to form a granulation tissue embedded in loose connective tissue. Fibroblasts and periosteal cells then deposit dense collagen fibers and a cartilage matrix to form the soft callus that is subsequently replaced by a bony callus.
Keywords: Bone fracture, callus

50 **The answer is E: Woven.** The fibrocartilaginous, soft callus helps stabilize and bind together the fractured bone. Osteoprogenitor stem cells from the periosteum then differentiate into metabolically active osteoblasts. Osteoblasts synthesize new bone matrix surrounding the fracture site and form a bony sheath around the soft callus. This newly deposited bone enters the soft callus and eventually replaces it with a new bony callus. Within the bony callus, the newly formed immature bone tissue is the primary tissue type. Immature or woven bone contains randomly deposited collagen fibers and exhibits poor mineralization. It soon will be replaced by mature bone or lamellar bone (choice C), where the collagen fibers are organized into lamellae. Compact bone (choice B) refers to the outer layer of mature dense bone tissue of a bone where the collagen fibers organize into parallel or concentric lamellae around blood vessels. The interior of a bone consists of thin anastomosing bone spicules or trabeculae, so-called cancellous or spongy bone (choices A and D).
Keywords: Bone fracture, woven bone

Chapter 5

Blood and Hematopoiesis

QUESTIONS

Select the single best answer.

1 A 40-year-old woman complains of swelling of her eyelids, abdomen, and ankles. Her vital signs are normal. If this patient's soft tissue edema is caused by decreased plasma oncotic pressure, then routine blood work would show a significant decrease in which of the following plasma proteins?
(A) Albumin
(B) Clotting factors
(C) Complement proteins
(D) Immunoglobulins
(E) α-2-Macroglobulin

2 The patient described in Question 1 may have a chronic disease that affects which of the following internal organs?
(A) Adrenals
(B) Kidneys
(C) Lungs
(D) Pituitary
(E) Spleen

3 During a 4th year elective rotation in blood bank/transfusion medicine, you are asked to discuss differences between blood, plasma, and serum. You explain that blood plasma is converted to serum using which of the following laboratory procedures?
(A) Addition of heparin anticoagulant
(B) Centrifugation to remove the buffy coat
(C) Heat inactivation of complement
(D) Precipitation of immunoglobulins
(E) Removal of the insoluble fibrin clot

4 Microscopic examination of soft tissue reveals a vein embedded in adipose connective tissue (shown in the image). The tan-colored material within the lumen of the vessel, indicated by the asterisk, represents a precipitate of plasma protein. Which of the following proteins is most abundant in this fluid precipitate?

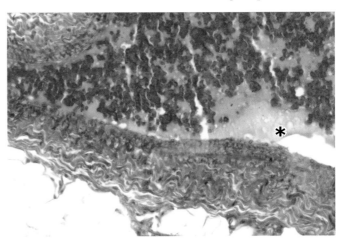

(A) Albumin
(B) Fibrinogen
(C) Immunoglobulin
(D) Plasmin
(E) Thrombin

5 An 18-year-old woman complains of fever and severe diarrhea for 3 days. Her temperature is 38°C (101°F). The CBC reveals an increased hematocrit, most likely caused by dehydration and hemoconcentration, secondary to diarrhea. Which of the following represents a normal hematocrit reading for this patient?
(A) 10%
(B) 20%
(C) 40%
(D) 60%
(E) 80%

6 A peripheral blood smear from a 20-year-old woman is examined in the clinical laboratory. Which of the following describes the primary function of the leukocyte shown in the image?

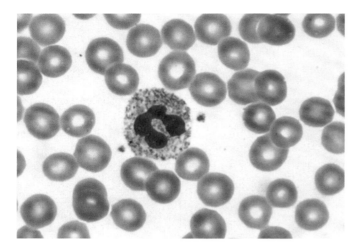

(A) Antibody production
(B) Coagulation and hemostasis
(C) Collagen biosynthesis
(D) Histamine release
(E) Phagocytosis

7 What is the average size (in microns) of the erythrocytes that are visible in the peripheral blood smear shown for Question 6?
(A) 2
(B) 4
(C) 6
(D) 8
(E) 10

8 A 26-year-old man is involved in a hunting accident and requires a blood transfusion. Five hours later, he becomes febrile (feverish) and has severe back pain. Laboratory studies show evidence of intravascular hemolysis. It is discovered that type A blood was given by mistake to this type B patient. Which of the following best describes the chemical nature of the antigens responsible for this patient's adverse transfusion reaction?
(A) Glycosaminoglycans
(B) Oligosaccharides
(C) Phospholipids
(D) Polypeptides
(E) Polysaccharides

9 A 25-year-old woman with a history of heavy menstrual periods complains of chronic fatigue. Examination of a peripheral blood smear suggests iron deficiency anemia (shown in the image). Which of the following terms

appropriately describes the morphology of the patient's erythrocytes?

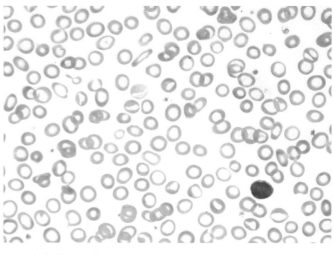

(A) Hyperchromic
(B) Macrocytic
(C) Microcytic
(D) Normocytic
(E) Poikilocytic

10 During clinical rounds, the attending physician asks you to discuss basic principles of hematology. Which of the following is the most abundant formed element in the blood?
(A) Erythrocytes
(B) Granulocytes
(C) Lymphocytes
(D) Monocytes
(E) Platelets

11 A 55-year-old woman with autoimmune hemolytic anemia presents with increasing fatigue. Which of the following serum components is expected to be elevated in this patient with antibody-mediated hemolysis?
(A) Albumin
(B) Bilirubin
(C) Fibrinogen
(D) Hageman factor
(E) Transferrin

12 Which of the following hematologic findings is expected for the patient described in Question 11?
(A) Leukemoid reaction
(B) Lymphocytosis
(C) Neutrophilia
(D) Pancytopenia
(E) Reticulocytosis

13 A 56-year-old woman undergoing chemotherapy for malignant breast cancer develops septic shock and expires. The patient's red bone marrow is examined at autopsy (shown in the image). Which of the following peripheral blood findings would have been expected prior to the patient's death?

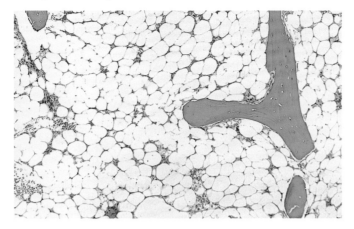

(A) Leukocytosis
(B) Pancytopenia
(C) Lymphocytosis
(D) Neutrophilia
(E) Thrombocytosis

14 You are engaged in basic research to identify novel markers for the isolation and long-term culture of hematopoietic stem cells. In addition to cord blood, hematopoietic stem cells have been isolated from which of the following fetal organs?
(A) Brain
(B) Gonads
(C) Liver
(D) Lungs
(E) Pancreas

15 A 75-year-old woman presents with a 3-day history of productive cough, fever, and shortness of breath. Her temperature is 38°C (101°F). An x-ray film of the chest shows consolidation of both the lungs, and sputum cultures are positive for *Streptococcus pneumoniae*. The patient develops respiratory insufficiency and expires. Her lungs are examined at autopsy (shown in the image). Which of the following inflammatory cells is most abundant in the alveolar air spaces of this patient?

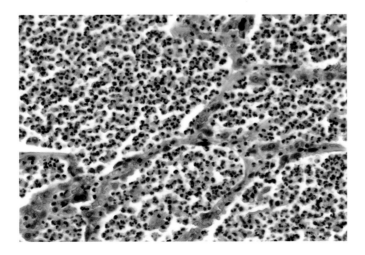

(A) Basophils
(B) Lymphocytes
(C) Macrophages
(D) Neutrophils
(E) Plasma cells

16 A 55-year-old alcoholic is brought to the emergency room with a fever (38.7°C/103°F) and foul-smelling breath. The patient subsequently develops broncho-pneumonia and dies of respiratory insufficiency. In addition to pneumonia, autopsy reveals a pulmonary abscess filled with acute inflammatory cells and necrotic debris. Which of the following terms best describes the creamy fluid (pus) within this patient's pulmonary abscess?
(A) Effusion
(B) Fibrinous exudate
(C) Purulent exudate
(D) Serous exudate
(E) Transudate

17 Examination of soft tissue at autopsy of a 50-year-old drug abuser shows evidence of vasodilation of a post-capillary venule (shown in the image). What additional finding is evident in this photomicrograph?

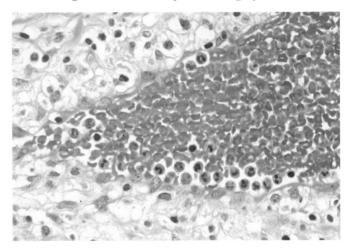

(A) Degranulation of tissue mast cells
(B) Differentiation of circulating monocytes
(C) Margination of segmented neutrophils
(D) Necrosis of capillary endothelial cells
(E) Proliferation of helper T lymphocytes

18 What glycoprotein mediates initial tethering of segmented neutrophils to endothelial cells in the autopsy specimen described in Question 17?
(A) Cadherin
(B) Entactin
(C) Integrin
(D) Laminin
(E) Selectin

19 A 19-year-old woman presents with 5 days of fever (38°C/101°F) and sore throat. She reports that she has felt fatigued for the past week and has difficulty swallowing. Physical examination reveals cervical lymphadenopathy. A peripheral blood smear is examined. Identify the leukocytes shown in the image.

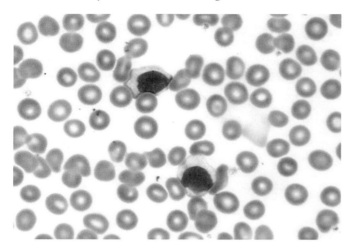

(A) Basophils
(B) Eosinophils
(C) Lymphocytes
(D) Monocytes
(E) Neutrophils

20 The patient described in Question 19 is shown to have serum antibodies directed against the Epstein-Barr virus (the monospot test is positive). This patient's CBC with differential will most likely show which of the following hematologic findings?
(A) Eosinophilia
(B) Leukopenia
(C) Lymphocytosis
(D) Neutropenia
(E) Neutrophilia

21 A 70-year-old man presents with fever, shaking chills, and shortness of breath. The patient exhibits grunting respirations, 30 to 35 breaths per minute, with flaring of the nares. The sputum is rusty yellow and displays polymorphonuclear leukocytes (neutrophils). The patient is successfully treated with antibiotics. Which of the following inflammatory cells will infiltrate the patient's respiratory alveoli during the recovery to remove necrotic debris?
(A) Basophils
(B) Eosinophils
(C) Lymphocytes
(D) Macrophages
(E) Plasma cells

22 A peripheral blood smear from a 30-year-old man is examined in the pathology department. Which of the following describes the primary function of the leukocyte shown in the image?

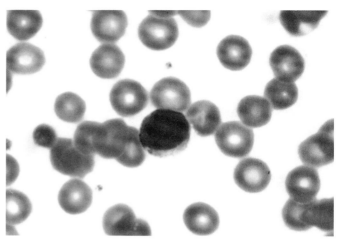

(A) Collagen biosynthesis
(B) Complement activation
(C) Cytokine secretion
(D) Histamine release
(E) Phagocytosis

23 A 38-year-old man presents with myalgia (muscle pain), low-grade fever, and swelling of the right calf. The patient reports recently attending a Fireman's pig roast. Laboratory data show elevated serum levels of creatine kinase. The peripheral blood smear is shown in the image. Identify the leukocyte in the center of this field.

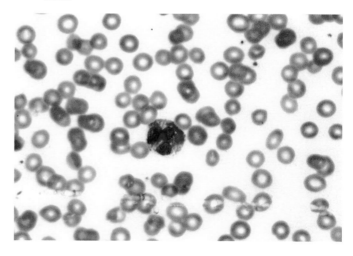

(A) Basophil
(B) Eosinophil
(C) Monocyte
(D) Neutrophil
(E) Plasma cell

24 An 8-year-old boy with a history of recurrent bacterial infections presents with fever and a productive cough. Biochemical analysis of his neutrophils demonstrates that he has an impaired ability to generate reactive oxygen species. Which of the following describes the normal function of reactive oxygen species (ROS) generated by segmented neutrophils during acute inflammation?

(A) Degradation of pathogens
(B) Formation of phagolysosomes
(C) Neutrophil margination and diapedesis
(D) Opsonization of pathogens
(E) Transmembrane signaling

25 A 78-year-old man with prostate cancer and bone metastases presents with shaking chills and fever. The peripheral WBC count is 1,000/µL (normal reference range = 4,000 to 11,000/µL). Which of the following terms describes this hematologic finding?

(A) Leukocytosis
(B) Leukopenia
(C) Neutropenia
(D) Pancytopenia
(E) Thrombocytopenia

26 A 54-year-old woman smoker complains of intermittent blood in her urine. Urinalysis confirms hematuria. The CBC reveals increased hematocrit. A CT scan of the abdomen reveals a 3-cm renal mass, and a CT-guided biopsy demonstrates a renal cell carcinoma. Which of the following tumor-derived hormones is responsible for increased hematocrit in this patient?

(A) Aldosterone
(B) Angiotensin
(C) Erythropoietin
(D) Renin
(E) Thrombopoietin

27 A 24-year-old mountain climber suffers massive trauma during an expedition to the Himalayan Mountains and expires. Examination of the patient's bone marrow at autopsy reveals colonies of hematopoietic stem cells (arrows, shown in the image). These proliferative "burst-forming units" are committed to which of the following pathways of stem cell differentiation?

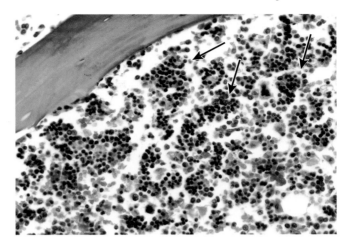

(A) Erythrocyte
(B) Granulocyte
(C) Lymphocyte
(D) Megakaryocyte
(E) Monocyte

28 A 38-year-old man with an iron overload disease presents with increasing abdominal girth and yellow discoloration of his skin and sclera. Physical examination reveals hepatomegaly (enlargement of liver) and jaundice. A Prussian blue stain of a liver biopsy reveals large deposits of iron. Which of the following is the principal iron transport protein in this patient's serum?

(A) Bilirubin
(B) Ceruloplasmin
(C) Ferritin
(D) Hemosiderin
(E) Transferrin

29 A 35-year-old construction worker sustains a laceration on the palmar surface of her left hand. The wound is cleaned, sutured, and wrapped with sterile gauze. Which of the following formed elements of the blood initiates thrombosis and hemostasis in this patient's wound?

(A) Erythrocytes
(B) Granulocytes
(C) Lymphocytes
(D) Monocytes
(E) Platelets

30 Which of the following cell adhesion proteins mediates the transendothelial migration (diapedesis) of leukocytes in the wound of the patient described in Question 29?

(A) Cadherins
(B) Fibronectins
(C) Integrins
(D) Laminins
(E) Selectins

31 A 4-year-old girl presents with fatigue, fever, and night sweats. Physical examination reveals marked pallor.

Palpation of her sternum demonstrates diffuse tenderness. Laboratory studies disclose anemia, thrombocytopenia, and leukocytosis. A bone marrow biopsy is obtained (shown in the image). Which of the following characterizes the patient's bone marrow?

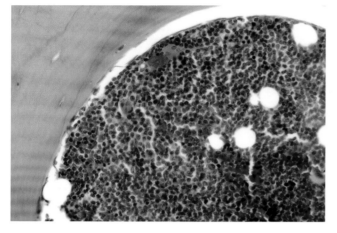

(A) Active hematopoiesis (red bone marrow)
(B) Expansion of marrow sinusoids
(C) Hypercellularity of the bone marrow
(D) Inactive hematopoiesis (yellow bone marrow)
(E) Proliferation of adipose tissue

32 A 58-year-old woman with a 3-day history of pneumococcal pneumonia develops a purulent effusion involving her right pleural cavity. Aspiration of this fluid will reveal an abundance of which of the following inflammatory cells?
(A) Basophils
(B) Eosinophils
(C) Lymphocytes
(D) Monocytes
(E) Neutrophils

33 A 28-year-old man with a recent history of infectious mononucleosis complains of intermittent pain and tingling in the tips of his fingers, particularly in cold weather. A peripheral blood smear is shown in the image. Red blood cell clumping (arrow) in this patient is most likely due to the action of which of the following plasma proteins?

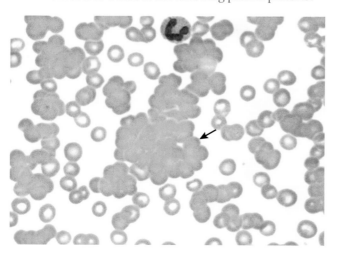

(A) α-1-Antitrypsin
(B) Clotting factors
(C) Complement proteins
(D) Immunoglobulins
(E) α-2-Macroglobulin

34 A 12-year-old boy cuts his thumb while chopping vegetables in the kitchen. The wound is cleaned and closed with sterile gauze and adhesive tape. Which of the following mediators of inflammation cleaves fibrinogen to yield insoluble fibrin in this patient's wound?
(A) Kinins
(B) Leukotrienes
(C) Plasmin
(D) Prostaglandins
(E) Thrombin

35 Which of the following proteases degrades intravascular thrombi during healing of the wound described in Question 34?
(A) Caspase
(B) Elastase
(C) Plasmin
(D) Thrombin
(E) Trypsin

36 A bone marrow aspirate is obtained from a 50-year-old woman with B-cell lymphoma (shown in the image). Identify the hematopoietic cells indicated by the arrows.

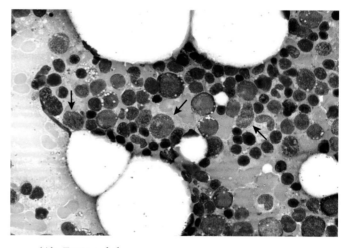

(A) Eosinophils
(B) Lymphocytes
(C) Macrophages
(D) Monocytes
(E) Neutrophils

37 A 69-year-old woman with a history of ischemic heart disease is hospitalized for shortness of breath. Physical examination shows marked jugular venous distension, hepatomegaly, ascites, and pitting edema. The patient subsequently dies of cardiorespiratory failure. Histologic examination of the lungs at autopsy reveals iron-laden macrophages filled with the remnants of extravasated erythrocytes. These so-called "heart failure" cells are derived from which of the following peripheral blood cells?

(A) Basophils
(B) Eosinophils
(C) Lymphocytes
(D) Monocytes
(E) Neutrophils

38 A peripheral blood smear from a 28-year-old woman is examined in the clinical laboratory (shown in the image). Which of the following describes the primary function of the leukocyte indicated by the arrow after it exists the blood?

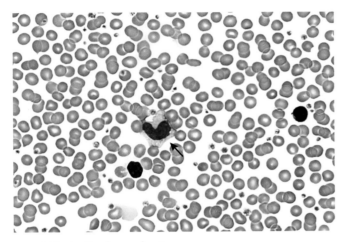

(A) Antibody production
(B) Collagen biosynthesis
(C) Complement activation
(D) Histamine release
(E) Phagocytosis

39 A 6-year-old girl is brought into the physician's office with mild respiratory distress. She has a history of allergies to cats and wool, and her parents state that she has recurrent episodes of upper respiratory tract infections. Physical examination shows expiratory wheezes, with use of accessory respiratory muscles. This patient's CBC with differential will most likely show an absolute increase in which of the following cells?

(A) Eosinophils
(B) Lymphocytes
(C) Monocytes
(D) Neutrophils
(E) Plasma cells

40 A peripheral blood smear from a 22-year-old man is examined in the clinical laboratory (shown in the image). The leukocyte identified by the arrow has cell surface receptors for which of the following types of immunoglobulin?

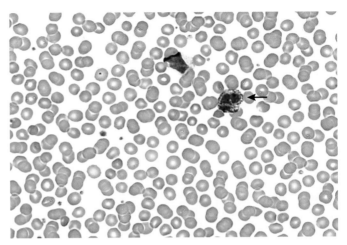

(A) IgA
(B) IgD
(C) IgE
(D) IgG
(E) IgM

41 A section of a glomerulus that was stained with phosphotungstic acid hematoxylin demonstrates several purple-colored microthrombi (shown in the image). These small blood clots are composed primarily of which of the following proteins?

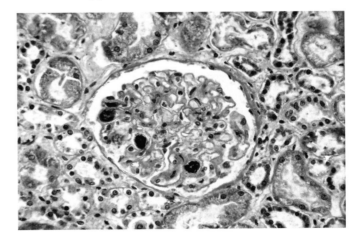

(A) Collagen
(B) Elastin
(C) Fibrin
(D) Keratin
(E) Laminin

42 A 70-year-old woman with a history of diabetes mellitus presents with poor vision, peripheral vascular disease, and mild proteinuria. Which of the following hemoglobin subtypes provides the best monitor of the control of blood sugar levels in this patient?
(A) HbA1c
(B) HbA2
(C) HbAS
(D) HbF
(E) HbH

43 A bone marrow biopsy is obtained from a 5-year-old boy recently diagnosed with lymphoblastic leukemia (shown in the image). Identify the normal hematopoietic cell indicated by the arrow.

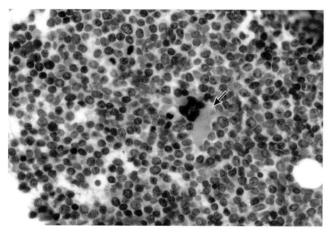

(A) Macrophage
(B) Megakaryocyte
(C) Monocyte
(D) Myelocyte
(E) Reticulocyte

44 A 25-year-old pregnant woman comes to the obstetrician for a prenatal check up. Routine laboratory testing reveals a mild anemia with serum hemoglobin of 9.4 g/dL (normal reference range = 12 to 15 g/dL). Examination of a peripheral blood smear reveals elliptical erythrocytes (shown in the image). The pathologist asks you to identify the normal leukocyte in the center of the field.

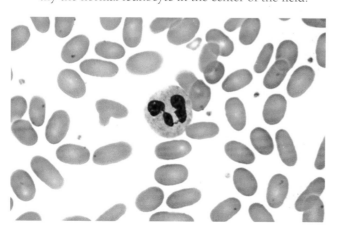

(A) Eosinophil
(B) Monocyte
(C) Basophil
(D) Neutrophil
(E) Lymphocyte

45 A 58-year-old man presents with fever, shaking chills, shortness of breath, and chest pain. Sputum cultures are positive for *Streptococcus pneumoniae*. Which of the following terms describes the process of coating bacteria, with antibodies and complement proteins, to facilitate their binding and uptake by phagocytic cells?
(A) Acute-phase response
(B) Coagulation
(C) Granulation
(D) Haptotaxis
(E) Opsonization

46 A 90-year-old woman is brought to the emergency room. Her blood pressure is 70/30 mm Hg. She is febrile (38°C/100.5°F). Laboratory studies demonstrate a WBC count of 22×10^9/L with 92% neutrophils (neutrophilia). Which of the following most likely accounts for this patient's clinical signs and symptoms?
(A) Chronic bronchitis
(B) Chronic renal failure
(C) Congestive heart failure
(D) Hepatic cirrhosis
(E) Septic shock

47 A 12-year-old boy presents with flank pain that developed shortly after playing a game of soccer. Physical examination demonstrates an area of soft tissue bleeding (ecchymosis) in the right flank that is tender to palpation. The patient has a lifelong history of easy bruising. His brother shows the same tendency. Laboratory studies would most likely reveal a deficiency of which of the following plasma proteins?
(A) Albumin
(B) Clotting factor
(C) Complement protein
(D) Immunoglobulin
(E) α-2-Macroglobulin

ANSWERS

1 **The answer is A: Albumin.** The forces that regulate the balance of vascular and tissue fluids include (1) hydrostatic pressure, (2) oncotic pressure, and (3) lymph flow. Plasma oncotic pressure (also referred to as colloidal osmotic pressure) is largely determined by the concentration of plasma proteins, especially albumin. Albumin is the principal protein in the blood (normal reference range = 3 to 5 g/dL). Any condition that lowers plasma albumin levels promotes generalized edema. By contrast, increased vascular permeability during inflammation results in local edema. Noninflammatory edema is referred to as a transudate, whereas inflammatory edema is referred to as an exudate. The other proteins (choices B to E) are less abundant in plasma than albumin, and a decrease in their levels would not lead to generalized edema.
Keywords: Edema, plasma

2 **The answer is B: Kidneys.** Albumin is synthesized in the liver; therefore, patients with chronic liver disease will exhibit hypoalbuminemia and generalized edema. Hypoalbuminemia is also seen in patients with kidney disease (nephrotic syndrome). Nephrotic syndrome is characterized by heavy proteinuria (greater than 3.5 g protein/24 hours), hypoalbuminemia, hyperlipidemia, and generalized edema. Chronic diseases of the other internal organs (choices A, C, D, and E) would not significantly alter the colloidal osmotic (oncotic) pressure of the patient's blood.
Keywords: Nephrotic syndrome

3 **The answer is E: Removal of the insoluble fibrin clot.** Blood is an amazing connective tissue that delivers nutrients and oxygen to cells and removes metabolic waste. Blood also provides a transport mechanism for hormones and other signaling molecules. Blood consists of formed elements (cells and platelets) and a protein-rich fluid termed plasma. Most plasma proteins are synthesized in the liver. In addition to albumin and immunoglobulins (e.g., IgG and IgM), plasma contains numerous clotting factors. During blood coagulation, fibrinogen (a 340-kDa glycoprotein) is converted to insoluble fibrin, forming an adherent intravascular clot (thrombus). Without anticoagulants, blood removed from the circulation will clot spontaneously. Once the fibrin clot is removed, the fluid that remains is referred to as serum. None of the other laboratory procedures describe a method for converting plasma to serum.
Keywords: Plasma, serum, coagulation

4 **The answer is A: Albumin.** This trichrome stain of a vein highlights connective tissue in blue and smooth muscle cells and erythrocytes in red. The tan area identified by the asterisk on the slide represents a protein precipitate. Plasma proteins include albumin, immunoglobulins, nonimmune globulins, clotting factors (e.g., Hageman factor and fibrinogen), complement proteins, and various enzymes and hormones. Albumin accounts for approximately half of the total plasma protein. The principal function of albumin is maintenance of plasma oncotic pressure. However, albumin also binds and transports hormones (e.g., thyroxine) and lipids. The other proteins are less abundant components of plasma.
Keywords: Plasma, blood, oncotic pressure

5 **The answer is C: 40%.** When a sample of blood to which anticoagulants have been added is centrifuged, the volume of packed erythrocytes is referred to as the hematocrit. The normal hematocrit for women is 35% to 45% (v/v). The normal hematocrit for men is slightly higher (39% to 50%). Increased hematocrit in this patient reflects hemoconcentration, secondary to fluid loss (severe diarrhea). This hematologic condition, termed relative polycythemia, is characterized by decreased plasma volume with a normal red cell mass. When patients suffer from burns, vomiting, excessive sweating, or diarrhea, they not only lose fluid but also suffer electrolyte disturbances. Systemic blood pressure falls with continuous dehydration, and declining perfusion eventually leads to death. None of the other percentages falls within the reference range for normal hematocrit in women.
Keywords: Dehydration, hematocrit, polycythemia

6 **The answer is E: Phagocytosis.** The peripheral blood smear shows a maturing neutrophil surrounded by erythrocytes (red blood cells). Neutrophils are the most abundant white blood cells (WBC, leukocyte) found in the peripheral blood. These acute inflammatory cells are phagocytes (cells that devour); they exit the circulatory system at sites of tissue injury or infection to remove pathogens and necrotic debris. Neutrophils exhibit variation in size and nuclear morphology. As they leave the bone marrow, neutrophils exhibit a horseshoe-shaped nucleus and are referred to as "band cells." As they mature in the peripheral blood, their nuclei become lobulated (segmented). Mature, segmented neutrophils are commonly referred to as polymorphonuclear leukocytes. The nuclei of mature segmented neutrophils have two to four lobes joined by thin strands of chromatin. Neutrophils are loaded with granules that contain enzymes (e.g., myeloperoxidase and collagenase) and antimicrobial peptides (e.g., lysozyme and defensin). B lymphocytes produce antibodies (choice A). Platelets regulate coagulation and hemostasis (choice B). Fibroblasts synthesize collagen (choice C). Upon degranulation, mast cells release histamine (choice D).
Keywords: Neutrophils, granulocytes

7 **The answer is D: 8.** Erythrocytes are approximately 7 to 8 μm in diameter. They are about the same size as the nuclei of small lymphocytes. Red blood cells (RBCs) can be used as a "histologic ruler," because their size is not significantly affected by fixation. Because of their

biconcave disc shape, erythrocytes display an area of central pallor that is approximately one-third the diameter of the cells. The red color of blood is imparted by hemoglobin. Erythrocytes carry oxygen to tissues. The average life span of erythrocytes in the blood is 120 days. Senescent RBCs are removed by the mononuclear phagocyte system present in the spleen, liver, and bone marrow. None of the other sizes accurately describes the diameter of normal circulating erythrocytes.
Keywords: Erythrocytes, hemoglobin

8 **The answer is B: Oligosaccharides.**   The addition of specific oligosaccharides to surface glycoproteins and glycolipids leads to the formation of red cell antigens. The ABO blood group system reflects alternative patterns of oligosaccharide chain modification (e.g., galactose vs. N-acetylgalactosamine). Variations in ABO antigen expression in the general population reflect genetic polymorphism for the expression of glycosyltransferase enzymes. In this case, preformed anti-A antibodies in the patient's blood attached to foreign antigens (A oligosaccharides) on the membranes of transfused erythrocytes. At sufficient density, bound immunoglobulins activate the complement system (i.e., fix complement). Once activated, the complement cascade leads to the destruction of the target cell through formation of a membrane attack complex. This type of complement-mediated cell lysis also occurs in patients with autoimmune hemolytic anemia. Although the ABO antigens are carried on membrane sphingolipids and proteins, the antigens are best described as oligosaccharides composed of four to six monosaccharides. None of the other choices describe the biochemistry of ABO blood group antigens.
Keywords: Hemolytic anemia, transfusion reaction

9 **The answer is C: Microcytic.**   In addition to having central pallor, the patient's red blood cells appear significantly smaller than the nucleus of a small lymphocyte (visible in the image). The blood smear shows microcytic, hypochromic (pale) erythrocytes that are characteristic of iron deficiency anemia caused by inadequate uptake or, more often, excessive loss of iron. Women who have menorrhagia, especially those who consume restricted diets, are especially prone to iron deficiency anemia. Hyperchromic cells (choice A) display increased pigmentation. Macrocytic cells are larger than normal (choice B). Normocytic cells (choice D) display normal size and shape. Poikilocytes (choice E) are abnormally shaped erythrocytes.
Keywords: Anemia, iron deficiency

10 **The answer is A: Erythrocytes.**   Formed elements in the blood include platelets, red blood cells (erythrocytes), and white blood cells (leukocytes). Of these, erythrocytes are the most abundant formed elements in the peripheral blood (normal reference range = 3.7 to 5.2 × 10^{12}/L). There are approximately 1,000 times more RBCs

than WBCs (choices B, C, and D). RBCs are 10 times more abundant than platelets (choice E). Platelets are nonnucleated (anucleate) cytoplasmic fragments derived from megakaryocytes in the bone marrow. RBCs are anucleate cells devoid of common intracellular organelles. Basophils are the least abundant leukocytes in the peripheral blood.
Keywords: Hematopoiesis, erythropoiesis

11 **The answer is B: Bilirubin.**   Hemolysis refers to the premature elimination of circulating erythrocytes. Immune hemolytic anemias are characterized by increased red cell destruction (hemolysis), secondary to antibodies directed against antigens on the erythrocyte surface. Antibody-mediated hemolysis liberates free hemoglobin that is degraded by proteases to peptides and heme (the porphyrin ring that binds iron). Heme is further degraded to bilirubin by reticuloendothelial cells of the spleen. Laboratory findings commonly associated with hemolysis include increased levels of bilirubin and hemoglobin in the blood and urine. The other serum components are not elevated in patients with hemolytic anemia.
Keywords: Hemolytic anemia, bilirubin

12 **The answer is E: Reticulocytosis.**   Hemolytic anemias are characterized by a compensatory increase in the production and release of red cells by the bone marrow. This accelerated release of red cells from the bone marrow is manifested in the blood by an increased reticulocyte count (normal reference range = 0.5% to 1.5%). Reticulocytes are anucleate red cells that represent the last stage of differentiation before the mature erythrocyte. The nucleus is extruded from orthochromatic erythroblasts, leaving mitochondria and polyribosomes in the reticulocyte. After release from the bone marrow, reticulocytes lose their capacity for aerobic metabolism and hemoglobin synthesis, and become a mature erythrocyte after 1 to 2 days. Circulating levels of leukocytes and their precursors may occasionally reach very high levels (greater than 50,000 WBC/μL). This leukemoid reaction (choice A) is sometimes difficult to differentiate from leukemia. Lymphocytosis (choice B) refers to increased numbers of B or T lymphocytes in the peripheral blood. None of the other hematologic findings are expected in a patient with hemolytic anemia.
Keywords: Hemolytic anemia, reticulocytes

13 **The answer is B: Pancytopenia.**   The patient's bone marrow consists largely of fat cells and lacks normal hematopoietic activity. This condition is termed aplastic anemia. In brief, aplastic anemia is a disorder of pluripotential stem cells that leads to bone marrow failure. The disorder features hypocellular bone marrow and pancytopenia (decreased circulating levels of all formed elements in the blood). Depending on the underlying cause, the stem cell injury may not be reversible. Cytotoxic

chemotherapy is known to cause a transient aplastic anemia. Leukocytosis (choice A), lymphocytosis (choice C), and neutrophilia (choice D) are all characterized by an increase in the number of circulating white blood cells. Thrombocytosis (choice E) refers to an increase in circulating blood platelets.
Keywords: Aplastic anemia, pancytopenia

14 **The answer is C: Liver.** Hematopoietic stem cells arise from mesoderm associated with the aorta/gonad/mesonephros (AGM) region of the embryo. Hematopoiesis also occurs in blood islands within mesoderm of the extraembryonic yolk sac. Hematopoiesis switches from the yolk sac to the fetal liver around the 3rd month of embryogenesis, and switches to bone marrow after the second trimester of gestation. From birth until 4 years of age, all bone cavities are densely packed with hematopoietic tissue. After that time, the size of the bone cavities outgrows the volume required for hematopoiesis, and in adults, fat cells are intermixed in the available space. None of the other organs provide a hospitable environment (niche) for hematopoiesis during fetal development.
Keywords: Hematopoiesis, hematopoietic stem cells

15 **The answer is D: Neutrophils.** Inflammation is the response of the microvasculature to a pathologic insult. It is characterized by the movement of (1) fluid and (2) leukocytes from blood into the injured tissue. Neutrophils are the cellular hallmark of acute inflammation. These phagocytes exit the blood to clear debris and begin the process of wound healing. Lobar pneumonia refers to consolidation of an entire lobe, whereas bronchopneumonia signifies scattered solid foci in the same or several lobes. Basophils (choice A) are precursors of tissue mast cells. Lymphocytes (choice B) and plasma cells (choice E) are mediators of chronic inflammation; they provide antigen-specific immunity to infectious diseases. Tissue macrophages (choice C) are chronic inflammatory cells derived from circulating blood monocytes; they secrete numerous cytokines to regulate wound healing.
Keywords: Bacterial pneumonia, *Streptococcus pneumonia*

16 **The answer is C: Purulent exudate.** Lung abscess is a localized accumulation of pus accompanied by the destruction of pulmonary parenchyma. The most common cause of pulmonary abscess is aspiration, often in the setting of depressed consciousness (e.g., the patient is an alcoholic). The creamy fluid (pus) within the abscess represents a purulent exudate. Purulent exudates and effusions are associated with pathologic conditions such as bacterial infections, in which the predominant cell type is the segmented neutrophil (polymorphonuclear leukocyte). Effusions (choice A) represent excess fluid in a body cavity. Fibrinous exudates (choice B) contain large amounts of fibrin. Serous exudates (choice D) have

a yellow, strawlike color. A transudate (choice E) is noninflammatory edema with low protein content.
Keywords: Pulmonary abscess, exudates, purulent

17 **The answer is C: Margination of segmented neutrophils.** An essential feature of inflammation is the accumulation of leukocytes within injured tissue. During acute inflammation, segmented neutrophils recognize vascular endothelial cells bearing appropriate receptors. This process of cell recognition and cell adhesion is termed neutrophil margination. After rolling to a stop, activated neutrophils flatten and migrate through the endothelial wall to enter the surrounding connective tissue (diapedesis). The photomicrograph shows the attachment of several neutrophils to endothelium. None of the other choices describe the behavior of intravascular segmented neutrophils.
Keywords: Margination, acute inflammation

18 **The answer is E: Selectin.** Selectins are sugar-binding glycoproteins that mediate the initial adhesion of leukocytes to endothelial cells at sites of inflammation. E-selectins are found on endothelial cells; P selectins are found on platelets; and L-selectins are found on leukocytes. E selectins are stored in Weibel Palade bodies of resting endothelial cells. Upon activation, E-selectins are redistributed along the luminal surface of the endothelial cells, where they mediate the initial adhesion (tethering) and rolling of leukocytes. After leukocytes come to a stop, integrins (choice C) mediate transendothelial cell migration and subsequent chemotaxis to sites of injury. Cadherins (choice A) are not involved in neutrophil adhesion to vascular endothelium. Entactin (choice B) and laminin (choice D) are basement membrane glycoproteins.
Keywords: Margination, acute inflammation

19 **The answer is C: Lymphocytes.** The peripheral blood smear shows reactive (antigen-stimulated) large lymphocytes. Naïve lymphocytes encounter antigen-presenting cells (macrophages and dendritic cells) in the secondary lymphoid organs. In response to this cell–cell interaction, they become activated and circulate in the vascular system, before they are recruited to a peripheral tissue. The lymphocytes in the peripheral smear shown in the image appear reactive, because they are larger than normal circulating lymphocytes and have more cytoplasm. They are commonly seen in viral infections, including infectious mononucleosis, and they are usually of T-cell lineage. None of the other leukocytes display the distinctive nuclear and cytoplasmic features of activated lymphocytes.
Keywords: Infectious mononucleosis, lymphocytes

20 **The answer is C: Lymphocytosis.** In contrast to bacterial infections, viral infections (including infectious mononucleosis) are characterized by lymphocytosis, an absolute increase in the number of circulating lymphocytes.

Lymphocytosis is defined as an increase in the absolute peripheral blood lymphocyte count above the normal reference range (greater than 4,000/μL in children and greater than 9,000/μL in infants). The principal causes of absolute peripheral blood lymphocytosis are (1) acute infections (infectious mononucleosis, whooping cough), (2) chronic bacterial infections (tuberculosis, brucellosis), and (3) lymphoproliferative diseases. Parasitic infestations and certain allergic reactions cause eosinophilia (choice A), an increase in the number of circulating eosinophils. Leukopenia (choice B) and neutropenia (choice D) represent a decrease in the circulating WBC count. Neutrophilia (choice E) represents an increase in the number of circulating neutrophils.

Keywords: Infectious mononucleosis, lymphocytosis

21 **The answer is D: Macrophages.** Inflammation has historically been referred to as either acute or chronic, depending on the persistence of the injury, clinical symptoms, and the nature of the inflammatory response. The cellular components of chronic inflammation are lymphocytes, antibody-producing plasma cells, and macrophages. Macrophages are a principal source of growth factors and are recognized for their phagocytic functions. During healing of the lung, macrophages enter the alveolar air spaces to remove inflammatory debris. The chronic inflammatory response is often prolonged and may be associated with aberrant repair (i.e., fibrosis). Basophils (choice A) and eosinophils (choice B) do not respond to *S. Pneumoniae*. Lymphocytes (choice C) and plasma cells (choice E) are not phagocytes.

Keywords: Bacterial pneumonia, *Streptococcal pneumoniae*

22 **The answer is C: Cytokine secretion.** The peripheral blood smear shows a small lymphocyte with a dark spherical nucleus and scant blue cytoplasm. Lymphocytes are the principal mediators of antigen-specific immunity. B and T lymphocytes originate in the bone marrow. T cells are educated as to self-/nonself-antigenicity in the thymus. Together, B and T lymphocytes constitute about 30% of total peripheral blood leukocytes. Most lymphocytes in the peripheral blood are immunocompetent; they have been sensitized to a target and are in transit from one tissue to another. T and B cells are indistinguishable by light microscopy. B cells secrete immunoglobulins (antibodies), whereas T cells either lyse target cells or secrete cytokines. Cytokines (signaling molecules) produced by helper T lymphocytes include interferon-γ, TGF-β, and a variety of interleukins. None of the other immunological responses describe the principal function of lymphocytes.

Keywords: Lymphocytes, T cells

23 **The answer is B: Eosinophil.** The peripheral blood smear shows a mature eosinophil, with a trilobed nucleus and numerous red (eosinophilic) cytoplasmic granules. Eosinophils are granulocytes that are derived from a common myeloid progenitor cell in the bone marrow. They are particularly evident during allergic-type reactions and parasitic infestations. For example, infections with *Trichinella* are accompanied by eosinophilia, and skeletal muscle is typically infiltrated by eosinophils. Trichinosis is produced by the roundworm *Trichinella spiralis*. After mating, the females liberate larvae into the circulation. The larvae can invade almost any tissue but survive only in skeletal muscle in an encapsulated form. Elevated serum levels of creatine kinase indicate muscle cell necrosis. The other cells do not exhibit distinctive red granules that are the cytologic hallmark of eosinophilic granulocytes.

Keywords: Trichinosis, granulocytes, eosinophils

24 **The answer is A: Degradation of pathogens.** The importance of oxygen-dependent mechanisms in the bacterial killing by phagocytic cells is exemplified in chronic granulomatous disease of childhood. Children with this disease suffer from a hereditary deficiency of NADPH oxidase, resulting in a failure to produce superoxide anion and hydrogen peroxide during phagocytosis. Persons with this disorder are susceptible to recurrent bacterial infections, because they are unable to generate toxic oxygen species that are required for pathogen degradation. These reactive oxygen species include O_2^- and H_2O_2. None of the other cellular functions is mediated by reactive oxygen species.

Keywords: Chronic granulomatous disease, phagocytosis

25 **The answer is B: Leukopenia.** Leukopenia refers to an absolute decrease in circulating WBCs. It is occasionally encountered under conditions of chronic inflammation, especially in patients who are malnourished or who suffer from a chronic debilitating disease. Leukopenia may also be caused by typhoid fever and certain viral and rickettsial infections. Leukocytosis (choice A) is an absolute increase in circulating WBCs. Neutropenia (choice C) is an absolute decrease in circulating neutrophils. Pancytopenia (choice D) refers to decreased circulating levels of all formed elements in the blood. Thrombocytopenia is an absolute decrease in circulating platelets. In 1990, prostatic adenocarcinoma became the most frequently diagnosed cancer in American men, surpassing the incidence of lung cancer. Prostatic adenocarcinomas, which account for 98% of all prostatic tumors, are commonly located in the peripheral zone of the prostate gland.

Keywords: Prostate cancer, leukopenia

26 **The answer is C: Erythropoietin.** Renal cell carcinomas often secrete erythropoietin, a 34-kDa glycoprotein that regulates erythropoiesis. This hormone stimulates the growth of erythrocyte progenitors in the bone marrow by inhibiting a default pathway of programmed cell death (apoptosis). Increased hematocrit in this patient is the result of bone marrow hyperplasia affecting burst-forming and colony-forming units of the erythroid lineage. The cellular and molecular mechanisms responsible for hyperplasia relate to the control of stem cell viability and cell proliferation. The other hormones do not regulate erythropoiesis.

Keywords: Renal cell carcinoma, erythropoiesis

27 **The answer is A: Erythrocyte.** These proliferative stem cell colonies are committed to the erythrocyte pathway of differentiation. Erythroid hyperplasia is typically seen in people living (or climbing) at high altitude. Low oxygen tension evokes the production of erythropoietin by the kidneys, which promotes the survival and proliferation of erythroid progenitor cells in the bone marrow. Hyperplasia is defined as an increase in the number of cells in an organ or tissue. Like hypertrophy, it is often a response to trophic signals or increased functional demand and is commonly a normal process. None of the other cells undergo physiological hyperplasia in response to low oxygen tension.

Keywords: Renal cell carcinoma, erythropoietin

28 **The answer is E: Transferrin.** Free iron is carried in the blood by transferrin, an 80-kDa glycoprotein with two high-affinity binding sites for Fe^{3+}. Transferrin receptors on cells throughout the body import transferrin via receptor-mediated endocytosis. Bilirubin (choice A) is a product of heme catabolism that may accumulate in liver cells but does not transport iron. Ceruloplasmin (choice B) carries copper in the blood. Ferritin (choice C) is an intracellular iron-storage protein. About 25% of the body's total iron content is bound by ferritin. Hemosiderin (choice D) is a partially denatured form of ferritin that aggregates and is recognized microscopically as yellow brown granules within the cytoplasm. Hereditary hemochromatosis (HH) is a common, autosomal recessive, genetic disorder that is characterized by excessive iron absorption and the toxic accumulation of iron in parenchymal cells, particularly of the liver, heart, and pancreas. In the liver, HH leads to cirrhosis and a high incidence of primary hepatocellular carcinoma. The Prussian blue stain binds iron and provides histologic evidence for iron overload.

Keywords: Hereditary hemochromatosis, transferrin

29 **The answer is E: Platelets.** Thrombosis and hemostasis are regulated by the activation of circulating platelets and plasma clotting factors. Platelets are small cytoplasmic fragments of megakaryocytes with a life span of about 10 days. They play a critical role in maintaining the integrity of the cardiovascular system. Platelets bind to exposed fibrillar collagen at sites of endothelial cell injury and degranulate, releasing growth factors (PDGF) and vasoactive mediators (serotonin and thromboxane A_2). Activated platelets also provide a substrate for the conversion of fibrinogen to insoluble fibrin. The fibrin strands are cross-linked to form a mesh that traps platelets and cells. This intravascular hemostatic plug is appropriately referred to as a thrombus.

Keywords: Hemostasis, platelets, thrombosis

30 **The answer is C: Integrins.** Leukocytes leave the intravascular space and follow gradients of chemotactic factors to sites of tissue injury during inflammation. Selectins (choice E) provide an initial tether for leukocytes. Once they have come to a stop (margination), leukocytes respond to signals from activated endothelial cells, express new cell adhesion molecules (e.g., integrins), and move through small gaps between vascular endothelial cells. These tight junction gaps form in response to histamine and other vasoactive mediators that are released by tissue mast cells. Leukocytes use integrins to modulate cell adhesion during transendothelial migration. Cadherins (choice A) mediate cell adhesion between epithelial cells. Fibronectin and laminin (choices B and D) are extracellular matrix proteins that provide ligands for integrin binding during cell migration.

Keywords: Inflammation, endothelial cells

31 **The answer is C: Hypercellularity of the bone marrow.** Normal bone marrow consists stromal and hematopoietic cells separated by sinusoids. Stromal cells include endothelial cells, reticular adventitial cells, adipocytes, and fibroblasts. Hematopoietic cells include progenitor cells at various stages of differentiation. This patient's biopsy is best described as hypercellular. It shows densely packed, malignant B lymphoblasts. Most precursor B-cell malignancies involve primarily bone marrow and peripheral blood and are termed B-cell acute lymphoblastic leukemias (B ALL). Approximately 75% of B ALL cases occur in children under the age of 6 years. B ALL features numerical aberrations and chromosomal translocations, including the Philadelphia chromosome. The Philadelphia chromosome is a 9;22 reciprocal translocation that produces an oncogenic *bcr/abl* fusion protein. None of the other choices describe histopathologic features of lymphoblastic leukemia.

Keywords: Acute lymphoblastic leukemia, bone marrow

32 **The answer is E: Neutrophils.** An effusion represents excess fluid in a body cavity. Purulent effusions (and exudates) contain a prominent cellular component. Neutrophils respond to bacterial infections and would be expected in this patient's pleural effusion. Basophils (choice A) are the least numerous WBC in the peripheral blood. Eosinophils (choice B) respond to parasitic infestations and certain allergies. Lymphocytes (choice C) and monocytes (choice D) are chronic inflammatory cells.

Keywords: Bacterial pneumonia, pleural effusion

33 The answer is D: Immunoglobulins. The peripheral blood smear from this patient shows clumped red cells caused by serum autoantibodies. Antibodies are multivalent immunoglobulins that cross-link target antigens. Cold agglutinins are mostly IgM antibodies. They are directed against the I/i antigen system and act optimally at 4°C. Cold agglutinins may be idiopathic or develop secondary to an underlying condition, most frequently infections (EBV) or lymphoproliferative disorders. α-1-Antitrypsin (choice A) and α-2-macroglobulin (choice E) are protease inhibitors produced by the liver. None of the other plasma proteins are agglutinins.
Keywords: Autoimmune hemolytic anemia

34 The answer is E: Thrombin. Coagulation factors are present in the blood in an inactive (zymogen) state. Clotting factor XII (Hageman factor) provides a key source of vasoactive mediators. It is activated by exposure to negatively charged surfaces, such as basement membranes, proteolytic enzymes, bacterial lipopolysaccharide, and foreign materials. Activated Hageman factor initiates a coagulation cascade that culminates in the formation of thrombin—a serine protease that converts fibrinogen (clotting factor I) to insoluble fibrin strands. Thrombin also activates platelets to amplify the coagulation cascade. None of the other mediators of inflammation regulate the formation of intravascular fibrin plugs (thrombi) at sites of tissue injury.
Keywords: Hemostasis, thrombosis

35 The answer is C: Plasmin. Activation of Hageman factor sets in motion the following: (1) Conversion of plasminogen to plasmin; (2) conversion of prekallikrein to kallikrein; (3) activation of the complement system; and (4) activation of the coagulation system. Plasmin generated by activated Hageman factor is a serine protease that induces fibrinolysis. The products of fibrin degradation (fibrin split products) augment vascular permeability. Plasmin also cleaves components of the complement system, generating biologically active products, including the anaphylatoxins C3a and C5a. Caspases (choice A) are cysteine proteases that regulate apoptosis. Elastase (choice B) is a protease that degrades elastin. Thrombin (choice D) and trypsin (choice E) are proteases, but they do not specifically degrade intravascular thrombi.
Keywords: Thrombosis, fibrinolysis

36 The answer is A: Eosinophils. The bone marrow aspirate shows progenitor cells at various stages of differentiation and maturation. The arrows identify three large cells filled with red (eosinophilic) granules. These eosinophils will leave the bone marrow and circulate with a life span of 8 to 12 hours but may survive for days within target tissues. They are characteristic of hypersensitivity reactions, as well as allergic and asthmatic responses. Eosinophils contain preformed mediators of inflammation. They express cell surface IgA receptors and contain intracellular granules filled with eosinophil major basic protein (MBP), a carbohydrate-binding protein that provides a powerful defense against worm-like parasitic infestations (helminths). None of the other hematopoietic cells exhibit large eosinophilic granules.
Keywords: Lymphoma, granulocytes, eosinophils

37 The answer is D: Monocytes. Failure of the left ventricle leads to chronic passive congestion of the lungs. Blood leaks from the congested pulmonary capillaries into the alveoli. Alveolar macrophages degrade these extravasated RBCs and accumulate intracellular hemosiderin (ferritin-derived iron storage pigment). These hemosiderin-laden phagocytes are called "heart failure" cells. They can be identified in histologic sections using the Prussian blue stain for iron. In addition to removing pathogens and necrotic debris, macrophages take up and process microbes and present antigens to lymphocytes. These cells can also differentiate into dendritic cells, which are highly efficient antigen-presenting cells. Macrophages are derived from circulating blood monocytes. None of the other cells are progenitors for the mononuclear phagocyte system.
Keywords: Congestive heart failure, heart failure cells

38 The answer is E: Phagocytosis. The peripheral blood smear shows a large, agranular cell with a markedly indented nucleus. This kidney-shaped nuclear morphology is the hallmark of circulating monocytes. The nuclear indentation is filled with membranes of the Golgi apparatus and centrioles. Monocytes are the progenitors of the mononuclear phagocyte system. Monocytes exit the circulation and migrate into all tissues and organs to become resident macrophages. Examples include alveolar macrophages, bone osteoclasts, and liver Kupffer cells. In response to inflammatory mediators, they also accumulate at sites of acute and chronic inflammation. Macrophages recognize, internalize, and digest foreign materials, microorganisms, and cellular debris. This process is termed phagocytosis, and the effector cells are known as phagocytes. None of the other mechanisms of inflammation describe the primary function of macrophages. The peripheral blood smear shown in the image also reveals numerous platelets.
Keywords: Monocytes, macrophages

39 The answer is A: Eosinophils. Asthma is a chronic lung disease caused by increased responsiveness of the airways to a variety of stimuli. Patients typically have paroxysms of wheezing, dyspnea, and cough. Bronchial hyperresponsiveness in asthma is believed to be an inflammatory reaction to diverse stimuli, either extrinsic (e.g., pollen) or intrinsic (e.g., exercise). Histologic examination of lung from a patient who died in status asthmaticus often shows increased numbers of eosinophils. Eosinophils participate in allergic responses, and their peripheral blood count may be elevated in patients with severe asthma. The peripheral blood count of the other cells would not be expected to change significantly in patients with bronchial asthma.

Keywords: Bronchial asthma

40 The answer is C: IgE. The peripheral blood smear shows a large lymphocyte and a basophilic granulocyte (arrow, shown on the image). The basophil has a bilobed nucleus and contains large, basophilic granules. Basophils and tissue mast cells express cell surface receptors for the Fc domain of IgE. When IgE-primed basophils and mast cells encounter multivalent antigens, their Fc receptors are clustered in the plane of the membrane. This clustering event triggers degranulation and the release of a variety of inflammatory mediators (e.g., histamine). Histamine is a primary mediator of increased vascular permeability during inflammation. Histamine binds specific H1 receptors in the vascular wall, inducing endothelial cell contraction, gap formation, and local edema. Basophils do not have cell surface receptors for the other immunoglobulin classes.

Keywords: Granulocytes, basophils

41 The answer is C: Fibrin. A thrombus is an aggregate of clotted blood that contains platelets, fibrin, and trapped blood cells. By definition, thrombi are adherent to the vascular wall. Detachment and movement of a thrombus through the circulatory system (arterial or venous) is referred to as thromboembolism. The process of generating an intravascular thrombus is termed thrombosis. Collagen (choice A), elastin (choice B), and laminin (choice E) are extracellular matrix proteins. Keratin (choice D) is an intermediate filament protein synthesized by epidermal cells of the skin, nails, and hair.

Keywords: Coagulation, thrombosis

42 The answer is A: HbA1c. About 96% of hemoglobin found in adults is referred to as hemoglobin A (HbA). A specific fraction of HbA in circulating erythrocytes is modified by the addition of carbohydrate. This glycosylated subtype of hemoglobin (hemoglobin A1c) is measured routinely to monitor the overall degree of hyperglycemia that occurred during the preceding 6 to 8 weeks. Nonenzymatic glycosylation (glycation) of hemoglobin is irreversible, and the level of hemoglobin A1c, therefore, serves as a marker for glycemic control. Glycemic control is essential, because complications of diabetes are related to the severity and chronicity of hyperglycemia. None of the other choices are quantitative measures of serum glucose levels.

Keywords: Diabetes mellitus, hemoglobin

43 The answer is B: Megakaryocyte. Megakaryocytes in the bone marrow mature into multilobed giant cells by a number of endomitotic cell divisions. After reaching a certain size and ploidy, megakaryocyte cytoplasm is released into bone marrow sinusoids in long, platelet-containing ribbons. After their release from the bone marrow, platelets circulate with a life span of about 10 days. They help maintain the integrity of the vascular endothelium by initiating thrombosis and delivering growth factors that stimulate tissue regeneration and repair. Platelets can be observed in a peripheral blood smear (examined at high magnification) as small (2 to 3 μm) anucleate particles. Platelets can be readily observed in the blood smear shown for Questions 6 and 38). None of the other cells undergo endomitotic divisions or appear as multinucleated giant cells.

Keywords: Megakaryocyte, lymphoblastic leukemia

44 The answer is D: Neutrophil. The blood smear displays elliptical erythrocytes, as well as a normal segmented neutrophil. Neutrophils are the most abundant leukocyte present in the peripheral blood (40 to 73 relative %). Hereditary elliptocytosis (HE) refers to a heterogeneous group of inherited disorders involving the erythrocyte cytoskeleton, all of which feature an abnormality within the cytoskeleton. HE usually manifests as a mild normocytic anemia; however, many patients are asymptomatic. None of the other cells display the distinctive polymorphonuclear morphology of segmented neutrophils.

Keywords: Hereditary elliptocytosis

45 The answer is E: Opsonization. The recognition, binding, and internalization of pathogens by phagocytes are greatly enhanced by coating the pathogens with specific plasma components, particularly immunoglobulins and the C3b fragment of complement. These plasma components are termed opsonins. None of the other mechanisms of inflammation are enhanced by opsonization.

Keywords: Bacterial pneumonia, phagocytosis

46 The answer is E: Septic shock. The clinical and laboratory data suggest that this patient has a systemic blood infection. Septicemia (bacteremia) denotes the clinical condition in which bacteria are found in the circulation. In patients with endotoxic shock, lipopolysaccharide (LPS) released from gram-negative bacteria stimulates monocytes/macrophages to secrete large quantities of tumor necrosis factor–α (TNF-α). This glycoprotein causes direct cytotoxic damage to capillary endothelial cells resulting in a failure to maintain adequate blood supply to the microcirculation (shock). Sepsis often leads to multiple organ dysfunction in critically ill patients. Fever and neutrophilia are systemic manifestations of

acute inflammation. The other diseases are not typically associated with hypotension, fever, and neutrophilia.
Keywords: Septic shock

47 **The answer is B: Clotting factor.**   Classic hemophilia results from mutations in the gene encoding factor VIII (hemophilia A). Hemophilia A is the most frequently encountered inherited bleeding disorder (1 per 5,000 to 10,000 males). It is an X-linked recessive disorder of blood clotting that results in spontaneous bleeding, particularly into joints, muscles, and internal organs. A deficiency of the other plasma proteins would not cause a familial bleeding disorder.
Keywords: Hemophilia

Chapter 6
Muscle Tissue

QUESTIONS

Select the single best answer.

1 A portion of the sartorius muscle, obtained at autopsy, is prepared using routine H&E staining and examined by light microscopy (shown in the image). Identify the structures indicated by the arrows.

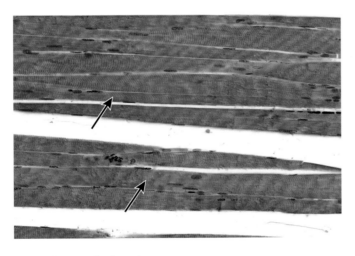

(A) Muscle fascicles
(B) Muscle fibers
(C) Myofibrils
(D) Myofilaments
(E) Sarcomeres

2 A section of the lip that shows transverse sections of skeletal muscle is examined by a group of first-year medical students (shown in the image). Identify the structure indicated by the oval line.

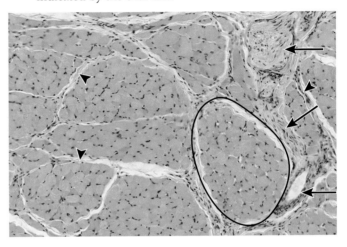

(A) Muscle fascicle
(B) Muscle fiber
(C) Myofibril
(D) Myofilament
(E) Sarcomere

3 Examination of a thin section of striated muscle at high magnification reveals longitudinal muscle fibers and cross sections of muscle fibers (shown in the image).

Identify the structure that forms the space indicated by the arrowheads.

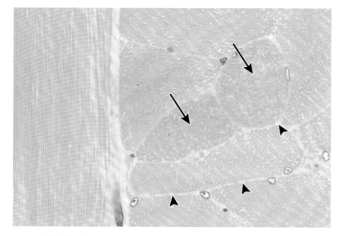

(A) Endomysium
(B) Epimysium
(C) Myofibril
(D) Perimysium
(E) Sarcoplasmic reticulum

4 For the muscle fibers described in Question 3, which of the following terms describes the pink-stained dots visible in cross sections, and the longitudinal lines visible in longitudinal sections?
(A) A bands
(B) Myofibrils
(C) Myofilaments
(D) Myosins
(E) Thin filaments

5 A thin plastic section of skeletal muscle is examined at high magnification in the histology laboratory. Identify the lines that bisect the light-stained I bands (arrows, shown in the image).

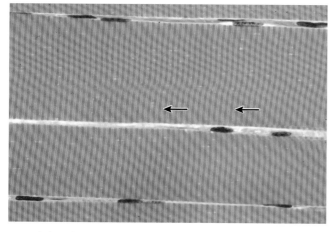

(A) A bands
(B) H zones
(C) I bands
(D) M lines
(E) Z lines

6 During a small group seminar, you are asked to discuss the physiology of muscle contraction. The sarcomere is the basic contractile unit of skeletal muscle. It lies between which of the following paired structures in myofibrils?
(A) Adjacent A bands
(B) Adjacent I bands
(C) Adjacent M lines
(D) Adjacent Z lines
(E) Z line and M line

7 Which of the following portions of the sarcomere contains both thick and thin filaments?
(A) A band
(B) H zone
(C) I band
(D) M line
(E) Z line

8 A frozen section of a skeletal muscle biopsy is stained by enzyme histochemistry using an alkaline pH reaction for myosin ATPase. Identify the structures indicated by the arrows (shown in the image).

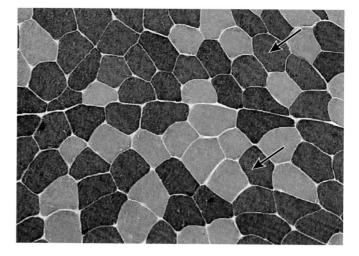

(A) Intermediate fibers
(B) Myofibrils
(C) Myofilaments
(D) Type I fibers
(E) Type II fibers

9 Which of the following muscles is composed primarily of slow-twitch (type I) fibers?
(A) Adductor pollicis
(B) Erector spinae
(C) Flexor digitorum profundus
(D) Lateral rectus
(E) Superior oblique

10 A 30-year-old woman begins a vigorous program of bodybuilding. After 6 months, her muscles have become prominent and strong. Which of the following physiologic changes underlies muscle enlargement in this woman?

(A) Deposition of newly formed adipocytes

(B) Increase in the diameter of individual muscle fibers

(C) Increase in the number of muscle fibers

(D) Thickening of the endomysium

(E) Thickening of the perimysium

11 The parents of a 5-year-old boy are concerned that their son tires easily. Physical examination reveals enlargement of the child's calf muscles. Serum levels of creatine kinase are elevated. A biopsy of calf muscle reveals muscle fiber necrosis, regenerating fibers, and fibrosis. The child is subsequently diagnosed with Duchenne muscular dystrophy. This X-linked recessive disease is caused by mutations in the gene for which of the following muscle proteins?

(A) Creatine kinase

(B) Desmin

(C) Dystrophin

(D) Glycogen phosphorylase

(E) Myosin

12 A biopsy of the biceps brachii muscle is prepared using a special stain and examined in the pathology department (shown in the image). Identify the structure indicated by the arrows.

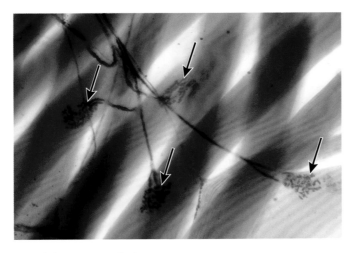

(A) Motor end plates

(B) Motor unit

(C) Muscle spindles

(D) Myelinated axons

(E) Tendon organs

13 During a clinical conference, you are asked to discuss skeletal muscle anatomy and physiology. Which of the following best describes histologic features of a "motor unit"?

(A) A single axonal branch and the muscle fibers it innervates

(B) A single nerve axon and the muscle fiber(s) it innervates

(C) A single peripheral nerve and the muscle(s) it innervates

(D) The muscle spindle and the muscle fibers it innervates

(E) The nerve fiber(s) that innervate a single muscle fascicle

14 Physical examination of a 10-year-old boy reveals a displaced left nipple and partial absence of the left pectoralis muscle. The parents of the boy ask you to explain muscle formation during embryogenesis. Which of the following tissues in the embryo provides stem cells for the development of limb musculature?

(A) Intermediate mesoderm

(B) Lateral plate parietal mesoderm

(C) Lateral plate visceral mesoderm

(D) Neural crest–derived mesenchyme

(E) Paraxial mesoderm

15 A 36-year-old woman complains of impaired speech and frequent aspiration of food. Physical examination reveals double vision (diplopia) and drooping eyelids (ptosis). The patient is subsequently diagnosed with myasthenia gravis. The symptoms of muscle weakness in this patient are caused by autoantibodies directed against which of the following cellular components?

(A) Acetylcholine

(B) Acetylcholine receptor

(C) Calcium channel

(D) Rheumatoid factor

(E) Thyroid-stimulating hormone receptor

16 Skeletal muscle patterns in the developing embryo (e.g., shape, origin, insertion) are regulated by interactions between undifferentiated myoblasts and which of the following cells or tissues?

(A) Connective tissue

(B) Endothelial cells

(C) Neural tube

(D) Notochord

(E) Peripheral nerves

17 A section of skeletal muscle is examined in the histology laboratory (shown in the image). Identify the structure indicated by the arrow.

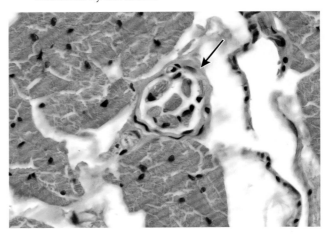

(A) Muscle fascicle

(B) Muscle fiber

(C) Muscle spindle

(D) Myofibril

(E) Perimysium

18 The myocardium of a woman who died of a cardiac arrhythmia is examined in the pathology department (shown in the image). Which of the following statements describes an important feature of cardiac muscle that helps distinguish cardiac from skeletal muscle in routine H&E slide preparations?

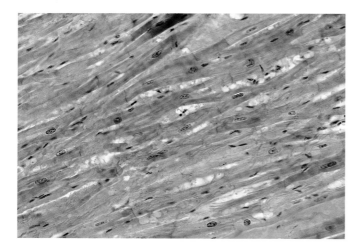

(A) Connective tissue contains a rich capillary network.
(B) Muscle fibers are composed of multiple cells.
(C) Muscle fibers exhibit cross-striations.
(D) Sarcomeres are located between adjacent Z lines.
(E) Thin filaments contain actin.

19 Thin sections of the cardiac muscle described in Question 18 are examined at high magnification (shown in the image). Identify the structures indicated by the arrows.

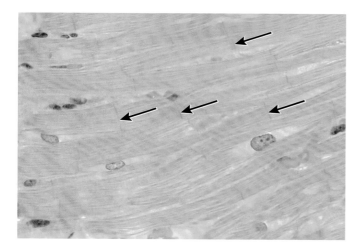

(A) A bands
(B) I bands
(C) Intercalated disks
(D) M lines
(E) Z lines

20 A 21-year-old man is discovered on routine physical examination to have a cardiac arrhythmia. Which of the following structures initiates cardiac muscle contraction?
(A) Motor end plates
(B) Muscle spindles
(C) Parasympathetic nerve fibers
(D) Purkinje fibers
(E) Sympathetic nerve fibers

21 In addition to Purkinje fibers, which of the following cellular structures distributes electrochemical signals between cardiac myocytes to ensure a normal heart rhythm?
(A) Endomysium
(B) Fascia adherens
(C) Gap junctions
(D) Macula adherens
(E) Sarcomere

22 The wall of the colon is examined at autopsy (shown in the image). Identify the tissue.

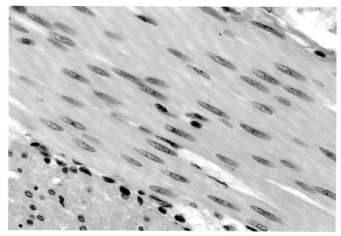

(A) Dense regular connective tissue
(B) Elastic connective tissue
(C) Nerve fibers
(D) Skeletal muscle
(E) Smooth muscle

23 Which of the following cells synthesizes the basal lamina and endomysium that surrounds smooth muscle fibers?
(A) Endothelial cells of capillaries
(B) Epithelial cells
(C) Fibroblasts in the perimysium
(D) Schwann cells of peripheral nerves
(E) Smooth muscle cells

24 Smooth muscle fibers in the wall of the gastrointestinal tract are derived from which of the following tissues during embryonic development?
(A) Embryonic endoderm
(B) Intermediate mesoderm
(C) Lateral plate somatic mesoderm
(D) Lateral plate visceral mesoderm
(E) Paraxial mesoderm

ANSWERS

1 **The answer is B: Muscle fibers.** Unlike connective tissue fibers (e.g., collagenous fibers, elastic fibers, reticular fibers), a muscle fiber is actually a muscle cell. These elongated cells (myocytes) are organized into parallel arrays to form muscle tissue. In skeletal muscle, a muscle fiber is a multinucleated syncytium formed by the fusion of several embryonic myoblasts. In longitudinal sections, skeletal muscle cells appear as long cylindrical fibers with multiple, long oval nuclei located at the periphery of the cells. Myofibrils (choice C) are longitudinal arrays of contractile filaments in the cytoplasm of muscle cells. Myofibrils are composed of thick (myosin) and thin (actin) myofilaments (choice D). A sarcomere (choice E) is the segment of a myofibril that forms the basic functional unit of skeletal muscle. Muscle fascicles (choice A) are bundles of muscle fibers bound together by a connective tissue sheath.
Keywords: Muscle fibers

2 **The answer is A: Muscle fascicle.** Skeletal muscles are invested with distinct layers of connective tissue: (1) endomysium surrounds individual muscle fibers; (2) perimysium surrounds bundles of muscle fibers; and (3) epimysium surrounds the external surface of muscles. Groups of muscle fibers surrounded by perimysium are referred to as muscle fascicles or muscle bundles. As shown in the image, large blood vessels and nerves (indicated by arrows) travel within the perimysium (indicated by arrowheads) to supply the muscle fascicles. Muscle fibers (choice B) exhibit a polygonal shape in cross section and feature multiple peripheral nuclei. None of the other structures exhibit the distinctive histologic features of muscle fascicles.
Keywords: Muscle fascicles

3 **The answer is A: Endomysium.** A delicate connective tissue (indicated by the arrowheads) composed of a basal lamina and reticular fibers surrounds individual muscle fibers (indicated by the arrows). This connective tissue layer is endomysium. Numerous capillaries travel through the endomysium to supply muscle fibers with oxygen and nutrients. Epimysium (choice B) is the dense connective tissue sheath that envelops an entire muscle. It provides the investing fascia that is described in gross anatomy. It is continuous with the tendon or aponeurosis that anchors a muscle to its attachment site. Thin connective tissue septa arising from the epimysium extend into the muscle and surround muscle fascicles. These connective septa form the perimysium (choice D). Sarcoplasmic reticulum (choice E) is a highly organized, tubular network of smooth endoplasmic reticulum that separates bundles of myofilaments into myofibrils (choice C).
Keywords: Endomysium

4 **The answer is B: Myofibrils.** When examined in cross section at high magnification, skeletal muscle fibers appear stippled because of the presence of numerous myofibrils in the cytoplasm. In longitudinal sections, myofibrils demonstrate cross-striations with alternating regions of light-stained I bands and dark-stained A bands. The precise lateral alignment of light- and dark-stained bands gives skeletal muscle its distinctive striated appearance; hence the term "striated muscle." Myofibrils are bundles of the actin and myosin myofilaments (choice C) that produce muscle fiber contraction. Two types of myofilaments are found in skeletal muscle cells: thick filaments contain myosin (choice D), whereas thin filaments (choice E) contain primarily actin.
Keywords: Myofibrils

5 **The answer is E: Z lines.** As described above, alternating A and I bands form cross-striations that are a characteristic feature of skeletal muscle fibers. When examined by polarized light microscopy, the dark A bands (anisotropic bands) exhibit birefringence, whereas the light I bands (isotropic bands) exhibit monorefringence. When examined at high magnification, dense Z lines (Z disks) are observed to bisect the light-stained I bands. The Z lines appear as zigzag lines in longitudinal sections. The major protein found in Z lines is the actin-binding protein, α-actinin. α-Actinin anchors thin filaments to Z lines. A less dense region, termed the H zone (H band), is observed to bisect the dark-stained A bands. A narrow dense line, the M line, is located at the center point of the H zone. H zones and M lines are not visible by light microscopy, but they are revealed when skeletal muscle fibers are examined by electron microscopy.
Keywords: Myofibrils

6 **The answer is D: Adjacent Z lines.** Sarcomeres are the repetitive functional units of striated muscle fibers. They are defined as the segments of myofibrils that lie between adjacent Z lines. Sarcomeres extend about 2.5 μm in resting muscle, but the length of a sarcomere is reduced to about 1 μm during muscle contraction. The explanation for this observation is that during muscle contraction, thin filaments in I bands slide into A bands. Thus, the length of I bands becomes shorter during muscle contraction, whereas the length of A bands remains unchanged. A single skeletal muscle fiber may contain over 100,000 sarcomeres.
Keywords: Sarcomeres

7 **The answer is A: A band.** Thick filaments composed of myosin extend along the entire length of the A band. The center point of the A band is the dense M line that contains a myosin-binding protein, myomesin. This protein links thick filaments together, forming the M line. The less-dense H zone that flanks the M line consists exclusively of thick filaments. The thin filament anchored to the Z line extends over one-half of the I band and, therefore, overlaps with a portion of the A band. Thus, portions of the A band that flank the H zone contain both thin and thick filaments. These thin and thick filaments are organized so that each thick filament is in contact with six thin filaments. During muscle contraction, longer portions of the thin filaments slide into the A bands. As result of these molecular changes, H zones become thinner and I bands become shorter during muscle contraction.

Keywords: Sarcomeres

8 **The answer is E: Type II fibers.**   Three types of muscle fibers are found in skeletal muscle, namely red, white, and intermediate. These muscle fibers differ in their color, diameter, and enzyme biochemistry. Histochemical reactions detecting myosin ATPase can be used to distinguish type I (slow-twitch) fibers from type II (fast-twitch) fibers. The rationale for this observation is that myosin ATPase activity is positively correlated with muscle contraction velocity. When stained for myosin ATPase, type I fibers appear pale and type II fibers appear dark (shown in the image). In fresh tissue, type I fibers are small and red. They tend to have more mitochondria and more myoglobin. Type I fibers are characterized by a slow velocity of the myosin ATPase reaction, which results in slow/prolonged contractions (i.e., slow-twitch fibers). By contrast, type II fibers exhibit high anaerobic enzyme activity and they produce faster, shorter, and stronger contractions than do type I fibers (fast-twitch fibers). An intermediate muscle fiber was recently identified. Intermediate (type IIa) fibers are fast-twitch, fatigue-resistant motor units. They are not identified in this muscle biopsy. Myofibrils and myofilaments (choices B and C) cannot be resolved in frozen sections examined at low magnification.

Keywords: Skeletal muscle, slow-twitch and fast-twitch fibers

9 **The answer is B: Erector spinae.**   The three types of muscle fibers described above (slow-twitch, fast-twitch, and intermediate) are present in all skeletal muscles; however, the relative proportions vary depending on the function of the particular muscle. Type I fibers are the principal fibers found in the long back muscles that support an erect body posture. These slow-twitch fibers are small and red in fresh tissue. They generate prolonged contractions with lower tension and are resistant to fatigue. Type II fibers (also referred to as type IIb fibers) are large fast-twitch fatigue-prone motor units that exhibit the fastest myosin ATPase velocity. These muscle fibers are richly innervated. They produce rapid contractions and regulate precise movements. For example, type IIb fibers are abundant myofibers in muscles of the forearm and hand (choices B and C), and in the extraocular muscles that control eye movements (choices D and E). As mentioned above, intermediated fibers are fast-twitch and fatigue-resistant. Intermediate fibers are most abundant in the limb muscles of 400 m/800 m runners and middle-distance swimmers.

Keywords: Skeletal muscle, slow-twitch and fast-twitch fibers

10 **The answer is B: Increase in the diameter of individual muscle fibers.**   Muscle fiber diameter varies according to physiologic demand. The size of muscle fibers also varies as a function of age, sex, and nutrition. It is commonly known that physical training and exercise leads to muscle enlargement. This enlargement is caused by increased diameter of individual muscle fibers (i.e., increased cell volume). Exercise stimulates the production of new intracellular myofibrils that increase the diameter of individual muscle fibers. This process, growth by increased cell size, is referred as hypertrophy. Skeletal muscle has limited capacity to regenerate in response to injury, and does not respond to increased workload by increasing the number of muscle fibers (hyperplasia, choice C). Exercise *reduces* fat deposition in muscles (choice A) and does not increase the abundance of interstitial connective tissue (choices D and E).

Keywords: Skeletal muscle hypertrophy

11 **The answer is C: Dystrophin.**   Dystrophin is a rod-shaped cytoplasmic protein located beneath the sarcolemma (plasma membrane). It links actin filaments of the outmost layer of the myofilaments to the inner surface of the plasma membrane (sarcolemma). It interacts with many other muscle proteins and forms a dystrophin-associated protein complex that links cytoplasmic proteins with extracellular structural proteins. Duchenne muscular dystrophy is a severe, progressive, X-linked, inherited condition characterized by progressive degeneration of muscles, particularly those of the pelvic and shoulder girdles. Dystrophin deficiency leads to impaired force transmission from thin filaments to the sarcolemma. The resulting weakness is noted mainly around the pelvic and shoulder girdles (proximal muscle weakness) and is progressive. Enlargement of the patient's calf muscles is referred to as "pseudohypertrophy." Healthy muscle tissue is replaced gradually with an abundance of fibrofatty connective tissue. None of the other proteins are associated with pathogenesis of Duchenne muscular dystrophy.

Keywords: Duchenne muscular dystrophy

12 **The answer is A: Motor end plates.**   Neuromuscular junctions (or motor end plates) are functional contacts between a motor nerve fiber and a muscle fiber. At this junction, the terminal end of an axon (or terminal twig of an axon) forms a synapse with the plasma membrane (sarcolemma) of the target muscle fiber. Synaptic vesicles stored in the terminal axon bulb contain acetylcholine. Nerve impulses cause acetylcholine to be released into the synaptic cleft. Binding of this neurotransmitter to its receptor initiates muscle cell contraction. Motor nerves containing myelinated axons travel within the perimysium. The axons lose their myelin sheath at the neuromuscular junction. None of the other structures exhibit histologic features of a motor end plate.

Keywords: Motor end plate

13 The answer is B: A single nerve axon and the muscle fiber(s) it innervates. Muscles that control precise and delicate movements (e.g., extraocular muscles and intrinsic hand muscles) are richly innervated. In these muscles, a single nerve fiber usually innervates a single muscle fiber. By contrast, muscles that produce large and coarse movements (e.g., back and limb muscles) are typically innervated by nerve fibers with hundreds of terminal branches (twigs). In these muscles, axon twigs (not individual axons) form synapses with myofibers. Thus, a motor unit is best described as a single nerve axon and the muscle fiber or fibers that it innervates. None of the other choices describe histologic features of a motor unit.
Keywords: Motor unit, neuromuscular junction

14 The answer is E: Paraxial mesoderm. This patient shows signs of Poland sequence anomaly, a rare congenital birth defect associated with underdevelopment of the chest muscles. During development, skeletal muscles of the axial and appendicular skeleton are derived from blocks of paraxial mesoderm. Paraxial mesoderm forms somites that are further subdivided into sclerotome, myotome, and dermatome. Myotome stem cells (myoblasts) migrate through the embryo and form skeletal muscle. Intermediate mesoderm (choice A) gives rise to the genitourinary system. Lateral plate parietal mesoderm (choice B) forms the axial skeleton. Lateral plate visceral mesoderm (choice C) forms smooth muscle of the gastrointestinal system. Neural crest cells give rise to a wide variety of tissues, including the autonomic nervous system.
Keywords: Poland anomaly, paraxial mesoderm

15 The answer is B: Acetylcholine receptor. Myasthenia gravis is a type II hypersensitivity disorder caused by autoantibodies that bind to the acetylcholine receptor. These antibodies interfere with the transmission of neural impulses at the neuromuscular junction, causing muscle weakness and easy fatigability. External ocular and eyelid muscles are most often affected, but the disease is often progressive and may cause death, owing to respiratory muscle paralysis.
Keywords: Myasthenia gravis

16 The answer is A: Connective tissue. As mentioned above, skeletal muscle develops from myoblasts that migrate throughout the embryo. During migration, myoblasts receive biochemical signals and cues from the surrounding connective tissue. In the head region of the embryo, connective tissue is primarily of neural crest origin. In the limbs, the connective tissue is derived from lateral plate parietal (somatic) mesoderm. The cellular and molecular mechanisms that pattern the size, shape, and attachments of muscles are largely unknown. None of the other cells or tissues are known to regulate the patterning of skeletal muscles during embryonic development.
Keywords: Skeletal muscle, development

17 The answer is C: Muscle spindle. Muscle spindles are encapsulated sensory receptors that are situated among muscle fascicles. They are proprioceptors that continuously monitor changes in muscle fiber length during body movement. As shown in the image, muscle spindles consist of a connective tissue capsule that surrounds a few small muscle fibers. These small fibers are said to be "intrafusal," whereas the surrounding large muscle fibers are said to be "extrafusal." Unlike extrafusal fibers, intrafusal fibers are not striated. Sensory nerve fibers penetrate the capsule and synapse with individual intrafusal fibers. Muscle spindles constantly monitor muscle stretching and relay this information to the spinal cord for processing. Muscle spindles generate essential reflexes that maintain posture and coordinate the actions of opposing muscle groups during body movement.
Keywords: Muscle spindles

18 The answer is B: Muscle fibers are composed of multiple cells. Unlike skeletal muscle, where muscle fibers are multinucleated cells, cardiac muscle fibers are composed of multiple cells that make tight end-to-end connections. Cardiac muscle cells may split and unite, giving cardiac muscle a typical "branching" morphology. Cardiac and skeletal muscles both exhibit cross-striations—their thick and thin contractile filaments exhibit the same organization (choices C, D, E). The nuclei of cardiac and skeletal muscle are, however, distinctly different. The nuclei of skeletal muscle cells are located at the periphery of the fiber, whereas the nucleus of a cardiac myocyte is located in the center of the cell (shown in the image). This difference in nuclear location provides a useful means for distinguishing cardiac from skeletal muscle. Cardiac and skeletal muscle fibers are both invested with connective tissue that conveys nerves and capillaries (choice A).
Keywords: Cardiac muscle

19 The answer is C: Intercalated disks. Intercalated disks are a distinctive histologic feature of cardiac muscle. In routine H&E histologic preparations, intercalated disks appear as darker-stained lines that cross the muscle fibers. They represent highly specialized regions of cell–cell adhesion. They are composed of junctional complexes that form strong molecular bridges between cardiac myocytes. When examined by scanning electron microscopy, intercalated disks appear as steplike disks with transverse and lateral regions. In the transverse region, fascia adherens (the equivalent of zonula adherens in epithelial cells) and desmosomes mediate cell adhesion. Gap junctions and desmosomes are found in the lateral region of the intercalated disk. The other structures (lines and bands) are present in cardiac myocytes, but they do not contribute to the morphology of intercalated disks, and they would not be visible at this magnification.
Keywords: Intercalated disks

20 The answer is D: Purkinje fibers. As mentioned above, skeletal muscle contraction is initiated by the release of acetylcholine from motor neurons at neuromuscular junctions (motor end plates). By contrast, cardiac muscle contractions are initiated, regulated, and coordinated by a cardiac conducting system. This conducting system is composed of specialized cardiac muscle cells. It includes nodal tissue that generates intrinsic cardiac contractile impulses and conducting fibers. Purkinje fibers are the terminal conducting fibers. They are located in the sub-endocardium of the heart. Purkinje fibers transmit contractile impulses to heart muscle in a rapid and precise sequence, leading to spontaneous and rhythmic cardiac contractions (heart beats).
Keywords: Purkinje fibers

21 The answer is C: Gap junctions. Gap junctions are molecular pores that permit ions and other small molecules to pass between adjacent cells. Gap junctions are found in the lateral regions of the intercalated disks in cardiac muscle. They permit electrochemical signals to move between cardiac myocytes (ionic coupling). Gap junction communication enables cardiac muscle cells to form an electrochemical syncytium that helps maintain a normal heart rhythm.
Keywords: Gap junctions

22 The answer is E: Smooth muscle. Smooth muscle is an involuntary and nonstriated muscle that is widely distributed in the body. For example, smooth muscle is found in the gastrointestinal tract, blood vessels, urinary bladder, uterus, male/female reproductive tracts, and iris of the eye. In longitudinal sections, smooth muscle fibers appear as elongated fusiform cells with central nuclei and uniformly eosinophilic cytoplasm (illustrated in the image). Depending on location, the length of smooth muscle fibers varies from 20 µm (media of small blood vessel) to 500 µm (myometrium of pregnant uterus). Smooth muscle fibers are typically arranged into bundles or sheets. None of the other tissues exhibit the distinctive histologic features of smooth muscle.
Keywords: Smooth muscle

23 The answer is E: Smooth muscle cells. In addition to their contractile properties, smooth muscle cells demonstrate the characteristic features of secretory cells. For example, endomysium, a thin layer of connective tissue, and the basal lamina that surrounds smooth muscle fibers are produced and deposited by smooth muscle cells. Reticular fibers in the endomysium form an intricate network that supports the parenchymal cells and binds them together. In large blood vessels, smooth muscle cells secrete type I collagen and elastic tissue components.
Keywords: Smooth muscle

24 The answer is D: Lateral plate visceral mesoderm. During gastrulation, the embryo generates several types of mesoderm with different developmental fates. These types of mesoderm include notochord, cardiac, paraxial, intermediate, and lateral plate. The visceral (splanchnic) layer of lateral plate mesoderm becomes intimately associated with the primitive gut tube (choice A). Here, visceral mesoderm forms the investing layers of the gastrointestinal (GI) tract, namely lamina propria, muscularis mucosae, submucosa, and muscularis externa. Smooth muscle in the muscularis externa provides the GI tract with motility to facilitate the passage of food. Intermediate mesoderm (choice A) gives rise to the genitourinary system. Lateral plate somatic mesoderm (choice B) forms the axial skeleton and soft tissues of the limbs. Skeletal muscles are derived from paraxial mesoderm (choice E).
Keywords: Somatic mesoderm

Chapter 7

Nerve Tissue

QUESTIONS

Select the single best answer.

1 A 48-year-old man died in a motor vehicle accident and a spinal cord specimen is harvested at autopsy. A smear preparation of the patient's gray matter is stained with H&E and examined by light microscopy (shown in the image). The arrow identifies which of the following cells of the central nervous system?

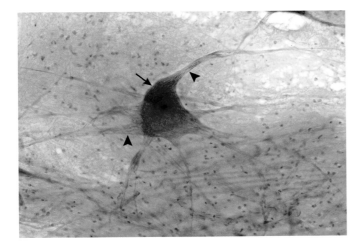

(A) Astrocyte
(B) Microglial cell
(C) Neuron
(D) Oligodendrocyte
(E) Satellite cell

2 For the spinal cord preparation described in Question 1, the indicated cell is classified as which of the following?
(A) Bipolar
(B) Multipolar
(C) Pseudounipolar
(D) Purkinje
(E) Pyramidal

3 Which of the following tissues/structures is most likely innervated by the cell identified in Questions 1 and 2?
(A) Cardiac muscle
(B) Skeletal muscle
(C) Skin
(D) Smooth muscle
(E) Sweat glands

4 For the spinal cord preparation described in Question 1, the arrowheads identify which of the following cellular/subcellular structures?
(A) Axons
(B) Dendrites
(C) Nissl bodies
(D) Nucleoli
(E) Synaptic junctions

5 A section of a spinal cord specimen at autopsy is stained with Luxol fast blue and cresyl violet (shown in the image). Cell bodies of large neurons are observed in this section. Which of the following best describes the dark-stained structures indicated by lines within the neuronal cell bodies?

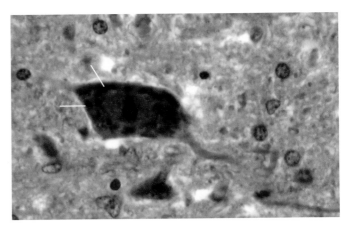

(A) Heterochromatin
(B) Lysosomes
(C) Nissl bodies
(D) Peroxisomes
(E) Segmented nuclei

6 A 35-year-old woman injures her common fibular nerve in a motorcycle accident. Which of the following best describes the *primary function* of neuronal axons within this major division of the sciatic nerve?
(A) Convey signals to dendrites
(B) Receive signals from other neurons
(C) Synthesize structural proteins
(D) Transmit signals to other cells
(E) Uptake of neurotransmitters

7 Which of the following cellular structures gives rise (origin) to the cell projection that conducts impulses away from the cell body?
(A) Axon hillock
(B) Centromere
(C) Centrosome
(D) Kinetochore
(E) Nissl body

8 Which of the following structures of a neuron is responsible for the generation of an action potential that is conducted from one neuron to another neuron?
(A) Dendritic tree
(B) Initial segment
(C) Myelin sheath
(D) Nissl body
(E) Synapse

9 A 46-year-old woman is diagnosed with colon cancer and undergoes surgery. The resected colon segment contains a margin of normal colon tissue that is examined by light microscopy (shown in the image). Which of the following best describes the structure located within the oval?

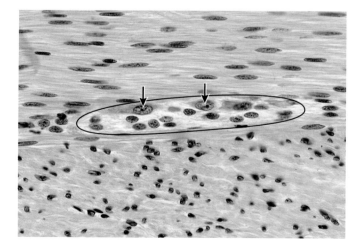

(A) Muscle spindle
(B) Myenteric plexus
(C) Peripheral nerve fiber
(D) Smooth muscle bundle
(E) Sympathetic ganglion

10 For the patient described in Question 9, the arrows identify which of the following types of cells?
(A) Interneurons
(B) Somatic afferent neurons
(C) Somatic efferent neurons
(D) Visceral afferent neurons
(E) Visceral efferent neurons

11 A 72-year-old man complains of balance problems. Physical examination reveals reduced facial expression, resting tremor, and slowness of voluntary movements (bradykinesia). The patient is subsequently diagnosed with Parkinson disease. The patient's symptoms are caused by a deficiency of which of the following neurotransmitters?
(A) Acetylcholine
(B) Dopamine
(C) Nitric oxide
(D) Norepinephrine
(E) Serotonin

12 A chemical synapse is typically composed of a presynaptic element, as well as a synaptic cleft and postsynaptic membrane. Which of the following represents a presynaptic element of a chemical synapse?
(A) Axon
(B) Cell body
(C) Dendrite
(D) Golgi apparatus
(E) Plasma membrane of target cell

13 A 53-year-old woman presents to the emergency room complaining of blurred vision and difficulty speaking (dysarthria). She reports eating a large quantity of home-canned vegetables. The patient subsequently progresses to respiratory arrest and expires. Inhibition of the release of which of the following neurotransmitters most likely caused paralysis of respiratory muscles in this patient?
(A) Acetylcholine
(B) Dopamine
(C) Epinephrine
(D) Norepinephrine
(E) Serotonin

14 For the patient described in Question 13, the neurotransmitter that stimulates contraction of the thoracic diaphragm is normally released from which of the following terminal end-bulb structures?
(A) Golgi membranes
(B) Herring bodies
(C) Nissl bodies
(D) Nuclear pores
(E) Synaptic vesicles

15 An 80-year-old woman with a history of diabetic neuropathy suffers a stroke and expires. At autopsy, a peripheral nerve is stained with osmium tetroxide (OsO_4), sectioned, and examined by electron microscopy (shown in the image). Which of the following best describes the structures that are indicated by the arrowheads?

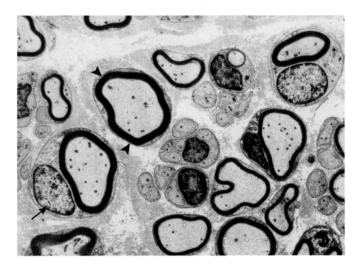

(A) Endoneurium
(B) Epineurium
(C) Glycocalyx
(D) Myelin sheath
(E) Perineurium

16 For the nerve specimen described in Question 15, the arrow identifies the nucleus of which of the following glial/stromal cells?
(A) Astrocyte
(B) Fibroblast
(C) Oligodendrocyte
(D) Satellite cell
(E) Schwann cell

17 The cell identified in Question 16 was derived from which of the following stem cell populations during embryonic and fetal development?
(A) Glioblasts
(B) Monocytes
(C) Neural crest cells
(D) Neuroblasts
(E) Neuroepithelial cells

18 A 35-year-old woman complains of blurred vision. Two months later, the patient develops double vision and numbness in the fingers of her left hand. MRI shows scattered plaques in the patient's brain and spinal cord. The patient is diagnosed with multiple sclerosis. The plaques observed in this patient represent selective loss of which of the following proteins of the central nervous system?
(A) Acetylcholine receptors
(B) Alpha-synuclein
(C) Beta-amyloid protein
(D) Myelin
(E) Tubulin

19 In the central nervous system, myelin is produced and maintained by which of the following types of cells?
(A) Astrocytes
(B) Microglial cells
(C) Neurons
(D) Oligodendrocytes
(E) Schwann cells

20 A peripheral nerve collected at autopsy is teased apart, fixed to a slide, and stained with H&E (shown in the image). The arrows identify which of the following nerve-associated structures?

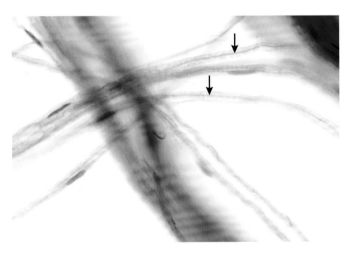

(A) Axon
(B) Collagen fiber
(C) Myelin sheath
(D) Node of Ranvier
(E) Nucleus of Schwann cell

21 Another peripheral nerve specimen is fixed and stained with OsO_4 and examined by light microscopy (shown in the image). The arrow identifies which of the following nerve-associated structures?

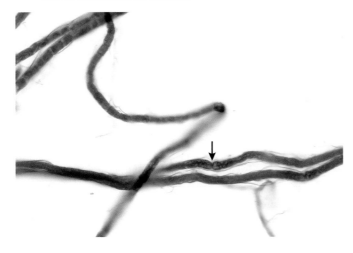

(A) Endoneurium
(B) Internodal segment
(C) Node of Ranvier
(D) Perineurium
(E) Schmidt-Lanterman clefts

22 A 27-year-old man suffers a gunshot wound to the thorax and expires. A dorsal root ganglion near the bullet track is examined at autopsy (shown in the image). The arrows identify the nuclei of which of the following types of cells?

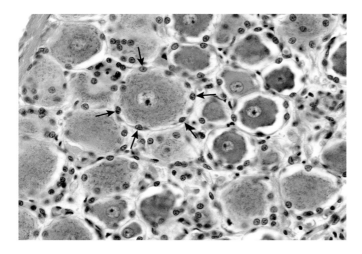

(A) Astrocytes
(B) Neurons
(C) Oligodendrocytes
(D) Satellite cells
(E) Schwann cells

23 Which of the following best describes the neurons that are present in the ganglion described in Question 22?
(A) Bipolar
(B) Interneuron
(C) Motor
(D) Multipolar
(E) Pseudounipolar

24 Which of the following describes the function of neurons that are located in dorsal root ganglia of the nervous system?
(A) Autonomic motor
(B) Interneuron communicating
(C) Somatic motor
(D) Visceral motor
(E) Visceral sensory

25 A 36-year-old woman suffers a concussion while skiing. CT scan of the brain reveals a massive cerebral contusion of the left frontal lobe. The woman lies comatose for 20 days but then expires. A section of the patient's brain is stained at autopsy using an antibody directed against an intermediate filament protein (shown in the image). This immunohistochemical labeling technique identifies which of the following cells?

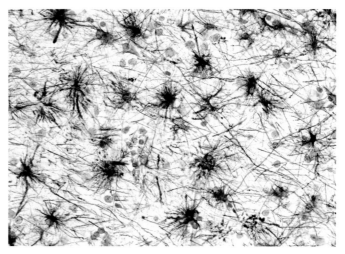

(A) Astrocytes
(B) Endothelial cells
(C) Microglial cells
(D) Neurons
(E) Oligodendrocytes

26 Which of the following best describes the primary function of the cells that are identified in the brain of the patient described in Question 25?
(A) Defense against pathogens and neoplastic cells
(B) Generation of cerebrospinal fluid
(C) Myelination of neuronal axons
(D) Phagocytosis of senescent neurons
(E) Support and nourishment of neurons

27 Another section of brain from the patient described in Question 25 is stained with H&E and examined by light microscopy (shown in the image). The cells with elongated nuclei indicated by the arrows are best described as which of the following?

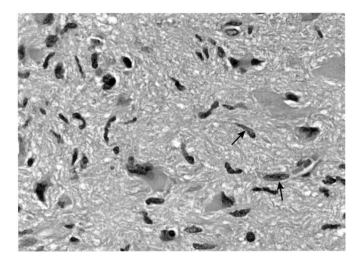

(A) Astrocytes
(B) Endothelial cells
(C) Microglial cells
(D) Oligodendrocytes
(E) Sensory neurons

28 The cells identified in Question 27 are derived from which of the following stem cell populations during development of the nervous system?
(A) Glioblasts
(B) Granulocyte/monocyte progenitor cells
(C) Neural crest cells
(D) Neuroblasts
(E) Neuroepithelial cells

29 Which of the following best describes the function of microglia in the central nervous system?
(A) Establishment of blood–brain barrier
(B) Myelination of neuronal axons
(C) Phagocytosis and defense against injury
(D) Production of cerebrospinal fluid
(E) Support and nourishment of neurons

30 A 68-year-old man with dementia suffers a massive stroke and expires. At autopsy, a section of the patient's brain is stained with H&E and examined by light microscopy (shown in the image). The large cells with

pale cytoplasm and central nuclei represent which of the following types of cells?

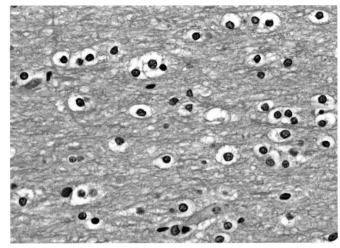

(A) Astrocytes
(B) Ependymal cells
(C) Microglial cells
(D) Oligodendrocytes
(E) Sensory neurons

31 A 46-year-old man with malignant glioblastoma develops cardiorespiratory failure and expires. A section of the patient's brain near the lateral ventricle is examined by light microscopy (shown in the image). The arrows identify which of the following cells?

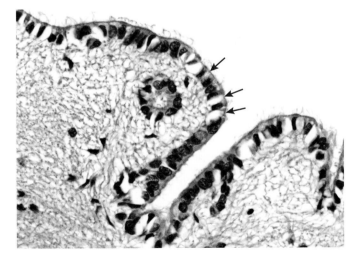

(A) Astrocytes
(B) Endothelial cells
(C) Ependymal cells
(D) Microglial cells
(E) Oligodendrocytes

32 A longitudinal section of the median nerve obtained at autopsy is stained with H&E and examined by light microscopy (shown in the image). The asterisk identify which of the following nerve-associated structures?

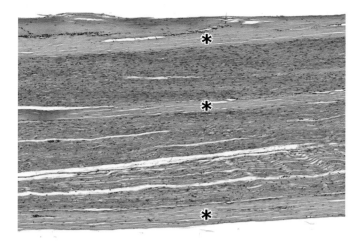

(A) Endoneurium
(B) Epineurium
(C) Nerve fascicles
(D) Nerve fibers
(E) Perineurium

33 A transverse section of the nerve described in Question 32 is stained with Mallory trichrome and examined by light microscopy (shown in the image). Which of the numbered lines indicates perineurium?

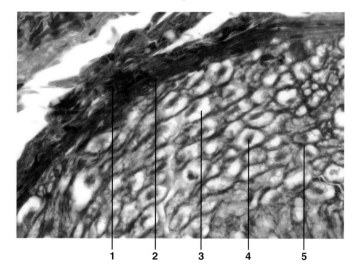

(A) Line 1
(B) Line 2
(C) Line 3
(D) Line 4
(E) Line 5

34 The red-stained central dot indicated by Line 4 in the image shown for Question 33 represents which of the following structures?
(A) Axon
(B) Endoneurium
(C) Fibroblast nucleus
(D) Myelin sheath
(E) Schwann cell nucleus

35 A peripheral nerve is collected at autopsy of a 70-year-old woman with a history of diabetes and hypertension. A transverse section of a nerve fascicle is fixed and stained with osmium tetroxide (OsO_4) in order to identify membrane lipids (shown in the image). The arrows identify which of the following nerve-associated structures?

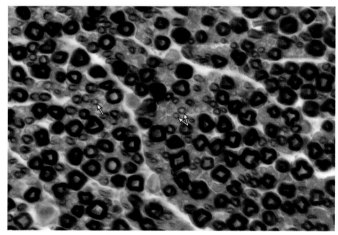

(A) Endoneurium
(B) Myelinated nerve fiber
(C) Perineurium
(D) Poorly myelinated nerve fiber
(E) Schwann cell nucleus

36 A longitudinal section of the nerve fascicle described in Question 35 is stained with H&E and examined by light microscopy (shown in the image). The arrows identify which of the following nerve-associated structures?

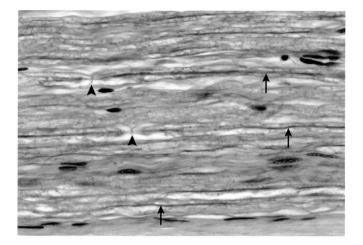

(A) Axon
(B) Collagen fiber
(C) Cytoplasm of Schwann cell
(D) Endoneurium
(E) Myelin sheath

37 Arrowheads on the image shown for Question 36 identify which of the following nerve-associated structures?
(A) Axon terminal
(B) Capillary
(C) Internodal segment
(D) Node of Ranvier
(E) Synapse

38 Which of the following best describes the function of nodes of Ranvier in the peripheral nervous system?
(A) Release and degradation of neurotransmitters
(B) Saltatory conduction of nerve impulse
(C) Uptake of oxygen and nutrients
(D) Formation of neuromuscular junctions
(E) Location of satellite cells for repair of nerve injury

39 Which of the following structures contributes to the formation of a blood–nerve barrier in the peripheral nervous system?
(A) Endoneurium
(B) Epineurium
(C) Myelin sheath
(D) Node of Ranvier
(E) Perineurium

40 A 62-year-old woman presents with a small mass on the upper surface of her lip. Physical examination reveals a pearly nodule with rolled borders and central ulceration. The nodule is subsequently removed and examined by light microscopy. Which of the following tissues is located within the circle?

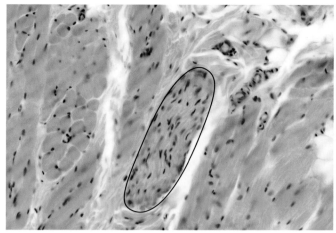

(A) Dense regular connective tissue
(B) Loose connective tissue
(C) Peripheral nerve
(D) Skeletal muscle
(E) Smooth muscle

41 A 68-year-old man with a history of hyperlipidemia suffers a ruptured abdominal aneurysm and expires. During the autopsy, ganglia are collected from different locations and examined by light microscopy (shown in the image). Which of the following best characterizes this particular ganglion?

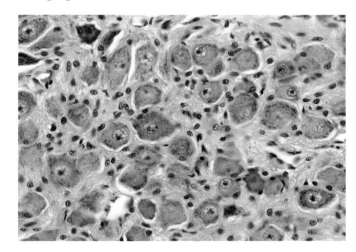

(A) Dorsal root ganglion
(B) Enteric ganglion
(C) Parasympathetic ganglion
(D) Sympathetic ganglion
(E) Ventral horn of the spinal cord

42 Which of the following best characterizes neurons present in the ganglion described in Question 41?
(A) Interneurons
(B) Somatic efferent neurons
(C) Somatic sensory neurons
(D) Visceral efferent neurons
(E) Visceral sensory neurons

43 Considering their essential and diverse functions, enteric glial cells most closely resemble which of the following cells of the central nervous system?
(A) Astrocyte
(B) Endothelial cell
(C) Ependymal cell
(D) Microglial cell
(E) Oligodendrocyte

44 Which of the following structures is a component of the central nervous system?
(A) Brainstem
(B) Dorsal root ganglion
(C) Enteric nervous system
(D) Paravertebral sympathetic chain
(E) Postsynaptic parasympathetic ganglion

45 In the central nervous system, the term "nucleus" refers to which of the following?
(A) Aggregate of pyramidal cells in the cerebral cortex
(B) Bundle of functionally related axons
(C) Bundle of functionally related dendrites
(D) Cluster of functionally related neuronal cell bodies
(E) Collection of Purkinje cells in the cerebellum

46 A segment of spinal cord (C5-C6) is collected at autopsy and stained for myelin with Luxol fast blue and cresyl violet (shown in the image). Which of the numbered lines points to the dorsal horn of gray matter?

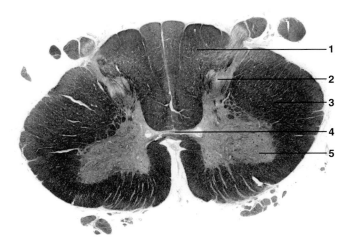

(A) Line 1
(B) Line 2
(C) Line 3
(D) Line 4
(E) Line 5

47 For the spinal cord segment described in Question 46, which of the following is the predominant component of the lateral funiculus in the white matter indicated by Line 3?

(A) Axons
(B) Blood vessels
(C) Cell bodies of neurons
(D) Dendrites
(E) Glial cells

48 A higher magnification view of the dorsal horn of the spinal cord segment described in Question 46 is shown in the image. Which of the following neurons are located in this region of the spinal cord?

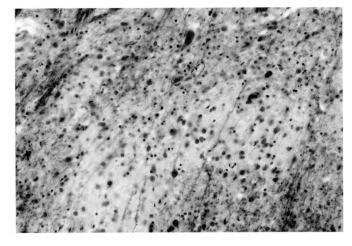

(A) Motor neurons
(B) Postsynaptic sympathetic neurons
(C) Presynaptic parasympathetic neurons
(D) Presynaptic sympathetic neurons
(E) Sensory interneurons

49 Another area of the spinal cord segment described in Question 46 is examined at high magnification (shown in the image). This region of spinal cord is appropriately described as which of the following?

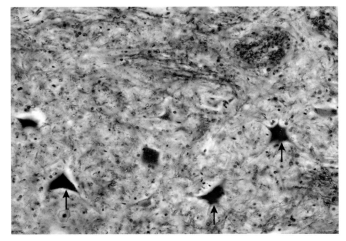

(A) Anterior funiculus
(B) Central canal
(C) Dorsal horn
(D) Posterior funiculus
(E) Ventral horn

50 Regarding the spinal cord section observed in Question 49, which of the following tissues/structures is innervated directly by the neurons that are indicated by the arrows?

(A) Adipose tissue
(B) Skeletal muscle
(C) Skin
(D) Smooth muscle
(E) Sweat gland

51 A 7-year-old girl is brought to the emergency room with fever, vomiting, and convulsions. The patient is febrile to 39.5°C (104°F). Physical examination reveals cervical pain and rigidity. A lumbar spinal puncture is performed to obtain cerebrospinal fluid to help make a diagnosis. The enlarged subarachnoid space that your needle enters (lumbar cistern) is formed (lined) by which of the following tissues/structures?

(A) Arachnoid mater and pia mater
(B) Dura mater and arachnoid mater
(C) Periosteum of vertebral body and dura mater
(D) Pia mater and spinal cord proper
(E) Vertebral body and its periosteum

52 The arachnoid mater of the central nervous system is primarily composed of which of the following types of tissue?

(A) Dense irregular collagenous connective tissue
(B) Elastic connective tissue
(C) Loose collagenous connective tissue
(D) Reticular connective tissue
(E) Simple columnar epithelial tissue

53 A 25-year-old man is rushed to the emergency room in a coma following an accident at work. MRI shows an expanding subdural hematoma over the left hemisphere. From your knowledge of basic histology you understand that this patient's subdural hematoma formed between which of the following pairs of tissues/structures?

(A) Arachnoid mater and pia mater
(B) Dura mater and arachnoid mater
(C) Periosteum and dura mater
(D) Pia mater and brain proper
(E) Skull and its periosteum

54 Which of the following intercellular junctions is essential for maintaining the integrity of the blood–brain barrier?

(A) Gap junctions
(B) Hemidesmosomes
(C) Macula adherens
(D) Zonula adherens
(E) Zonula occludens

55 Which of the following glial cells contributes to the formation of the blood–brain barrier in the central nervous system?

(A) Astrocytes
(B) Ependymal cells
(C) Microglial cells
(D) Oligodendrocytes
(E) Schwann cells

56 A 76-year-old man suffers a stroke and can no longer move his upper and lower limbs on the right side. MRI of the brain reveals a large plaque composed of cellular scar tissue. Which of the following cells is the principal mediator of scar formation in the brain of this patient?

(A) Astrocyte
(B) Ependymal cell
(C) Injured neuron
(D) Microglia
(E) Oligodendrocyte

ANSWERS

1 **The answer is C: Neuron.** The human nervous system contains over 10 billion neurons that serve as the major functional units of the nervous system. From an anatomic and functional point of view, the nervous system is the most complex organ system in the body. In this smear preparation of spinal cord gray matter, the large cell bodies are neurons with multiple cellular extensions (processes). The nuclei of various neuroglial cells (choices A, B, and D) are visible as small dark-stained dots in the background and are indistinguishable from one another in this preparation. Satellite cells (choice E) surround and support neurons located in ganglia of the peripheral nervous system.
Keywords: Spinal cord, neuron

2 **The answer is B: Multipolar.** The functional components of neurons include axon, dendrite, cell body (soma), and synaptic junction. Axons and dendrites provide the core "circuitry" for the nervous system. Axons carry nerve signals away from neuronal cell bodies, whereas dendrites convey signals inward toward neuronal cell bodies. Based on the number of processes extending from the cell body, neurons can be classified as pseudounipolar (unipolar), bipolar, or multipolar. Motor neurons and communicating interneurons are common examples of multipolar neurons. The multipolar neuron identified in this patient's spinal cord shows multiple cellular processes. Bipolar neurons (choice A) have one axon and one dendrite. They are usually associated with special sensory organs, such as those for sight, taste, smell, and hearing. Pseudounipolar neurons (choice C) are commonly sensory neurons, whose cell bodies are located in dorsal root ganglia. Purkinje and pyramidal cells (choices D and E) are multipolar neurons located in the cerebellum and cerebral cortex, respectively.
Keywords: Spinal cord, motor neuron

3 **The answer is B: Skeletal muscle.** Multipolar motor neurons in the spinal cord are situated in the ventral horn. Their axons constitute the periphery nerves that innervate and activate contraction of voluntary skeletal muscle. Cardiac muscle (choice A), smooth muscle (choice D), and sweat glands (choice E) are innervated by autonomic nerve fibers. Skin (choice C) is innervated by sensory nerve fibers.
Keywords: Motor neuron, skeletal muscle

4 **The answer is B: Dendrites.** Dendrites are shorter processes than axons. A neuron typically has many dendrites that receive impulses from other neurons. Because they are often highly branched, it is common to refer to neurons as having a dendritic "tree." Signals from the dendritic tree are summed in the cell body and axon hillock resulting in various outcomes, including initiation of a new action potential. Neurons only have one axon.

The image shown here (see Question 1) does not provide enough detail to unambiguously identify an axon. None of the other choices show the distinctive features of neuronal dendrites.
Keywords: Spinal cord, dendrite

5 **The answer is C: Nissl bodies.** The cell body (soma) of a neuron contains a large nucleus and prominent nucleolus, as well as perinuclear cytoplasm. The small perinuclear structures that stain intensely blue in this preparation are termed Nissl bodies. Electron microscopy has demonstrated that Nissl bodies are composed of rough endoplasmic reticulum and aggregates of free ribosomes. Thus, Nissl bodies are sites of active protein synthesis and posttranslational modification. Lysosomes and peroxisomes (choices B and D) are intracellular organelles that may be present in the perinuclear region of some neurons; however, these organelles cannot be identified at this magnification. Heterochromatin (choice A) and segmented nuclei (choice E) are not cytoplasmic organelles.
Keywords: Spinal cord, Nissl body

6 **The answer is D: Transmit signals to other cells.** Each neuron has one axon that conveys electrical and chemical information away from the cell body to other neurons or to target cells (e.g., muscle fiber). Axons can be very long, such as those originating from first-order motor neurons located in the ventral horn of the spinal cord. They may travel a long distance to reach the skeletal muscle that they innervate (greater than 1 m). Axons that originate from interneurons are typically short. Protein synthesis (choice C) is the major function of the neuronal cell body. Dendrites and cell bodies receive impulses from other neurons (choices A and B). Uptake and degradation of neurotransmitters (choice E) takes place at synaptic junctions.
Keywords: Axon, action potential

7 **The answer is A: Axon hillock.** Neuronal axons arise from a pyramidal-shaped area of the cell body that is referred to as the axon hillock (small hill). The axon hillock lacks Nissl bodies and a Golgi complex but does contain microtubules, neurofilaments, mitochondria, and various intracellular vesicles. Centromeres, centrosomes, and kinetochores (choices B, C, and D) help organize microtubules in the mitotic spindle apparatus. Centrosomes (choice C) are also organizing centers in cilia and flagella.
Keywords: Axon hillock

8 **The answer is B: Initial segment.** Between the apex of the axon hillock and the beginning of the myelinated nerve axon, there is a short, unmyelinated segment that is referred as the initial segment. Recent research has demonstrated that the action potential of a nerve axon is summed in the axon hillock and then generated within

the initial axon segment. The other choices do not generate new action potentials.
Keywords: Axon, initial segment, action potential

9 The answer is B: Myenteric plexus. Myenteric plexus (also referred to as Auerbach plexus) refers to postsynaptic ganglion cells and their unmyelinated nerve fibers that are located between smooth muscle layers in the wall of the GI tract. Myenteric plexus and Meissner plexus (located in the submucosa) are components of the enteric division of the autonomic nervous system. The enteric nervous system is perhaps the best example of "autonomic self-regulating function" of the entire autonomic nervous system. It contains sensory neurons, interneurons, and visceral motor neurons, whose functions are independent of input from the CNS. It is often referred to as the "brain of the gut." Indeed, near-normal gut motility is observed in the absence of connections from the CNS. On the other hand, sympathetic and parasympathetic input from the CNS serves to modulate the enteric nervous system. Muscle spindles (choice A) are neuromechanical sensory receptors located within skeletal muscle. Longitudinal and transverse smooth muscle layers (choice D) are observed to sandwich the myenteric nerve plexus shown in this image. None of the other choices displays this distinctive tissue morphology.
Keywords: Colon cancer, myenteric nerve plexus

10 The answer is E: Visceral efferent neurons. The large, pale-stained nuclei belong to neurons located within Auerbach plexus. Their axons innervate smooth muscle fibers in the muscularis externa and initiate peristaltic movements of the GI tract. Cell bodies of visceral afferent neurons (choice D) and somatic afferent neurons (choice B) are located within dorsal root ganglia. Somatic efferent neurons (choice C) are motor neurons that are located within the ventral horn of the spinal cord. Most interneurons (choice A) are located within the CNS and provide connections between sensory and motor neurons.
Keywords: Colon cancer, myenteric plexus, Visceral efferent neuron

11 The answer is B: Dopamine. Neurotransmitters are small endogenous chemicals that are released at synaptic junctions and bind to receptors on postsynaptic membranes. They serve to transmit signals from one neuron to another neuron or target cell. Parkinson disease (PD) is a common movement disorder characterized pathologically by the loss of dopamine-producing neurons in the midbrain (substantia nigra). Clinically, PD features tremors at rest, muscular (cogwheel) rigidity, expressionless countenance, emotional lability, and dementia late in the course of the disease.
Keywords: Parkinson disease, neurotransmitter

12 The answer is A: Axon. Synapses are specialized structures that permit rapid neuron–neuron or neuron–target communication. Synapses occur between axons and many other structures, including dendrites, cell bodies, axons of other neurons, and the plasma membranes of target cells. Since each neuron has only one axon that conducts the action potential (impulse) away from the neuronal cell body, the presynaptic element in a synapse is typically an axon terminal. The axon terminal at the synapse usually appears as an enlarged tip (referred to as bouton or end-bulb). Neurotransmitters are released from end-bulbs into the synaptic cleft. Golgi apparatus (choice D) is an intracellular organelle that regulates protein and lipid glycosylation. None of the other choices represents a presynaptic element.
Keywords: Synapse, axon, end-bulb

13 The answer is A: Acetylcholine. Botulinum toxin is associated with improperly canned foods that are stored without refrigeration. Ingested toxin from the bacterium *Clostridium botulinum* is rapidly absorbed into the blood from the small intestine. Circulating toxin binds presynaptic nerve terminals and inhibits the release of acetylcholine (ACh), resulting in the paralysis of all skeletal muscles including the respiratory muscles. ACh is the neurotransmitter at the neuromuscular junction. The ACh receptors on the skeletal muscle cells are transmitter-gated Na⁺ channels. The released ACh at the nerve impulse at the neuromuscular junction interact with the ACh receptors and initiate the contraction of the muscle. Neurons using ACh as their neurotransmitter are referred as cholinergic neurons, including presynaptic sympathetic and parasympathetic neurons. None of the other neurotransmitters listed as choices activates skeletal muscle of the thoracic diaphragm.
Keywords: Botulism, acetylcholine

14 The answer is E: Synaptic vesicles. Synaptic vesicles are characterized features of the presynaptic bouton terminals. They are membrane-bound structures containing neurotransmitters. At a nerve impulse, the membrane of synaptic vesicles fuse with the plasma membrane of the presynaptic axon end bulb, thereby release the neurotransmitter into the synaptic cleft. Herring bodies (choice B) are dilated nerve endings of unmyelinated nerves in the posterior pituitary. These nerves store oxytocin and antidiuretic hormone. None of the other structures listed release neurotransmitters.
Keywords: Synapse, synaptic vesicles

15 The answer is D: Myelin sheath. The electron micrograph shows myelinated nerve fibers interspersed with groups of unmyelinated nerve fibers. Myelin sheaths are concentric layers of lipid-rich Schwann cell membrane that wrap around axons in the peripheral nervous system. Myelination serves to isolate axons from their surrounding extracellular environment, thereby enabling rapid, salutatory conduction of nerve impulses. Endoneurium (choice A) and perineurium (choice E) are connective tissues that surround nerve fibers and nerve fascicles, respectively. Epineurium (choice B) is connective tissue that binds nerve fascicles together and contains nutrient arteries.

Keywords: Diabetes, myelin sheath

16 The answer is E: Schwann cell.   Schwann cells are neuroglial cells that support peripheral nerves. Schwann cell membranes form myelin sheaths that envelope many nerves. Unmyelinated nerve fibers are also enveloped and supported by Schwann cells (though they lack myelin sheaths). Astrocytes (choice A) and oligodendrocytes (choice C) are neuroglial cells of the central nervous system. Fibroblasts (choice B) form endo-, peri-, and epineurium. Satellite cells (choice D) nourish and support ganglion cells (neurons) of the peripheral nervous system.

Keywords: Schwann cell, myelin sheath

17 The answer is C: Neural crest cells.   Neural crest cells originate from neuroectoderm along the margins of neural folds during early development. Neural crest cells undergo an epithelial–mesenchymal transition and migrate extensively throughout the embryo giving rise to many structures including Schwann cells, autonomic nervous system, and head mesenchyme. Glioblasts (choice A) and neuroblasts (choice D) are precursor cells for macroglial cells (e.g., astrocytes and oligodendrocytes) and neurons, respectively. Monocytes (choice B) are derived from hematopoietic stem cells; they enter the CNS as it becomes vascularized and differentiate as microglial cells. Neuroepithelial cells (choice E) are stem cells for all neurons and macroglial cells of the CNS.

Keywords: Neural crest, Schwann cells

18 The answer is D: Myelin.   Multiple sclerosis (MS) is a chronic demyelinating disease. It is the most common chronic CNS disease of young adults in the United States. The disorder affects sensory and motor functions and is characterized by exacerbations and remissions over years. Forty percent of cases are marked by eye problems, such as loss of visual fields, blindness in one eye, or diplopia. The demyelinated plaque is the hallmark of MS. Evolving plaques are marked by selective loss of myelin, influx of chronic inflammatory cells, and accumulation of edema fluid. Intracellular deposits of alpha-synuclein (choice B) are observed in patients with Parkinson disease. Beta-amyloid protein (choice C) accumulates in the cerebral cortex as extracellular plaques in patients with Alzheimer disease.

Keywords: Multiple sclerosis, myelin

19 The answer is D: Oligodendrocytes.   Myelin surrounding nerve fibers in the white matter of the brain and spinal cord is composed of concentric layers of oligodendrocyte

cell membrane. Multiple, tongue-like processes of individual oligodendrocytes are able to myelinate multiple nearby axons. Schwann cells (choice E) produce myelin for axons in the peripheral nervous system.

Keywords: Oligodendrocytes, myelin sheath

20 The answer is A: Axon.   In this teased preparation of a peripheral nerve, the axon is visible as the dark red line within the myelinated nerve fiber. Axons (also referred to as nerve fibers) are cell processes that conduct action potentials away from neuronal cell bodies. In this slide preparation, the myelin sheath was removed by solvent extraction and appears as empty (or foamy) space surrounding the axons. Numerous Schwann cell nuclei (choice E) are observed in this image residing along the myelin sheath.

Keywords: Peripheral nerve, axon

21 The answer is C: Node of Ranvier.   Long axons within a peripheral nerve are myelinated by multiple Schwann cells, resulting in a segmented myelin sheath. The junction where two successive Schwann cells meet is referred to as a node of Ranvier, and the myelin sheath between two sequential nodes of Ranvier is referred as an internodal segment (choice B). These segments are approximately 1 mm in length. Thus, a 1-m nerve leaving the spinal cord is associated with over 1,000 Schwann cells. The axon at the node of Ranvier is not myelinated but is covered by interdigitating processes arising from adjacent Schwann cell membranes. Nodes of Ranvier appear as small gaps in the myelin sheath (shown in the image). Schmidt-Lanterman clefts (choice E), also termed myelin clefts, are spaces containing Schwann cell cytoplasm that lies between adjacent myelin membrane lamellae. Schmidt-Lanterman clefts, endoneurium, and perineurium (choices E, A, and D) are also not visible in this preparation.

Keywords: Node of Ranvier, peripheral nerve

22 The answer is D: Satellite cells.   Neuronal cell bodies that cluster together in the peripheral nervous system are referred to as ganglia. Homologous structures in the CNS are referred to as nuclei. Neuroglial cells that surround neurons in a ganglion are termed satellite cells. Satellite cells are small, cuboidal cells. Satellite cells in dorsal root ganglia form a complete monolayer surrounding the central neurons. Astrocytes and oligodendrocytes (choices A and C) are neuroglial cells found in the CNS. Schwann cells (choice E) nourish and support peripheral nerve fibers.

Keywords: Dorsal root ganglion, satellite cells

23 The answer is E: Pseudounipolar.   Sensory neurons located in dorsal root ganglia are pseudounipolar neurons. They possess a single axon that leaves the neuronal cell body and forms two axonal branches: peripheral and central. These neurons are described as being pseudounipolar

because their two axonal processes arise from a single process. The peripheral axon travels to receptors in target organs such as skin or muscle. The central axon reaches the CNS where the impulse is further processed. Bipolar neurons (choice A) have two processes: one axon and one dendrite. They are typically found in special sensory organs. Interneurons (choice B) are located in the CNS, where they form a complex communicating and integrating neuronal network. Interneurons and motor neurons (choice C) are both multipolar neurons that contain one axon and a various number of dendrites (dendritic tree).
Keywords: Dorsal root ganglion, pseudounipolar neuron

24 **The answer is E: Visceral sensory.**   Cell bodies of both somatic and visceral sensory neurons are located within dorsal root ganglia (DRG). Thus, pseudounipolar neurons in DRG may process somatic sensation from the body wall or visceral sensory information arising from internal organs. Visceral motor and autonomic motor neurons (choices A and D) typically provide motor innervation to the viscera and glands; their postsynaptic neurons are located in the sympathetic or parasympathetic ganglia. Multipolar neurons located in the ventral horn of the spinal cord provide somatic motor innervation to skeletal muscle (choice C). Interneurons (choice B) are in the CNS.
Keywords: Dorsal root ganglion, sensory neuron

25 **The answer is A: Astrocytes.**   Astrocytes contain bundles of intermediate filaments that are composed primarily of glial fibrillary acidic protein (GFAP). The image shows the results of immunostaining using antibodies directed against GFAP. Astrocytes are identified as large cells with "stellate" processes projecting in all directions. Astrocytes have been called the "fibroblast" of the CNS because of their critical role in supporting neurons in the brain and spinal cord. Proliferation of astrocytes and microglia in response to injury is referred to as gliosis. Gliosis in the central nervous system is the equivalent of scar formation elsewhere in the body. In spinal cord injuries, axonal regeneration can be seen up to 2 weeks. However, after 2 weeks, gliosis has taken place and attempts at axonal regeneration come to an end. Axonal regeneration in the central nervous system occurs only in the hypothalamo-hypophysial region, where glial and capillary barriers do not inhibit directed cell migration (axonal path finding). Axonal regeneration appears to require intimate contact with extracellular fluids containing plasma proteins. The other cells listed as choices do not proliferate in response to injury, and they do not stain with antibodies against GFAP.
Keywords: Cerebral contusion, gliosis, astrocytes

26 **The answer is E: Support and nourishment of neurons.**
Astrocytes are the most numerous glial cells in the CNS. Two kinds of astrocytes have been identified: fibrous and protoplasmic. Fibrous astrocytes are primarily located in the white matter and have relatively few but long processes. Some of the processes can be very long and even span the entire thickness of the brain. Protoplasmic astrocytes possessing a large number of short and branched processes are found in the gray matter of the CNS. Astrocytes with their radiating processes form a network within the CNS that supports and modulates neuronal activities. The expanded "perivascular feet" of some of the processes of protoplasmic astrocytes terminate on capillaries and contribute to the formation of the "blood–brain barrier." The "perineural feet" of protoplasmic astrocytes cover bare areas of myelinated axons at synapses and at the nodes of Ranvier. Defense against pathogens and phagocytosis (choices A and D) are important functions of microglial cells. Myelination of axons (choice C) and production of cerebrospinal fluid (choice B) are the principal functions of oligodendrocytes and ependymal cells, respectively.
Keywords: Astrocytes

27 **The answer is C: Microglial cells.**   Microglia are the smallest neuroglial cells in the CNS, and they are inconspicuous healthy tissue. Microglia respond quickly to CNS injury (e.g., ischemia, trauma, or infection) and proliferate to become reactive microglial cells. In regions of injury or infectious disease, microglia accumulate in large numbers and demonstrate an infiltrative phenotype with characteristic thin elongated nuclei. This distinctive nuclear morphology makes them readily visible in routine H&E preparations (shown in the image). None of the other choices show this nuclear morphology.
Keywords: Microglia

28 **The answer is B: Granulocyte/monocyte progenitor cells.**
Microglia are representatives of the distributed monocyte–macrophage system. They are derived from monocytes that migrate into the brain as it becomes vascularized during embryonic and fetal development. Microglia are the only type of neuroglial cell that is not derived from glioblasts of neuroectodermal origin. Glioblasts (choice A) and neuroblasts (choice D) are precursors for macroglial cells and neurons, respectively. These stem cell populations are derived themselves from neuroepithelial cells (choice E) that are present in the wall of the neural tube during early development.
Keywords: Microglia

29 **The answer is C: Phagocytosis and defense against injury.**
Microglia are the bone marrow–derived mononuclear phagocytes of the CNS. They respond quickly to pathogens and insults to mediate repair and healing. Microglia play critical role in defense against infectious microorganisms and neoplastic cells. As macrophage-like phagocytic cells, they function to remove injured cells and necrotic debris. However, they are not as efficient as tissue macrophages present in other locations throughout the body. None of the other choices describes the function of microglia.
Keywords: Microglia, phagocytosis

30 **The answer is D: Oligodendrocytes.**   Oligodendrocytes are the myelin-forming cells in the CNS. Concentric layers of oligodendrocyte plasma membrane form the myelin sheath surrounding axons. In contrast to the peripheral nervous system, where a single Schwann cell envelopes an axon to form an internodal segment, each of the many tongue-like processes of a single oligodendrocyte in the CNS wraps a portion of an axon to form an internodal segment. Thus, a single oligodendrocyte can form multiple internodal segments surrounding one or more neuronal axons. On routine H&E-stained slides, oligodendrocytes exhibit a memorable "fried egg" appearance with central, small, dark round nuclei surrounded by a halo of vacuolated cytoplasm. None of the other choices show this distinctive cellular morphology.
Keywords: Oligodendrocyte

31 **The answer is C: Ependymal cells.**   The ciliated, cuboidal-columnar cells that line the brain ventricles and spinal canal are termed ependymal cells. The epithelial-like ependymal cell layer forms a barrier between the cerebrospinal fluid and brain parenchyma and regulates fluid transport between these two compartments. At specific locations within the ventricular system, ependymal cells are modified to form a choroid plexus with associated capillaries that secrete cerebrospinal fluid. None of the other cells listed as choices displays a low columnar epithelial morphology.
Keywords: Ependymal cells, cerebrospinal fluid

32 **The answer is B: Epineurium.**   Connective tissue is an important component of peripheral nerves. Nerve axons, along with their myelin sheaths and associated Schwann cells, are enveloped within several layers of connective tissue. The outermost irregular connective tissue layer wrapping a peripheral nerve is termed epineurium. It is continuous with dura mater in the CNS. It binds nerve fascicles together and contains nutrient arteries. Epineurium is lost near the termination of nerve fibers with free nerve endings but contributes to the capsules of encapsulated nerve endings. The collagen bundles in the epineurium are largely responsible for the remarkable tensile strength of peripheral nerves. Endoneurium and perineurium (choices A and E) are not readily identifiable at this magnification.
Keywords: Peripheral nerve, epineurium

33 **The answer is B: Line 2.**   Groups of nerve fibers bundled together are referred to as nerve fascicles. Nerve fascicles are surrounded by perineurium—a thin sheath composed of concentric layers of specialized epithelial-like connective tissue cells. Collagen fibers may be present between layers of the perineurial cells surrounding large nerve fascicles. Perineurium is continuous with the arachnoid layer of the meninges in the CNS. Distally, perineurium contributes to the capsule of many terminal nerve endings and receptors, including Pacinian and Meissner corpuscles, as well as muscle spindles and Golgi tendon organs. Perineurium

may be open-ended in certain locations (e.g., near neuro-muscular junctions), where the endoneurial space communicates freely with the interstitial fluid compartment of the body. On this trichrome-stained section, collagen fibers appear blue, whereas cells and axons appear red. Perineurium (Line 2) is seen as a thin red layer with interspersed collagen fibers. This layer surrounds the nerve fascicle that occupies the lower right-hand corner of the image. Collagen bundles within the epineurium (Line 1) also appear blue. The very thin, blue-stained layer indicated by Line 5 represents endoneurium—a fine layer of loose connective tissue surrounding individual nerve fibers.
Keywords: Peripheral nerve, perineurium

34 **The answer is A: Axon.**   In this transverse section of a peripheral nerve, axons appear as red-stained dots surrounded by a clear halo. This "empty space" indicated by Line 3 represents the myelin sheath in living tissue that is removed during tissue embedding and processing. An individual axon and its associated myelin sheath are enclosed by endoneurium (Line 5).
Keywords: Peripheral nerve, axon

35 **The answer is D: Poorly myelinated nerve fiber.**   Axons in the peripheral nervous system may be myelinated, poorly myelinated, or unmyelinated. Thickness of the myelin sheath is determined largely by the axon's diameter. The diameters of peripheral nerve fibers may differ widely. Larger fibers, with thicker myelin sheaths, typically conduct action potentials faster than the smaller nerve fibers. Most of the small fibers in the peripheral nervous system are poorly myelinated or unmyelinated. These axons are, however, still in direct contact with Schwann cells. The lack of myelination combined with the small axon diameter results in a relatively slow conduction of nerve action potentials. Osmium tetroxide (OsO_4) is a heavy metal salt that is commonly used to fix lipids and identify lipid-rich myelin membranes. In this transverse section of a peripheral nerve, most fibers exhibit a dark-stained myelin sheath. Other nerve fibers (e.g., those indicated by arrows in this image) are poorly myelinated. None of the other choices show this morphology.
Keywords: Peripheral nerve, myelin sheath

36 **The answer is A: Axon.**   In this high-magnification photomicrograph, axons appear as dark-stained lines. The myelin sheath (choice E) that surrounds axons has been extracted during tissue processing and is represented here as a clear halo. The numerous nuclei visible in this image belong to either Schwann cells or fibroblasts. It is not always possible to distinguish these cells based on nuclear morphology. The pink-stained area surrounding individual nerve fibers represents endoneurium (choice D). Endoneurium is composed of a thin layer of connective tissue containing collagen fibers (choice B). The cytoplasm of Schwann cells (choice C) is poorly visible.
Keywords: Peripheral nerve

37 **The answer is D: Node of Ranvier.** Nodes of Ranvier represent gaps or interruptions in the myelin sheath of axons. At these gaps, axons are separated from the extracellular (interstitial) space by finger-like projections of Schwann cell membranes and cytoplasm. Two adjacent nodes mark an internodal segment of the sheath. This makes nerve fibers appear as a "string of sausages." None of the other choices shows this distinctive morphology.
Keywords: Node of Ranvier, peripheral nerve

38 **The answer is B: Saltatory conduction of nerve impulse.** Nodes of Ranvier represent gaps in the myelin sheath. Here, the axon is covered by thin cell membranes with a high concentration of voltage-gated Na^+ and K^+ channels. Action potentials spread rapidly along the internodal segments of the myelinated axon. They jump (are regenerated) from one node of Ranvier to the next. This discontinuous impulse conduction along the axons is referred to as saltatory conduction. In unmyelinated axons, Na^+ and K^+ channels are uniformly distributed, and impulses are conveyed continuously and more slowly. None of the other choices describe the function of nodes of Ranvier.
Keywords: Node of Ranvier, nerve, action potential

39 **The answer is E: Perineurium.** Perineurium envelops nerve fiber bundles (fascicles) and is composed of concentric layers of perineurial cells and sparse collagen fibers. Perineurial cells connect to one another via tight junctions (zonula occludens), creating an effective blood–nerve barrier that ensures isolation of peripheral nerve fibers from the interstitial fluid compartment of the body. The role of perineurium as a blood–nerve barrier in the peripheral nervous system is analogous to the role of arachnoid mater in establishing a blood–brain barrier in the CNS. Endoneurium (choice A), a layer of loose connective tissue, wraps individual nerve fibers. Epineurium (choice B) is composed of irregular connective tissue and provides considerable tensile strength to the peripheral nerve. Myelin (choice C) is composed of concentric layers of Schwann cell membranes and ensures rapid conduction of action potentials. Node of Ranvier (choice D) provides saltatory conduction of nerve impulses.
Keywords: Peripheral nerve, perineurium

40 **The answer is C: Peripheral nerve.** The image shown is a section of normal lip. The structure indicated by the arrow demonstrates high cellularity and a wavy appearance. It is weakly basophilic compared to the surrounding structures and reveals wavy darker-stained nerve axons. Transverse and oblique sections of skeletal muscle fibers (choice D) occupy most of the field. These fibers have eosinophilic cytoplasm and peripheral nuclei. Dense regular connective tissue (choice A) and smooth muscle (choice E) are not present. Loose connective

tissue (choice B) with small blood vessels fills out space between skeletal muscle fibers and the peripheral nerve.
Keywords: Skin, peripheral nerve

41 **The answer is D: Sympathetic ganglion.** Large neurons with eccentric nuclei are visible in this image. The satellite cells do not form a continuous circle surrounding the neurons. These are the characteristic features of autonomic ganglia. Other than connective tissue, the image does not show any particular target tissue that would suggest a parasympathetic ganglion (choice C). Dorsal root ganglion (choice A) neurons have centrally located nuclei and are surrounded by a continuous layer of satellite cells. Enteric ganglia (choice B) are situated between smooth muscle layers in the gastrointestinal wall (not visible in this preparation). Ventral horn of the spinal cord (choice E) is characterized by large multipolar motor neurons.
Keywords: Sympathetic ganglion, autonomic nervous system

42 **The answer is D: Visceral efferent neurons.** Neurons in paravertebral and prevertebral ganglia are postsynaptic, sympathetic neuronal cell bodies. Their axons conduct visceral motor information to various target tissues, including visceral organs, blood vessels, and sweat glands. Visceral afferent nerve fibers (choice E) from thoracic and abdominal viscera travel with sympathetic efferent fibers, but their cell bodies are located in dorsal root ganglia. Interneurons (choice A) and somatic efferent neurons (choice B) are located in the CNS. Somatic sensory neurons (choice C) are located in the dorsal root ganglia.
Keywords: Sympathetic ganglion, autonomic nervous system

43 **The answer is A: Astrocyte.** Enteric glial cells are neuroglia found in the enteric ganglia. These cells are associated with enteric neurons, and they resemble astrocytes. They provide structural and metabolic support to enteric neurons. Schwann cells provide myelin to peripheral nerve fibers. Satellite cells in peripheral nerve ganglia are variants of neural crest–derived Schwann cells. The general functions of the Schwann cells and satellite cells are to provide metabolic support and electrical insulation. The other neuroglial cells listed as choices are found in the CNS and do not primarily function as structural and metabolic support to neurons.
Keywords: Neuroglia, enteric glial cells

44 **The answer is A: Brainstem.** The nervous system is divided anatomically into central nervous system (CNS) and periphery nervous system (PNS). The CNS is composed of the brain and spinal cord. It is situated within the cranial cavity and spinal canal of the vertebral column. The brain itself consists of the cerebrum, cerebellum, and brainstem. The PNS distributes cranial and spinal nerves to every part of the body, conducting impulses to-and-from the CNS. The other structures listed as choices are components of the PNS.

Keywords: Central nervous system

45 **The answer is D: Cluster of functionally related neuronal cell bodies.** Functionally related nerve cell bodies are usually clustered together in the CNS and are referred as a nucleus. Examples include facial nucleus, pontine nucleus, and nucleus ambiguous. Functionally related axons are bundled together (choice B) and form subdivisions within the white matter. There are a variety of names for bundled axons, including fasciculus, funiculus, lemniscus, peduncle, and tract. None of the other choices describes nuclei within the CNS.

Keywords: Central nervous system

46 **The answer is B: Line 2.** In this spinal cord preparation, myelin is stained dark blue. Therefore, the peripheral white matter appears darker than the central gray matter. The butterfly-shaped gray matter is clearly apparent in this section. Line 5 denotes the ventral horn of gray matter. Line 1 denotes a subdivision within the white matter that is termed the posterior funiculus. The area indicated by Line 4 is the central canal. Line 3 points to the lateral funiculus, another subdivision within the white matter.

Keywords: Spinal cord

47 **The answer is A: Axons.** In a transverse section of the spinal cord, the peripheral white matter can be subdivided into the posterior, lateral, and anterior funiculus. These regions contain ascending and descending tracts of axons of varying lengths. The longest axons extend all the way from the brain (brainstem and cerebrum) to the most caudal portion of the spinal cord. The other components listed as choices are supporting structures found in white matter, but they do not represent major functional components in this location.

Keywords: Spinal cord

48 **The answer is E: Sensory interneurons.** The dorsal horn of the spinal cord gray matter processes sensory information. The cell bodies of the sensory neurons are located in dorsal root ganglia (also refer as primary sensory neurons). Sensory interneurons and projection neurons are the major neurons found in the dorsal horn of the spinal cord. Sensory interneurons receive and process impulse conveyed by collateral fibers from the central processes of some primary sensory neurons. The central processes of some other primary sensory neurons synapse with projection neurons. Long axonal processes arise from the projection neurons and form ascending sensory pathways. Motor neurons (choice A) are located in the ventral horn of the spinal cord. Postsynaptic sympathetic neurons (choice B) are found in paravertebral and prevertebral sympathetic ganglia. Presynaptic

parasympathetic neurons (choice C) are located in the brainstem and the intermediolateral gray of sacral spinal cord segments S2-S4 (craniosacral flow). Presynaptic sympathetic neurons (choice D) are situated in the intermediolateral horn of the thoracic and upper lumbar spinal cord segments (T1-L2).

Keywords: Spinal cord, dorsal horn

49 **The answer is E: Ventral horn.** Large neurons (arrows) are the most prominent structures observed in this section of spinal cord. These neurons are characteristic features of the ventral horn of the spinal cord. As described previously, the dorsal horn of the spinal cord (choice C) contains smaller sensory interneurons. Anterior funiculus (choice A) and posterior funiculus (choice D) are located in the white matter. The central canal (choice B) is lined by low columnar cells.

Keywords: Spinal cord, ventral horn

50 **The answer is B: Skeletal muscle.** The large neurons present in the ventral horn of the spinal cord are lower motor neurons that provide somatic innervation to skeletal muscle. Adipose tissue, smooth muscle, and sweat glands (choices A, D, and E) are innervated by autonomic nerves, whose cell bodies are located in the peripheral nervous system. Skin (choice C) is innervated by sensory nerve fibers, whose cell bodies are located in dorsal root ganglia.

Keywords: CNS, spinal cord, motor neurons

51 **The answer is A: Arachnoid mater and pia mater.** Three connective tissue layers (meninges) cover the brain and spinal cord. The outmost layer is the tough dura mater, composed of dense connective tissue. Arachnoid mater adheres to the inner surface of the dura and extends web-like trabeculae to the pia mater on the surface of the CNS. The arachnoid and pia are collectively termed leptomeninges. The space between arachnoid and pia mater contains CSF and is referred to as the subarachnoid space. Meningitis is a dangerous infection caused by a variety of microorganisms. Leptomeningitis denotes an inflammatory process that is localized to the pia/arachnoid. This compartment holds the cerebrospinal fluid—an excellent culture medium for most pathogens. In untreated cases of bacterial meningitis, delirium gives way to coma and death.

Keywords: Meningitis, meninges, cerebrospinal fluid

52 **The answer is C: Loose collagenous connective tissue.** Arachnoid mater and pia mater are both composed of thin layers of loose connective tissue. The pia invests immediately on and follows the contour of the surface of the brain and spinal cord. The arachnoid bridges the dura and pia and exhibits delicate extensions (trabeculae) within the subarachnoid space.

Keywords: Meninges

53 **The answer is B: Dura mater and arachnoid mater.** Under normal conditions, a space does not exist between the dura and the arachnoid. However, the dural border cell layer (the innermost part of the dura) is composed of flattened fibroblasts and constitutes a plane of structural weakness. A subdural space may develop following blunt force trauma to the head, with the tearing of bridging veins. In contrast to the epidural space, the subdural space can expand. Because hematomas represent venous hemorrhage, they usually stop bleeding after 25 to 50 mL have accumulated, owing to local compression of affected veins. However, this tamponade may lead to venous thrombosis (intravascular coagulation of blood), which may prove fatal. Blunt force applied in the mid-sagittal plane will typically affect both cerebral hemispheres. Therefore, it is not surprising that subdural hematomas are frequently bilateral.
Keywords: Subdural hematoma, concussion, meninges

54 **The answer is E: Zonula occludens.** The blood–brain barrier effectively separates the nervous system from the rest of the body. It controls the passage of substances from the blood into the CNS and protects the brain and spinal cord from fluctuating levels of electrolytes and hormones, as well as potential toxins of microorganisms. The blood–brain barrier is also instrumental in providing a stable balance of electrolytes in the interstitial environment surrounding CNS tissue. The blood–brain barrier forms and is maintained by continuous-type capillaries that are sealed together by zonula occludens. These tight junctions efficiently prevent the diffusion of solutes and fluid components from blood into neural tissue. A complete and continuous basal lamina surrounding the endothelial cells further ensures the elimination of gaps. None of the other choices form tight junctions between cells.
Keywords: Blood–brain barrier

55 **The answer is A: Astrocytes.** The perivascular feet of astrocytes also contribute to the formation of the blood–brain barrier. Neuroglial astrocytes send out foot processes that terminate on capillaries and help maintain tight junctions between the endothelial cells. Recent research has shown that the integrity of endothelial tight junctions in the CNS depends on the normal function of astrocytes. None of the other cells listed contribute to the development or function of the blood–brain barrier.
Keywords: Blood–brain barrier, astrocyte

56 **The answer is A: Astrocyte.** Astrocytes are the ubiquitous supporting glial cells of the CNS, and they react to pathologic insults. When damage occurs in the CNS, astrocytes become activated and proliferate to eventually form cellular scar tissue. The process is referred as reactive gliosis, and the resulting permanent scar is termed a plaque. Many CNS diseases and injuries cause reactive gliosis. Current research is aimed at discovering methods for limiting gliosis in stroke patients. Microglial cells (choice D) are involved in removing necrotic debris from sites of injury, but they do not form glial scars. None of the other cells listed are involved in reactive gliosis.
Keywords: Reactive gliosis, astrocyte

Chapter 8
Skin and Epidermal Appendages

QUESTIONS

Select the single best answer.

1 A 3-day-old neonate suffers extensive blisters in his oral mucosa and skin. Laboratory studies reveal a mutation in the gene encoding type XVII collagen, and the patient is diagnosed with junctional epidermolysis bullosa. A skin biopsy taken from the back of the neonate reveals normal tissue at the margin of a blister (shown in the image). Identify the layer indicated by the arrow.

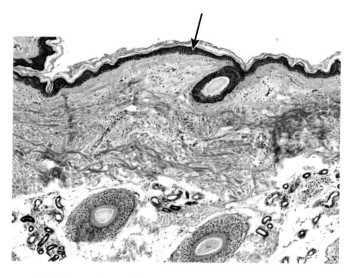

(A) Dermal papilla
(B) Dermis
(C) Epidermis
(D) Hypodermis
(E) Reticular dermis

2 The skin biopsy described in Question 1 is examined at higher magnification (shown in the image). The area indicated by the asterisk is best described as which of the following?

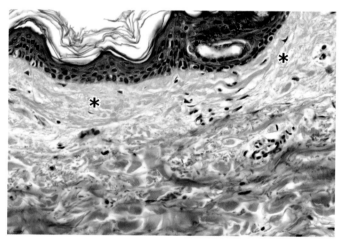

(A) Epidermis
(B) Hypodermis
(C) Papillary dermis
(D) Reticular dermis
(E) Subcutis

3 The congenital blistering disease described in Question 1 is caused by loss of cohesion between which of the following layers of the patient's skin?
(A) Basement membrane and papillary dermis
(B) Epidermis and basement membrane
(C) Papillary dermis and reticular dermis
(D) Reticular dermis and hypodermis
(E) Stratum spinosum and stratum basale of epidermis

4 A section of thick skin from the palm of the hand is examined in the histology laboratory. Multiple cell layers in the epidermis are evident at high magnification (shown in the image). Identify the layer indicated by the arrows.

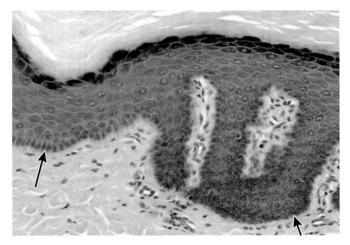

(A) Stratum basale
(B) Stratum corneum
(C) Stratum granulosum
(D) Stratum lucidum
(E) Stratum spinosum

5 The specimen described in Question 4 is examined at higher magnification (shown in the image). The intraepidermal cells indicated by the large arrows are derived from which of the following precursor cells?

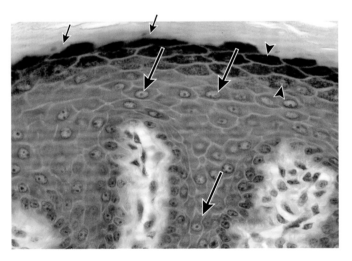

(A) Basal cells
(B) Langerhans cells
(C) Melanocytes
(D) Merkel cells
(E) Monocytes

6 Further examination of the specimen described in Question 5 reveals a population of epidermal cells containing dark, cytoplasmic granules (arrowheads, shown

in the image). These large granules are filled with which of the following essential biomolecules?
(A) Cathepsin
(B) Filaggrin
(C) Hyaluronan
(D) Keratin
(E) Melanin

7 During a dermatopathology conference, you are asked about differences between thick and thin skin. Which of the following epidermal layers is a unique feature of thick skin?
(A) Stratum basale
(B) Stratum corneum
(C) Stratum granulosum
(D) Stratum lucidum
(E) Stratum spinosum

8 The skin of the palm is examined at low magnification in the pathology department (shown in image). Identify the epidermal layer indicated by the arrow.

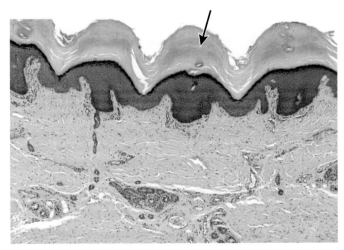

(A) Stratum basale
(B) Stratum corneum
(C) Stratum granulosum
(D) Stratum lucidum
(E) Stratum spinosum

9 The parents of a 2-year-old girl are concerned about their daughter's white scaly skin. Physical examination reveals coarse, fish-like scales on the child's forearms. The patient's father is afflicted with the same condition (ichthyosis vulgaris). A skin biopsy from this child would most likely show which of the following histopathologic findings?
(A) Accumulation of nucleated cells in the stratum corneum
(B) Acute inflammation of the papillary dermis
(C) Chronic inflammation of the reticular dermis
(D) Excessive thickening of the stratum corneum
(E) Hyperplasia of stem cells in the stratum basale

10 A 48-year-old man presents with numerous large blisters on his scalp, around his umbilicus, and in his oral cavity. The patient states that his blisters rupture easily leaving behind large denuded areas. Examination of a skin biopsy suggests the diagnosis of pemphigus vulgaris (shown in the image). The biopsy shows loss of cohesion between which of the following two layers of the patient's skin?

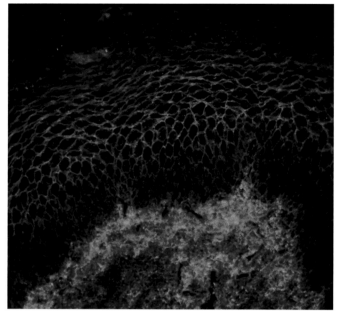

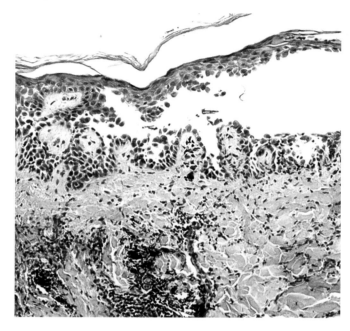

(A) Basement membrane and papillary dermis
(B) Epidermis and basement membrane
(C) Papillary dermis and reticular dermis
(D) Reticular dermis and hypodermis
(E) Stratum basale and stratum spinosum of epidermis

11 Another section of lesional skin from the patient described in Question 10 is stained with fluorescein-conjugated goat anti–human IgG antibody. The results of this direct immunolabeling assay demonstrate the presence of autoantibodies bound to junctions between keratinocytes (shown in the image). These autoantibodies bind to which of the following membrane-associated structures?

(A) ABO antigens
(B) Desmosomes
(C) Gap junctions
(D) Integrins
(E) Tight junctions

12 A 2-day-old neonate cries violently whenever she is breast-fed. Physical examination of the neonate reveals numerous blisters in the oral mucosa and on the skin. Microscopic examination of a skin biopsy reveals separation between upper and lower portions of basal cells in the epidermis. The results of immunolabeling assays are negative (i.e., they do not show evidence of immune complex deposition in the skin). Which of the following is the most likely diagnosis?
(A) Bullous pemphigoid
(B) Contact dermatitis
(C) Epidermolysis bullosa simplex
(D) Pemphigus vulgaris
(E) Psoriasis

13 A 64-year-old farmer presents with multiple patches of discoloration on his face. Biopsy of lesional skin reveals "actinic keratosis." This pathologic condition represents abnormal maturation of which of the following skin cells?
(A) Dermal fibroblasts
(B) Keratinocytes
(C) Langerhans cells
(D) Mast cells
(E) Melanocytes

14 A 16-year-old girl on the high school athletic swim team is concerned about the effects of water on her skin. She asks you whether she should apply creams or lotions to waterproof her skin before entering the pool. You explain to her that the skin itself serves as an effective water barrier to protect the body. Which of the following components of the skin is most important in establishing an effective water barrier?

(A) Cell and lipid envelopes
(B) Desmosomes between keratinocytes
(C) Thick epidermal basement membrane
(D) Thick stratum corneum
(E) Tight junctions between basal cells

15 You are invited to talk to elementary school students about your interest in biology and medicine. One of the students asks you to explain why his best friend has dark skin. Which of the following biological processes is responsible for darker pigmentation of the skin in those of African descent?

(A) Decreased thickness of the stratum spinosum
(B) Increased number of melanocytes
(C) Increased production of melanin
(D) Increased thickness of the stratum granulosum
(E) Slower degradation of melanin

16 A 28-year-old white woman returns home following a 4-week summer vacation at the beach. Her friends and family comment that her skin has become much darker in color. Which of the following biological processes accounts for this change in skin coloration?

(A) Increased number of granular keratinocytes
(B) Increased production of melanin
(C) Increased thickness of the stratum corneum
(D) Migration of melanocytes into the stratum corneum
(E) Slower degradation of melanin

17 A 68-year-old man from Africa presents with dark-colored lesions on his left heel. The center of the primary lesion is elevated and ulcerated (the patient's foot is shown in the image). Based on these observations, the patient's skin tumor is derived from which of the following cells?

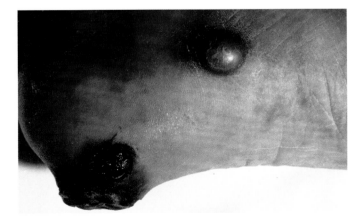

(A) Basal keratinocyte
(B) Langerhans cell
(C) Macrophage
(D) Melanocyte
(E) Merkel cell

18 A 48-year-old man complains of "poison ivy." Physical examination reveals skin rashes and blisters on his upper limb and trunk. Which of the following cells internalize and present "poison ivy" antigens to lymphatic cells of the immune system in this patient?

(A) Basal cells
(B) Granular keratinocytes
(C) Langerhans cells
(D) Merkel cells
(E) Spinous keratinocytes

19 A 12-year-old boy complains of mild pain in his skull. Radiologic examination of the patient's skull reveals a large, lytic lesion in the occipital bone (shown in the image). Biopsy of the lytic lesion reveals collections of large, phagocytic cells with pale, eosinophilic cytoplasm. By electron microscopy, these large cells are discovered to have racquet-shaped intracellular structures known as "Birbeck granules." These granules are an ultrastructural feature of which of the following cells?

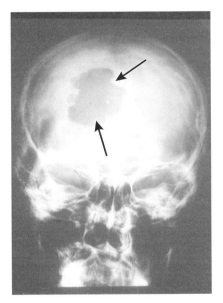

(A) Fibroblasts
(B) Keratinocytes
(C) Langerhans cells
(D) Lymphocytes
(E) Osteoblasts

20 The skin is richly innervated by sensory nerve fibers and contains a variety of sensory receptors. Which of the following epidermal cells is closely associated with terminal nerve fibers and serves as a mechanoreceptor in the skin?

(A) Basal cell
(B) Langerhans cell
(C) Melanocyte
(D) Merkel cell
(E) Spinous keratinocyte

21 The deep dermis of a skin biopsy from the tip of a finger is examined in the pathology department (shown in the image). Identify the structure indicated by the arrow.

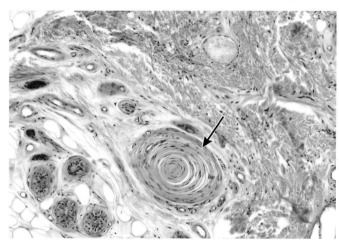

(A) Free nerve ending
(B) Meissner corpuscle
(C) Merkel disk
(D) Nerve fiber
(E) Pacinian corpuscle

22 The papillary dermis from the skin biopsy described in Question 21 is examined at higher magnification (shown in the image). Identify the structure indicated by the arrow.

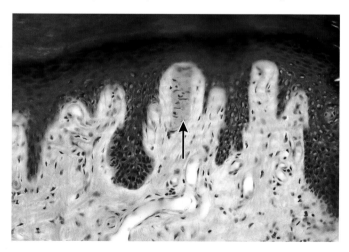

(A) Capillary loop
(B) Meissner corpuscle
(C) Merkel disk
(D) Myelinated nerve fiber
(E) Pacinian corpuscle

23 The papillary dermis of the skin biopsy described in Question 21 is examined further (shown in the image). Identify the structures indicated by the arrows.

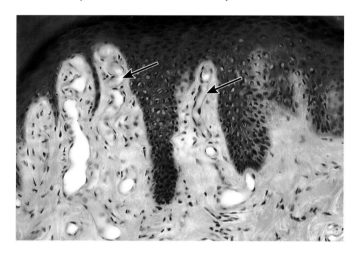

(A) Capillary loops
(B) Free nerve ending
(C) Meissner corpuscles
(D) Small arteries
(E) Small veins

24 A 4-year-old girl is rescued after becoming lost outdoors during a winter snowstorm. Physical examination indicates that the child is fine, except for exhaustion and a few skin sores related to hypothermia. Which of the following biological processes was chiefly responsible for conserving this child's core body temperature during her winter trek?

(A) Closing of arteriovenous anastomoses
(B) Decreased blood supply to the subcutaneous plexus
(C) Increased blood supply to the subpapillary plexus
(D) Opening of arteriovenous anastomoses
(E) Vasodilation of the microvascular bed in the skin

25 A 25-year-old woman with a recent history of "strep throat" presents with numerous tender, red papules on her legs. Histological examination of a skin biopsy reveals pink fibrin deposits and remnants of neutrophils surrounding small blood vessels (shown in the image). The patient is subsequently diagnosed with cutaneous necrotizing vasculitis. This inflammatory/immune reaction typically affects which of the following blood vessels?

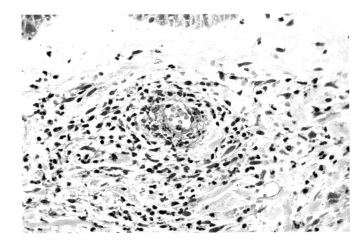

(A) Arteries in the subcutaneous plexus
(B) Arterioles in the deep reticular dermis
(C) Arteriovenous anastomoses in the hypodermis
(D) Postcapillary venules in the subpapillary plexus
(E) Veins in the subcutaneous plexus

26 A 38-year-old woman complains stiff and tense skin over her face and hands. Physical examination reveals radial furrows around the patient's mouth. The patient does not display facial expression during her visit. A skin biopsy is obtained (shown in the image). The patient is subsequently diagnosed with scleroderma. The histopathologic findings in this biopsy are consistent with excess collagen deposition in which of the following cutaneous locations?

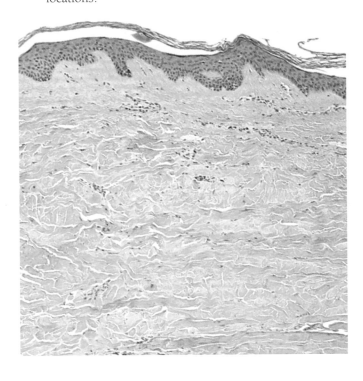

(A) Basement membrane
(B) Hypodermis
(C) Reticular dermis
(D) Stratum basale
(E) Stratum corneum

27 A scalp biopsy is examined in the pathology department (shown in the image). Identify the structures indicated by the arrows.

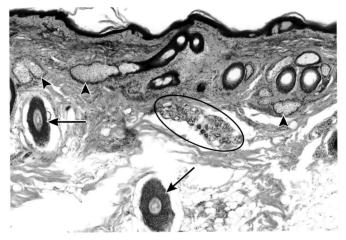

(A) Apocrine sweat glands
(B) Arteries
(C) Eccrine sweat glands
(D) Hair follicles
(E) Sebaceous glands

28 Further examination of the specimen described in Question 27 reveals a vertical section through a hair follicle (shown in the image). Identify the tuft of connective tissue demarcated by the dotted line.

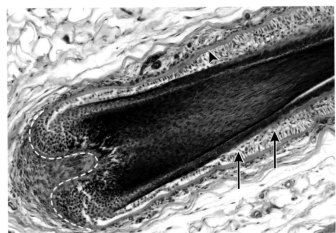

(A) Dermal papilla
(B) External root sheath
(C) Hair bulb
(D) Hair follicle
(E) Hair matrix

29 In the image shown for Question 28, the red-stained, acellular hyaline layer indicated by the arrowhead is continuous with which of the following cutaneous structures?
(A) Basement membrane
(B) Collagen bundles in reticular dermis
(C) Collagen fibers in papillary dermis
(D) Hypodermis
(E) Stratum corneum

30 A 32-year-old Asian man notices that he is losing hair and is concerned about becoming bald. You talk to him about the mechanisms that regulate hair growth. Cells in which of the following regions of the hair follicle are directly responsible for the growth of hair?
(A) Dermal papilla
(B) External root sheath
(C) Hair matrix
(D) Internal root sheath
(E) Stratum basale in epidermis

31 A section of thin skin is examined in the histology laboratory (shown in image). Identify the structure indicated by the arrows.

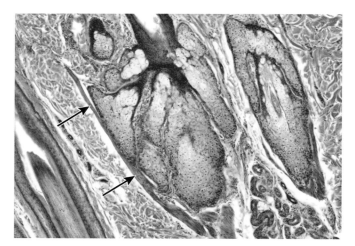

(A) Arrector pili muscle
(B) Collagen bundles
(C) Connective tissue sheath
(D) External root sheath
(E) Glassy membrane

32 A 12-year-old girl suffers second-degree burns on her left arm while helping her father in the kitchen. Regenerative stem cells that migrate extensively to resurface this patient's skin wound originate from which of the following cutaneous structures?
(A) Dermal papilla
(B) External root sheath
(C) Hair matrix
(D) Internal root sheath
(E) Stratum basale of epidermis

33 A 15-year-old girl presents with severe acne. Physical examination reveals many discrete papules and pustules on her face and neck. Acne is a chronic inflammatory disorder that principally affects which of the following cutaneous structures?
(A) Bulb of hair follicles
(B) Capillary loops within papillary dermis
(C) Dermal papillae of hair follicles
(D) Sebaceous glands
(E) Stratum basale of epidermis

34 A skin biopsy is obtained from a 34-year-old man. Formalin-fixed tissue is stained with H&E and examined by light microscopy (shown in the image). Identify the structure indicated by the arrow.

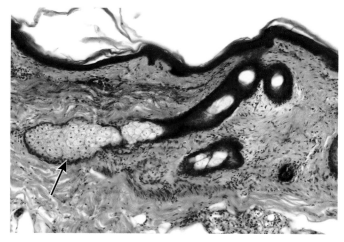

(A) Blood vessel
(B) External root sheath
(C) Hair follicle
(D) Sebaceous gland
(E) Sweat gland

35 A section of palm skin is examined in the histology laboratory. Distinctive clusters of cells are seen embedded in the dermis and hypodermis (shown in the image). Identify the structures indicated by the arrows.

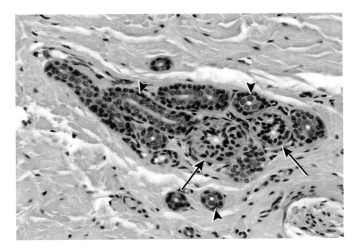

(A) Apocrine sweat glands
(B) Ducts of eccrine sweat glands
(C) Hair follicles
(D) Sebaceous glands
(E) Secretory portion of eccrine sweat glands

36 The secretory portion of the eccrine sweat gland described in Question 35 is examined at higher magnification (shown in the image). Identify the cells indicated by the arrows.

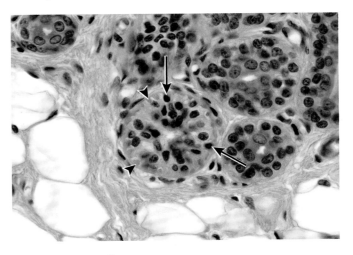

(A) Clear cells
(B) Dark cells
(C) Fibroblasts
(D) Myoepithelial cells
(E) Smooth muscle cells

37 A sample of skin from the axillary region is collected at autopsy and examined in the pathology department (shown in image). Identify the structures indicated by the arrows.

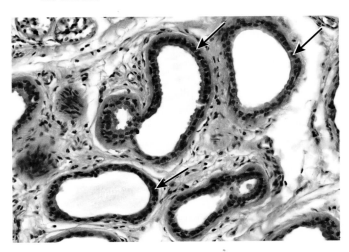

(A) Apocrine sweat gland, excretory portion
(B) Apocrine sweat gland, secretory portion
(C) Eccrine sweat gland, excretory portion
(D) Eccrine sweat gland, secretory portion
(E) Subcutaneous vascular plexus

38 During a 3rd year clinical rotation, you are asked to discuss the biological functions of the skin. Thermoregulation is the primary function of which of the following epidermal appendages?
(A) Apocrine sweat glands
(B) Arrector pili muscles
(C) Eccrine sweat glands
(D) Hair follicles
(E) Sebaceous glands

39 During small group seminar, you are asked to discuss the metabolism and function of vitamin D. You mention that the skin synthesizes vitamin D_3 when exposed to sunlight. Which of the following cells in the skin is responsible for the production of vitamin D_3?
(A) Fibroblasts in the dermis
(B) Keratinocytes in strata basale and spinosum
(C) Keratinocytes in the stratum granulosum
(D) Melanocytes in the epidermis
(E) Merkel cells in the epidermis

ANSWERS

1 **The answer is C: Epidermis.** The skin consists of two firmly adherent tissue layers, namely epidermis and dermis. Epidermis, the most superficial layer, is composed of a keratinized, stratified squamous epithelium. The basal cell layer of this stratified epithelium is firmly anchored to an underlying basement membrane. Dermis (choice B) represents connective tissue beneath the epidermis. This layer is subdivided into papillary and reticular dermis. Epidermis is derived from embryonic ectoderm, whereas dermis is derived from embryonic mesoderm. Hypodermis (choice D) represents the layer of adipose connective tissue located deep to the skin. This subcutaneous tissue represents the layer of superficial fascia that is identified in gross anatomy.

Keywords: Epidermolysis bullosa, epidermis

2 **The answer is C: Papillary dermis.** The dermis is composed of a superficial papillary layer and a deep reticular layer. The papillary layer, located immediately beneath the epidermis, is composed of loose connective tissue. Type I and type III collagen fibers and thread-like elastic fibers form an irregular network. This layer is more cellular than the reticular dermis. It contains numerous blood vessels, lymphatic vessels, and sensory nerve endings. The papillary dermis also forms finger-like protrusions into the overlying epidermis (referred to as dermal papillae). The deeper reticular layer of the dermis (choice D) is composed of dense, irregular connective tissue. It is less cellular than papillary dermis and contains an abundance of thick type I collagen fiber bundles and coarse elastic fibers (see Chapter 3). Hypodermis and subcutis (choices B and E) describe adipose connective tissue that is located deep to the reticular dermis.

Keywords: Dermis, papillary dermis

3 **The answer is B: Epidermis and basement membrane.** Epidermolysis bullosa (EB) refers to a heterogeneous group of inherited connective tissue disorders that cause blisters in the skin and mucosal membranes. Over 300 mutations in genes encoding extracellular macromolecules have been detected in patients with EB. Junctional EB is associated with mutations in the gene for type XVII collagen, as well as genes for laminins and integrins. Type XVII collagen is a transmembrane protein and a component of hemidesmosomes at the epidermal–basement membrane junction. It anchors keratinocytes to the underlying basement membrane. Mutations in the collagen XVII gene lead to diminished epidermal adhesion and blistering following minimal shearing forces. Loss of cohesion between the basement membrane and papillary dermis (choice A) is associated with dermolytic EB, a blistering skin disease caused by mutations in the gene for type VII collagen. Disintegration within the basal layer of epidermal cells is seen in patients with epidermolytic EB. None of the other choices are related to the pathogenesis of EB.

Keywords: Epidermolysis bullosa, type XVII collagen

4 **The answer is A: Stratum basale.** Skin is classified as thick or thin based on the relative thickness of the epidermis. Thick skin on the palm of the hand and sole of the foot lacks hair and has a much thicker epidermal layer than does thin skin covering other regions of the body. Keratinocytes composing the epidermis are arranged into five layers (strata) in thick skin and four layers in thin skin. Stratum basale, the deepest layer, consists of a single layer of cuboidal/low columnar epithelial cells. This basal layer contains proliferative stem cells that give rise to new keratinocytes. For this reason, the stratum basale is also referred to as the stratum germinativum. Basal cells in this photomicrograph appear small, and their nuclei are closely spaced and aligned in a row. Melanocytes are interspersed within the stratum basale. These neural crest–derived cells synthesize a melanin pigment that is transferred into the cytoplasm of neighboring basal cells—many of which appear dark brown in this image. Basal cells are connected to one another and to the upper layer of keratinocytes through desmosomes. They are connected to the underlying basement membrane through hemidesmosomes.

Keywords: Epidermis, thick skin

5 **The answer is A: Basal cells.** The arrows identify large keratinocytes with numerous cytoplasmic extensions. These cells form the stratum spinosum. This layer is so named, because of the "spinous" appearance of keratinocytes at this stage of maturation. The spinous processes provide focal contact points for adhesion between adjacent cells. Keratinocytes originate from proliferative stem cells in the stratum basale. Newly formed keratinocytes are lifted toward the surface of the skin. As they move, they mature; they develop cytoplasmic extensions (spinous processes), increase in size, and become flattened (shown in the image). The stratum spinosum is several cell layers thick. The other cells do not give rise to keratinocytes.

Keywords: Epidermis, thick skin

6 **The answer is B: Filaggrin.** As keratinocytes move up through the stratum spinosum, they accumulate intracellular "keratohyalin" granules. These most superficial cells of the nonkeratinized portion of the epidermis constitute the stratum granulosum. This layer is about one-to-three cells thick. Keratohyalin granules become more abundant as keratinocytes approach the surface of the skin. The granules contain two major intermediate filament–associated proteins, namely filaggrin and trichohyalin. These proteins are released into the cytoplasm, where they promote the aggregation of keratin filaments (choice D) in cornified cells of the stratum corneum. These proteins are intensely basophilic, and they acquire a dark blue color when stained with H&E. Melanin (choice E) is synthesized by melanocytes. None

of the other biomolecules are stored in keratohyalin granules.
Keywords: Epidermis, keratins

7   The answer is D: Stratum lucidum.   The stratum lucidum is composed of eosinophilic and refractile cells that are only visible in thick skin. These cells are located between the stratum granulosum and the stratum corneum. They represent an intermediate stage in the transformation of nucleated granular cells to form flattened, desiccated anucleate cells. When keratinocytes in the stratum spinosum release filaggrin and trichohyalin, their keratin filaments aggregate to form bundles that are referred to as tonofibrils. Thus, filaggrin and trichohyalin initiate the transformation of granular cells to cornified cells. This process is termed keratinization. During keratinization, cell nuclei and cytoplasmic organelles are degraded, and plasma membranes are thickened. The stratum lucidum is identified in the image associated with Question 5 (small arrows, shown in the image). The cells in this layer appear pink, because the tonofibrils are eosinophilic when stained with H&E.
Keywords: Epidermis, keratins

8   The answer is B: Stratum corneum.   With the formation of tonofibrils, granular cells are converted into cornified (keratinized) cells that leave the stratum granulosum and enter the stratum corneum. The stratum corneum is composed of mature squamous epithelial cells. The cytoplasm of these anucleated cells is filled with keratin filaments. Superficial cells are continuously sloughed off from the surface of the skin (exfoliation). The stratum corneum is constantly renewed by keratinocytes arising from deeper layers of the epidermis. The thickness of the stratum corneum varies depending on anatomic location. It is the thickest in the palm of the hand and the sole of the foot, where the skin is subject to constant abrasion ("wear and tear"). None of the other strata constitute the superficial layer of the epidermis.
Keywords: Epidermis, stratum corneum

9   The answer is D: Excessive thickening of the stratum corneum.   Ichthyosis vulgaris is a relatively common, autosomal dominant genetic disease (afflicting 1/250). It is characterized by a striking thickening of the stratum corneum. Hyperkeratosis in the stratum corneum and reduced or absent keratohyalin granules are the characteristic pathologic features of this congenital disease. Increased cohesiveness between keratinocytes causes scaling of the skin. Although cosmetically disfiguring, this condition is not life threatening. None of the other mechanisms of disease describe the pathogenesis of ichthyosis vulgaris.
Keywords: Ichthyosis vulgaris, epidermis, stratum corneum

10   The answer is E: Stratum basale and stratum spinosum of epidermis.   Pemphigus vulgaris is a chronic blistering skin disorder, secondary to diminished cohesion between keratinocytes. The blisters are suprabasal, meaning that the stratum basale separates from outer layers of the epidermis (shown in the image). The basal layer is intact and remains adherent to the basement membrane that forms the floor of the blister. The remaining epidermal layers form the roof of the blister. Acute and chronic inflammatory cells may be present within the vesicle. Distinctive, rounded keratinocytes are also shed into the lumen of the vesicle (acantholytic keratinocytes). None of the other layers of the skin exhibit physical separation in patients with pemphigus vulgaris.
Keywords: Pemphigus vulgaris

11   The answer is B: Desmosomes.   Direct immunofluorescence analysis of the patient's skin reveals a lace-like pattern that outlines individual keratinocytes (shown in the image). This experimental result is consistent with the deposition of immune complexes at points of contact between keratinocytes. The autoantibody formed in patients with pemphigus vulgaris has been shown to recognize desmoglein 3—a major structural protein found in desmosomes (zonula adherens). Desmosomes mediate adhesion between keratinocytes. Desmoglein 3 is more concentrated in the lower portion of the epidermis—a finding that explains loss of cohesion between basal cells and cells in upper layers of the epidermis. None of the other membrane-associated structures serve as primary adhesive junctions between keratinocytes.
Keywords: Pemphigus vulgaris

12   The answer is C: Epidermolysis bullosa simplex (EB simplex).   EB simplex, also known as epidermolytic EB, is a group of autosomal dominant skin disorders. The blister in EB simplex is caused by lysis of individual keratinocytes. The lowermost portion of the basal cell cytoplasm separates from the upper portion of the cells. Small pieces of basal cell cytoplasm remain attached to the basement membrane and form the floor of the vesicle. A nearly intact epidermis forms the roof of the blister. EB simplex is caused by mutations in the genes that encode cytokeratins. Keratin intermediate filament proteins provide essential mechanical stability to keratinocytes. Bullous pemphigoid (choice A) and pemphigus vulgaris (choice D) are autoimmune blistering skin diseases that are caused by autoantibodies to normal skin proteins. Psoriasis (choice E) is a proliferative skin disease of unknown etiology. Patients with psoriasis do not present with oral mucosal blisters at birth.
Keywords: Epidermolysis bullosa

13   The answer is B: Keratinocytes.   Actinic keratosis is a form of dysplasia in sun-exposed skin (actin meaning rays). Histologically, such lesions are composed of atypical squamous cells that vary in size and shape. Patches of epidermal dysplasia do not exhibit regular maturation as keratinocytes move from the basal layer of the epidermis to the surface. Dysplasia is a preneoplastic lesion, in the sense that it is a necessary stage in the multistep evolution to cancer. However, unlike cancer cells, dysplastic cells are not entirely autonomous. The histologic appearance of dysplastic tissue may still revert to normal. Adaptive changes in the other cells do not cause epidermal dysplasia.

Keywords: Actinic keratosis, dysplasia

14 **The answer is A: Cell and lipid envelopes.** One of the major functions of the skin is to provide a water barrier to maintain water homeostasis. In addition to keratohyalin granules, keratinocytes in the stratum spinosum and granulosum produce small membrane-bounded granules with a lamellar core (so-called lamellar bodies). Lamellar bodies contain a mixture of hydrophobic barrier lipids that are released into pericellular spaces. These lipids are organized into wide sheets of multilayered structures. These wide sheets form an outer protective coating that is referred to as a lipid envelope. A thick layer of insoluble protein is also deposited on the inner surface of the keratinocyte plasma membrane. This intracellular structure is referred to as a cell envelope. Together, thick insoluble cell and lipid envelopes form an effective epidermal water barrier.

Keywords: Epidermis, lamellar bodies

15 **The answer is E: Slower degradation of melanin.** The most significant factor in determining skin color is the content of melanin—a product of tyrosine metabolism. Melanocytes are neural crest–derived dendritic cells that are scattered among basal epidermal cells. They produce melanin within melanosomes and distribute these melanin granules to neighboring keratinocytes. The ratio of melanocytes to keratinocytes in the basal layer of the epidermis is referred to as the epidermal melanin unit. This ratio differs between different parts of the body but is essentially the same in all races. Skin color differences between the races are related primarily to the fate of melanin. In individuals with darker skin, the degradation of melanin within lysosomes proceeds at a slower rate than in light-skinned individuals. As a result of slower degradation in dark-skinned individuals, melanosomes are more widely distributed throughout the epidermis. As a result of faster degradation in light-skinned individuals, melanosomes are sparse in the upper layers of the epidermis. Increased number of melanocytes and increased synthesis of melanin (choices B and C) are biological responses to ultraviolet radiation. The other listed choices do not reflect variations in skin coloration.

Keywords: Melanocytes, melanosomes

16 **The answer is B: Increased production of melanin.** Melanin absorbs ultraviolet radiation and protects the skin from the harmful effects of sunlight. Harmful effects of sunlight exposure on the skin include inhibition of metabolism, generation of reactive oxygen species, activation of programmed cell death, mutagenesis, and cancer. Cancers linked to ultraviolet radiation including basal cell carcinoma, squamous cell carcinoma, and melanoma. Tanning, therefore, is a highly beneficial, reversible cellular adaptation. As a response to ultraviolet radiation exposure, melanocytes increase in cell number (hyperplasia) and accelerate their production of melanin. Increased pigmentation protects the skin against the harmful effects of sunlight. None of the other biological processes are related to the development of a suntan.

Keywords: Ultraviolet radiation, melanin

17 **The answer is D: Melanocyte.** Melanomas are neoplasms of melanocytes. If not diagnosed and removed at an early stage of tumor progression, melanomas can be deadly. Acral lentiginous melanoma is the most common type of melanoma in the dark-skinned population. This melanoma typically arises in the palm of the hand, sole of the foot, or in a subungual (nail bed) location. During the early radial growth phase, the tumor appears as an irregular, brown-to-black patch. As the disease progresses, neoplastic cells invade the deep dermal layer of the skin (vertical growth phase). These lesions appear as elevated rounded black nodules. Some tumors exhibit ulceration. Basal keratinocytes (choice A) are progenitor cells for basal cell carcinomas. None of the other cells give rise to melanomas.

Keywords: Melanoma, acral lentiginous, melanocytes

18 **The answer is C: Langerhans cells.** Langerhans cells are mononuclear phagocytes derived from bone marrow precursor cells. Monocytes in the bloodstream migrate into the epidermis where they differentiate into Langerhans dendritic cells. Langerhans cells are antigen-presenting cells in the epidermis. They phagocytose foreign substances that break through the skin barrier. Langerhans cells do not form zonula adherens junctions with neighboring keratinocytes. They move freely in the epidermis. Once an antigen is internalized, processed, and presented at the cell surface, Langerhans cells leave the epidermis and migrate to a regional lymph node. Here, Langerhans cells present foreign antigens to B and T lymphocytes (immunocytes). In routine H&E preparations, the nuclei of Langerhans cells stain intensely with hematoxylin, and the cytoplasm is clear. Keratinocytes (choices A, B, and E) are not involved in activating immune responses. Merkel cells (choice D) are mechanoreceptors in the skin.

Keywords: Langerhans cell

19 **The answer is C: Langerhans cells.** Birbeck granules are cytologic markers of Langerhans cells. By electron microscopy, these granules look like miniature tennis racquets. Malignant transformation of a Langerhans cell is referred to as Langerhans cell histiocytosis (LCH). LCH is a generic term for a group of rare diseases characterized by clonal proliferation of Langerhans cells. LCH includes three pathologic entities, namely, eosinophilic granuloma, Hand-Schüller-Christian disease, and Letterer-Siwe disease. A typical LCH lesion contains collections of abnormal Langerhans dendritic cells, as well as lymphocytes, eosinophils, and macrophages. LCH may occur anywhere in the body, ranging from isolated bone lesions to multisystem disease. None of the other cells exhibit intracellular Birbeck granules.

Keywords: Langerhans cell histiocytosis, Langerhans cell

20 The answer is D: Merkel cell.   The skin is the largest organ in the body and, as such, provides an extensive surface area for the processing external stimuli. A rich supply of terminal nerve fibers and a variety of sensory receptors are found in the dermis and epidermis. Some myelinated afferent (sensory) nerve fibers lose their myelin sheath when penetrating the epidermal basement membrane. These nerve endings expand into a disc or plate that is closely associated with the base of a Merkel cell, forming a Merkel disk or tactile disc. The Merkel disk serves as tactile mechanoreceptor. Merkel cells are derived from the neural crest. They are situated among basal keratinocytes in the stratum basale. Uncontrolled malignant proliferation of Merkel cells is referred to as a Merkel cell carcinoma. None of the other cells serve as neural receptors in the skin.

Keywords: Mechanoreceptor, Merkel disk, Merkel cell

21 The answer is E: Pacinian corpuscle.   Pacinian corpuscles are encapsulated tactile mechanoreceptors embedded in the deep dermis and hypodermis. They are large oval "onion-like" structures, with an outer capsule and numerous thin, concentric lamellae. A highly branched unmyelinated axon ending is present in the center of the corpuscle. The cellular concentric lamellae consist primarily of flattened Schwann cells. Collagen fibers and capillaries may be seen in the spaces between lamellae. Pacinian corpuscles are specialized for sensation of deep pressure and transient vibrations via displacement of capsular lamellae. Free nerve endings (choice A) are axon terminals that lack a Schwann cell or connective tissue covering. Free nerve endings are found in the epidermis and cornea of the eye. Nerve fibers (choice D) are seen throughout the dermis as a collection of myelinated nerve axons. None of the other choices describe the distinctive features of a pacinian corpuscle.

Keywords: Pacinian corpuscle

22 The answer is B: Meissner corpuscle.   Meissner corpuscles are encapsulated receptors specialized for the detection of shape and texture during active touch. They are found primarily in the fingertips and toes. These elliptical structures are situated within the cores of dermal papillae, with their long axis perpendicular to the surface of the skin. The "twisted skein of wool" appearance is due

to a spiral arrangement of Schwann cells. Several unmyelinated endings of myelinated axons course through the Schwann cell corpuscle. Capillary loops (choice A) are found in dermal papillae; however, these tubular structures usually exhibit a lumen. None of the other structures exhibit the distinctive features of a Meissner corpuscle.

Keywords: Meissner corpuscle

23 The answer is A: Capillary loops.   The skin is richly supplied with blood through two major vascular plexuses: deep and superficial. Cutaneous arteries and veins traveling in the hypodermis form a deep subcutaneous (hypodermic) plexus. Ascending arterioles arising from arteries in the hypodermis cross the reticular dermis. Near the border of the papillary dermis, neighboring ascending arterioles anastomose to form a superficial or subpapillary plexus. Terminal arterioles extend from the subpapillary plexus into each dermal papilla, forming a single capillary loop that supplies the epidermis via passive diffusion. Postcapillary venules return to the venous plexus in the subpapillary plexus. Small arteries and veins (choices D and E) are not present in dermal papillae. None of the other structures are characterized by the presence of a lumen.

Keywords: Capillaries, dermis, papillary dermis

24 The answer is D: Opening of arteriovenous anastomoses.   The arteriovenous anastomoses in the skin are referred as glomus bodies or AV shunts. The AV shunts serve as thermoregulators of the body. When AV shunts are open, blood flows directly from arterioles into venules and bypasses the capillary microcirculation. Numerous AV shunts are located in the dermis, between subcutaneous and subpapillary plexuses. In cold weather, the AV shunts open to decrease blood flow in the skin and thereby minimize heat loss. In warm/hot weather, the AV shunts close to increase blood flow through the capillary bed to facilitate heat loss. Together, AV shunts help maintain a constant body temperature.

Keywords: Arteriovenous shunts, Glomus body, temperature regulation

25 The answer is D: Postcapillary venules in the subpapillary plexus.   The skin biopsy shows a postcapillary venule that is nearly obliterated by a neutrophilic infiltrate. These histopathologic findings suggest a diagnosis of cutaneous necrotizing vasculitis. Damage to the vessel wall is associated with fibrin deposition and extravasation of erythrocytes (shown in the image). The lesions usually develop in the postcapillary venules that drain from capillary loops to the subpapillary venous plexus. Postcapillary venules are known to regulate the movement of inflammatory cells from the vascular space to regions of tissue injury during inflammation (see Chapters 5 and 9). Cutaneous necrotizing vasculitis may be primary (without a known cause) or secondary (e.g., caused by deposition of immune complexes). None of the other blood vessels are principal targets for immune complex–mediated inflammation in patients with cutaneous necrotizing vasculitis.

Keywords: Cutaneous necrotizing vasculitis

26 The answer is C: Reticular dermis. Scleroderma is a chronic autoimmune disease characterized by excessive collagen deposition in the skin and internal organs. Initial cutaneous lesions of scleroderma affect the lower reticular dermis. The entire dermis is eventually affected. Large, tightly packed collagen bundles parallel to the skin surface are a characteristic histologic finding in patients with scleroderma. Sweat glands and hair follicles are eventually destroyed, owing to the lack of adequate arterial blood supply. The affected skin becomes hard, stiff, and tense. The skin over the face becomes mask-like and patients appear expressionless. The hypodermis (choice B) is usually not involved in early stages of this disease. The other regions/structures are typically spared in patients with scleroderma.

Keywords: Scleroderma, dermis, reticular dermis

27 The answer is D: Hair follicles. Hair is present over most of the body surface, except for the skin of the palms, soles, lips, glans penis, clitoris, and labia minora. Hairs are filamentous keratinized structures derived from follicles. Hair follicles are invaginations of the epidermis that extend from the surface of the epidermis to the deep reticular dermis and/or hypodermis. Follicles are responsible for the continuous growth of hair. In this low-magnification image, transverse sections of several hair follicles exhibit epidermal epithelial cell sheaths surrounding centrally located hair shafts. Sebaceous glands (choice E) are associated with hair follicles (arrowheads, shown in the image). Eccrine sweat glands (choice C) are indicated by the oval in the image. Apocrine sweat glands (choice A) are not present in the scalp.

Keywords: Hair follicles

28 The answer is A: Dermal papilla. Dermal papilla refers to a tuft of vascularized loose connective tissue that is invaginated into the base of a hair bulb. A hair bulb (choice C) is the dilated proximal portion of a hair follicle. The dermal papilla is continuous with the surrounding dermal connective tissue and contains a capillary network that nourishes and sustains the living hair follicle. Disruption of this blood flow results in death of the hair follicle. Hair matrix (choice E) refers to the layer of epithelial cells covering the dermal papilla. External root sheath (choice B) is a continuation of the epidermis that covers the hair follicle (indicated by arrows in the image).

Keywords: Hair follicles, dermal papilla

29 The answer is A: Basement membrane. Down growth of epidermal epithelial cells (particularly the basal and spinous layers) into the dermis is referred to as the external root sheath. The invaginating epidermis is accompanied by its basement membrane deep into the dermis. Here, the basement membrane becomes thickened and is referred to as the "glassy membrane." Dense, irregular connective tissue surrounding the follicle forms a connective tissue sheath. The glassy membrane separates the hair follicle from the surrounding connective tissue sheath. None of the other cutaneous structures are continuous with the glassy membrane of the hair follicle.

Keywords: Hair follicles

30 The answer is C: Hair matrix. Epithelial cells surrounding the dermal papilla are collectively referred as the hair matrix. Matrix cells represent the proliferative (germinative) layer of the hair follicle, comparable to cells of the stratum basale of the epidermis. Matrix cells differentiate into keratin-producing cells of the hair. Continuous proliferation and division of these cells account for the growth of hair. Melanocytes are scattered among the matrix cells and pass melanin to the developing hair cells, thereby providing the hair with its natural color. Matrix cells also differentiate to form cells making up the internal root sheath (choice D). The internal root sheath consists of multiple cell layers and completely covers the initial part of the hair shaft. It degenerates near the level of the associated sebaceous glands. Dermal papilla (choice A) is composed of connective tissue whose primary function is to provide the vascular supply to the growing hair follicle. Inductive interactions between dermal papillae and matrix cells within the hair bulb are believed to regulate the size and shape of hair. The external root sheath (choice B) contains stem cells resembling epidermal basal cells (choice E); however, these cells do not contribute directly to the growth of hair.

Keywords: Hair follicles

31 The answer is A: Arrector pili muscle. Arrector pili are small bundles of smooth muscle fibers extending from the midpoint of the external root sheath to the papillary dermis. Contraction of these muscles causes hair shafts to become erect resulting in the formation of tiny skin bumps (so-called goose bumps). Arrector pili muscle is innervated by sympathetic nerve fibers. Stresses such as cold and fear can stimulate contraction of these small muscles. None of the other cutaneous structures exhibit the distinctive histologic features of arrector pili muscle.

Keywords: Arrector pili

32 The answer is B: External root sheath. The region of the external root sheath near the insertion site of the arrector pili muscle and the origin of the sebaceous gland is referred to as the follicular bulge. This small structure is home to clusters of undifferentiated epithelial stem cells. Thus, the bulge region of the external root sheath is believed to serve as an epidermal stem cell (ES cell) niche. ES cells are multipotential stem cells that develop into components of the hair follicle (internal root sheath,

cortex, medulla), as well as secretory cells lining the sebaceous glands. ES cells do not normally populate the stratum basale of the epidermis. However, when the epidermis is lost due to superficial abrasions or burns, ES cells migrate along the hair follicle glassy membrane toward the wound. Here, they proliferate and differentiate to resurface (regenerate) the skin lesion. The cellular and molecular signals that control ES cell differentiation and directed motility are important topics for basic research.
Keywords: Epidermal stem cells, hair follicles, follicular bulge

33 **The answer is D: Sebaceous glands.** Acne vulgaris is chronic inflammation within obstructed sebaceous glands. It commonly occurs in individuals during or after puberty. Sebaceous gland secretions increase greatly at the time of puberty under the influence of circulating sex hormones. These hormonal changes also induce abnormal cornification of epithelial cells near the neck of the sebaceous glands. Together, (1) excessive production of sebum (secretory product of sebaceous glands) and (2) abnormal cornification lead to the dilation of the sebaceous follicle. This provides a rich environment for the growth of *Propionibacterium acnes*. This bacterium proliferates in the affected glands, leading to an intense chronic inflammatory response. None of the other cutaneous structures are related to the pathogenesis of acne.
Keywords: Acne, sebaceous glands

34 **The answer is D: Sebaceous gland.** Sebaceous glands are branched acinar glands embedded in the dermis. A short duct delivers the secretory products of several acini to the upper portion of the hair follicle. Sebaceous glands develop as an outgrowth of the external root sheath of the hair follicle (shown in the image). Undifferentiated, flattened epithelial cells surround the periphery of glandular acini. The epithelial cells constantly proliferate, move toward the center of the acinus, and differentiate into large lipid-producing cells with fat droplets in their cytoplasm. Sebum, the oily product of the sebaceous gland, is released following rupture of the cells. This process is referred to as holocrine secretion. Sebum moves to the skin surface by following the path of the hair follicle. Sebum has antimicrobial and proinflammatory activities and serves to protect the stratum corneum of the epidermis.
Keywords: Sebaceous glands, sebum

35 **The answer is E: Secretory portion of eccrine sweat glands.** Eccrine sweat glands are widely distributed over the body surface, but they are lacking in the skin of the lips and parts of the external genitalia. Eccrine sweat glands are epidermal appendages that are independent of hair follicles. They are embedded in the dermis and hypodermis, and their excretory ducts open to the skin surface. Eccrine sweat glands are simple, coiled tubular structures consisting of two segments (or portions),

namely secretory and excretory. When stained with H&E, the secretory portions appear more pale stained than do excretory portions. They are composed of a pseudostratified epithelium with a small lumen. By contrast, excretory ducts (choice B) are lined by a distinctive, stratified cuboidal epithelium (arrowheads, shown in the image). Ductal epithelial cells are smaller and darker than secretory cells. Apocrine sweat glands (choice A) feature large secretory acini. They are present in the axilla, mons pubis, and perianal area. Hair follicles and sebaceous glands (choices C and D) do not exhibit the histological features of eccrine sweat glands.
Keywords: Eccrine sweat glands

36 **The answer is D: Myoepithelial cells.** The secretory epithelium of eccrine sweat glands consists of three cell types: (1) clear cells, (2) dark cells, and (3) myoepithelial cells. Myoepithelial cells are stellate cells with long processes. These cells are limited to the basal aspect of the secretory portion of the gland. They are located between the secretory cells. Myoepithelial cells are contractile cells that help propel sweat into the excretory duct for transport to the surface of the skin. Numerous contractile filaments in the cytoplasm of myoepithelial cells stain deeply with eosin, making these cells readily identifiable in H&E preparations. In the cross section of a secretory portion shown in the image, small cross sections of myoepithelial cytoplasm are evidently stained with eosin (indicated by the arrowheads). Clear cells (choice A) rest on the basal lamina. They store abundant glycogen in their cytoplasm and, therefore, appear pale stained in routine H&E preparations. Clear cells secrete most of the water and electrolytes in sweat. Dark cells (choice B) are located on top of the clear cells and line the luminal surface. Dark cells secrete glycoproteins. Fibroblasts (choice C) can be seen in the surrounding connective tissue (shown in the image). In longitudinal sections, myoepithelial cells may exhibit features of smooth muscle cells.
Keywords: Myoepithelial cells, eccrine sweat glands

37 **The answer is B: Apocrine sweat gland, secretory portion.** Apocrine sweat glands are tubular glands with large lumens. Like eccrine sweat glands, the secretory portions of apocrine sweat glands are embedded in the dermis and hypodermis. However, unlike eccrine sweat glands, their ducts open into hair follicles. Apocrine sweat glands are limited in distribution to axillary and perineal regions of the body and do not develop fully until puberty. The feature that distinguishes apocrine from eccrine sweat glands is the large size of their lumens. The secretory cells in apocrine sweat glands are simple cuboidal and eosinophilic. Myoepithelial cells are located between secretory cells and the basal lamina. The secretions of apocrine sweat glands contain proteins, carbohydrates, lipids, ammonia, and other organic compounds. These odorless secretions develop an acrid odor, through the action of microbes at the skin surface. The excretory ducts of apocrine sweat glands (choice A) are similar to those of eccrine sweat glands, but they take a more direct course and empty into hair follicle canals. The secretory portions of eccrine sweat glands (choice D) exhibit a pseudostratified epithelium and have a much smaller lumen. None of the other structures describe the histological features of apocrine sweat glands.

Keywords: Apocrine sweat glands

38 **The answer is C: Eccrine sweat glands.** Eccrine sweat glands produce as much as 10 L of sweat per day. The initial sweat produced by the secretory portions of the glands is similar in composition to an ultrafiltrate of the blood. Reabsorption of sodium and water occurs in the excretory ducts. This results in a hypotonic sweat that is released to the skin surface. Evaporation of sweat from the body surface serves to cool the skin. Sweating is a physical response to (1) elevated body temperature during exercise or fever and (2) high ambient temperature. Eccrine sweat glands are innervated by sympathetic nerve fibers and are stimulated by cholinergic neurotransmitters. In response to thermal stress, eccrine sweat glands are the most effective temperature regulator in the body. Emotional stress (e.g., fear) is associated with the release of adrenergic neurotransmitters that stimulate sweating from the palms and soles. None of the other epidermal appendages are involved in thermoregulation.

Keywords: Eccrine sweat glands, thermoregulation

39 **The answer is B: Keratinocytes in strata basale and spinosum.** When exposed to sunlight (ultraviolet light), the skin can rapidly produce vitamin D_3 (cholecalciferol) from the precursor molecule, 7-dehydrocholesterol. Synthesis of vitamin D_3 occurs primarily in the stratum basale and stratum spinosum of the epidermis. The skin is the major source of vitamin D_3, particularly in areas where dietary sources of vitamin D_3 are lacking. Vitamin D_3 enhances the intestinal absorption of calcium and phosphate, which are essential for the development of healthy bones and teeth. Deficiency of vitamin D_3 leads to osteomalacia in adults and rickets in children. None of the other skin cells synthesize vitamin D_3 when exposed to sunlight.

Keywords: Vitamin D_3

Chapter 9

Immune System and Lymphoid Organs

QUESTIONS

Select the single best answer.

1 During a research seminar, you are asked to explain the differences between innate and adaptive immunity. Which of the following biological processes best accounts for the vast antigenic repertoire of the adaptive immune system?
(A) Alternative splicing of receptor pre-mRNAs
(B) Gene segment class and isotype switching
(C) Germ line diversity of receptor variable domains
(D) Polymorphism of major histocompatibility complex
(E) Random somatic mutation and gene recombination

2 A neonate develops severe muscle cramps on the 2nd day postpartum. Laboratory studies show hypocalcemia. The neonate is subsequently diagnosed with DiGeorge syndrome. In addition to hypoparathyroidism, this neonate will be expected to have a congenital deficiency of which of the following cells?
(A) B lymphocytes
(B) Basophils/mast cells
(C) Bone marrow stem cells
(D) Monocytes/histiocytes
(E) T lymphocytes

3 Primary and secondary lymphoid organs are examined in the histology laboratory. Identify the organ shown in the image (low magnification).

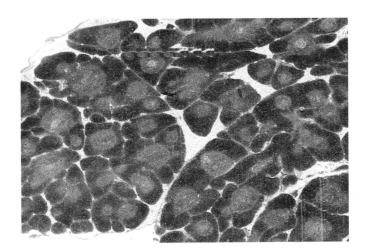

(A) Bone marrow
(B) Lingual tonsil
(C) Lymph node
(D) Spleen
(E) Thymus

4 You are invited to give a research seminar on current topics in immunology. During your presentation, you are asked to explain key steps in lymphocyte differentiation. T-cell receptor gene rearrangement takes place in which of the following anatomic locations?
(A) Bone marrow
(B) Cortex of the thymus
(C) Fetal liver
(D) Mantle zone of secondary lymphoid follicles
(E) Medulla of the thymus

5 A neonate with TORCH syndrome develops respiratory insufficiency and expires. A lobule of the thymus is examined at autopsy (shown in the image). What crucial T-cell maturation step takes place within the region indicated by the circle?

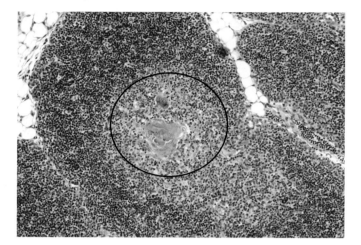

(A) Negative selection for foreign antigen recognition
(B) Negative selection for MHC recognition
(C) Negative selection for self-antigen recognition
(D) Positive selection for foreign antigen recognition
(E) Positive selection for MHC recognition

6 The tissue described in Question 5 is examined at higher magnification (shown in the image). The structure indicated by the arrow shows concentric layers of epithelial cells derived from pharyngeal pouches during embryogenesis. Name this distinctive histologic feature of the medulla of the thymus.

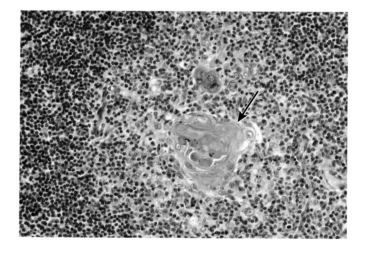

(A) Hassall corpuscle
(B) Herring body
(C) Mallory body
(D) Meissner corpuscle
(E) Pacinian corpuscle

7 Which of the following proteins provides an immunohistochemical marker for differentiated epithelial cells that form the structure identified in Question 6?
(A) Fibronectin
(B) Keratin
(C) Laminin
(D) Perlecan
(E) Vimentin

8 During a hematopathology conference, you are asked to discuss mechanisms of T-cell "education" in the prepubertal thymus. Which of the following cells regulates negative selection of self-reactive thymocytes in the medulla of the thymus by expressing a wide variety of tissue-specific genes?
(A) Dendritic cells
(B) Epithelioreticular cells
(C) Langerhans cells
(D) Macrophages
(E) Reticular cells

9 Cortical thymocytes are examined at high magnification in the histology laboratory (shown in the image). What crucial step in T-cell maturation takes place in this region of the prepubertal thymus?

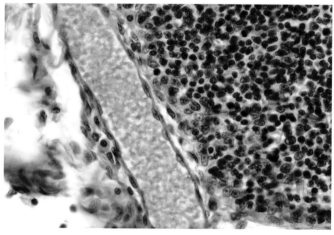

(A) Negative selection for foreign antigen recognition
(B) Negative selection for MHC recognition
(C) Negative selection for self-antigen recognition
(D) Positive selection for foreign antigen recognition
(E) Positive selection for MHC recognition

10 Further examination of the specimen described in Question 9 reveals numerous thymocytes clustered within a channel that courses through connective tissue between adjacent lobules (shown in the image). What is the appropriate name for this channel?

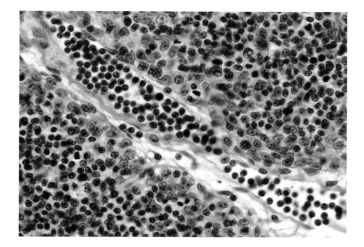

(A) Afferent lymphatic vessel
(B) Efferent lymphatic vessel
(C) Medullary sinus
(D) Postcapillary venule
(E) Precapillary arteriole

11 You are involved in a translational medicine research project designed to test the efficacy of vaccine delivery using a microneedle skin patch. The premise for your experimental approach is targeted delivery of foreign proteins to which of the following antigen-presenting cells?
(A) Epithelioreticular cells
(B) Follicular dendritic cells
(C) Kupffer cells
(D) Langerhans cells
(E) Reticular cells

12 What is the fate of the antigen-presenting cells identified in Question 11 after they have ingested the foreign proteins that were delivered by your microneedle skin patch?
(A) Formation of multinucleated giant cells
(B) Migration into lymphatic vessels
(C) Migration into postcapillary venules
(D) Proliferation within the papillary dermis
(E) Proliferation within the reticular dermis

13 A 43-year-old woman complains of chronic constipation and anovulatory menstrual cycles. Physical examination reveals a diffusely enlarged thyroid gland. Serum levels of T_3 and T_4 are low. A thyroid biopsy reveals chronic inflammatory cells (shown in the image). The germinal center of this lymphoid follicle is largely composed of which of the following cells?

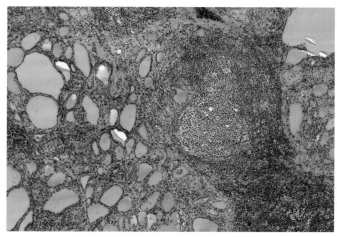

(A) B lymphocytes
(B) Macrophages
(C) Natural killer cells
(D) Th1 lymphocytes
(E) Th2 lymphocytes

14 A 34-year-old woman complains of excessive menstrual bleeding and pelvic pain of 6 months' duration. An endometrial biopsy is obtained (shown in the image). Identify the cells marked by the arrows.

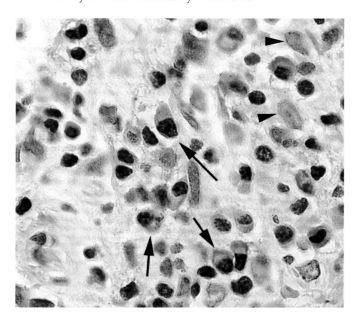

(A) Basophils
(B) Eosinophils
(C) Macrophages
(D) Monocytes
(E) Plasma cells

15 A 59-year-old man with adenocarcinoma of the large intestine undergoes a right hemicolectomy. Microscopic examination of the surgical specimen reveals lymphatic tissue in the lamina propria of the distal ileum (shown in the image). Identify the area indicated by the arrows.

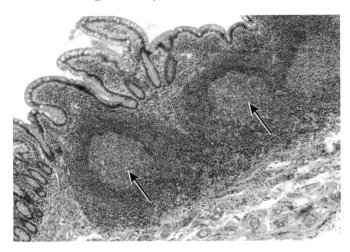

(A) Diffuse lymphatic tissue
(B) Germinal center
(C) Medullary sinus
(D) Periarteriolar sheath
(E) Primary lymphoid follicle

16 For the surgical specimen described in Question 15, what is the appropriate name for the corona of lymphocytes that surrounds the germinal centers of these lymphoid follicles?
(A) Cortical matrix
(B) Lymphoid sheath
(C) Mantle zone
(D) Primary cortex
(E) Secondary center

17 As you examine the surgical specimen described in Questions 15 and 16, the pathologist asks you to discuss trafficking of blood-borne lymphocytes to Peyer patches in the distal ileum. Which of the following lymphocyte proteins binds oligosaccharide ligands (addressins) on the luminal surface of high endothelial venules to initiate extravasation at this location in the gastrointestinal tract?
(A) E-selectin
(B) GlyCAM-1
(C) L-selectin
(D) LFA-1
(E) P-selectin

18 A 15-year-old girl presents with 5 days of fever (38°C/101°F) and sore throat. She reports that she has felt fatigued for the past week and has difficulty swallowing. Physical examination reveals generalized lymphadenopathy. The monospot test is positive. Which of the following best explains the development of swollen "glands" in this patient with infectious mononucleosis?

(A) Bone marrow stem cell hyperplasia
(B) Decreased lymphocyte trafficking
(C) Hypertrophy of follicular dendritic cells
(D) Obstruction of efferent lymphatic channels
(E) Reactive follicular hyperplasia

19 Primary and secondary lymphoid organs are examined in the histology laboratory. Identify the organ shown in the image (low magnification).

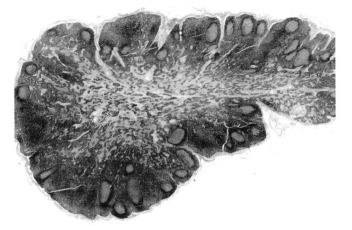

(A) Bone marrow
(B) Lingual tonsil
(C) Lymph node
(D) Spleen
(E) Thymus

20 A 56-year-old man with a history of cigarette smoking presents with a 5-month history of chest pain and cough. A chest x-ray reveals a peripheral mass in the left upper lobe. A CT scan of the thorax demonstrates hilar lymphadenopathy (arrow, shown in the image). Which of the following cells synthesize type III collagen fibers that helped trap metastatic cells in this patient's hilar lymph nodes?

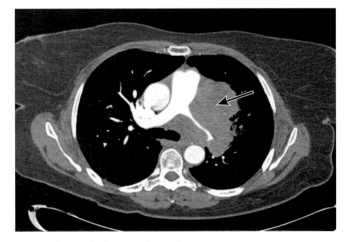

(A) Epithelioreticular cells
(B) Fibroblasts
(C) Follicular dendritic cells
(D) Macrophages
(E) Reticular cells

21 A mediastinal lymph node is collected at autopsy and examined in the pathology department (shown in the image). The germinal centers of these secondary lymphoid follicles contain nonimmune cells with thin, hairlike processes that intercalate maturing B lymphocytes. Name these nonimmune cells of the reticular meshwork.

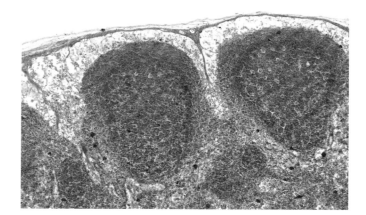

(A) Dendritic cells
(B) Follicular dendritic cells
(C) Langerhans cells
(D) Macrophages
(E) Reticular cells

22 A 55-year-old woman with breast cancer undergoes a modified radical mastectomy with axillary lymph node dissection. The resected lymph nodes are carefully examined for evidence of malignant disease (shown in the image). Identify the region of the lymph node indicated by the arrows.

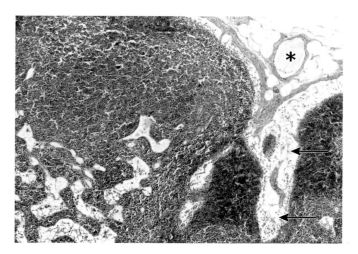

(A) Lymphatic vessel
(B) Medullary cord
(C) Medullary sinus
(D) Subcapsular sinus
(E) Trabecular sinus

23 For the surgical specimen described in Question 22, identify the structure indicated by the asterisk.
(A) Afferent lymphatic vessel
(B) Cortical sinus
(C) Efferent lymphatic vessel
(D) Precapillary arteriole
(E) Precapillary venule

24 Another axillary lymph node obtained from the patient described in Questions 22 and 23 is examined in the pathology department. What is the appropriate name for the region indicated by the asterisk?

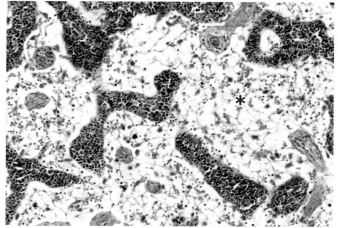

(A) Cortical sinus
(B) Efferent lymphatic vessel
(C) Medullary cord
(D) Medullary sinus
(E) Trabecular sinus

25 A 20-year-old woman with systemic lupus erythematosus complains of joint pain, weight loss, and sporadic fever. Physical examination reveals a butterfly rash over the patient's cheeks (malar skin rash). The antinuclear antibody test is positive. Polyclonal activation of B cells in this patient requires costimulatory signals from helper T cells. Which of the following B-cell surface proteins presents antigenic peptides to helper T cells during B-cell activation?
(A) B-cell receptor
(B) CD4
(C) CD40
(D) MHC class I
(E) MHC class II

26 A 22-year-old woman presents with a 3-day history of sore throat. Her temperature is 38.7°C (103°F). Physical examination reveals inflamed tonsils and swollen cervical lymph nodes. Trafficking of blood-borne lymphocytes to regional lymph nodes in this patient involves cell migration through high endothelial venules (HEVs). These specialized postcapillary venules are located primarily in which of the following regions of the patient's lymph nodes?

(A) Deep cortex
(B) Medullary sinus
(C) Nodular cortex
(D) Subcapsular sinus
(E) Trabecular sinus

27 A 69-year-old man with high-grade prostatic adenocarcinoma receives radiation and chemotherapy, but eventually expires. The patient's para-aortic lymph nodes are examined at autopsy for evidence of malignant disease (shown in the image). Identify the channel/space indicated by the arrows.

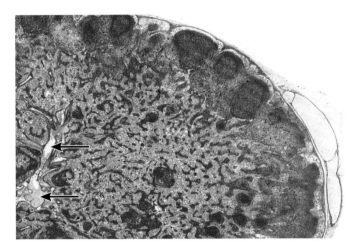

(A) Afferent lymphatic vessel
(B) Efferent lymphatic vessel
(C) Medullary sinus
(D) Precapillary arteriole
(E) Precapillary venule

28 A 45-year-old woman presents with a 2-month history of fatigue and recurrent fever. She also complains of tenderness below the right costal margin and dark urine. Physical examination reveals jaundice and mild hepatomegaly. The serum is positive for hepatitis B virus (HBV) antigens. Which of the following hepatocyte membrane proteins presents viral peptides to cytotoxic T lymphocytes in this patient?

(A) CD4
(B) CD8
(C) MHC class I
(D) MHC class II
(E) T-cell receptor

29 For the patient described in Question 28, which of the following enzymes is essential for generating viral peptides for display on the surface of HBV-infected cells?

(A) Alanine aminotransferase
(B) Glucuronyl transferase
(C) Glycogen phosphorylase
(D) Plasminogen activator
(E) Ubiquitin ligase

30 A 55-year-old woman with end-stage renal disease is transplanted with a cadaver kidney. Two weeks later, the patient develops mild fever, lymphocytosis, and elevated blood urea nitrogen (BUN). A kidney biopsy shows evidence of acute graft rejection. Which of the following antigens is the principal target for cell-mediated immune destruction of this patient's renal allograft?

(A) ABO
(B) CD8
(C) HLA
(D) LFA-1
(E) Rh

31 A 68-year-old woman undergoing chemotherapy for breast cancer presents with a 3-day history of chest pain, fever, and swelling of her feet. Cardiac catheterization reveals a markedly reduced ejection fraction with normal coronary blood flow. A myocardial biopsy reveals chronic inflammation (shown in the image). PCR studies demonstrate a coxsackievirus infection. Which of the following membrane glycoproteins provides an immunohistochemical marker for identifying killer T cells in this patient's heart biopsy?

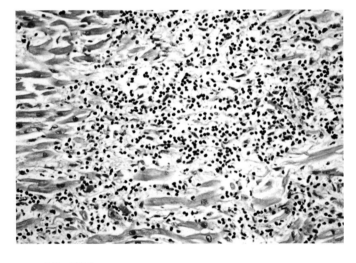

(A) CD4
(B) CD8
(C) CD20
(D) CD40
(E) CD94

32 Primary and secondary lymphoid organs are examined in the histology laboratory. Identify the organ shown in the image (low magnification).

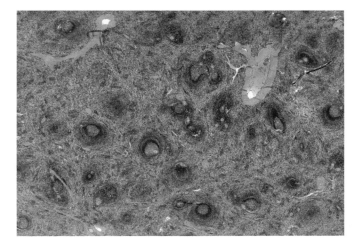

(A) Bone marrow
(B) Lymph node
(C) Peyer patch
(D) Spleen
(E) Thymus

33 You are invited to lead a discussion on the pathophysiology of maternal–fetal interactions during pregnancy. Which of the following classes of maternal antibody crosses the placenta to provide the fetus and neonate with passive humoral immunity?
(A) IgA
(B) IgD
(C) IgE
(D) IgG
(E) IgM

34 A 26-year-old man ruptures his spleen in a motorcycle accident and requires an emergency splenectomy to control internal bleeding. The surgical specimen is examined in the pathology department (shown in the image). Which of the following histologic features best characterizes the region of the spleen indicated by the oval?

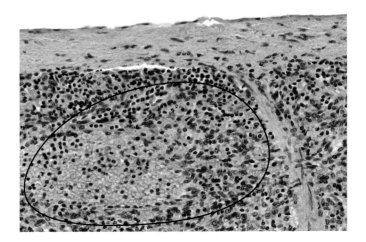

(A) Cords and venous sinuses (red pulp)
(B) Periarteriolar lymphoid sheath (PALS)
(C) Splenic capsule and visceral peritoneum
(D) Splenic lymphoid nodules (white pulp)
(E) Trabecular connective tissue

35 The capsule of the organ described in Question 34 is known to contain which of the following connective tissue cells?
(A) Dendritic cells
(B) Epithelioreticular cells
(C) Follicular dendritic cells
(D) Myofibroblasts
(E) Reticular cells

36 During a hematopathology conference you are asked to list and discuss functions of the spleen. Which of the following cells removes senescent and defective RBCs from the circulation in the spleen?
(A) Dendritic cells
(B) Endothelial cells
(C) Kupffer cells
(D) Macrophages
(E) Reticular cells

37 A 35-year-old woman with systemic lupus erythematosus undergoes a partial splenectomy to control her autoimmune hemolytic anemia. The surgical specimen is examined by a multiheaded microscope in the pathology department. Which of the following cells is expected to be most abundant in the region of the white pulp indicated by the double arrow (shown in the image)?

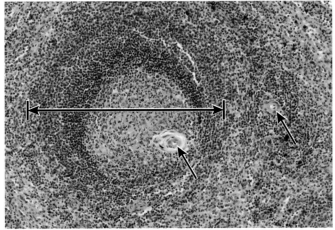

(A) B lymphocytes
(B) Dendritic cells
(C) Macrophages
(D) Th1 lymphocytes
(E) Th2 lymphocytes

38 For the surgical specimen described in Question 37, identify the blood vessels indicated by the arrows.
(A) Central
(B) Cortical
(C) Penicillar
(D) Splenic
(E) Trabecular

39 Another microscopic field of the specimen described in Questions 37 and 38 reveals a diffuse halo of cells surrounding a central arteriole (shown in the image). Identify the cells that constitute this periarteriolar lymphoid sheath.

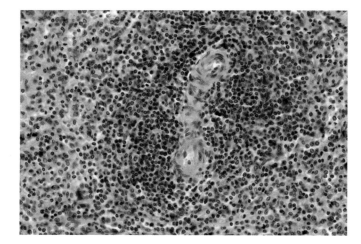

(A) B lymphocytes
(B) Macrophages
(C) Memory B lymphocytes
(D) Plasma B cells
(E) T lymphocytes

40 During a clinical conference, you are asked to discuss mechanisms of hypersensitivity in patients with conditions such as bronchial asthma, myasthenia gravis, and Graves disease. Which of the following components of the immune system is believed to play a crucial role in preventing hypersensitivity reactions and autoimmune diseases?
(A) B lymphocytes
(B) Dendritic cells
(C) Macrophages
(D) Natural killer (NK) cells
(E) T lymphocytes

41 A 24-year-old man complains of seasonal red eyes and runny nose ("hay fever"). Which of the following explains the pathogenesis of allergic rhinitis in this patient?
(A) Antibody-dependent cellular cytotoxicity
(B) Cytokine-mediated endothelial cell injury
(C) Deposition of immune complexes
(D) Generation of anaphylatoxins
(E) IgE-mediated mast cell degranulation

42 A 15-year-old girl with a history of allergies undergoes skin testing to identify potential allergens in her environment. Immediate swelling at the site of a positive skin reaction is caused by the release of which of the following mediators of inflammation from mast cells?
(A) Anaphylatoxins
(B) Histamine
(C) Kinins
(D) Leukotrienes
(E) Prostaglandins

43 An 18-year-old military recruit is given a Mantoux (tuberculin) screening test for tuberculosis. Forty-eight hours later, the intradermal injection site on the anterior surface of the forearm is raised and hardened (indurated). What is the principal function of helper T lymphocytes that have massively infiltrated the dermis in this patient?
(A) Antigen presentation
(B) Cytokine secretion
(C) Immune suppression
(D) Phagocytosis
(E) Target cell killing

44 A 30-year-old woman with a history of infertility is discovered to have a high titer of antisperm antibodies. Which of the following immunoglobulin classes most likely provides acquired "immunity" against spermatozoa in the reproductive tract of this patient?
(A) IgA
(B) IgD
(C) IgE
(D) IgG
(E) IgM

45 A 25-year-old woman complains of a poison ivy rash that she developed after working in her garden. The patient's arms and hands are red and covered with oozing blisters. Which of the following best explains the pathogenesis of these skin lesions?
(A) Antibody-dependent cellular cytotoxicity
(B) Cell-mediated immunity
(C) Cytotoxic humoral immune response
(D) IgE-mediated mast cell degranulation
(E) Immune complex disease

46 A 35-year-old woman with a history of drug abuse presents with an infectious mononucleosis-like syndrome and lymphadenopathy. Blood tests subsequently indicate that she is HIV positive. Which of the following membrane glycoproteins serves as a coreceptor on CD4$^+$ T cells for HIV entry?

(A) β-Chemokine receptor-5

(B) GlyCAM-1

(C) Integrin αvβ$_3$

(D) L-selectin

(E) LFA-1

47 For the patient described in Question 47, cytolysis of HIV-infected lymphocytes is mediated, in part, by the release of which of the following proteins from killer T cells?

(A) Gamma interferon

(B) Granzyme

(C) Lysozyme

(D) Major basic protein

(E) Tumor necrosis factor-α

48 A 55-year-old woman presents with a 3-day history of fever, night sweats, and chest pain. Her temperature is 38.7°C (103°F). Which of the following mediators of inflammation induces fever in this patient with bronchopneumonia?

(A) Gamma interferon

(B) Histamine

(C) Prostacyclin

(D) Thromboxane A$_2$

(E) Tumor necrosis factor–α

ANSWERS

1 The answer is E: Random somatic mutation and gene recombination.   The vast repertoire of the adaptive (acquired) immune system is based primarily on random gene recombination and somatic mutation events that occur in B and T lymphocytes. Antigen receptors on lymphocytes are encoded by the immunoglobulin gene superfamily. Immunoglobulin receptors on B cells are composed of heavy chains and light chains, each of which have constant and variable domains. During B-cell maturation, specific variable domain gene segments are spliced together. This intricate process of gene splicing is termed V(D)J recombination. Variable domain genes are modified further through somatic hypermutation. Cells that generate high-affinity antipathogen receptors and receive appropriate costimulatory signals undergo clonal expansion. Although T lymphocytes have different antigen receptors ($\alpha\beta$ heterodimers), they utilize the same process of somatic gene recombination and mutation to generate a vast diversity of antigen-binding sites. Gene mutation and clonal selection enable lymphocytes to respond to ever-changing microbial flora and pathogens. The other processes contribute to the complexity and diversity of immune response, but they do not provide a fundamental basis for generating de novo the vast antigenic repertoire of the adaptive immune system.
Keywords: Immune system, adaptive immunity

2 The answer is E: T lymphocytes.   DiGeorge syndrome is a congenital T-cell immunodeficiency disorder caused by failure of the third and fourth pharyngeal pouches to develop during embryogenesis. Patients with DiGeorge syndrome exhibit agenesis (or hypoplasia) of the thymus and parathyroid glands, congenital heart defects, dysmorphic facies, and a variety of other congenital anomalies. Parathyroid agenesis results in hypocalcemia that manifests as increased neuromuscular excitability. Thymic aplasia results in a congenital immune deficiency syndrome characterized by the loss of helper and killer (cytotoxic) T lymphocytes. Patients exhibit a deficiency of cell-mediated immunity, with a particular susceptibility to recurrent viral and fungal infections. None of the other choices are associated with thymic aplasia.
Keywords: DiGeorge syndrome, thymus

3 The answer is E: Thymus.   Primary lymphoid organs generate immature B and T lymphocytes; these organs include the bone marrow and thymus. Secondary lymphoid organs provide an environment for antigen stimulation and clonal selection; these organs include (1) diffuse and nodular lymphoid tissue; (2) lymph nodes, and (3) spleen. The image shows the distinctive lobular architecture of the thymus. The lobules are separated by connective tissue trabeculae that originate from a thin capsule. Each lobule is composed of a dark-stained cortex (cortical cap) and a light-stained medulla. The medullary regions are continuous. The cortex

and medulla are populated by T lymphocytes (thymocytes) at various stages of differentiation. Reticuloepithelial cells form an extensive meshwork that organizes thymocytes and regulates their growth and development. At low magnification, thymic lobules look like secondary lymphoid follicles with germinal centers (choices B and C); however, lymphoid follicles in mucosa-associated lymphoid tissue are not separated by trabeculae, and lymph nodes have subcapsular, trabecular, and medullary sinuses. The thymus undergoes atrophy after puberty and is replaced by adipose tissue (thymic involution). None of the other lymphoid tissues/organs exhibit the distinctive lobular morphology of the prepubertal thymus.
Keywords: Thymus, primary lymphoid organ

4 The answer is B: Cortex of the thymus.   T-lymphocyte precursors arise in the bone marrow, enter the circulatory system, and populate the thymus during fetal development. These multipotential lymphoid stem cells migrate to the cortical region of the thymic lobules. Here, they undergo T-cell receptor gene segment recombination and mutation to generate a heterogeneous population of thymocytes—each bearing a unique cell surface antigen receptor. Unlike surface immunoglobulins on B lymphocytes, T-cell receptors bind antigens that are presented by proteins encoded by the major histocompatibility complex (MHC). None of the other lymphoid organs provide a microenvironment (niche) for T-cell receptor gene assembly.
Keywords: Thymus, thymocytes

5 The answer is C: Negative selection for self-antigen recognition.   The circle on the image identifies the medulla of a thymic lobule. This region appears pale compared to the cortex owing to the larger size of the maturing thymocytes. In this niche, immature T cells complete their "education." In brief, thymocytes bearing MHC-restricted receptors are "tested" for their ability to recognize self-antigens. Self-reactive thymocytes undergo programmed cell death, and the residual apoptotic bodies are removed by macrophages. Cells that survive this test leave the thymus as naïve helper or killer T lymphocytes. The acronym TORCH, mentioned in the vignette, refers to a complex of similar signs and symptoms produced by fetal or neonatal infection with a variety of microorganisms, including Toxoplasma (T), Rubella (R), Cytomegalovirus (C), and Herpes (H). The letter "O" represents "others" including congenital syphilis. Negative selection for foreign antigens and MHC molecules (choices A and B) does not happen. The other selection processes listed are essential for developing an acquired immune response, but they do not take place in the medulla of the thymus.
Keywords: TORCH syndrome, programmed cell death

6 The answer is A: Hassall corpuscle.   The histologic feature identified in the image represents a remnant of epithelial tissue derived from third and fourth pharyngeal pouches during embryonic development. These structures are referred to as Hassall corpuscles. They are a distinguishing feature of the medulla of the thymus. Hassall corpuscles are composed of concentric whorls of type VI epithelioreticular cells. Six functionally distinct populations of epithelioreticular cells have been described. These cells provide a framework for thymocytes and regulate crucial aspects of T-cell education. Herring bodies (choice B) are dilated terminal axons of neurons in the posterior pituitary. Mallory bodies (choice C) represent precipitated intermediate filament protein in the hepatocytes of chronic alcoholics. Meissner and Pacinian corpuscles (choices D and E) are tactile receptors in the dermis of the skin.

Keywords: Thymus, Hassall corpuscle

7 The answer is B: Keratin. Epithelioreticular cells comprising Hassall corpuscles express keratin proteins. Keratins are a family of intermediate filament proteins expressed by stratified squamous epithelial cells in the skin and epidermal appendages (e.g., hair and nails). Their presence in the thymus is, perhaps, not surprising given the origin of reticuloepithelial cells from epithelial cells lining the embryonic oropharynx. The concentric whorls of keratinized cells shown in the image resemble keratin pearls—an important histologic feature of neoplastic squamous epithelial cells. Hassall corpuscles are believed to synthesize and secrete interleukins (e.g., IL-4 and IL-7) that help regulate the differentiation of thymocytes. The other proteins are markers of *mesenchymal* cells.

Keywords: Thymus, Hassall corpuscle

8 The answer is B: Epithelioreticular cells. As mentioned above, negative selection of immature T lymphocytes takes place in the medulla of the thymus during infancy and childhood. In this protected environment, MHC-restricted thymocytes encounter a variety of self-antigens that are displayed on the surface membranes of epithelioreticular cells. Up-regulation of self-antigens (e.g., insulin) on the surface of thymic reticuloepithelial cells is controlled by the autoimmune regulator (AIRE) gene product—a transcription factor. Thymocytes that are self-reactive undergo programmed cell death (negative selection). Macrophages (choice D) remove the residual apoptotic bodies of these self-reactive thymocytes. None of the other cells regulate T-cell education in the thymus.

Keywords: Thymus, epithelioreticular cells

9 The answer is E: Positive selection for MHC recognition. The image shows cortical thymocytes in close proximity to a postcapillary venule that is located within trabecular connective tissue. After lymphoid stem cells enter the thymus and migrate to the cortex of thymic lobules, they undergo T-cell receptor gene segment recombination. T-cell receptors on helper and killer T lymphocytes bind peptide antigens presented (carried) by MHC proteins (HLA antigens in humans). Thus, the first step in T-cell education in the thymus is positive selection for MHC recognition. Thymocytes with receptors that fail to bind MHC proteins undergo programmed cell death. Thymocytes in the cortical region of thymic lobules are protected from self-antigens by an impermeable blood-thymic barrier. This barrier is composed of (1) capillary endothelial cells, (2) macrophages, and (3) type I epithelioreticular cells. Negative selection for foreign antigens and MHC molecules (choices A and B) does not happen. The other selection processes listed are essential for developing an acquired immune response, but they do not take place in the cortex of the thymus.

Keywords: Thymus, thymocyte education

10 The answer is B: Efferent lymphatic vessel. The image shows a channel embedded in connective tissue between thymic lobules. The channel is filled with a monomorphic population of small lymphocytes (presumably thymocytes). The absence of red blood cells within the vessel lumen (see image of Question 9 for comparison) suggests that it is a lymphatic channel. Because the thymus lacks afferent lymphatic channels, this channel most likely represents an efferent channel. Efferent lymphatic vessels accompany blood vessels and nerves through the subcapsular and trabecular connective tissue. None of the other channels describe the morphology of lymphatic vessels in the thymus.

Keywords: Thymus, Lymphatic vessels

11 The answer is D: Langerhans cells. Microneedle patches have been shown to provide an efficient method for delivering immunogens (vaccines) to antigen-presenting cells in the skin. Langerhans cells are antigen uptake and presenting cells that reside in the epidermis and papillary dermis. They are derived from the bone marrow and are members of the mononuclear phagocytic system. Their cellular processes provide an efficient system for trapping pathogens and other foreign antigens that enter the body through the skin. Langerhans cells play an important role in cutaneous hypersensitivity reactions (i.e., contact dermatitis). Reticular cells (choice E) synthesize type III collagen fibers and contribute to the architecture of lymph nodes. The other cells process and/or present antigens, but they are not located in the skin. For example, Kupffer cells are perisinusoidal macrophages found in the liver.

Keywords: Langerhans cells, microneedle patch

12 The answer is B: Migration into lymphatic vessels. After encountering a pathogen, Langerhans cells alter their metabolism and modulate patterns of gene expression. They retract their cellular processes, enter lymphatic channels in the dermis, and migrate to regional lymph nodes where they display antigenic peptides to B and T lymphocytes. Langerhans cells (like other professional antigen-presenting cells) degrade pathogenic proteins to 8 to 10 residue amino acid peptides within phagolysosomes. Foreign peptides are bound by MHC class II molecules in the endosome compartment of the cell and then transported to the cell surface. Here, MHC–peptide complexes are "evaluated" by receptors on B and T lymphocytes. None of the other developmental pathways describe the fate of Langerhans cells upon activation.

Keywords: Langerhans cells

13 **The answer is A: B lymphocytes.** Diffuse and nodule lymphatic tissue is commonly found in the respiratory system, urogenital organs, and wall of the gastrointestinal tract. In this case, however, nodular lymphatic tissue is evident in the thyroid gland of a patient with autoimmune thyroiditis. When primary collections of small lymphocytes (primary follicles) develop a germinal center, they are referred to as secondary lymphoid follicles. The germinal centers of secondary lymphoid follicles are sites of B-cell proliferation and maturation. Because these cells are larger, the germinal centers appear pale stained, compared to the surrounding diffuse lymphoid tissue. B cells within germinal centers (plasmablasts) give rise to mature plasma cells that secrete antibody (e.g., IgM, IgG, IgA). Chronic autoimmune thyroiditis (Hashimoto thyroiditis) is a common cause of goitrous hypothyroidism. The disease is characterized by the presence of circulating antibodies to thyroid antigens. As shown in the image, chronic inflammatory infiltrates in patients with Hashimoto thyroiditis form lymphoid follicles with germinal centers. Although the other cells are found in diffuse and nodular lymphatic tissue, they do not form germinal centers in secondary lymphoid follicles.

Keywords: Hashimoto thyroiditis, lymphoid follicles

14 **The answer is E: Plasma cells.** This photomicrograph reveals plasma cells (arrows) and macrophages within stromal connective tissue of the endometrium. Plasma cells are mature antibody-producing B lymphocytes. They are much larger than resting lymphocytes and frequently oval in shape. A few macrophages are also visible (arrowheads). The presence of plasma cells and macrophages in a surgical biopsy or autopsy specimen provides histologic evidence of chronic inflammation. Inflammation has historically been referred to as either acute or chronic, depending on the persistence of the injury, clinical symptoms, and the nature of the inflammatory response. The cellular components of chronic inflammation are lymphocytes, antibody-producing plasma cells, and macrophages. The chronic inflammatory response is often prolonged and may be associated with aberrant repair (i.e., fibrosis). None of the other inflammatory cells exhibit the distinctive cytologic features of plasma cells.

Keywords: Endometritis, inflammation

15 **The answer is B: Germinal center.** The lymphoid nodules shown in the image exhibit central, pale stained germinal centers that are filled with proliferating B lymphocytes

(plasmablasts). These secondary lymphoid follicles (nodules) are similar in morphology to the nodule present in the thyroid gland of the patient described in Question 13. The distal ileum is characterized by the presence of multiple lymphatic nodules, referred to as Peyer patches. These aggregates of nodular lymphoid tissue play a crucial role in regulating immune surveillance of the gut flora. Specialized epithelial microfold (M) cells sample antigens present in the lumen of the gut and transport them to the underlying lymphoid tissue to stimulate immune activation or anergy (tolerance). None of the other structures exhibit the morphology of a germinal center in a secondary lymphoid follicle.

Keywords: Peyer patch, M cells

16 **The answer is C: Mantle zone.** The corona of small lymphocytes that surrounds the germinal centers in secondary lymphoid follicles is referred to as the mantle zone. These small lymphocytes include resting T and B cells. Immunohistochemical labeling assays are used to distinguish between these lymphocyte subpopulations. In addition to lymphocytes, nodular lymphatic tissue is characterized by the presence of follicular dendritic cells that trap antigenic debris for uptake by antigen-presenting cells. None of the other histologic features exhibit the morphology of the mantle zone in a secondary lymphoid nodule.

Keywords: Peyer patch, nodular lymphatic tissue

17 **The answer is C: L-selectin.** Homing (trafficking) of lymphocytes to diffuse and nodular lymphatic tissue is mediated, in part, by L-selectin. This carbohydrate-binding protein is expressed on the surface of lymphocytes. Ligands for L-selectin are N-linked oligosaccharide side chains carried primarily by GlycCAM-1 (choice B). This glycoprotein is expressed on the luminal (apical) surface of epithelial cells that line high endothelial venules. E-selectin (choice A) and P-selectin (choice E) regulate margination and diapedesis of leukocytes during acute inflammation. LFA-1 (choice D) is a cell adhesion molecule that mediates attachment of lymphocytes to antigen-presenting cells.

Keywords: Peyer patch, selectins, high endothelial venules

18 **The answer is E: Reactive follicular hyperplasia.** Enlarged lymph nodes (swollen glands) are a common symptom of infection. Lymph nodes become swollen due to a combination of factors, including (1) *increased* proliferation of lymphocytes (reactive hyperplasia), (2) *increased* delivery of lymph fluid (lymphedema), and (3) *increased* leukocyte trafficking. Infectious mononucleosis is characterized by fever, pharyngitis, and lymphadenopathy (i.e., swollen glands). This viral infection is caused by Epstein-Barr virus (EBV), a herpes virus that is transmitted through respiratory droplets and saliva. T cells proliferate in response to activated B lymphocytes and appear in the peripheral blood as atypical lymphocytes.

None of the other biological responses listed as choices are associated with the pathogenesis of swollen glands in a patient with infectious mononucleosis.
Keywords: Infectious mononucleosis, Epstein-Barr virus

19 The answer is C: Lymph node.   The photomicrograph provides a low magnification view of a lymph node. This secondary lymphoid organ is composed of a peripheral cortex and a pale stained, central medulla. Numerous lymphatic nodules are present in the cortex. The hilum, seen on the lower right side of the image, provides a region for blood vessels and an efferent lymphatic channel to enter and/or exit the lymph node. Lymph nodes filter the lymph, removing macromolecular antigens, and they provide a microenvironment for antigen-driven activation of B and T lymphocytes. None of the other lymphoid organs exhibit the distinctive morphology of a lymph node.
Keywords: Lymph nodes, lymph

20 The answer is E: Reticular cells.   Lymph is continuously generated as a filtrate of the microcirculation and moved through delicate lymphatic channels, before returning to the circulatory system by joining large veins in the neck. Along the way, lymph passes through multiple lymph nodes that serve as filters. Lymph enters a node through afferent channels and percolates through lymphatic sinuses that are spanned by a fine meshwork of extracellular reticular fibers, reticular cells, and macrophages. Reticular cells synthesize and organize type III collagen reticular fibers. Special silver stains can be used to visualize reticular fibers. Together, reticular cells and fibers filter the lymph to retain pathogens and cellular debris. In patients with malignant neoplasms, reticular fibers may trap tumor cells, resulting in the formation of metastatic tumor colonies. For this reason, lymph node dissection and histologic examination are essential elements of cancer staging. Lymph drains from a common efferent lymphatic channel at the hilum of the node. None of the other cells synthesize reticular fibers.
Keywords: Lymph nodes, metastatic lung cancer

21 The answer is B: Follicular dendritic cells.   The image shows secondary lymphoid follicles near the periphery of a lymph node. The follicles are separated from the capsule by a subcapsular sinus. Germinal centers within secondary lymphoid follicles frequently contain follicular dendritic cells. These large cells have multiple, hair-like processes that intercalate B lymphocytes to support their maturation. Follicular dendritic cells express cell surface Fc receptors that bind antigen–antibody (immune) complexes and store them for weeks (and even years). Follicular dendritic cells do not qualify as antigen-presenting cells (APCs), because the antigens they trap are not internalized and processed for display by MHC molecules; rather, the antigens are merely retained at the cell surface for "inspection" by passing lymphocytes. Dendritic cells (choice A) are typically located in T-cell–rich areas of the deep cortex. None of the other cells display histologic features of follicular dendritic cells.
Keywords: Lymph nodes, follicular dendritic cells

22 The answer is E: Trabecular sinus.   Lymph nodes are characterized by the presence of subcapsular, trabecular, and medullary sinuses that provide channels for the circulation of lymph. The arrows identify a trabecular sinus that appears to be penetrating the cortex of the node (shown in the image). Trabecular sinuses drain to central medullary sinuses. Trabeculae are composed of dense connective tissue. They are continuous with the capsule and provide a framework for lymph node architecture. None of the other regions/structures exhibit histologic features of a trabecular sinus.
Keywords: Breast cancer, axillary lymph nodes

23 The answer is A: Afferent lymphatic vessel.   Multiple afferent lymphatic vessels penetrate the capsule of lymph node. Lymph that is delivered to the subcapsular sinus flows through trabecular and medullary sinuses, before being drained by an efferent lymphatic vessel located at the hilum of the lymph node. The image shows an afferent lymphatic vessel located outside the capsule. None of the other structures exhibit the morphology of afferent lymphatic vessels near the periphery of a lymph node.
Keywords: Lymph nodes, lymphatic vessels

24 The answer is D: Medullary sinus.   Examination of the photomicrograph reveals medullary cords within an open medullary sinus. A fine meshwork of reticular fibers and reticular cell processes crisscrosses this lymphatic sinus. As lymph filters through the lymph node, antigens and antigen-presenting cells provide signals to lymphocytes to coordinate their activation, proliferation, and maturation. Mature plasma cells leave the cortex of the node. They populate medullary cords and secrete antibodies. Antibodies (immunoglobulins) are subsequently delivered to the blood through the right lymphatic trunk or the left thoracic duct. Antibodies are targeting molecules that initiate humoral and/or cellular mechanisms of cytotoxicity. None of the other regions/structures exhibit histologic features of a medullary sinus.
Keywords: Lymph nodes, plasma cells

25 The answer is E: MHC class II.   Naive (immature) B cells are stimulated by exposure to antigens that are either soluble or presented by antigen-presenting cells (APCs) such as macrophages and dendritic cells. B-cell receptors (choice A) facilitate receptor-mediated endocytosis of antigens. Recent studies indicate that B cells also pinch off and internalize small fragments of antigen-bearing plasma membranes. Protein antigens are degraded by proteases within phagolysosomes to yield a collection of 8 to 10 amino acid peptides. Immunogenic peptides are carried by MHC class II molecules to the surface of

B cells for activation of helper T lymphocytes. MHC class I molecules (choice D) activate cytotoxic (killer) T lymphocytes. None of the other proteins present antigenic peptides to helper T cells during B-cell activation.

Keywords: Systemic lupus erythematosus, major histocompatibility complex

26 **The answer is A: Deep cortex.**   Most lymphocytes (about 90%) enter lymph nodes and diffuse/nodular lymphatic tissue through specialized postcapillary venules termed high endothelial venules (HEVs). HEVs are lined by cuboidal endothelial cells. They express an array of cell adhesion molecules (selectins and addressins) that mediate leukocyte binding and transendothelial migration (diabedesis). In lymph nodes, HEVs are located primarily in the deep cortex, a T-cell–rich region of the lymph node. Upon arrival in a lymph node, T cells meander in the deep cortex, while B cells migrate to the cortex. Immunohistochemical assays are used routinely to localize B- and T-cell populations in primary and secondary lymphoid organs. None of the other regions of the lymph node are characterized by the presence of HEVs.

Keywords: Lymphadenopathy, high endothelial venules

27 **The answer is B: Efferent lymphatic vessel.**   The image shows an efferent lymphatic vessel in the medulla near the hilum of a lymph node. Most lymphocytes leave lymph nodes through a common efferent lymphatic channel. Afferent lymphatic vessels (choice A) enter lymph nodes by penetrating the outer capsule. A large afferent lymphatic vessel is visible along the right side of this specimen (shown in the image). Unlike lymphatic channels, a medullary sinus (choice C) would contain medullary cords. Similarly, blood vessels (choices D and E) would contain WBCs and RBCs.

Keywords: Lymph nodes, lymphatic vessels

28 **The answer is C: MHC class I.**   Viral peptides are presented to the immune system by MHC class I molecules. These proteins bind endogenous protein fragments and "show" them at the cell surface to cytotoxic T lymphocytes (CTLs) during graft rejection and during cell-mediated killing of virus-infected cells. All tissues express class I molecules, whereas class II molecules (choice D) are displayed primarily on antigen-presenting cells and B lymphocytes. CD4 and CD8 (choices A and B) are surface markers of helper and killer T lymphocytes, respectively. They bind MHC proteins, but they do not bind viral peptides. Hepatocytes do not express T-cell receptors (choice E).

Keywords: Hepatitis, major histocompatibility complex

29 **The answer is E: Ubiquitin ligase.**   Peptides carried by MHC class I or class II molecules are generated through different processing pathways. MHC class I molecules interact with fragments of endogenous proteins that are degraded in the cytosol by proteasomes. By contrast, MHC class II molecules interact with exogenous proteins

that are degraded by proteases within phagolysosomes. Viral proteins synthesized in the liver of this patient are degraded by proteasomes—large protein complexes that hydrolyze proteins to yield small peptides. Endogenous proteins are targeted for proteasomal degradation by the covalent attachment of ubiquitin—a small regulatory protein. Enzymes that add ubiquitin to proteins targeted for destruction are termed ubiquitin ligases. Small peptides generated by proteasomes enter the rough endoplasmic reticulum where they interact with newly synthesized MHC class I proteins. Plasminogen activator (choice D) is a plasma protease that regulates hemostasis. None of the other enzymes target proteins for proteolytic degradation.

Keywords: Proteasomes, viral hepatitis

30 **The answer is C: HLA.**   Acute graft rejection is caused primarily by donor-recipient differences in HLA molecules encoded by the major histocompatibility complex (MHC). These molecules are expressed on most cell surface membranes. MHC genes are highly polymorphic. This leads to allograft rejection, because the host immune system interprets MHC alleles as evidence of loading with a viral or foreign peptide. Preformed antibodies directed against ABO antigens constitute an absolute barrier to successful transplantation. Preformed anti-ABO antibodies bind endothelial cells in the graft and cause immediate (hyperacute) graft rejection. However, ABO antigens are carbohydrates, and they do not elicit a cellular immune response. None of the other antigens mediates acute or chronic graft rejection.

Keywords: Transplantation medicine

31 **The answer is B: CD8.**   Two populations of lymphocytes are generated in the thymus, namely helper and killer T cells. These populations can be identified by flow cytometry or immunohistochemistry using monoclonal antibodies directed against specific cluster of differentiation (CD) antigens. Helper T lymphocytes express CD4, whereas killer T lymphocytes express CD8. These phenotypic differences are crucial for regulating adaptive immunity. CD4 binds MHC class II molecules, and so helper T cells are described as being "class II restricted." CD8 binds MHC class I molecules, and so killer T cells are described as being "class I restricted." Patients with viral myocarditis show an accumulation of lymphocytes in their affected heart muscle (shown in the image). Killer T lymphocytes bind and destroy virus-infected cells. None of the other CD antigens provide markers for identifying killer T lymphocytes.

Keywords: Myocarditis, CD antigens

32 **The answer is D: Spleen.**   The image shows a low magnification section through the spleen. Examination of the specimen reveals scattered splenic lymphoid nodules (white pulp) surrounded by small venous sinuses (red pulp). A dense connective tissue capsule encloses the

spleen from which numerous trabeculae penetrate the parenchymal tissue. The spleen filters the blood, removing aged and defective RBCs. The spleen also provides a microenvironment for generating immune responses to blood-borne antigens. None of the other lymphoid organs display red and white pulp.
Keywords: Spleen

33 **The answer is D: IgG.** Immunoglobulins are antigen-binding proteins that are found in all fluid compartments of the body including blood, lymph, interstitial fluid, and bodily secretions (e.g., tears, saliva, breast milk). During maturation, B cells select one of five different heavy chain genes for immunoglobulin assembly. These heavy-chain isotypes (also referred to as classes) include IgA, IgD, IgE, IgG, and IgM. These five isotypes have different biochemical properties and biological functions. IgG is the most abundant immunoglobulin in serum (about 1,200 mg/dL). IgG crosses the placenta during pregnancy to provide the fetus with passive humoral immunity. IgA (choice A) is found in bodily secretions (tears, saliva, milk). IgD (choice B) serves as an antigen receptor. IgE (choice C) binds mast cells and mediates type I hypersensitivity reactions. IgM (choice E) serves as an antigen receptor and is most efficient in fixing complement.
Keywords: Immunoglobulins, pregnancy

34 **The answer is A: Cords and venous sinuses (red pulp).** The oval identifies a region of the spleen that is filled with venous sinuses separated by thin cords. The splenic cords are difficult to visualize by light microscopy; they are composed of reticular cells and reticular fibers and may include a variety of acute and chronic inflammatory cells. Together, splenic cords and sinuses are referred to as red pulp. Circulation of blood through red pulp allows macrophages to remove senescent or defective RBCs and filter the blood for pathogens. None of the other choices describe histologic features of red pulp in the spleen.
Keywords: Spleen, red pulp

35 **The answer is D: Myofibroblasts.** The arrow identifies dense connective tissue in the capsule of the spleen. The capsule and associated trabeculae of the spleen are populated by myofibroblasts. These contractile cells are believed to provide tension on the red pulp to accommodate changes in blood flow and discharge reserves of RBCs as needed. Myofibroblasts also synthesize a variety of extracellular matrix molecules. None of the other cells have been identified in the capsule of the spleen.
Keywords: Spleen, myofibroblasts

36 **The answer is D: Macrophages.** The spleen filters the blood. It removes pathogens and initiates immune response. The spleen also removes senescent and defective RBCs and retrieves iron from hemoglobin. The average life span of circulating RBCs is 120 days. With each pass through the red pulp of the spleen, RBCs must deform so as to

squeeze through parallel stacks of long endothelial cells (so-called stave cells) that line the venous sinuses. This open circulation (from sheathed capillaries, to splenic cords, to venous sinuses) provides an opportunity for macrophages to remove RBCs that may be fragile or stiff. Macrophages also have receptors for phosphatidylserine molecules that appear on the outer leaflet of the RBC lipid bilayer following membrane damage. Kupffer cells (choice C) are resident macrophages in the liver. None of the other cells remove defective RBCs from the circulation in the spleen.
Keywords: Spleen, red pulp, macrophages

37 **The answer is A: B lymphocytes.** The double arrow identifies a secondary lymphoid nodule within the white pulp of the spleen. The germinal center is surrounded by a *mantle* of small lymphocytes. Red pulp immediately adjacent to the white pulp is referred to as the *marginal* zone. Th1 lymphocytes (choice D) interact with B cells and mediate delayed hypersensitivity reactions (e.g., poison ivy). Th2 lymphocytes (choice E) interact with eosinophils and mast cells, and mediate hypersensitivity responses to parasitic infestations and allergens. Although the other cells are found in diffuse and nodular lymphatic tissue, they do not form germinal centers in lymphoid follicles.
Keywords: Spleen, white pulp

38 **The answer is A: Central.** Blood flow through the spleen is complex. In brief, the branches of splenic and trabecular arteries that enter the white pulp of the spleen are termed central arteries. Lymphocytes surround the central artery and its branches, forming a periarteriolar lymphatic sheath (PALS). The central artery continues into the red pulp of the spleen where it gives rise to multiple, small penicillar arterioles. These arterioles form sheathed capillaries that empty blood directly into splenic cords. As discussed above (Question 36), the open circulation of blood in the spleen, from sheathed capillaries to splenic cords to venous sinuses, provides an opportunity for macrophages to remove senescent RBCs.
Keywords: Spleen, white pulp

39 **The answer is E: T lymphocytes.** Most lymphocytes in the periarteriolar lymphoid sheath (PALS) are T cells. Thus, PALS are similar in function to the deep cortical region in lymph nodes; both are said to be thymus-dependent lymphoid zones. The mechanisms whereby T lymphocytes exit the blood and congregate around the central artery and its branches are poorly understood. Although the other cells listed are found in diffuse and nodular lymphatic tissue, they are not the principal component of PALS in the spleen.
Keywords: Spleen, white pulp, PALS

40 **The answer is E: T lymphocytes.** Immunity is a powerful system for defense against invasion by foreign pathogens, but defects in immune regulation can lead to serious tissue

injury. Congenital or acquired defects in suppressor/regulator T-cell function are believed to contribute to the pathogenesis of many hypersensitivity reactions (e.g., allergic rhinitis, bronchial asthma) and autoimmune diseases (systemic lupus erythematosus, Graves disease). Suppressor/regulatory T lymphocytes have been shown to modulate immune responses. They (1) terminate cycles of immune cell activation, (2) maintain tolerance to self-antigens, and (3) prevent autoimmunity. Natural killer cells (choice D) recognize and kill transformed and virus-infected cells. None of the other cells regulates the immune system by suppressing the activation and maturation of lymphocytes.
Keywords: Autoimmune disease, hypersensitivity reactions

41 **The answer is E: IgE-mediated mast cell degranulation.**
Allergies are type I hypersensitivity reactions that occur within minutes after exposure to an "allergen" to which the person has been previously sensitized. Immediate hypersensitivity reactions may be associated with bronchoconstriction, airway obstruction, and circulatory collapse (anaphylactic shock). Allergic rhinitis (hay fever) is the most common type I hypersensitivity disease in adults. It is caused by pollen, house dust, animal dandruff, and other allergens. Inhaled antigens react with IgE antibodies attached to basophils and mast cells in the nasal mucosa, thereby triggering the release of vasoactive substances. These vasoactive mediators increase the permeability of mucosal vessels, causing runny nose and sneezing. None of the other mechanisms of inflammation and immunity cause seasonal allergies.
Keywords: Hay fever, hypersensitivity reactions

42 **The answer is B: Histamine.** Soft tissue swelling at the site of a positive skin reaction is caused by increased vascular permeability and the accumulation of extravascular edema fluid. Type I hypersensitivity reactions feature the formation of IgE antibodies that bind avidly to mast cells and basophils. Subsequent exposure to the allergen induces an immediate release of histamine from stored cytoplasmic granules (degranulation). Histamine stimulates smooth muscle contraction, edema formation, and the recruitment of eosinophils. Immediate hypersensitivity affecting the skin is appropriately referred to as allergic contact dermatitis. None of the other mediators of inflammation are stored in cytoplasmic granules and released by tissue mast cells upon activation.
Keywords: Contact dermatitis, mast cells

43 **The answer is B: Cytokine secretion.** Delayed hypersensitivity is a tissue reaction involving lymphocytes and mononuclear phagocytes that occurs in response to a soluble protein antigen and reaches greatest intensity 24 to 48 hours after exposure. In the initial phase, foreign protein antigens or chemical ligands interact with antigen-presenting cells bearing MHC class II molecules. Protein antigens are actively processed into short peptides

within phagolysosomes and are presented on the cell surface in conjunction with MHC class II molecules. The latter are recognized by CD4+ T cells, which become activated to synthesize an array of cytokines (signaling proteins). The cytokines recruit and activate lymphocytes, monocytes, fibroblasts, and other chronic inflammatory cells. Induration at the site of injection indicates that this patient had prior exposure to *Mycobacterium tuberculosis*. None of the other choices describe the function of helper T lymphocytes in delayed hypersensitivity.
Keywords: Cellular immunity, tuberculosis

44 **The answer is A: IgA.** Bodily secretions are protected from microbes and pathogens by secretory IgA antibody. IgA antibodies are present in tears, breast milk (colostrum), saliva, and vaginal fluid. They are also present in secretions of the prostate, nasal cavity, bronchi, and gastrointestinal tract. For unknown reasons, rarely, some women become sensitized to sperm antigens and become infertile. None of the other immunoglobulin classes (heavy chain isotypes) is transported across epithelial boundaries into body fluid secretions.
Keywords: Infertility, immunoglobulins

45 **The answer is B: Cell-mediated immunity.** Poison ivy is perhaps the most common example of cell-mediated, delayed-type hypersensitivity. Chemical ligands from the poison ivy plant (urushiol) interact with antigen-presenting cells (Langerhans cells, macrophages) to form immunogenic cell surface HLA molecules. These structures are recognized by CD4+ T cells, which become activated to synthesize cytokines (signaling proteins) that recruit other chronic inflammatory cells. Mast cell degranulation (choice D) may contribute to increased vascular permeability in patients with poison ivy; however, the principal activation pathway involves cytokine secretion by helper T lymphocytes. None of the other mechanisms of inflammation and immunity explain the pathogenesis of delayed-type hypersensitivity.
Keywords: Hypersensitivity, poison ivy

46 **The answer is A: β-Chemokine receptor-5.** HIV-1 infections and acquired immunodeficiency syndrome (AIDS) affect tens of millions of people worldwide (worldwide pandemic). Specific target cells for HIV-1 infection are CD4+ helper T lymphocytes and mononuclear phagocytes. The HIV envelope glycoprotein gp120 binds CD4 on the surface of helper T lymphocytes. Binding of gp120 to CD4 allows gp41 to insert into the plasma membrane of the lymphocyte, thereby promoting fusion of the viral envelope with the lymphocyte. Entry of HIV-1 into a target cell in vivo also requires viral binding to a coreceptor, namely β-chemokine receptor-5 (CCR-5). Rare individuals who lack CCR-5 are resistant to HIV infection, and bone marrow transplants from these individuals have provided functional cures for a few patients with AIDS. GlyCAM-1 and L-selectin (choices B and D) mediate leukocyte homing. Integrin $\alpha v \beta_3$ and LFA-1 (choices C and E) are members of the integrin family of proteins that mediate cell–cell adhesion.

Keywords: Acquired immunodeficiency

47 **The answer is B: Granzyme.**   Cytolytic T lymphocytes recognize immunogenic viral peptides carried by MHC class I molecules on the surface of virus-infected cells. CD8+ cytolytic T cells are class I restricted. After binding to a target cell, killer T cells release activators of apoptosis, including perforins and granzymes. Perforins form membrane pores that contribute to cell death and also facilitate the entry of granzymes into target cells. Granzymes are serine proteases. Once inside a target cell, granzymes activate other proteases (caspases) that initiate apoptosis. Residual apoptotic bodies are engulfed by macrophages. Major basic protein (choice D) is stored in the cytoplasmic granules of eosinophils and is toxic to parasitic infestations. None of the other proteins mediates killing of HIV-infected cells by CD8+ T lymphocytes.

Keywords: Acquired immunodeficiency, T cells

48 **The answer is E: Tumor necrosis factor–α.**   Fever is an important systemic manifestation of acute and chronic inflammation. Elevation of body temperature is caused by the release of specific cytokines (termed pyrogens), primarily from activated macrophages. These pyrogens include interleukin-1 (IL-1) and tumor necrosis factor–α (TNF-α). Pyrogens act on the hypothalamus of the brain to alter the central "thermostat." Chills (sensation of cold), rigor (profound chills with shivering and piloerection), and sweats (to allow heat dissipation) are symptoms associated with fever. Prostacyclin and thromboxane A$_2$ (choices C and D) are prostaglandins that have direct effects on the microcirculation. The other choices are mediators of inflammation, but they do not directly control body temperature.

Keywords: Bacterial pneumonia, pyrogens

Chapter 10

Cardiovascular System

QUESTIONS

Select the single best answer.

1 A 68-year-old man develops sudden, severe substernal chest pain. Laboratory studies and ECG confirm an acute myocardial infarction (heart attack). The patient cannot maintain his blood pressure and expires 4 hours later. Which of the following was the most likely cause of the patient's death?

(A) Cardiogenic shock
(B) Hypovolemic shock
(C) Neurogenic shock
(D) Respiratory insufficiency
(E) Septic shock

2 The heart of the patient described in Question 1 is examined at autopsy. Routine H&E staining reveals layered structures within the wall of the heart (shown in the image). Identify the indicated layer.

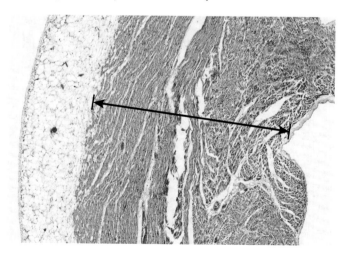

(A) Endocardium
(B) Epicardium
(C) Myocardium
(D) Parietal layer of the pericardium
(E) Visceral layer of the pericardium

3 The autopsy specimen described in Question 2 is examined at higher magnification (shown in the image). Identify the indicated structure.

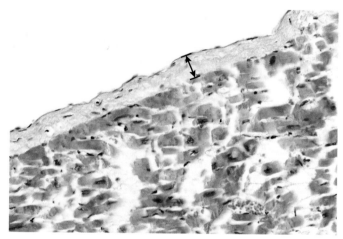

(A) Endocardium
(B) Epicardium
(C) Mesothelium
(D) Myocardium
(E) Purkinje fibers

4 Another region of the autopsy specimen described in Questions 2 and 3 is examined in the pathology department (shown in the image). Identify the indicated zone.

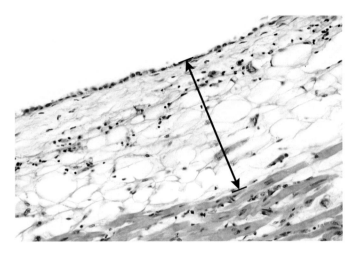

(A) Endocardium
(B) Epicardium
(C) Fibrous pericardium
(D) Myocardium
(E) Visceral pleura

5 Two weeks after suffering a massive heart attack, a 54-year-old man presents to the emergency room complaining of sharp pain on the left side of his chest. On physical examination, the patient is apprehensive and sweating. His blood pressure is 80/40 mm Hg, and the pulse rate is 100 per minute. The patient expires shortly after admission. At autopsy, the left ventricle shows a rupture in the myocardial wall. What was the most likely cause of the patient's death?
(A) Cardiac tamponade
(B) Dissecting aortic aneurysm
(C) Pulmonary edema
(D) Pulmonary thromboembolism
(E) Septic shock

6 Autopsy of the patient described in Question 5 reveals 400 mL of blood in the pericardial cavity. This blood is in direct contact with which of the following anatomic structures?
(A) Endocardium
(B) Epicardium
(C) Fibrous pericardium
(D) Myocardium
(E) Parietal pleura

7 A 52-year-old man with a history of active pulmonary tuberculosis presents with difficulty breathing, chest pain, and abdominal discomfort. Physical examination reveals hepatomegaly, ascites, and pitting edema of the legs (signs of right-sided heart failure). Cardiac auscultation demonstrates a pericardial friction rub. The patient is subsequently diagnosed with constrictive pericarditis caused by spread of his mycobacterial infection to the pericardial cavity. Which of the following structures of the heart was most directly and severely affected by this patient's infectious disease?
(A) Conducting system of the heart
(B) Coronary arteries
(C) Endocardium
(D) Myocardium
(E) Pericardium

8 Heart tissue obtained at autopsy is embedded, sectioned at 6 μm, and stained with H&E (shown in the image). Identify the structure within the rectangular box.

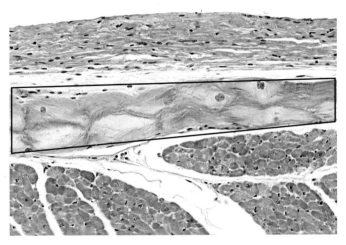

(A) Adipose tissue
(B) Cardiac muscle fibers
(C) Loose connective tissue
(D) Purkinje fibers
(E) Smooth muscle fibers

9 A 56-year-old man complains of recurring heart palpitations and is subsequently diagnosed with a cardiac arrhythmia. Which of the following cardiac structures functions as the "pacemaker" of the heart?
(A) Atrioventricular bundle of His
(B) Atrioventricular node
(C) Purkinje fibers
(D) Sinoatrial node
(E) Sympathetic fibers

10 A 13-year-old girl is discovered to have a left-sided heart murmur during her annual physical examination. One year ago, the girl presented with bacterial pharyngitis (strep throat). Her symptoms included fever, malaise, joint swelling, and a diffuse skin rash. She was treated with an antibiotic and recovered. Based on the patient's past medical history, the recent heart murmur is most likely associated with which of the following underlying conditions?
(A) Dilated cardiomyopathy
(B) Dissecting aortic aneurysm
(C) Myocardial infarction
(D) Pulmonary thromboembolism
(E) Rheumatic heart disease

11 For the patient described in Question 10, which of the following heart structures was most likely injured by episodes of rheumatic fever?
(A) Coronary arteries
(B) Interatrial septum
(C) Interventricular septum
(D) Mitral valve
(E) Purkinje fibers

12 You are asked to lead a problem-based learning session on valvular heart disease. Which of the following tissues forms the central core of heart valves?
(A) Avascular dense connective tissue
(B) Cardiac muscle fibers
(C) Elastic connective tissue
(D) Smooth muscle fibers
(E) Vascular loose connective tissue

13 A 56-year-old woman is diagnosed with a left atrial myxoma. The tumor is removed, and the surgical specimen is examined by light microscopy. The tumor margin shows normal heart tissue (shown in the image). The structure within the circle represents a branch of which of the following blood vessels?

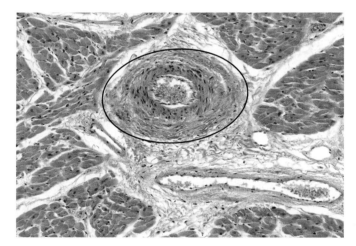

(A) Cardiac vein
(B) Coronary artery
(C) Coronary sinus
(D) Internal thoracic artery
(E) Supreme thoracic artery

14 The epicardium of the surgical specimen described in Question 13 is examined in the pathology department. Identify the structure indicated by the circle.

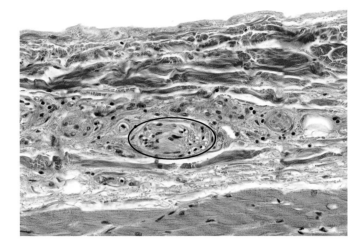

(A) Arteriole
(B) Cardiac muscle
(C) Connective tissue
(D) Nerve
(E) Venule

15 During a clinical rotation through the cardiac intensive care unit of the hospital, you are asked to discuss the control of heart rate by the autonomic nervous system. Which of the following best describes the primary function of sympathetic stimulation on the heart?
(A) Constriction of coronary arteries
(B) Decreases heart rate
(C) Increases heart rate
(D) Initiates cardiac muscle contraction
(E) Reduces the force of muscle contraction

16 A 68-year-old man with a history of smoking and hypertension suffers sudden cardiac arrest and expires. The patient's thoracic aorta is examined at autopsy. Identify layer "A" (shown in the image).

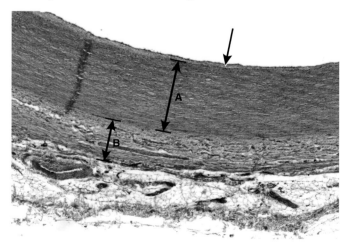

(A) Endothelium
(B) Myocardium
(C) Tunica adventitia
(D) Tunica intima
(E) Tunica media

17 The autopsy specimen described in Question 16 is examined at higher magnification (shown in the image). Identify the cells whose nuclei are indicated by the arrows.

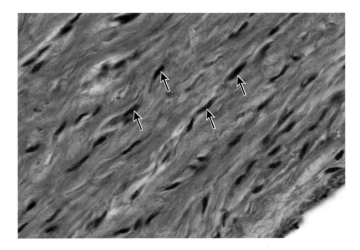

(A) Adipocytes
(B) Cardiac muscle cells
(C) Fibroblasts
(D) Macrophages
(E) Smooth muscle cells

18 A section of the aorta obtained from the patient described in Question 16 is treated with Verhoff van Gieson stain to visualize connective tissue elements in the tunica media (shown in the image). The dark wavy lines represent which of the following histologic structures?

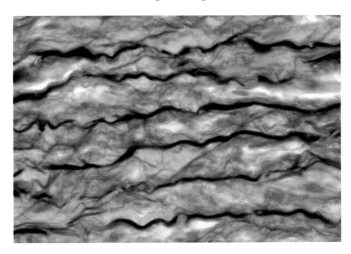

(A) Collagen fibers
(B) Elastic lamellae
(C) Nerve fibers
(D) Reticular fibers
(E) Smooth muscle fibers

19 A 73-year-old man with a history of hypertension presents to the emergency room with "tearing" chest pain. His blood pressure is 85/45 mm Hg, and his pulse rate is 100 per minute. The patient expires shortly after

admission. A dissecting aneurysm of the descending arch of the aorta is discovered at autopsy. Microscopic examination of the aortic wall reveals tearing/dissection along the outer third of the tunica media (shown in the image). This patient's dissecting aneurysm was most likely caused by chronic injury (and subsequent failure) to which of the following vascular structures?

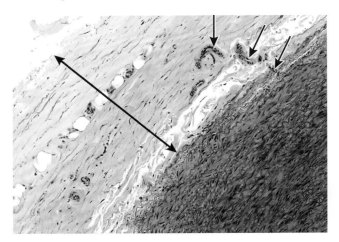

(A) Collagen fibers in the tunica adventitia
(B) Elastic lamellae in the tunica media
(C) Endothelial cells in the tunica intima
(D) Subintimal connective tissue
(E) Vasa vasorum in the tunica adventitia

20 A section of aorta is stained with an elastic stain and examined in the histology laboratory (shown in the image). Identify the structures indicated by the arrows.

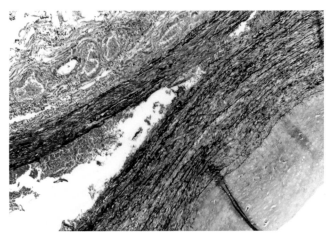

(A) Adipocytes
(B) Collagen fibers
(C) Elastic fibers
(D) Nervi vascularis
(E) Vasa vasorum

21 A 39-year-old immigrant presents to the emergency room with a rapid pulse and cold clammy skin. A CT scan of the thorax reveals dilation of the ascending aorta. The fluorescent treponemal antibody (FTA) test is positive.

The patient is subsequently diagnosed with a syphilitic aneurysm. Which of the following mechanisms of disease is the most likely cause of aortic aneurysm in this patient?

(A) Atherosclerosis
(B) Cystic medial necrosis
(C) Endarteritis of the vasa vasorum
(D) Fibrillin gene mutation
(E) Systemic hypertension

22 A section of the aorta is examined in the histology laboratory. The luminal surface of the vascular wall is shown at high magnification in the image. Which of the following describes the area indicated by the double arrow?

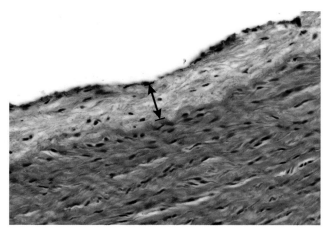

(A) Elastic lamella
(B) Endothelium
(C) Internal elastic membrane
(D) Subendothelium
(E) Tunica media

23 A 69-year-old woman presents with crushing substernal chest pain and nausea. She is treated with plasminogen activator, oxygen, and morphine sulfate. The patient subsequently becomes hypotensive and suffers cardiac arrest. A cross-section of the patient's anterior interventricular artery is examined at autopsy (shown in the image). Which of the following best describes the pathologic changes visible in this specimen?

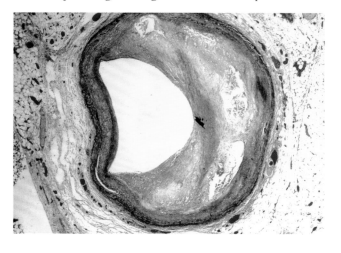

(A) Acute arteritis
(B) Aneurysmal dilation
(C) Atherosclerosis
(D) Thrombosis
(E) Vasodilation

24 Microscopic examination of the autopsy specimen described in Question 23 at high magnification would most likely reveal which of the following pathologic changes?

(A) Acute inflammation in the tunica adventitia
(B) Bacterial colonies in the tunica media
(C) Cystic medial necrosis in the tunica intima
(D) Lipid deposition and smooth muscle cell hyperplasia in the tunica intima
(E) Obliterative endarteritis of the vasa vasorum

25 Lipid accumulation in the atheroma described in Questions 23 and 24 was primarily related to chronic injury and dysfunction of which of the following vascular components?

(A) Adventitial connective tissue
(B) Elastic lamellae
(C) Endothelial cells
(D) Smooth muscle cells
(E) Subendothelial connective tissue

26 A neonate has a small, raised, strawberry-colored skin lesion on her forehead. A biopsy reveals benign vascular channels filled with blood (shown in the image). Which of the following types of cells lines these vascular channels?

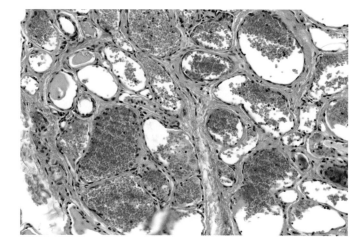

(A) Endothelial cells
(B) Fibroblasts
(C) Inflammatory cells
(D) Mesothelial cells
(E) Smooth muscle cells

27 A neurovascular bundle from the upper limb is collected at autopsy, and the tissue sections are processed using Weigert elastica staining reagent. The wall of a blood vessel is examined by light microscopy (shown in the image). Based on these histologic findings, this blood vessel is best identified as which of the following?

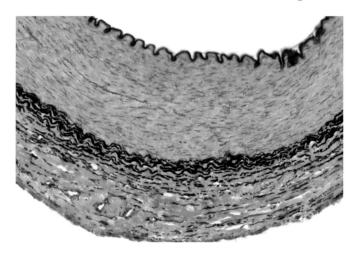

(A) Arteriole
(B) Elastic artery
(C) Large vein
(D) Muscular artery
(E) Small artery

28 Sections from the autopsy specimen described in Question 27 are processed using a different histochemical stain and examined by light microscopy (shown in the image). The layer of the artery indicated by the double arrow is primarily composed of which of the following vascular components?

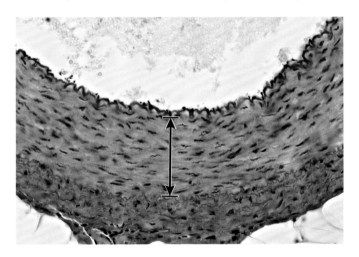

(A) Collagen fibers
(B) Elastic lamellae
(C) Fibroblasts
(D) Reticular fibers
(E) Smooth muscle cells

29 A 30-year-old man suffers a sudden and severe headache during a basketball game and loses consciousness. The patient is rushed to the hospital but expires 2 days later. Autopsy demonstrates a massive subarachnoid hemor-

rhage arising from a balloon-like outpouching near the origin of the posterior cerebral artery. Which of the following mechanisms of disease best explains the pathogenesis of this patient's saccular (berry) aneurysm?
(A) Cystic medial necrosis
(B) Deficiency of smooth muscle
(C) Endarteritis of the vasa vasorum
(D) Formation of atheromatous plaque
(E) Platelet aggregation and degranulation

30 A colon biopsy is examined in the pathology department (shown in the image). Identify the blood vessel located within the submucosa of the appendix.

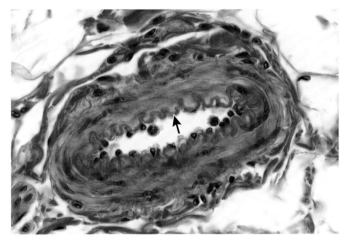

(A) Arteriole
(B) Elastic artery
(C) Medium artery
(D) Small artery
(E) Small vein

31 You watch a group of high school students playing football. Which of the following components of the circulatory system plays the most important role in directing increased blood flow to capillaries in the skeletal muscles of these young athletes?
(A) Aorta
(B) Arterioles
(C) Heart
(D) Medium arteries
(E) Pulmonary arteries

32 A 55-year-old man complains of recurring dizziness and nausea for about 1 year. His blood pressure is 170/110 mm Hg. Which of the following contributes the most to the pathogenesis of systemic hypertension in this patient?
(A) Arterial cystic medial necrosis
(B) Increased heart rate
(C) Increased peripheral vascular resistance
(D) Increased vascular permeability
(E) Vasodilation of arterioles

33 A section of the myocardium obtained at autopsy is stained with H&E and examined in the pathology department (shown in the image). Identify the structure indicated by the arrow.

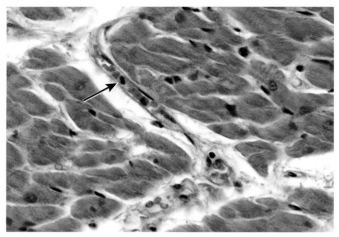

(A) Arteriole
(B) Capillary
(C) Lymphatic vessel
(D) Small artery
(E) Venule

34 A 68-year-old man with a history of smoking presents with chest pain and mild fever. The patient is subsequently diagnosed with lung cancer. Examination of the surgical specimen reveals normal tissue along the tumor margin (shown in image). Which of the following best describes structural features of the capillary indicated by the arrow?

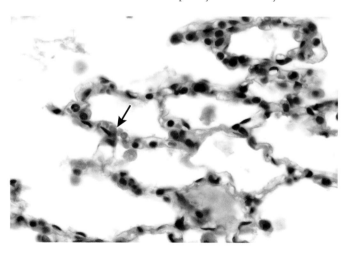

(A) Continuous endothelial cells with continuous basal lamina
(B) Discontinuous endothelial cells with discontinuous basal lamina
(C) Endothelial cells with fenestrations covered by diaphragms
(D) Fenestrated endothelial cells with continuous basal lamina
(E) Sinusoidal capillary with discontinuous basal lamina

35 A 59-year-old diabetic woman complains of declining visual acuity. Funduscopic examination of the patient's retina reveals capillary microaneurysms and small hemorrhage. Loss of which of the following components from the capillary wall is the most likely cause of early-stage diabetic retinopathy in this patient?
(A) Basal lamina
(B) Elastic fibers
(C) Endothelial cells
(D) Pericytes
(E) Smooth muscle cells

36 A 48-year-old woman presents with a painful, raised, red lesion on the dorsal surface of her right hand. Histologic examination of a skin biopsy reveals a benign tumor of the glomus body. Which of the following best describes the structure of a normal glomus body in the dermis of the skin?
(A) Arteriovenous shunt
(B) Capillary loop in the dermal papillae
(C) Deep dermal venous plexus
(D) Dilated lymphatic channel
(E) Vascularized skin wart

37 You are asked to lead a small group discussion on topics related to the histology and physiology of the cardiovascular system. Which of the following best describes the biological function of arteriovenous shunts in the skin?
(A) Activation of coagulation and hemostasis
(B) Drainage of extravascular lymphedema
(C) Regulation of capillary permeability
(D) Regulation of granulocyte diapedesis during acute inflammation
(E) Temperature-dependent regulation of blood flow

38 During your group discussion, you are asked to discuss mechanisms that regulate blood flow through the heart in response to physiologic needs for oxygen and nutrients. Which of the following structures directly regulates blood flow to the microvascular bed in the heart?
(A) Arteriole endothelial cells
(B) Capillary endothelial cells
(C) Connective tissue capsule of AV shunts
(D) Postcapillary venules
(E) Precapillary sphincters

39 A 38-year-old man develops a painful femoral hernia, and the herniated intestinal segment is removed surgically. Microscopic examination of the submucosa reveals a series of small blood vessels (shown in the image). Identify the vessel indicated by the arrow.

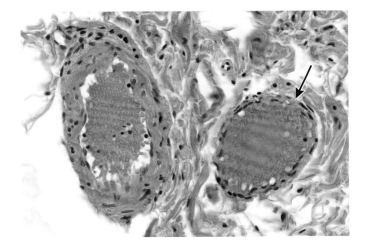

(A) Arteriole
(B) Capillary
(C) Muscular artery
(D) Small vein
(E) Venule

40 A 17-year-old wrestler presents with a painful sore on his right shoulder. Physical examination reveals a 0.7-cm abscess that drains thick, purulent material. Diapedesis of leukocytes into and around this patient's infected wound occurs primarily at which of the following locations?

(A) Capillary bed
(B) Lymphatic capillary
(C) Postcapillary venule
(D) Precapillary arteriole
(E) Proximal lymph node

41 A 56-year-old man presents with painful dilated knots in both legs. Ulcers are noted over some of the knots. A photograph of the patient is shown. Which of the following structures in the legs is most likely affected in this patient?

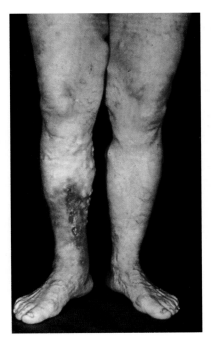

(A) Cutaneous nerves
(B) Deep veins
(C) Small arteries
(D) Superficial lymphatic vessels
(E) Superficial veins

42 A skin biopsy is taken from the patient described in Question 41. Microscopic examination reveals blood vessels in the subcutaneous tissue (shown in the image). Identify the structures indicated by the arrows.

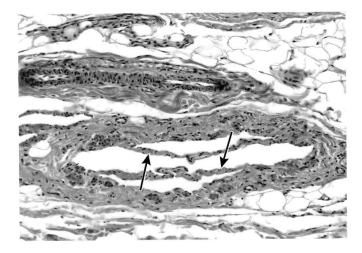

(A) Arteriovenous shunt
(B) Lymphatic vessels
(C) Smooth muscle fibers
(D) Subendothelial connective tissue
(E) Venous valves

43 An ulnar neurovascular bundle is harvested at autopsy and examined using the trichrome stain to help distinguish between collagenous connective tissue, red blood cells, and smooth muscle (shown in the image). Identify this patient's blood vessel.

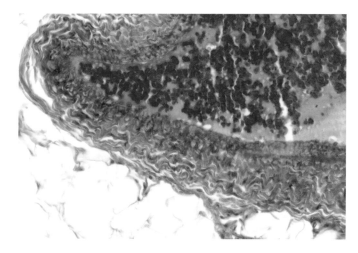

(A) Large vein
(B) Muscular artery
(C) Medium vein
(D) Small artery
(E) Venule

44 A segment of the inferior vena cava is obtained at autopsy and examined by routine H&E staining (shown in the image). Identify the structures indicated by the arrows.

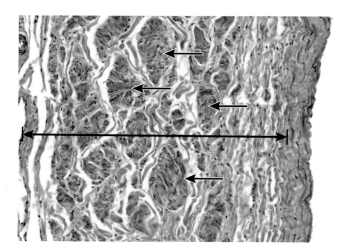

(A) Bundles of elastic fibers
(B) Collagen fibers
(C) Nervi vascularis
(D) Smooth muscle fibers
(E) Vasa vasorum

45 A kidney biopsy is stained with the trichrome reagent and examined in the pathology department (shown in the image). Blood that circulates through the glomerular capillary tuft within the renal corpuscle (indicated by the arrow) drains into which of the following renal blood vessels?

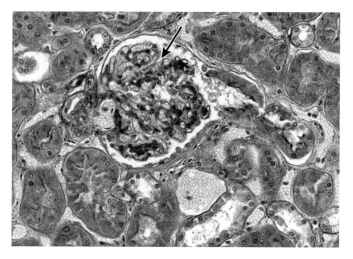

(A) Afferent arteriole
(B) Efferent arteriole
(C) Peritubular capillary
(D) Vasa recta
(E) Venule

46 A 48-year-old man is rushed to the emergency room after he began to vomit blood and experienced bloody stools. The patient develops hypovolemic shock and expires shortly after admission. The patient was an alcoholic and was diagnosed with alcoholic cirrhosis 2 years ago. Which of the following pathologic conditions is the most likely underlying cause of death in this patient?
(A) Alcoholic hepatitis
(B) Esophageal varices
(C) Ischemia of the gastric mucosa
(D) Mallory-Weiss syndrome
(E) Peptic ulcer disease

47 A 28-year-old woman experiences sudden chest pain and is rushed to the emergency room. The patient is unable to maintain cardiac output and expires the following day. Autopsy reveals a thromboembolus at the bifurcation of the right pulmonary artery. Which of the following mechanisms of disease is the most likely cause of pulmonary thromboembolism in this patient?
(A) Bacterial endocarditis
(B) Complicated atherosclerotic plaque
(C) Deep vein thrombosis
(D) Paradoxical embolization
(E) Right ventricular mural thrombus

48 A lymph node from the patient described in Question 47 is examined by light microscopy. At the hilum of the lymph node, a series of vascular structures are observed. Identify the vessels indicated by the asterisk.

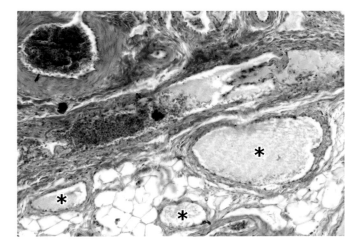

(A) Arterioles
(B) Lymphatic vessels
(C) Small arteries
(D) Veins
(E) Venules

49 A biopsy of the jejunum is examined in the histology laboratory. A section through an intestinal villus is shown in image. Identify the channel indicated by the arrow.

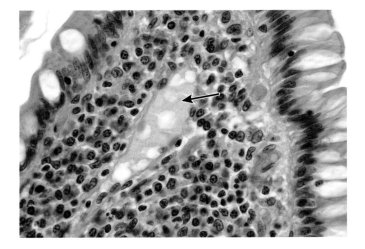

(A) Arteriole
(B) Capillary
(C) Lymphatic capillary
(D) Small vein
(E) Venule

50 You are part of a medical team that is visiting small villages in several South Asian countries. A 33-year-old man presents with massive edema of the scrotum and left lower extremity. The patient is shown in the image. He is diagnosed with a filarial roundworm infestation. The parasites have lodged in and obstructed which of the following vessels in this patient?

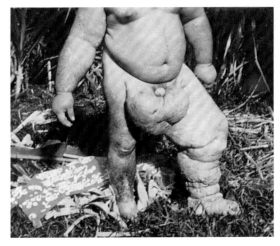

(A) Capillaries in the mesentery
(B) Capillaries in the skin
(C) Lower limb arteries
(D) Lower limb veins
(E) Lymphatic vessels

ANSWERS

1 **The answer is A: Cardiogenic shock.** A myocardial infarct is a geographic area of necrosis in the heart that is caused by acute blockage of a coronary artery. Patients suffering a myocardial infarction are at risk of developing shock related to pump failure. The end result is an inability of the heart to adequately perfuse tissues and organs with blood. Cardiogenic shock typically arises as a complication of myocardial infarction but may be caused by several other conditions, including arrhythmias, pulmonary embolism, cardiac tamponade, myocarditis, dissecting aneurysm, and hypertrophic cardiomyopathy. These medical conditions either prevent heart filling or reduce cardiac output. None of the other medical conditions are associated with reduced cardiac output in a patient with a recent history of myocardial infarction.
Keywords: Myocardial infarction, shock

2 **The answer is C: Myocardium.** The heart is a folded endothelial tube with a thickened muscular wall that pumps blood through the circulatory system. The principal functional component of the heart is the myocardial layer (myocardium) that is composed of cardiac muscle. The myocardium is covered externally by an epicardium (choice B), consisting of a layer of mesothelium and associated adipose connective tissue. The inner (luminal) surface of the myocardium is lined by endocardium (choice A), consisting of a layer of endothelium and associated connective tissue. Parietal layer of pericardium (choice D) lines the fibrous pericardial sac and is not visible in this section. Visceral layer of pericardium (choice E) refers to the mesothelial cell layer of epicardium. The myocardium is considerably thicker in the ventricles, than in the atria, reflecting the needs of the ventricles to propel blood through pulmonary and systemic circulations.
Keywords: Heart, myocardium

3 **The answer is A: Endocardium.** Endocardium lines the luminal surface of the heart chambers. It is composed of a layer of endothelium and subendothelial connective tissue. Smooth muscle fibers can be found in the subendothelial connective tissue. Purkinje fibers (choice E) are specialized cardiomyocytes that conduct action potentials in the heart. None of the other tissue layers describe histologic features of the endocardium.
Keywords: Heart, endocardium

4 **The answer is B: Epicardium.** Epicardium covers the external surface of the heart and is in direct contact with the potential space provided by the pericardial cavity. Epicardium is composed of (1) a layer of the mesothelium (visceral layer of serous pericardium) and (2) an underlying adipose connective tissue. The adipose tissue functions as a cushion for the heart as it moves within the pericardial sac. Blood vessels and nerves supplying the heart travel through the epicardium. Endocardium (choice A) lines the luminal surface of the heart and is typically devoid of adipose tissue. Fibrous pericardium (choice C) is composed of dense connective tissue and is not visible in this image. Visceral pleura (choice E) represents a layer of mesothelium that is adherent to the surface of the lungs.
Keywords: Heart, epicardium

5 **The answer is A: Cardiac tamponade.** Rupture of a myocardial infarct causes blood to fill the peritoneal cavity (hemopericardium). This medical catastrophe restricts the motion of the heart and is referred to as cardiac tamponade. When it happens, it typically occurs within the first 3 weeks following myocardial infarction. Pulsus paradoxus (>10 mm Hg drop in arterial blood pressure with inspiration) is commonly observed in patients with hemopericardium. Although aortic dissections (choice B) can break through to the pericardium, they do not rupture the heart wall. None of the other cardiovascular diseases are associated with rupture of the heart wall and cardiac tamponade.
Keywords: Hemopericardium, cardiac tamponade

6 **The answer is B: Epicardium.** The pericardial sac is lined by visceral and parietal mesothelia that together are referred to as serous pericardium. The visceral layer of serous pericardium represents the mesothelial layer of the epicardium. The parietal layer of serous pericardium lines the inner surface of the fibrous pericardium (choice C). The space between the visceral and parietal layers of serous pericardium defines the pericardial cavity. In normal condition, a thin layer of serous fluid within the pericardial cavity (about 50 mL) provides lubrication for movement of the heart during contraction. Myocardial rupture, pericarditis, or chest injuries can cause excess fluid or blood to accumulate in the pericardial cavity. Accumulation of excess fluid or blood restricts ventricular filling, a life-threatening condition referred to as cardiac tamponade. Pericardiocentesis is often required to drain excess pericardial fluid to relieve pressure on the heart. None of the other structures are in direct contact with the pericardial cavity.
Keywords: Cardiac tamponade, heart, epicardium

7 **The answer is E: Pericardium.** The pericardium is a sac that surrounds and protects the heart. It is composed of an outer fibrous pericardium and an inner serous pericardium. The potential space between visceral and parietal layers of the serous pericardium defines the pericardial cavity. Infections within the pericardial cavity cause acute or chronic pericarditis. An exuberant healing response to pericarditis can obliterate the pericardial cavity. In these patients, visceral and parietal layers of the pericardium are fused together by dense deposits of collagenous scar tissue. As a result, the heart is compressed and cardiac filling is restricted. This condition is referred to as constrictive pericarditis.
Keywords: Constrictive pericarditis, pericardium

8 **The answer is D: Purkinje fibers.** Purkinje fibers are components of the conducting system of the heart. They are found within the subendocardial connective tissue of the ventricles and along both sides of the interventricular septum. Purkinje fibers are modified cardiac myocytes that are specialized for the conduction of action potentials (impulses). They are considerably larger than typical cardiac muscle fibers. Their cytoplasm shows a sparse distribution of myofibrils, located primarily near the periphery of the cells. Abundant intracellular deposits of glycogen provide an important energy reserve for these metabolically active cells. Because the glycogen deposits are extracted during tissue processing, the cytoplasm of Purkinje fibers typically appears pale (washed-out). None of the other structures demonstrate histologic features of Purkinje cells.
Keywords: Heart, Purkinje fibers

9 **The answer is D: Sinoatrial node.** Rhythmic cardiac muscle contractions are initiated and propagated by the conducting system of the heart. The conducting system of the heart consists of the (1) sinoatrial (SA) node, (2) atrioventricular (AV) node, (3) AV bundle of His, and (4) right and left bundle branches. The SA node, situated at the junction of superior vena cava and the right atrium, is composed of specialized nodal cardiac muscle cells. Because the SA node generates electrical impulses and has the fastest depolarization rate, it is commonly referred to as the "pacemaker" of the heart. Impulses from the SA node are conducted to the AV node (choice B) through an internodal pathway. The AV node is located in the interatrial septum near the orifice of the coronary sinus. The AV node generates impulses at a considerably lower rate than the SA node and, therefore, cannot function as pacemaker of the heart. The AV bundle of His (choice A) and Purkinje fibers (choice C) transmit impulses from the AV node to ventricular cardiac muscle. Sympathetic fibers (choice E) regulate heart rate, but they do not initiate cardiac muscle contraction.
Keywords: Heart, sinoatrial node

10 **The answer is E: Rheumatic heart disease.** Rheumatic fever develops after antibodies to surface antigens of group A (beta hemolytic) streptococci cross-react with similar antigens found in the heart, joints, and connective tissue of the skin. Cardiac lesions caused by acute rheumatic fever include endocarditis, myocarditis, and pericarditis (or all three combined). Chronic rheumatic endocarditis causes fibrous scarring in the heart leading to murmurs and other functional defects. None of the other cardiopulmonary diseases are associated with streptococcal infections of the pharynx.
Keywords: Rheumatic heart disease

11 **The answer is D: Mitral valve.** Heart murmurs are signs of valvular heart disease. The inflammatory reaction following a streptococcal infection commonly involves heart valves (acute valvulitis). Inflammation induces neovascularization in the normally avascular central core of the heart valves. Repeated bouts of rheumatic endocarditis result in fibrous scarring and deformity of the cardiac valves, as well as insufficiency or stenosis of valvular orifices, leading to heart murmurs and functional defects. The mitral valve is the most commonly affected valve (65% to 70%) in patients with chronic rheumatic heart disease, in part, because it closes under greater blood pressure than the other valves. The other cardiac structures listed are less likely to be affected by reactive antibodies and T lymphocytes in patients with rheumatic heart disease.
Keywords: Mitral valve, rheumatic heart disease

12 **The answer is A: Avascular dense connective tissue.** Mitral, tricuspid, aortic, and pulmonary heart valves have an avascular, dense connective tissue core (termed fibrosa) that is continuous with collagen fibers forming the fibrous skeleton of the heart. These valves are covered by a layer of loose connective tissue on the atrial or blood vessel side and by endothelium on the ventricular side. Heart valves are normally lacking in blood vessels, since they are continuously exposed to oxygen and nutrients in the blood. None of the other tissues characterize the central core of heart valves.
Keywords: Heart, valves

13 **The answer is B: Coronary artery.** The photomicrograph shows an arteriole and an accompanying venule embedded in adipose connective tissue. The heart receives arterial blood supply from the right and left coronary arteries—branches off the initial part of the ascending aorta. The coronary arteries give rise to numerous branches that travel within the adipose tissue of the epicardium near the surface of the heart. Cardiac veins (choice A) accompany branches of the coronary arteries. These veins drain to the coronary sinus (choice C) on the posterior wall of the heart, which, in turn, empties into the right atrium. None of the other blood vessels supply the heart.
Keywords: Arteries, coronary arteries

14 **The answer is D: Nerve.** As mentioned above, the nerves and major blood vessels supplying the heart travel within the epicardium. Nerves innervating the heart contain sympathetic, parasympathetic, and visceral afferent (sensory) fibers. An arteriole (choice A) is visible to the right of the nerve. The walls of arterioles are thicker than venules (choice E). Red blood cells are seen within the lumens of the blood vessels. Cardiac muscle fibers (choice B) are seen at the lower portion of the image. Connective tissue fibers (choice C) are seen in longitudinal, cross-, and oblique sections throughout the epicardium.
Keywords: Heart, epicardium

15 **The answer is C: Increases heart rate.** The cardiac plexus innervating the heart is composed of (1) sympathetic nerve fibers originating from the lateral horn of spinal cord segments T1 to T6 and (2) parasympathetic nerve fibers from the vagus nerve (cranial nerve X). These autonomic nerve fibers terminate at the sinoatrial (SA) and atrioventricular (AV) nodes of the conducting system of the heart and extend onto the coronary arteries. Sympathetic stimulation increases heart rate, force of contraction, and blood flow through dilated coronary arteries (support for increased heart activity). By contrast, parasympathetic stimulation slows heart rate, reduces the force of muscle contraction, and reduces blood flow to the heart (vasoconstriction). None of the other choices describe the primary function of sympathetic stimulation on the heart.

Keywords: Autonomic nervous system, sympathetic division, cardiac nervous plexus

16 **The answer is E: Tunica media.** Large- and medium-sized blood vessels are composed of three major layers or tunics: intima, media, and adventitia. The tunica media is the middle layer. It is sandwiched between the tunica intima near the vessel lumen (arrow, shown in the image) and connective tissue of the tunica adventitia (layer "B," shown in the image). The tunica media is the thickest of these layers in the aorta and other large elastic arteries. None of the other structures describe histologic features of the tunica media.

Keywords: Arteries, tunica media

17 **The answer is E: Smooth muscle cells.** Smooth muscle fibers form circumferential layers within the tunica media of large elastic arteries. Smooth muscle fibers typically appear as linear arrays of cells in cross-section (shown in the image). In addition to their contractile function, smooth muscle cells synthesize and secrete extracellular matrix components of the tunica media. These extracellular matrix molecules provide structural support to the vessel wall and help to convert the pulsatile blood flow leaving the heart to more continuous flow of blood in the microcirculation. Fibroblasts and macrophages (choices C and D) may migrate through the tunica media, but they would be difficult to identify without the use of special stains. None of the other cells are present in the tunica media of the vessel wall.

Keywords: Arteries, tunica media, smooth muscle cell

18 **The answer is B: Elastic lamellae.** Elastic lamellae (sheets) are found in the tunica media of large elastic arteries. These lamellae are fenestrated to facilitate diffusion of oxygen and nutrients from the blood. Elastic lamellae are arranged in concentric layers. In cross section, these sheets appear as wavy bands, interspersed with layers of smooth muscle (not visible in this preparation). Collagen fibers and reticular fibers (choices A and D) may be present in the tunica media, but they are not visible in this preparation. Large elastic arteries buffer the pulsatile (intermittent) blood flow leaving the heart. None of the other structures exhibit histologic features of elastic lamellae in the tunica media.

Keywords: Arteries, elastic lamellae

19 **The answer is B: Elastic lamellae in the tunica media.** Elastic lamellae are the principal structural support in the tunica media of elastic arteries. Chronic injury caused by hypertension and/or atherosclerosis can disrupt elastic lamellae, leading to vascular dilations (aneurysms) and aneurysmal tears (dissections). Patients with Marfan syndrome are also at risk for dissecting aortic aneurysms. These patients have missense mutations in the gene coding for fibrillin-1 (*FBN1*). Fibrillins are a family of connective tissue proteins analogous to collagens. They are widely distributed in many tissues in the form of fiber systems termed microfibrils. Deposition of elastin on microfibrils produces the distinctive concentric rings of elastic lamellae found in the aortic wall. Defects in the other structures would not be expected to disrupt elastic tissue in the tunic media of the aorta.

Keywords: Dissecting aortic aneurysms, arteries, elastic lamellae

20 **The answer is E: Vasa vasorum.** The tunica adventitia is the outermost layer of the blood vessel wall (indicated by the double arrow in the image). It is composed of loose connective tissue. Arteries and veins that supply the adventitia and outer portions of the media are referred to as vasa vasorum. These blood vessels travel in the tunica adventitia and send branches into the outer layer of the tunica media (arrows, shown in the image). Nerves innervating the wall of large blood vessels are referred to as nervi vascularis (choice D). Nerves are present in the tunica adventitia, but they are not visible in this section. Adipocytes, collagen fibers, and elastic fibers (choices A, B, and C) are also present in the tunica adventitia, but these cells/structures do not exhibit the distinctive histologic features of the vasa vasorum.

Keywords: Arteries, tunica adventitia, vasa vasorum

21 **The answer is C: Endarteritis of the vasa vasorum.** Syphilis is a sexual transmitted disease caused by the bacterium *Treponema pallidum*. At one time, syphilis was the most common cause of aortic aneurysm. Syphilitic aneurysms typically affect the ascending aorta, where infection causes endarteritis of the vasa vasorum. Ischemia caused by obliterative endarteritis of the vasa vasorum causes focal necrosis and loss of structural integrity in the tunica media. Blood flow during systole eventually stretches the aorta to form an aneurysmal dilation. As mentioned above, patients with Marfan syndrome are also at risk for dissecting aortic aneurysm. They have fibrillin gene mutations (choice D) that cause cystic medial necrosis in the tunica media (choice B). Atherosclerosis (choice A) and systemic hypertension (choice E) are important risk factors for aneurysms, but they would not be the most likely cause of an aneurysm affecting the ascending aorta in a woman with a history of untreated syphilis.

Keywords: Syphilitic aneurysm, vasa vasorum

22 **The answer is D: Subendothelium.** The tunica intima is the innermost layer of arteries and veins. It is composed of endothelium with a basal lamina and an underlying (subendothelial) layer of connective tissue. Endothelial cells (choice B) form a physical barrier to the vascular compartment and help regulate coagulation, inflammation, and wound healing. Smooth muscle cells constitute the major cell type found in the subendothelial connective tissue and secrete a variety of extracellular matrix molecules, including collagen and elastin. The tunica intima of large elastic arteries is relatively thick compared to other arteries. Elastic lamellae (choice A) are components of the tunica media (choice E) visible in the lower part of the image. Internal elastic membrane (choice C) is an elastic lamella along the most external portion of the subendothelial layer. This membrane is more prominent in the tunica media of muscular arteries and arterioles. In large arteries, the internal elastic membrane is inconspicuous, since it is merely the inner layer of many elastic lamellae.
Keywords: Arteries, tunica intima

23 **The answer is C: Atherosclerosis.** Atherosclerosis is the most common acquired abnormality of large- and medium-sized arteries. Major complications of atherosclerosis, including intermittent claudication, abdominal aortic aneurysm, coronary artery disease, cerebrovascular disease, and peripheral vascular disease, account for more than half of the annual deaths in the United States. Chest pain is the major complaint of patients with coronary artery disease (also referred to as ischemic heart disease). The pain typically occurs in the substernal portion of the chest and may radiate to the left arm, jaw, and/or epigastrium. Diabetes mellitus and hyperlipidemia are risk factors for atherosclerosis. The image shows atherosclerosis in the narrowed lumen. Thrombosis of an atherosclerotic plaque can result in ischemic necrosis of the dependent cardiac muscle (myocardial infarction). None of the other choices describe histologic features of atherosclerosis.
Keywords: Atherosclerosis, myocardial infarction

24 **The answer is D: Lipid deposition and smooth muscle cell hyperplasia in the tunica intima.** The classic lesion of atherosclerosis is best described as a fibroinflammatory lipid plaque (atheroma) in the tunica intima. Inflammatory and immune cells, hyperplastic smooth muscle fibers, cholesterol crystals, and other connective tissue components accumulate progressively in the tunica intima of large elastic and medium-sized muscular arteries. Microscopic examination of the atheroma reveals pools of extracellular lipid and numerous lipid-laden macrophages (foam cells). Atherosclerosis is not an infectious disease process or an acute inflammatory reaction (choices A and B). Cystic medial necrosis (choice C) is present in the tunica media in cases of dissecting aortic aneurysm. Obliterative endarteritis (choice E) describes the effects of tertiary syphilis.
Keywords: Ischemic heart disease, atherosclerosis

25 **The answer is C: Endothelial cells.** Loss of integrity of the vascular endothelial cell barrier initiates plaque formation in atherosclerosis. Hyperlipidemia, hyperglycemia, hypertension, smoking, and certain infections can lead to chronic injury and disruption of the endothelial cell barrier. Low-density lipoproteins (LDLs) in the blood carry lipids and cholesterol into the developing atheroma. Injured endothelial cells show increased permeability to LDL and increased production of reactive oxygen species such as O_2^-, which oxidizes LDL. Oxidized LDL activates endothelial cells and recruits macrophages and other inflammatory cells into the tunica intima. Macrophages phagocytize oxidized LDL and become lipid-laden "foam" cells. Hyperplastic smooth muscle cells in the subendothelial layer of the tunica intima also participate in lipid accumulation.
Keywords: Atherosclerosis, endothelial cells

26 **The answer is A: Endothelial cells.** Hemangiomas are benign tumors composed of vascular channels lined by endothelial cells. These congenital lesions occur primarily in the skin, where they may be termed ruby spots, strawberry birthmarks, or port wine stains. The photomicrograph shows numerous, closely packed, blood-filled capillaries. Loose connective tissue fills the interstitial space between blood channels. None of the other cells line vascular or lymphatic channels.
Keywords: Hemangioma, endothelial cells

27 **The answer is D: Muscular artery.** The arteries that conduct oxygenated blood from the heart to the microcirculation are traditionally grouped into three types based on their size and wall morphology. These types include (1) large or elastic arteries, (2) medium or muscular arteries, and (3) small arteries. The aorta and its larger branches and the pulmonary arteries are classified as large elastic arteries, since elastic lamellae constitute the major structural component of their tunica media. As these arteries branch, they are referred to as medium or muscular arteries. Examples of medium arteries include ulnar, popliteal, splenic, renal, and mesenteric arteries. The tunica intima is thinner in muscular arteries compared to elastic arteries. The internal elastic membrane is a prominent and characteristic feature of medium artery. Owing to the contraction of smooth muscle cells after death, internal elastic membranes typically appear as a folded line in histologic sections (shown in the image). An external elastic membrane is observed as a wavy line separating the tunica media from the tunica adventitia. None of the other types of blood vessels exhibit histologic features of medium arteries.
Keywords: Arteries, muscular arteries

28 The answer is E: Smooth muscle cells. The tunica media in medium arteries is composed almost entirely of smooth muscle fibers. As large elastic arteries undergo branching morphogenesis and their diameter becomes smaller, the tunica media exhibits a gradual reduction in elastic tissue, and a corresponding increase in smooth muscle cells. Smooth muscle fibers are the predominant structural and functional component of the tunica media in medium-sized muscular arteries. Contraction of smooth muscle cells in medium arteries helps maintain systemic blood pressure. Collagen and reticular fibers (choices A and D) are interspersed between smooth muscle cells, but they are not the major structural component of the tunica media. Elastic lamellae (choice B) and fibroblasts (choice C) are not present in the tunica media of medium arteries. Smooth muscle cells synthesize the extracellular matrix components (including collagen and reticular fibers and ground substance) present in the tunica media of medium arteries. **Keywords:** Muscular arteries, tunica media, smooth muscle cells

29 The answer is B: Deficiency of smooth muscle. Saccular aneurysms, also referred to as berry aneurysms, are balloon-like outpouchings of the arterial wall. They are the most common type of aneurysm affecting cerebral arteries. Berry aneurysms typically occur at branch points in the circle of Willis. At these locations, the wall of the artery may be weak, owing to a congenital deficiency of smooth muscle. Rupture of a berry aneurysm leads to catastrophic subarachnoid hemorrhage. Cystic medial necrosis and formation of atheromatous plaque (choices A and D) are associated with aortic aneurysms. Endarteritis of the vasa vasorum (choice C) is associated with syphilitic aneurysms of the ascending aorta. **Keywords:** Saccular aneurysm

30 The answer is A: Arteriole. Medium arteries branch repeatedly into smaller arteries. The smallest and most terminal branches of the arterial system are termed arterioles. The diameter of an arteriole is generally smaller than 0.5 mm. The lumen is as wide as the wall is thick. There are only one to five layers of smooth muscle fibers in the media of an arteriole. These muscle fibers are oriented in concentric rings around the vascular lumen. Internal elastic membranes are present in larger arterioles (as shown in the image and indicated by the arrow), but they are lacking in smaller arterioles. The adventitia is rather inconspicuous and blends with surrounding connective tissue. Arterioles feed capillary beds and, therefore, represent the beginnings of the microvasculature. **Keywords:** Arterioles

31 The answer is B: Arterioles. Contraction and relaxation of smooth muscle fibers in arterioles regulate vasoconstriction and vasodilation, respectively. These structural changes enable arterioles to regulate (and redistribute) blood flow to capillary beds in regions of the body where arterial blood flow is most needed. Arterioles are commonly referred to as resistance vessels, because tonic contraction of their smooth muscle creates vascular resistance, which is considered to be the major determinant of systemic blood pressure. None of the other components of the circulatory system regulate regional blood flow. **Keywords:** Arterioles, vasoconstriction, vasodilation

32 The answer is C: Increased peripheral vascular resistance. Although different mechanisms may contribute to the pathogenesis of primary hypertension, the common end result for all of them is increased peripheral vascular resistance. In most cases of primary hypertension, small arteries and arterioles show structural narrowing and reduced luminal diameter, which may result from an increased number of smooth muscle cells in the vascular wall and/or increased active contraction of smooth muscle cells. Increased heart rate (choice B) does not necessarily lead to systemic hypertension. Vasodilation of arterioles (choice E) lowers blood pressure. Arterial cystic medial necrosis (choice A) and increased vascular permeability (choice D) may be consequences of hypertension, but they do not cause hypertension. **Keywords:** Systemic hypertension

33 The answer is B: Capillary. Capillaries are the smallest blood vessels. They are composed of a single layer of endothelial cells (a simple squamous epithelium) surrounded by a delicate basal lamina. These narrow endothelial channels are just large enough to allow erythrocytes to pass through, one at a time, and thin enough to allow for efficient transendothelial diffusion. Capillaries form fine networks that facilitate the exchange of fluids, electrolytes, gases, nutrients, and metabolic waste products between blood and interstitial tissues of organs. None of the other blood vessels exhibit the distinctive histologic features of capillaries. **Keywords:** Capillaries

34 The answer is A: Continuous endothelial cells with continuous basal lamina. Three types of capillaries can be distinguished on the basis of their ultrastructural morphology: continuous, fenestrated, and discontinuous. Continuous capillaries have an uninterrupted endothelial lining, surrounded by a continuous layer of basal lamina. Endothelial cells are linked by tight junctions (zonula occludens). Continuous capillaries are found in the lungs, CNS, thymus, skeletal muscle, and bone. Fenestrated capillaries (choices C and D) have many small windows (fenestra) that facilitate the diffusion of biological molecules across the endothelium. The fenestrations may, or may not, be covered by a thin "diaphragm." The basal lamina is continuous in fenestrated capillaries. Fenestrated capillaries with diaphragms are found in the intestines, endocrine organs, and kidney tubules (i.e., peritubular capillaries). Fenestrated capillaries without diaphragms facilitate the ultrafiltration of blood in the renal glomerulus. Discontinuous capillaries (also referred to as sinusoidal capillaries) display an incomplete endothelial lining and a fragmented basal lamina. These capillaries (choices B and E) facilitate communication between parenchymal cells and blood. Discontinuous capillaries are found in the liver, spleen, and bone marrow.

Keywords: Capillaries, endothelial cells

35 The answer is D: Pericytes. Pericytes are contractile cells associated with some continuous capillaries and postcapillary venules. Their branching cytoplasmic processes surround endothelial cells to provide support and stability. Loss of pericytes in patients with diabetes mellitus is believed to play a key role in the pathogenesis of early-stage diabetic retinopathy. Without the support of pericytes, the retinal capillaries form microaneurysms and small hemorrhages that are evident on funduscopic examination. These lesions do not usually impair vision. However, after many years, diabetic retinopathy becomes proliferative. Delicate new blood vessels grow toward the vitreous body, resulting in a reduction or loss of vision. Injury to the other vascular wall components does not lead to the development of diabetic retinopathy.

Keywords: Diabetic retinopathy, pericyte

36 The answer is A: Arteriovenous shunt. Glomus bodies are neuromyoarterial receptors that are sensitive to temperature and are involved in body temperature regulation. The glomus body consists of an arteriovenous (AV) shunt surrounded by a richly innervated connective tissue capsule. Sympathetic stimulation of the glomus apparatus (body) causes vasoconstriction of the AV shunt, forcing blood to flow through the adjoining capillary bed. A glomus tumor is a benign tumor of the glomus body that is often extremely painful. The lesions are small, usually smaller than 1 cm in diameter. None of the other choices describe histologic features of the glomus body.

Keywords: Glomus tumor, glomus body

37 The answer is E: Temperature-dependent regulation of blood flow. Precapillary arterioles generally convey blood into capillary networks that are drained by postcapillary venules. However, in many tissues, especially in the skin of the fingertips and in erectile tissues of the penis and clitoris, the capillary circulation can be bypassed via direct connections between terminal arterioles and postcapillary venules. These direct routes are termed arteriovenous anastomoses or arteriovenous shunts (AV shunts). AV shunts are enclosed in connective tissue capsules and are richly innervated. AV shunts in the skin are involved in thermoregulation at the body surface. When exposed to cold weather, AV shunts open and capillary beds are closed to prevent heat loss. In warm weather, AV shunts close, allowing blood to flow into capillary beds to augment heat dissipation.

Keywords: Arteriovenous shunts

38 The answer is E: Precapillary sphincters. The capillary network and associated precapillary arteriole and postcapillary venule form a functional unit, referred as the microcirculatory (microvascular) bed. Smooth muscle fibers of precapillary arterioles near the origins of capillaries are arranged into sphincters, termed precapillary sphincters. Contraction of these precapillary sphincters regulates the amount (volume) of the blood entering the microvascular bed. None of the other structures regulates blood flow into the capillary bed.

Keywords: Capillaries, precapillary sphincter

39 The answer is E: Venule. Venules connect the distal ends of capillary beds with the venous system. Venules are composed of a layer of endothelial cells with a basal lamina. A thin layer of adventitia supports the venule and binds it to the surrounding connective tissue. Venules continuous with the capillaries are referred as postcapillary venules. The more distal and larger venules that connect to small veins are termed muscular venules. Although venules lack a smooth muscle coat, postcapillary venules are invested with pericytes. Muscular venules are distal to postcapillary venules; they are approximately 0.1 mm in diameter. Larger muscular venules have one or two layers of smooth muscle cells that form a tunica media. Pericytes are not associated with muscular venules.

Keywords: Venules, pericytes

40 The answer is C: Postcapillary venule. Postcapillary venules are the principal site where endothelial cells respond to vasoactive molecules, such as histamine and serotonin. In response to tissue injury, endothelial cells alter their membrane properties to (1) permit leakage of fluid and plasma components from the intravascular compartment and (2) facilitate the emigration of leukocytes from the vascular space into the surrounding extravascular tissue. This complex process of transendothelial cell migration is referred to as diapedesis. Leukocyte recruitment in the postcapillary venule is initiated by interaction of leukocytes with endothelial cell surface molecules termed selectins. Leukocytes do not typically undergo diapedesis at the other anatomic locations listed.

Keywords: Postcapillary venule

41 The answer is E: Superficial veins. Superficial varicosities of the saphenous veins and their tributaries in the lower limb are very common, owing to upright posture. Varicose veins are common in the posteromedial portions of the lower limbs. The incidence of varicose veins is greater in individuals whose occupations require them to stand for long periods of time. Varicosities are enlarged and tortuous, due to incompetence of venous valves and/or dilation of the vessel. Blood flow in the varicose vein is turbulent and slow, and the capillary bed is engorged. Fluid leaks into the surrounding cutaneous tissue and causes stasis dermatitis. None of the other structures give rise to varicose leg veins.

Keywords: Varicose veins

42 **The answer is E: Venous valves.** Valves are characteristic features of medium-sized veins, in both superficial and deep veins. They are most numerous in the lower limb veins, because of the need to direct the flow of blood back to the heart against the force of gravity. Venous valves are cusp-like projections into the lumen of the vein. The valves are covered by endothelium, and they are strengthened by collagen and elastic fibers. They have cup-like valvular sinuses that fill from above. The valve cusps occlude the lumen of the vein when they are full, so as to prevent reflux of blood and ensure that the venous blood continues to flow in one direction back toward the heart.

Keywords: Varicose veins, venous valves

43 **The answer is C: Medium vein.** Medium-sized veins typically accompany muscular arteries in a common connective tissue sheath. Medium veins have a diameter range of 0.1 to 10 mm, and they exhibit all three vascular tunics. The tunica intima is composed of endothelium and a thin subendothelial layer. In larger medium-sized veins, a thin internal elastic membrane may be present. The tunica media is much thinner in medium veins compared to medium arteries. As shown in this image, there are only a few layers of circular smooth muscle fibers (red wavy lines) interspersed between blue-stained connective tissue fibers (collagen and elastin). The tunica adventitia is thicker than the tunica media, with an abundance of collagen and elastic fibers. None of the other vessels describe the characteristic structural features of the muscular vein.

Keywords: Veins, muscular

44 **The answer is D: Smooth muscle fibers.** The venae cavae, pulmonary, subclavian, and portal veins are considered large veins in the human body. As seen in the image, the tunica adventitia (indicated by the double arrow) is the thickest layer of the wall of large veins. It contains aggregates of bundles of longitudinally arranged smooth muscle fibers. The tunica media of large veins is thin, with a few layers of smooth muscle fibers and abundant connective tissue. The other structures are found in the tunica adventitia of large veins, but they do not show histologic features of smooth muscle fibers.

Keywords: Veins

45 **The answer is B: Efferent arteriole.** Capillary networks typically receive blood from precapillary arterioles and are drained by postcapillary venules. However, this standard arrangement is altered in the kidney. Here, an arteriole is interposed between two capillary networks. Afferent arterioles (choice A) supply blood to the glomerulus (the capillary network within the renal corpuscle)

and efferent arterioles drain blood away. The efferent arteriole leaves the renal corpuscle and branches into a secondary capillary network, either (1) peritubular capillaries (choice C) that envelope the tubules or (2) vasa recta (choice D) that surround the limbs of the loop of Henle. The peritubular capillaries and vasa recta are drained by venules (choice E). Another special capillary arrangement occurs in portal systems of the liver and pituitary. In the liver, the portal vein (containing blood from intestinal capillaries) branches into a sinusoid capillary network between cords of hepatocytes. Hepatic sinusoids drain via hepatic veins to the inferior vena cava.

Keywords: Kidney, glomerulus

46 **The answer is B: Esophageal varices.** Esophageal varices are dilated (varicose) veins located immediately beneath the mucosa. They are prone to rupture and hemorrhage in patients with portal hypertension, secondary to hepatic cirrhosis. Submucosal venous blood from the lower esophagus drains to the azygos vein through esophageal veins or drains to the portal vein by way of the left gastric vein. Portal–systemic anastomoses occur at this site. In patients with portal hypertension secondary to cirrhosis of the liver, these portal–systemic anastomoses become distended with blood. The submucosal veins become varicose. When these esophageal varices become greater than 5 mm in diameter, they are likely to rupture, in which case life-threatening hemorrhage may ensue. Alcoholic hepatitis (choice A) by itself does not cause varices; however, long-term alcohol abuse often leads to hepatic cirrhosis, portal hypertension, and the development of esophageal varices. None of the other pathologic conditions are associated with bleeding esophageal varices.

Keywords: Esophageal varices, cirrhosis

47 **The answer is C: Deep vein thrombosis.** A thrombus is an aggregation of coagulated blood (platelets, fibrin, and cells) that forms within a vascular lumen. Deep vein thrombosis (DVT) represents the formation of coagulated blood in a deep vein. Most DVTs occur in the deep veins of the lower limb. If a DVT of the lower limb dislodges, it can be carried up to the inferior vena cava, through the heart, to the pulmonary arteries. A large pulmonary thromboembolus causes acute obstruction of the pulmonary arterial tree. As a result, the patient develops severe hypotension (cardiogenic shock) and may die within minutes. The other mechanisms of disease cause arterial thrombosis.

Keywords: Pulmonary thromboembolism, deep vein thrombosis

48 **The answer is B: Lymphatic vessels.** Lymphatic vessels convey protein-rich fluid to the bloodstream. Lymphatic channels play a crucial role in regulating interstitial fluid volume and in providing tissue debris to regional lymph nodes for immune surveillance. The smallest lymphatic vessels are lymphatic capillaries. These simple endothelial tubes have closed ends that are in close proximity to blood capillaries. They are most abundant in the skin and gastrointestinal tract. Lymphatic vessels converge and, ultimately, unite to form the thoracic duct (the largest lymphatic vessel) and the right lymphatic trunk. The thoracic duct and right lymphatic trunk empty lymph into the venous circulatory system at the junction of the internal jugular vein and the subclavian vein bilaterally. None of the other vessels exhibit histologic features of efferent lymphatic vessels.

Keywords: Lymphatic system

49 **The answer is C: Lymphatic capillary.** Lymphatic capillaries are lined by a simple squamous endothelium, but they lack a continuous basal lamina. As a result, lymphatic capillaries are highly permeable. They convey large proteins, protein complexes, and large lipid micelles and chylomicrons. They are more efficient than blood capillaries in removing tissue fluid and necrotic debris. Lymphatic capillaries in the villi of the small intestine are referred as lacteals. Lacteals collect dietary fats absorbed by the intestinal villi. Emulsified triglycerides in the lumen of the small intestine pass through the simple columnar epithelial lining and enter the lamina propria of the intestinal villi. Here, triacylglycerol combines with phospholipids, cholesterol esters, and apolipoprotein B-48 to form chylomicrons. The chylomicrons are absorbed into the lacteals and form a milky substance known as chyle. Lacteals merge to form larger lymphatic vessels, which transport chyle to the bloodstream by way of the thoracic duct. None of the other channels exhibit histologic features of lymphatic capillaries.

Keywords: Lacteal, lymphatic capillary

50 **The answer is E: Lymphatic vessels.** This patient exhibits massive lymphedema caused by a roundworm infestation. Filariasis is an inflammatory infection of lymph nodes and lymph vessels caused by filarial nematodes. Microfilariae, the infectious larvae transmitted into human body by mosquito bites, migrate into and mature within lymphatic vessels and regional lymph nodes. The adult worms inhabit the lymphatic tissue. They cause acute lymphangitis and lymphatic obstruction, leading to severe lymphedema. Massive lymphedema is termed elephantiasis.

Keywords: Filariasis, elephantiasis

Chapter 11

Respiratory System

QUESTIONS

Select the single best answer.

1 A 5-year-old girl with cystic fibrosis is admitted to the hospital with pneumonia. As you examine the patient, you recall the anatomy and histology of the respiratory system. Which of the following air passages is the most distal part of the conducting portion of the patient's lungs?
(A) Alveolar ducts
(B) Respiratory bronchioles
(C) Secondary bronchi
(D) Segmental bronchi
(E) Terminal bronchioles

2 During a problem-based learning session, your facilitator asks about proper usage of the term "bronchial tree." Which of the following structures is a component of the bronchial tree in the respiratory system?
(A) Alveolar ducts
(B) Alveolar sacs
(C) Bronchioles
(D) Larynx
(E) Trachea

3 The respiratory portion of the respiratory system begins at which of the following locations in the lungs?
(A) Alveolar ducts
(B) Alveolar sacs
(C) Alveoli
(D) Respiratory bronchioles
(E) Terminal bronchioles

4 The parents of an 8-year-old boy with bronchial asthma ask about the anatomy and physiology of the lungs, to better understand their child's medical condition. Which of the following components of the respiratory system is the major site of gas exchange?
(A) Alveoli
(B) Respiratory bronchioles
(C) Secondary bronchi
(D) Segmental bronchi
(E) Terminal bronchioles

5 Which of the following anatomic relationships best describes the structural basis for gas exchange in the lungs?
(A) Association of pulmonary veins with the bronchial tree
(B) Close association of alveolar spaces and pulmonary capillaries
(C) Continuous branching of the bronchopulmonary tree
(D) Dual blood supply to the lungs
(E) Intimate relationship of pulmonary arteries and veins

6 A segment of trachea is obtained at autopsy. Paraffin sections are stained with H&E and examined by light microscopy (shown in the image). Identify the structure within the oval.

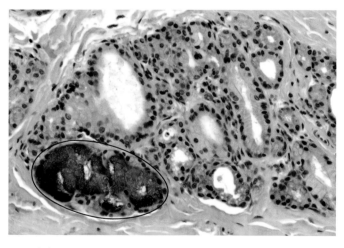

(A) Artery
(B) Lymphoid follicle
(C) Mucous gland
(D) Nerve
(E) Serous gland

7 Which of the following best describes the function of the structure identified in Question 6?
(A) Conditioning of inhaled air
(B) Polypeptide hormone secretion
(C) Production of secretory IgA antibody
(D) Source of pulmonary surfactant
(E) Substrate for inflammatory cell adhesion

8 A 14-year-old girl with the common cold presents with a "stuffy nose" due to nasal congestion. Which of the following represents a hallmark of the lamina propria in the nasal cavity?
(A) Elastic fibers
(B) Loose connective tissue
(C) Lymphocytes
(D) Reticular fibers
(E) Rich vascular plexus

9 Which of the following mechanisms of disease best describes the pathogenesis of nasal congestion in the patient described in Question 8?
(A) Increased secretion from mucous glands in the lamina propria
(B) Increased secretion from serous glands in the lamina propria
(C) Infiltration of the lamina propria with chronic inflammatory cells
(D) Overproduction of mucus by goblet cells in the respiratory epithelium
(E) Swelling of the lamina propria of the nasal mucosa

10 A 48-year-old woman with a 3-day history of an upper respiratory infection complains that she has lost her sense of smell. Her perception of smell recovers about 1 week later. The epithelial lining of which portion of the respiratory system was temporally affected in this patient?
(A) Larynx
(B) Nasal vestibule
(C) Nasopharynx
(D) Olfactory region of nasal cavity
(E) Respiratory region of nasal cavity

11 A biopsy of the olfactory mucosa is examined by light microscopy (shown in the image). Which of the following cells in the olfactory epithelium is responsible for the sense of smell?

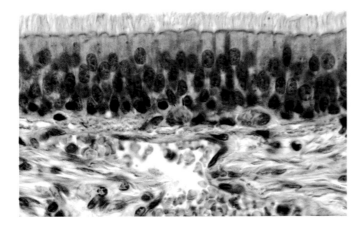

(A) Basal cells
(B) Brush cells
(C) Goblet cells
(D) Neurons
(E) Supporting cells

12 The cell described in Question 11 is best characterized as which of the following types of neurons?
(A) Bipolar
(B) Interneuron
(C) Motor
(D) Multipolar
(E) Pseudounipolar

13 Which of the following cells in the olfactory epithelium of the nasal cavity is responsible for the recovery of olfactory perception in the patient described in Question 10?
(A) Basal cells
(B) Brush cells
(C) Goblet cells
(D) Olfactory neurons
(E) Supporting cells

14 Which of the following cells of the olfactory epithelium is equivalent functionally to neuroglial cells of the central nervous system?
(A) Basal cells
(B) Brush cells
(C) Goblet cells
(D) Olfactory neurons
(E) Supporting cells

15 A portion of olfactory mucosa is obtained at autopsy and examined by light microscopy (shown in the image). Identify the structure indicated by the arrow.

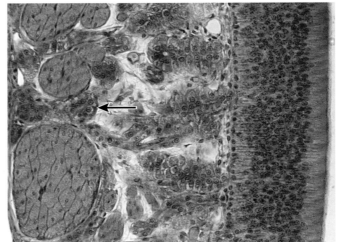

(A) Blood vessel
(B) Lymphatic nodule
(C) Mucous gland
(D) Nerve
(E) Olfactory gland

16 A 49-year-old woman with a history of recurrent para-nasal sinusitis presents with facial pain and fever. Which of the following types of epithelium normally lines the paranasal sinus cavities?
(A) Ciliated, pseudostratified columnar epithelium with goblet cells
(B) Keratinized, stratified squamous epithelium
(C) Nonkeratinized, stratified squamous epithelium
(D) Simple columnar epithelium
(E) Simple squamous epithelium

17 Loss of function of which of the following cells or subcel-lular structures is a likely cause of chronic sinusitis?
(A) Basal cells
(B) Cilia
(C) Goblet cells
(D) Microvilli
(E) Mucous glands

18 A 29-year-old opera singer complains about recent changes in the frequency of her vibrato and the quality of her vocal sound. Phonation in your patient is initiated and shaped by which of the following structures of the head and neck?
(A) Epiglottis
(B) Oropharynx
(C) Ventricle of the larynx
(D) Ventricular folds
(E) Vocal folds

19 Which of the following types of epithelium covers the vocal folds in the patient described in Question 18?
(A) Pseudostratified columnar
(B) Simple columnar
(C) Simple squamous
(D) Stratified columnar
(E) Stratified squamous

20 A 50-year-old woman with lung cancer develops respiratory insufficiency and expires. A transverse section of the trachea is examined at autopsy. The pos-terior aspect of the patient's trachea appears normal (shown in the image). Which of the following struc-tures is essential for maintaining an open tracheal air passage?

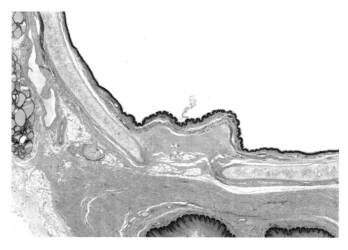

(A) Cartilaginous rings
(B) Connective tissue in the adventitia
(C) Dense connective tissue in the submucosa
(D) Proximity of the esophagus to the posterior tracheal wall
(E) Respiratory epithelium with elastic fibers in the lamina propria

21 The posterior aspect of the trachea described in Question 20 is examined at higher magnification (shown in the image). Identify the structure indicated by the arrow.

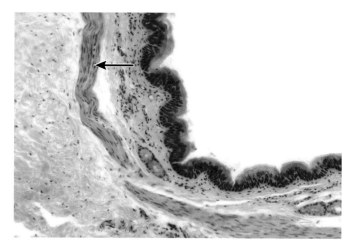

(A) Adventitia
(B) Dense regular connective tissue
(C) Hyaline cartilage
(D) Smooth muscle
(E) Submucosa

22 Respiratory epithelium of the trachea is examined at high magnification (shown in the image). Identify the cell indicated by the arrow.

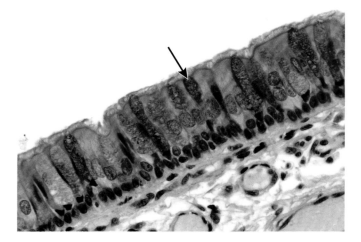

(A) Basal cell
(B) Brush cell
(C) Ciliated columnar cell
(D) Goblet cell
(E) Small granule cell

23 Which of the following describes the principal function of ciliated columnar epithelial cells in respiratory epithelium of the lungs?
(A) Coordinated motion of mucus
(B) Degradation of mucus polysaccharides
(C) Fluid uptake via pinocytosis
(D) Production of anti-inflammatory molecules
(E) Receptors for binding and internalization of inhaled pathogens

24 You are asked to give a seminar on the endocrine functions of the lungs. Which of the following cells in the respiratory system is a neuroendocrine cell?
(A) Basal cells
(B) Brush cells
(C) Ciliated cells
(D) Goblet cells
(E) Small granule cells

25 Various regions of the respiratory system are reviewed at autopsy for evidence of histopathology. Identify the component of the normal trachea that is indicated by arrowheads (shown in the image).

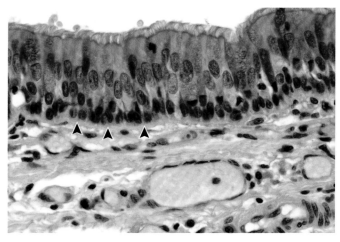

(A) Basement membrane
(B) Lamina propria
(C) Lymphatic vessel
(D) Mucosa
(E) Submucosa

26 You are part of a team that prepares to remove a tumor from the lung of a 68-year-old woman. Prior to surgery, you review the organization of bronchopulmonary segments. How many segmental bronchi arise from the right primary bronchus?
(A) 3 segments
(B) 6 segments
(C) 8 segments
(D) 10 segments
(E) 12 segments

27 A 54-year-old woman with a history of smoking presents with hemoptysis and chest pain. A CT scan of the thorax reveals a 5-cm mass in the middle lobe of the right lung. The mass is removed using a pulmonary segmentectomy. Which of the following pulmonary units best characterizes the structural basis for your surgical resection?

(A) Bronchopulmonary segment
(B) Pulmonary acinus
(C) Pulmonary lobe
(D) Pulmonary lobule
(E) Respiratory bronchiolar unit

28 The specimen obtained at surgery from the patient described in Question 27 reveals an adenocarcinoma, with a margin of normal lung parenchyma. Examination of the tumor margin shows an intrapulmonary bronchus (shown in the image). Which of the following histologic features distinguishes this intrapulmonary bronchus from an extrapulmonary primary bronchus?

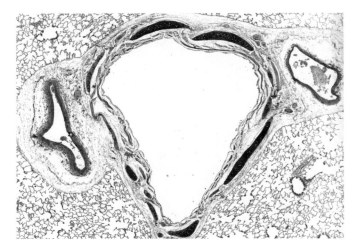

(A) Absence of submucosal glands
(B) Adventitia composed of connective tissue
(C) Lack of cartilage in the bronchial wall
(D) Loss of respiratory epithelium
(E) Presence of cartilage plates

29 The wall of the intrapulmonary bronchus described in Question 28 is examined at higher magnification (shown in the image). Identify the structure indicated by the arrow.

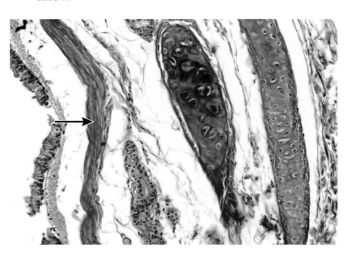

(A) Basement membrane
(B) Dense connective tissue
(C) Lamina propria
(D) Muscularis mucosa
(E) Submucosa

30 Sections through an intrapulmonary bronchus and a pulmonary artery (shown in the image) are examined in the pathology department. Which of the following tissue components is responsible for the folded appearance of the mucosa in this bronchus?

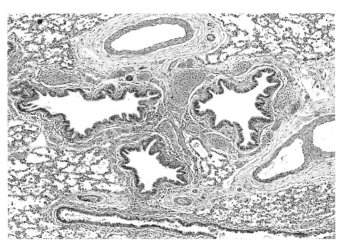

(A) Basement membrane
(B) Cartilaginous plates
(C) Elastic fibers in the adventitia
(D) Fibroelastic tissue in the lamina propria
(E) Muscularis mucosa

31 The parents of a 10-year-old boy with asthma ask you about the mechanisms that control airflow in the lungs. Which of the following nerve fibers stimulates contraction of smooth muscle fibers in the muscularis mucosa of the respiratory system and thereby reduces the diameter of the conducting air passages?
(A) Parasympathetic
(B) Somatic motor
(C) Somatic sensory
(D) Sympathetic
(E) Visceral afferent

32 A 49-year-old woman with bronchial asthma receives a prescription for an inhaler to help relieve her shortness of breath. This β2-adrenergic receptor agonist (salbutamol) has a direct effect on which of the following components of the conducting portion of the patient's respiratory system?
(A) Basement membranes
(B) Cartilage plates
(C) Cilia of the epithelium
(D) Smooth muscle
(E) Submucosal glands

33 A lung specimen (shown in the image) is examined in the pathology department. Identify the structure within the oval.

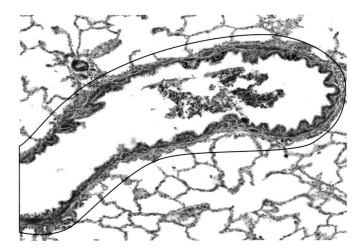

(A) Bronchiole
(B) Extrapulmonary bronchus
(C) Pulmonary artery
(D) Respiratory bronchiole
(E) Segmental bronchus

34 Another area from the specimen described in Question 33 is examined by light microscopy (shown in the image). Identify the structure within the oval line.

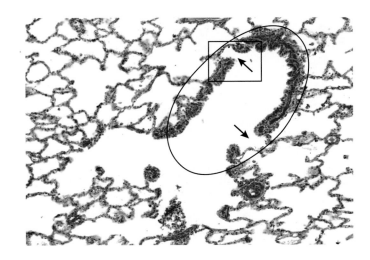

(A) Alveolar duct
(B) Bronchiole
(C) Intrapulmonary bronchus
(D) Respiratory bronchiole
(E) Terminal bronchiole

35 The area within the rectangular box shown in the image described in Question 34 is examined at higher magnification (shown in the image). Identify the cells indicated by the arrows.

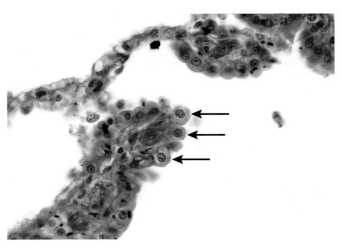

(A) Basal cells
(B) Brush cells
(C) Clara cells
(D) Goblet cells
(E) Small granule cells

36 You are involved in a research project to study the biology of Clara cells. As part of your research, you develop a monoclonal antibody that identifies these cells in paraffin-embedded sections. Immunohistochemical assays using your antibody confirm that Clara cells first appear in the epithelium of the bronchopulmonary tree at which of the following anatomic locations?
(A) Alveolar sacs
(B) Alveoli
(C) Large bronchioles
(D) Segmental bronchi
(E) Terminal bronchioles

37 Which of the following cellular activities best describes the principal function of Clara cells in terminal and respiratory bronchioles?
(A) Degradation of mucin
(B) Fluid uptake via pinocytosis
(C) Production of inflammatory cytokines
(D) Receptors for binding pathogens
(E) Secretion of surfactant

38 A section of normal lung tissue is examined by light microscopy at low magnification (shown in the image). Identify the space indicated by the asterisk.

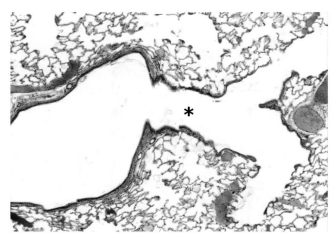

(A) Alveolar duct
(B) Alveolar sac
(C) Large-diameter bronchiole
(D) Respiratory bronchiole
(E) Terminal bronchiole

39 You are asked to discuss the physiology of pulmonary gas exchange during a laboratory meeting. Gas exchange begins at what point in the respiratory tree?
(A) Alveoli
(B) Large-diameter bronchioles
(C) Respiratory bronchioles
(D) Segmental bronchi
(E) Terminal bronchioles

40 Another area of the specimen described in Question 38 is examined at low magnification (shown in the image). Which of the numbered spaces represents an alveolar duct?

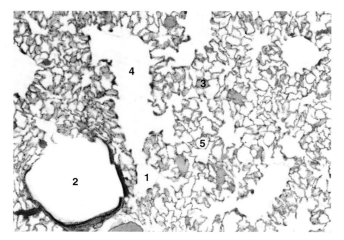

(A) Space 1
(B) Space 2
(C) Space 3
(D) Space 4
(E) Space 5

41 In the image shown for Question 40, the space indicated by number 1 is best identified as which of the following components of the respiratory system?
(A) Alveolar duct
(B) Alveolar sac
(C) Alveolus
(D) Respiratory bronchiole
(E) Terminal bronchiole

42 In the image shown for Question 40, which of the numbered spaces represents a respiratory alveolus?
(A) Space 1
(B) Space 2
(C) Space 3
(D) Space 4
(E) Space 5

43 A lung biopsy is examined at high magnification (shown in the image). Identify the cells indicated by the arrows.

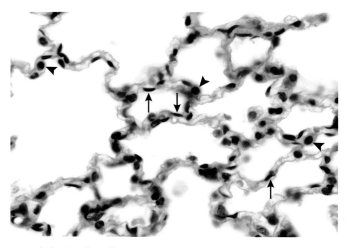

(A) Brush cells
(B) Macrophages
(C) Small granule cells
(D) Type I alveolar cells
(E) Type II alveolar cells

44 The squamous epithelial cells that cover most (95%) of the surface area of the pulmonary alveoli are connected to one another through junctions that prevent the leakage of interstitial fluid into the alveolar air spaces. Which of the following types of intercellular junctions serve this important biological function?
(A) Cadherins
(B) Hemidesmosomes
(C) Macula adherens
(D) Zonula adherens
(E) Zonula occludens

45 Identify the cells indicated by arrowheads in the image shown for Question 43.
(A) Alveolar macrophages
(B) Clara cells
(C) Kulchitsky cells
(D) Type I alveolar cells
(E) Type II alveolar cells

46 Which of the following best describes the function of type II alveolar cells?
(A) Cytokine production
(B) Fluid transport
(C) IgA antibody production
(D) Phagocytosis of pathogens
(E) Secretion of surfactant

47 A 50-year-old woman with leukemia undergoes chemotherapy. During treatment, she develops increasing cough and shortness of breath. Sputum cultures are negative, and the patient does not respond to antibiotic therapy. If this patient has acquired a viral pneumonia, with alveolar damage, which of the following cells can regenerate the alveolar epithelium during healing?
(A) Clara cells
(B) Enterochromaffin cells
(C) Small granular cells
(D) Type I alveolar cells
(E) Type II alveolar cells

48 An electron micrograph of the alveolus is examined for evidence of structural changes. The barrier that separates atmospheric gasses from blood features which of the following important biological adaptations?
(A) Fusion of epithelial and endothelial basal laminae
(B) Gap junctions between epithelial and endothelial cells
(C) Interdigitation of microvilli on adjacent epithelial and endothelial cells
(D) Sinusoidal alveolar capillaries
(E) Tight junctions between epithelial and endothelial cells

49 A 72-year-old woman with a history of heavy smoking dies of congestive heart failure. The patient's lungs (shown in the image) are examined at autopsy. Identify the cells indicated by the arrows.

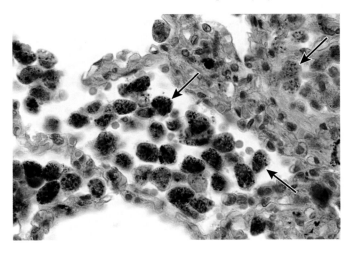

(A) Clara cells
(B) Macrophages
(C) Neutrophils
(D) Plasma cells
(E) Type II alveolar cells

50 During cadaver dissection, a student notices that the lymph nodes at the hilum of her cadaver's lungs appear black. Which of the following best explains the dark color of these hilar lymph nodes?
(A) Acute inflammatory cell infiltrate
(B) Aggregates of senescent red blood cells
(C) Carbon particles within macrophages
(D) Pollen and dust within the lymph fluid
(E) Primary and secondary lymphoid nodules

51 A 67-year-old smoker presents with increasing shortness of breath and dry cough. He is constantly "gasping for air" and walks with difficulty because he becomes breathless after only a few steps. A chest x-ray discloses hyperinflation of the lungs, and the patient is diagnosed with pulmonary emphysema. This disease is caused by smoking-related injury to which of the following components of the respiratory system?
(A) Alveolar septa
(B) Capillary endothelial cells
(C) Respiratory epithelial cells
(D) Submucosal cartilage plates
(E) Submucosal mucous glands

52 A 32-year-old woman delivers a baby prematurely at 25 weeks of gestation. Shortly after birth, the neonate becomes short of breath, with intercostal retraction and nasal flaring during respiration. The neonate is placed on a ventilator but dies of respiratory insufficiency. Respiratory distress in your patient is most likely caused by injury to which of the following components of the respiratory system?
(A) Alveoli
(B) Bronchioles
(C) Main stem bronchi
(D) Segmental bronchi
(E) Trachea

53 Respiratory distress syndrome described in Question 52 was most likely caused by lack of fetal development (immaturity) of which of the following cells?
(A) Brush cells
(B) Clara cells
(C) Goblet cells
(D) Type I alveolar cells
(E) Type II alveolar cells

54 A section of lung parenchyma is examined by light microscopy (shown in the image). Identify the tissue indicated by the arrows.

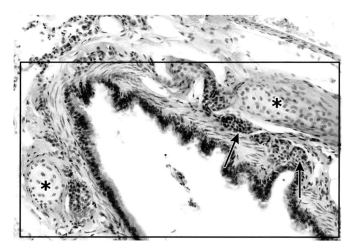

(A) Cartilage
(B) Connective tissue
(C) Lamina propria
(D) Mucous glands
(E) Smooth muscle

55 Identify the structure within the rectangular box in the image described in Question 54.
(A) Extrapulmonary bronchus
(B) Intrapulmonary bronchus
(C) Large bronchiole
(D) Small bronchiole
(E) Terminal bronchiole

56 A lung carcinoma is resected, and the tumor margin is carefully examined in the pathology department (shown in the image). The arteriole indicated by the arrow on the image is a branch from which of the following arteries?

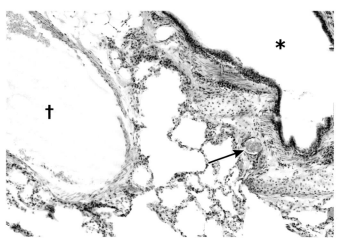

(A) Internal thoracic
(B) Lateral thoracic
(C) Pulmonary
(D) Thoracic aorta
(E) Thyrocervical trunk

57 The artery indicated by the dagger on the image shown in Question 56 supplies blood to which of the following structures of the respiratory system?
(A) Alveoli and alveolar septa
(B) Connective tissue at hilum of lungs
(C) Large-diameter bronchioles
(D) Segmental bronchi
(E) Terminal bronchioles

ANSWERS

1   **The answer is E: Terminal bronchioles.**   The respiratory system is composed of a conducting and a respiratory portion. The conducting portion includes air passages outside and inside the lungs. The nasal cavities, nasopharynx, larynx, trachea, and paired primary bronchi are air passages external to the lungs (extrapulmonary). Upon entering the lungs, the paired primary bronchi undergo branching to form the intrapulmonary bronchial tree. The branches become smaller and lead to the respiratory portion of the lungs, where gas exchange takes place. Components of the bronchial tree include the primary bronchi, lobar (secondary) bronchi, segmental (tertiary) bronchi, and bronchioles. Terminal bronchioles are the smallest components of the bronchial tree and the terminal part of the conducting portion of the respiratory system. Cystic fibrosis is an autosomal recessive disorder that affects children. It is characterized by (1) chronic pulmonary disease, (2) deficient exocrine pancreatic function, and (3) other complications of retained (inspissated) mucus in a number of organs, including the small intestine, the liver, and the reproductive tract. All of the pathologic consequences of cystic fibrosis can be attributed to the presence of abnormally thick mucus.
Keywords: Terminal bronchioles, cystic fibrosis

2   **The answer is C: Bronchioles.**   The term "bronchial tree" refers to intrapulmonary air conducting passages of the respiratory system. This tree is composed of internal bronchi that bifurcate from the primary bronchi and also the bronchioles. Larynx and trachea (choices D and E) are extrapulmonary air conducting passages. Alveolar ducts and sacs (choices A and B) are components of the respiratory portion of the lungs and are sites for gas exchange.
Keywords: Bronchioles

3   **The answer is D: Respiratory bronchioles.**   Respiratory bronchioles are branches from air conducting, terminal bronchioles. In turn, respiratory bronchioles give rise to alveolar ducts, alveolar sacs, and finally to alveoli where gas exchange occurs. Alveoli are small air cavities, approximately 200 μm in diameter, enveloped by a rich capillary bed. Respiratory bronchioles have discontinuous walls that open directly to numerous alveoli. Therefore, respiratory bronchioles are included in the respiratory portion of the respiratory system, along with the alveolar ducts, alveolar sacs, and terminal alveoli.
Keywords: Respiratory bronchioles

4   **The answer is A: Alveoli.**   Fresh air reaches the respiratory portion of the respiratory system through the extra- and intrapulmonary conducting ducts. Gas exchange begins within the respiratory bronchioles (choice B), because these air passages have alveoli connected to them. However, the major site of gas exchange in the lungs takes place within the smallest air spaces—the alveoli. Alveoli are organized as clusters. These clusters open to a common space that is referred to as the alveolar sac. Moving proximally in the respiratory tract, the alveoli and alveolar sacs are observed to open into larger, elongated spaces termed alveolar ducts. The other structures listed do not participate in gas exchange. Asthma in this patient is a chronic lung disease caused by increased responsiveness of the airways to a variety of stimuli. Patients typically exhibit paroxysms of wheezing, dyspnea, and cough.
Keywords: Asthma, alveolus

5   **The answer is B: Close association of alveolar spaces and pulmonary capillaries.**   The alveolar air spaces are separated from one another by alveolar septa. Capillaries arising from the pulmonary arteries travel within these very thin interstitial spaces. Fresh air in the alveolus is only several hundred nanometers removed from deoxygenated blood in the pulmonary capillaries. This intimate relationship of air and pulmonary capillaries provides the structural basis for gas exchange in the lungs. Dual blood supply to the lungs (choice D) explains the pathologic finding that geographic areas of pulmonary necrosis are typically red (hemorrhagic infarcts). None of the other choices describe or explain the structural basis for gas exchange.
Keywords: Alveoli

6   **The answer is C: Mucous gland.**   Mucous and serous glands are found along most of the conducting portion of the respiratory tract, within the mucosa and the submucosa. Goblet cells located within the respiratory epithelium also produce abundant mucus. Serous glands (choice E) would stain with eosin. None of the other choices exhibit the distinctive morphology of tracheal mucous glands.
Keywords: Mucous and serous glands

7   **The answer is A: Conditioning of inhaled air.**   The mucus, produced by glands and goblet cells, coats the luminal surface over most of the conducting portion of the respiratory tract. Mucous and serous secretions help moisten, warm, and clean the inhaled air, before it reaches the delicate and fragile alveolar air spaces. Small particles and pathogens become trapped within the mucus and are removed by the coordinated ciliary action of the respiratory epithelium. None of the other choices describe the function of serous and mucous glands in the mucosa and submucosa of the respiratory system.
Keywords: Mucous and serous glands

8   **The answer is E: Rich vascular plexus.**   The two nasal cavities, separated by a nasal septum, comprise the uppermost part of the respiratory system. The nasal cavities

communicate with nasopharynx posteriorly, as well as the paranasal sinuses and lacrimal sacs laterally and superiorly. The most anterior portion of the nasal cavity is the nasal vestibule, which is lined by skin. The nasal cavity posterior to the vestibule can be divided into two parts: (1) the inferior two-thirds represent the respiratory region and (2) the superior one-third represents the olfactory region. The respiratory region is covered by a ciliated, pseudostratified columnar epithelium (respiratory epithelium). The lamina propria is connected to periosteum or perichondrium of the underlying bone and cartilage. It exhibits an extensive vascular plexus with complex sets of capillary loops. This vascular latticework serves to warm the inhaled air to protect the lungs. The other choices are components of loose connective tissue that are found in many organs. Rhinovirus is the most frequent cause of the "common cold."
Keywords: Nasal cavity, nasal mucosa

9 **The answer is E: Swelling of the lamina propria of the nasal mucosa.** The nasal mucosa contains a rich vascular plexus. These venous sinusoids are known as "swell bodies." Allergic reactions and inflammation related to "colds" and "flu" can cause abnormal engorgement of the sinusoidal swell bodies. Increased hydrostatic pressure and increased vascular permeability lead to an accumulation of extravascular edema fluid in the lamina propria of the nasal mucosa, resulting in the sensation of "stuffy nose." Although the other choices describe changes associated with inflammation, they are not related to nasal congestion in patients with the common cold.
Keywords: Nasal cavity, swell body

10 **The answer is D: Olfactory region of nasal cavity.** Three bony plates in the nasal cavity (superior, middle, and inferior conchae) project inferomedially from the lateral wall. The middle and inferior conchae are covered by respiratory epithelium and form the lateral wall of the respiratory region of the nasal cavity. By contrast, the superior conchae in the olfactory region at the roof of the nasal cavity are covered by a specialized olfactory mucosa (epithelium and lamina propria). The olfactory epithelium contains olfactory chemoreceptors. Damage to the olfactory mucosa caused by inflammation can result in the loss of smell. Epithelia in the other anatomic regions listed are not specialized for olfactory perception.
Keywords: Nasal cavity, olfactory region

11 **The answer is D: Neurons.** The olfactory epithelium of the nasal cavity is a ciliated, pseudostratified columnar epithelium but includes many other cells that are not found in typical respiratory epithelium. Olfactory neurons, also referred to as olfactory cells or olfactory receptor cells, span the entire thickness of the olfactory epithelium. The dendrite extends above the surface of the epithelium and forms a knoblike swelling termed the olfactory vesicle. Long, nonmotile cilia that arise from the olfactory vesicle function as receptors for chemical odorants. Axonal processes of these neurons leave the epithelium, unite as small nerve bundles within the basal lamina, and pass through the cribriform plate of the ethmoid bone to form the olfactory nerve, which enters the brain. Toxic fumes and physical injury can damage olfactory neurons resulting in a temporary loss of the sense of smell. Fortunately, olfactory neurons can be replaced by regeneration from proliferative stem cells in the epithelium. Other cells found in the olfactory epithelium include basal cells, brush cells, and supporting cells (choices A, B, and E).
Keywords: Olfactory epithelium, olfactory neurons

12 **The answer is A: Bipolar.** Olfactory neurons have one dendritic process and an axon. Cilia arising from the dendritic process serve as chemoreceptors for odorants. The neuronal axon extends from the olfactory epithelium to the central nervous system. None of the other types of neurons listed show the distinctive features of olfactory neurons.
Keywords: Olfactory epithelium, olfactory neuron

13 **The answer is A: Basal cells.** Basal cells are small, round cells located along the basal aspect of the olfactory epithelium. These cells are capable of regeneration. They serve as progenitors for other types of cells in the olfactory epithelium. Damaged olfactory neurons are replaced quickly, owing to the regenerative capacity of the basal stem cells. None of the other cells listed are capable of regeneration.
Keywords: Olfactory epithelium, basal cells

14 **The answer is E: Supporting cells.** Supporting cells, also termed sustentacular cells, are similar to neuroglial cells of the central nervous system. They are the most numerous type of cell in the olfactory epithelium. These tall, columnar cells have nuclei that are located close to the apical surface of the epithelium. They provide mechanical and metabolic support to the olfactory neurons. Supporting cells secrete odorant-binding proteins (OBPs) that transport odorant chemicals to olfactory receptors (specialized proteins) that are present in the plasma membranes of cilia in the olfactory vesicles. None of the other choices provide structural and metabolic support to olfactory neurons.
Keywords: Olfactory epithelium, supporting cells

15 **The answer is E: Olfactory gland.** Olfactory glands, also referred to as Bowman glands, are a distinguishing hallmark of the olfactory mucosa. Their serous secretions are discharged to the surface of the olfactory epithelium where they provide a solvent for chemical odorants. Continuous secretion from the olfactory glands creates a constant flow of fluid that helps to clean and remove odorants, thereby allowing the olfactory neurons to detect new odorants as they arise. Nerve fibers and glands in a lamina propria serve as key hallmarks of olfactory mucosa. None of the other choices show these characteristic histologic features.

Keywords: Olfactory gland

16 The answer is A: Ciliated, pseudostratified columnar epithelium with goblet cells. The paranasal sinuses are bilateral open spaces within frontal, maxillary, ethmoid, and sphenoid bones. These spaces are lined by respiratory epithelium, and they communicate with nasal cavities through narrow openings. Other regions of the respiratory system that are covered by a respiratory epithelium include respiratory region of the nasal cavities, nasopharynx, larynx (excluding vocal folds and epiglottis), trachea, bronchi, and large bronchioles. Keratinized, stratified squamous epithelium (choice B) is found in the skin. Nonkeratinized, stratified squamous epithelium (choice C) is found in the esophagus and uterine cervix. None of the other choices describe the covering epithelium of the sinus cavities.

Keywords: Paranasal sinus

17 The answer is B: Cilia. Cilia are delicate projections of the plasma membrane that produce a coordinated, sweeping motion along the apical surface of an epithelium. Mucus that is produced by goblet cells and mucous glands in the respiratory system is swept into the nasal cavities by the coordinated motion of innumerable cilia. Defective ciliary action leads to an accumulation of mucus within the paranasal sinuses. Mucus accumulation in the sinuses leads to chronic obstruction of the drainage orifices and recurrent bouts of paranasal infections (chronic sinusitis). The other choices are unlikely causes of chronic sinusitis.

Keywords: Sinusitis, cilia

18 The answer is E: Vocal folds. The larynx is a short tubular structure located between the pharynx and the trachea. Its wall is composed of a series of cartilage plates connected by skeletal muscles and ligaments. Two anteroposterior mucosal folds, vocal folds, project toward the lumen of the larynx (voice box). Ligaments and skeletal muscles generate tension in these vocal folds and, thereby, control phonation. The vocal folds control the flow of air passing through the larynx, and they vibrate to produce sound. Injury or inflammation to the vocal folds may cause changes in phonation. None of the other choices are related to vocal sound.

Keywords: Larynx, vocal folds, phonation

19 The answer is E: Stratified squamous. Air moves rapidly through the opening formed between the two vocal folds (the rima glottidis) for respiration and phonation. To protect the mucosa from abrasion by the rapidly moving stream of air, the vocal folds are lined by a protective, stratified squamous epithelium. None of the other choices describe this histologic feature of the vocal folds.

Keywords: Larynx, vocal folds

20 The answer is A: Cartilaginous rings. The trachea is an air tube that extends from the larynx to the sternal angle, where it bifurcates into two primary bronchi. Approximately 15 to 20 C-shaped cartilaginous rings are embedded in the connective tissue that is present between the submucosa and adventitia of the trachea. These cartilaginous rings stack vertically to form a supporting skeleton for the trachea; they reinforce the anterior and lateral aspects of the tracheal wall to maintain an open passage for air conduction. The other choices are important histologic features of the trachea, but they do not create an open air passage.

Keywords: Trachea, cartilage rings, cartilage

21 The answer is D: Smooth muscle. Cartilaginous support is absent along the posterior aspect of the trachea adjacent to the esophagus. This histologic feature of the trachea facilitates the passage of food through the esophagus to the stomach. The gap between free ends of the two C-shaped cartilaginous rings is filled by smooth muscle and a connective tissue that is rich in both elastic and collagen fibers. The smooth muscle identified by the arrow in the image is termed the trachealis muscle. None of the other choices identify smooth muscle.

Keywords: Trachea, trachealis muscle

22 The answer is D: Goblet cell. As in other parts of the respiratory system, the lumen of the trachea is lined by a respiratory epithelium that is composed of goblet cells, brush cells, small granule cells, basal cells, and ciliated columnar cells. Goblet cells secrete mucus. Intracellular mucinogen granules are clearly visible in this slide preparation. Mucus produced by goblet cells, as well as mucous glands, coats the lumen of the trachea and bronchial tree. This mucus conditions the inspired air and helps trap particles and pathogens that move through the upper respiratory tree. None of the other choices show the distinctive morphology of goblet cells.

Keywords: Goblet cells, trachea

23 The answer is A: Coordinated motion of mucus. Ciliated columnar cells are the most numerous type of cell in the respiratory epithelium. Hairlike motile cilia arise from the apical surface of the columnar epithelial cells. The cilia move in a coordinated sweeping fashion to move mucus and entrapped particles up the respiratory tree, toward the oropharynx. This coordinated ciliary movement (commonly referred to as the mucociliary ladder) is an important protective mechanism for the respiratory system. None of the other choices are related to the function of ciliated cells in respiratory epithelium.

Keywords: Trachea, ciliated epithelial cells, cilia

24 The answer is E: Small granule cells. Small granule cells (also referred to as Kulchitsky cells or enterochromaffin cells) account for about 3% of cells in the respiratory epithelium. These neuroendocrine cells are difficult to distinguish from basal cells in routine histological preparations. Small granule cells are believed to be part of the "diffuse neuroendocrine system." They are not derived from neural crest but originate from the pulmonary anlage during development. Their secretions include catecholamines, serotonin, calcitonin, and gastrin-releasing peptide. None of the other cells listed are neuroendocrine cells.
Keywords: Trachea, small granule cells

25 The answer is A: Basement membrane. A characteristic feature of the trachea is the presence of a thick basement membrane visible by light microscopy. This membrane becomes thicker in smokers as a response to chronic mucosal irritation. Lamina propria (choice B) is the underlying loose connective tissue layer that contains lymphatic vessels (choice C). The submucosa (choice E) of the trachea is composed of loose connective tissue and is difficult to distinguish from the lamina propria in routine histological preparations. A thin layer of elastic tissue forms a boundary between the mucosa (choice D) and the submucosa.
Keywords: Trachea, basement membrane

26 The answer is D: 10 segments. Left and right primary bronchi enter the lung through the hilum and divide into lobar (secondary) bronchi. Thus, there are two lobar bronchi in the left lung and three lobar bronchi in the right lung. Each secondary bronchus supplies one lobe of the lungs. Lobar bronchi then bifurcate into segmental (tertiary) bronchi, forming 8 segmental bronchi in the left lung and 10 segmental bronchi in the right lung. Each segmental bronchus and the lung parenchyma that it supplies constitute one bronchopulmonary segment. Thus, there are 8 segments in the left lung and 10 segments in the right lung.
Keywords: Bronchi, bronchopulmonary segments

27 The answer is A: Bronchopulmonary segment. The lungs can be divided into lobes, and lobes are further divided into bronchopulmonary segments. The segments are pyramidal in shape, with their base at the pleural surface and their apex facing the hilum. Each segment is supplied by a segmental bronchus and a tertiary branch of the pulmonary artery. Each segment is drained by an intersegmental branch of the pulmonary veins that travel within septa that separate adjacent bronchopulmonary segments. Segments are the largest subdivisions of a pulmonary lobe and are, therefore, convenient anatomic structures for surgical resection. Surgical resection of a pulmonary lobe (choice C) is referred to as lobectomy. Pulmonary lobules (choice D) are subdivisions of bronchopulmonary segments, where each lobule is supplied

by a separate bronchiole. A terminal bronchiole and its associated lung parenchyma together constitute a pulmonary acinus (choice B). The smallest functional unit of the lung, the respiratory bronchiolar unit (choice E), consists of a respiratory bronchiole and its associated pulmonary alveoli.
Keywords: Bronchopulmonary segment, lung cancer

28 The answer is E: Presence of cartilage plates. The histologic features of extrapulmonary segments of the primary bronchi are similar to those of the trachea. However, once primary bronchi enter the lung and become intrapulmonary, their structure changes. The first major histologic change is that C-shaped cartilage rings are replaced by small cartilaginous plates. These irregular-shaped cartilage plates are distributed around the circumference of the bronchial wall to prevent collapse of the bronchial air passage. As the bronchi continue to branch and become smaller in diameter, these cartilage plates decrease significantly in size. They eventually disappear at the point where the most distal bronchi become bronchioles. None of the other choices distinguish extra- from intrapulmonary bronchi.
Keywords: Intrapulmonary bronchi

29 The answer is D: Muscularis mucosa. Another distinction between extra- and intrapulmonary bronchi is the appearance of a distinct layer of smooth muscle between the lamina propria and the submucosa in the intrapulmonary air passages. In larger bronchi, this muscularis mucosa forms a continuous layer. However, as the bronchi become smaller, the muscularis mucosa becomes discontinuous. This muscle layer characterizes the bronchopulmonary tree as far distally as the alveolar ducts, where smooth muscle fibers are observed as knoblike structures within interalveolar septa. Contractions of the muscularis mucosae regulate the diameter of the conducting airways of the respiratory system.
Keywords: Intrapulmonary bronchi

30 The answer is E: Muscularis mucosa. The mucosa of the conducting airways of the respiratory system appears folded in most histologic preparations, due to the contraction of the muscularis mucosa after death. None of the other choices would facilitate folding of the bronchial mucosa after death.
Keywords: Intrapulmonary bronchi

31 The answer is A: Parasympathetic. In addition to neuroendocrine signals, the musculature of the bronchial tree and bronchioles is regulated by the autonomic nervous system. Parasympathetic fibers of the vagus nerve (CN X) stimulate contraction of bronchial smooth muscle. This stimulation has the effect of decreasing the diameter of the conducting airways and thereby reducing the volume of airflow through the lungs to the respiratory alveoli. By contrast, sympathetic fibers (choice D) cause relaxation of bronchial smooth muscle and increase airflow to the

respiratory alveoli. None of the other nerve fibers stimulate contraction of bronchial smooth muscle.
Keywords: Innervation

32 The answer is D: Smooth muscle.   Chronic inflammation in the conductor portion of the respiratory system in a patient with asthma stimulates contraction of bronchial smooth muscle, particularly in the bronchioles, causing variable airflow obstruction. During an asthma attack, patients experience respiratory distress with symptoms of wheezing, dyspnea (shortness of breath), and coughing. Inhaled salbutamol and other sympathetic agonists relax bronchial smooth muscle, increase the diameter of bronchioles, and help to restore normal ventilation of the lungs. Salbutamol does not affect the other structures listed.
Keywords: Asthma

33 The answer is A: Bronchiole.   After about 10 generations of branching, the intrapulmonary bronchi become very small in diameter. Bronchioles arise from small terminal bronchi and supply specific pulmonary lobules. Cartilage plates and glands are no longer present in the walls of these bronchioles (shown in the image). The muscularis layer is present and becomes relatively thick in all bronchioles. The bronchioles continue branching. As these airways become progressively narrowed, the ciliated pseudostratified columnar epithelium that covers initial segments of the bronchioles gives way to a ciliated, simple columnar or cuboidal epithelium. Goblet cells are present in large bronchioles, but their number diminishes in the terminal bronchioles. None of the other choices shows the distinctive histologic features of pulmonary bronchioles.
Keywords: Bronchioles

34 The answer is D: Respiratory bronchiole.   Large bronchioles undergo continuous branching, before reaching the respiratory portion of the lungs. Respiratory bronchioles arise from terminal bronchioles. They serve as a transition between the conducting and the respiratory portions of the respiratory system. They are involved in both air conducting and gas exchange. The feature that distinguishes respiratory bronchioles from terminal bronchioles (choice E) is the presence of an incomplete wall that is interrupted by alveoli (arrows, shown in the image). A respiratory bronchiole, along with the alveolar ducts, alveolar sacs, and alveoli that it supplies, forms the smallest functional component of the respiratory system, termed respiratory bronchiolar unit.
Keywords: Respiratory bronchioles

35 The answer is C: Clara cells.   Clara cells are nonciliated, low-columnar, or cuboidal epithelial cells present in terminal and respiratory bronchioles. These cells feature a dome-shaped apical surface and a round centrally located nucleus. None of the other cells listed show these distinctive cytological features.
Keywords: Clara cells

36 The answer is E: Terminal bronchioles.   Larger bronchioles are lined by typical respiratory epithelium. However, with terminal bronchioles, the lining epithelium begins to assume a simple cuboidal morphology with Clara cells interspersed among ciliated cells. Clara cells increase in number as the bronchioles narrow to become respiratory bronchioles. Clara cells become the major cell population present in the epithelium of distal respiratory bronchioles. Clara cells are not typically found in other pulmonary locations listed.
Keywords: Clara cells

37 The answer is E: Secretion of surfactant.   Clara cells are also referred to as exocrine bronchiolar cells. These cells secrete a surface-active lipoprotein that helps prevent luminal adhesion and collapse of the bronchioles, particularly during expiration. Clara cells are also reserve stem cells that can repopulate respiratory bronchioles following injury (e.g., following smoke inhalation). None of the other cell biological activities listed describes the principal function of Clara cells.
Keywords: Clara cells

38 The answer is E: Terminal bronchiole.   The part of the conducting portion of the respiratory system is observed to originate from a large bronchiole on the left side of the image and give rise to two respiratory bronchioles on the right of the image. The wall of the terminal bronchiole is complete—without interruption. This feature distinguishes terminal bronchioles from respiratory bronchioles (choice D). Terminal bronchioles are lined by a simple cuboidal epithelium, with Clara cells scattered among the ciliated cells. Smooth muscle fibers are present in the walls of terminal bronchioles. Terminal bronchioles are the smallest and most distal conducting duct of the bronchial tree. The term "pulmonary acinus" refers to a terminal bronchiole and the lung tissue that it supplies.
Keywords: Terminal bronchioles

39 The answer is C: Respiratory bronchioles.   In this transitional zone, respiratory bronchioles function as both conducting passages (delivering air to and from alveoli) and sites of gas exchange. The anatomic basis for gas exchange at this location is that respiratory bronchioles open directly to alveoli, as well as alveolar ducts and sacs. It is not the major site for gas exchange, but it is the initial site for gas exchange in the lungs. Alveoli (choice A) are the primary site of gas exchange. Choices B, D, and E are not related to gas exchange.
Keywords: Respiratory bronchioles

40 The answer is D: Space 4.   Alveolar ducts are elongated tubes that branch from respiratory bronchioles. There is an increase in the number of alveolar openings along the walls of respiratory bronchioles as these air passages

move distally. The continuity of the wall of the respiratory bronchiole is all but lost at the point where alveolar ducts originate. Alveolar ducts are lined almost entirely by openings of the alveoli. Smooth muscle cells are present only at the rim of the alveoli. The other labeled spaces do not demonstrate features of alveolar ducts.
Keywords: Alveolar ducts

41 **The answer is B: Alveolar sac.** Clusters of alveoli surround and open into common air spaces termed alveolar sacs. Moving proximally in the respiratory system, alveolar sacs open into alveolar ducts that further connect to respiratory bronchioles. None of the other choices exhibit histologic features of alveolar sacs.
Keywords: Alveolar sacs

42 **The answer is E: Space 5.** Alveoli are sites of respiration in the lungs. They are terminal air spaces that form as pocket-like evaginations of the respiratory bronchioles, alveolar ducts, and alveolar sacs. These thin-walled cavities give the lungs a characteristic spongy texture and they dramatically increase the total surface area for gas exchange in the lungs. The alveoli are defined by alveolar septa (the scaffold for pulmonary architecture) that are composed of a very thin delicate connective tissue. Capillaries arising from the pulmonary arteries course through the alveolar septa, providing a rich blood supply to each alveolus. Alveolar septa contain elastin, collagen, and reticular fibers that provide support and mechanical strength to the lung. Loss of elasticity of alveolar septa underlies the pathogenesis of pulmonary emphysema. Emphysema is a chronic lung disease characterized by enlargement of air spaces distal to the terminal bronchioles, with destruction of their walls, but without fibrosis or inflammation. It is largely a disease of smokers.
Keywords: Alveoli

43 **The answer is D: Type I alveolar cells.** The lumen of the alveolus is lined by an epithelium consisting of type I and type II alveolar cells. Type I alveolar cells, also referred to as type I pneumocytes, are extremely thin, simple squamous epithelial cells. They cover most of the luminal surface of the pulmonary alveoli. By electron microscopy, the cytoplasm of type I alveolar cells is observed to be attenuated and virtually free of cytoplasmic organelles. The thin squamous epithelial lining of the alveoli by type I alveolar cells facilitates gas diffusion and exchange.
Keywords: Alveolus, type I alveolar cells

44 **The answer is E: Zonula occludens.** Tight junctions between type I alveolar cells form an effective barrier that prevents leakage of interstitial fluid into the air spaces of the lungs. Without this barrier, patients would develop pulmonary edema. Type I alveolar cells also form a blood–air barrier that is thin enough for efficient gas exchange. Cadherins (choice A) are Ca^{2+}-dependent cell adhesion molecules that localize to zonula adherens

(choice D); these junctions are found in type I alveolar cells, but they do not prevent fluid leakage. None of the other choices provide a barrier to the movement of interstitial fluid into the alveolar air spaces.
Keywords: Type I alveolar cells, zonula occludens

45 **The answer is E: Type II alveolar cells.** Type II alveolar cells, also termed type II pneumocytes, are rounded cells with rounded nuclei. They are interspersed among the type I alveolar cells and account for about 60% of cells in the alveolar wall. Type II alveolar cells tend to cluster at junctions between the alveolar septa and bulge into the alveolar lumen. None of the other cells listed show the distinctive histologic features of type II pneumocytes.
Keywords: Alveolus, type II alveolar cells

46 **The answer is E: Secretion of surfactant.** Although type II alveolar cells are the most numerous cells in the alveolar epithelium, they cover only less than 5% of the alveolar surface area. These cells secrete surfactant, a surface-active lipoprotein mixture that coats the alveolar lining epithelium. Surfactant lipids and proteins form a protective layer that reduces surface tension within the alveoli, to stabilize alveolar spaces and prevent their collapse.
Keywords: Alveolus, type II alveolar cells, surfactant

47 **The answer is E: Type II alveolar cells.** The alveolar surface is continuously exposed to inhaled pathogens and is vulnerable to many destabilizing forces. As described in this clinical vignette, viral infections of the pulmonary parenchyma produce interstitial pneumonia with diffuse alveolar damage. Necrosis of type I alveolar cells results in pathologic changes that are indistinguishable from diffuse alveolar damage in other settings (e.g., toxic smoke inhalation). Type I alveolar cells are mature cells that are not capable of proliferation and differentiation. By contrast, type II alveolar cells are pluripotent reserve cells that divide to repopulate the alveolar epithelium following injury. These stem cells are able to replace both type I and type II alveolar cells. Diffuse alveolar damage is characteristically associated with hyperplasia of type II alveolar cells (a key pathologic finding). None of the other cells listed are stem cells for regeneration of the alveolar epithelium.
Keywords: Alveolus, type II alveolar cells

48 **The answer is A: Fusion of epithelial and endothelial basal laminae.** Gas exchange occurs when (1) O_2 in the alveolus moves into capillary blood and (2) CO_2 moves in the opposite direction. The structural components that separate the alveolar air space from blood are collectively referred to as the "blood–air barrier." This physical barrier is remarkably thin and attenuated to permit efficient gas exchange. The thinnest portion of the blood–air barrier is composed of a layer of surfactant within the lumen of the alveolus, the type I alveolar cell and its basal lamina, and the capillary endothelial cell and its basal

lamina. EM studies demonstrate that the basal laminae of type I alveolar cells and endothelial cells are fused together in the thinnest portions of the air–blood barrier. Most gas exchange is believed to occur at this location. None of the other choices describe the blood–air barrier in the lungs.
Keywords: Alveoli, blood–air barrier

49 **The answer is B: Macrophages.** Macrophages in the lung are commonly referred to as "dust cells" because of their ability to ingest inhaled dust particles and pollen. Macrophages are part of the innate immune A system, and this protective mechanism of particle removal is termed phagocytosis. Alveolar macrophages are found in the alveolar air spaces and in alveolar septa. In addition to dust particle, macrophages phagocytose microorganisms and even red blood cells that enter the air spaces in patients with congestive heart failure. Macrophages with ingested red blood cells are referred to as "heart failure cells." Macrophages leave alveoli by migrating into bronchioles and then moving up the bronchial tree within the mucociliary ladder. Other macrophages remain in septal connective tissue—sometimes for the life span of the individual. None of the other cells listed exhibit morphologic features of alveolar macrophages.
Keywords: Lung cancer, alveolus, alveolar macrophages

50 **The answer is C: Carbon particles within macrophages.** Macrophages that have phagocytosed particles and pathogens typically aggregate, so as to move debris away from the respiratory portion of the lungs. These "dust cells" also migrate into the pulmonary lymphatic vessels and become concentrated at regional lymph nodes. During cadaver dissection, it is common to notice that the hilar lymph nodes appear black, owing to collections of pulmonary macrophages.
Keywords: Macrophages

51 **The answer is A: Alveolar septa.** Emphysema is a chronic obstructive pulmonary disease (COPD). It is characterized by enlargement of air spaces distal to the terminal bronchioles, with destruction of their walls, but without fibrosis or inflammation. The major cause of emphysema is cigarette smoking. Moderate to severe emphysema is rare in nonsmokers. Smokers develop squamous metaplasia of the respiratory epithelium (choice C) and hyperplasia of submucosal mucous glands (choice E); however, these pathologic changes do not explain the pathogenesis of respiratory distress in patients with emphysema. None of the other choices are related to the pathogenesis of pulmonary emphysema.
Keywords: Emphysema

52 **The answer is A: Alveoli.** The pathogenesis of respiratory distress syndrome (RDS) of the newborn is intimately linked to a deficiency of surfactant. Collapse of the alveoli (atelectasis) secondary to surfactant deficiency results in perfused but not ventilated alveoli, a situation that leads to hypoxia and acidosis. The leak of fibrin-rich fluid into the alveoli from the injured vascular bed contributes to the typical clinical and pathologic features of RDS. On gross examination, the lungs are dark red and airless. None of the other choices describe the pathogenesis of respiratory distress syndrome of the neonate.
Keywords: Respiratory distress syndrome of the neonate

53 **The answer is E: Type II alveolar cells.** Pulmonary surfactant is secreted by type II alveolar cells. However, these cells do not appear in fetal alveoli until late in pregnancy (typically after week 35). Pulmonary surfactant is released into amniotic fluid, where it can be sampled by amniocentesis to assess fetal lung maturity. Administration of exogenous surfactant to neonates that are born prematurely has greatly improved their survival. None of the other cells listed secrete pulmonary surfactant.
Keywords: Respiratory distress syndrome of the neonate, surfactant

54 **The answer is D: Mucous glands.** Mucous glands, and goblet cells, as well as serous glands are present in the wall of the conducting airways until the most distal bronchi. Glandular tissue disappears from the wall beginning at bronchioles. Mucus covers almost the entire luminal surface of the conducting passage. Mucus, as well as serous fluid, conditions the inhaled air, traps particles and pollens and protects the epithelial lining of the conducting airways.
Keywords: Mucous gland

55 **The answer is B: Intrapulmonary bronchus.** This lung specimen reveals the characteristic features of intrapulmonary bronchi, namely: discontinuous cartilage plates (indicated by asterisk), glandular tissue (indicated by arrows), and smooth muscle. Extrapulmonary bronchus (choice A) is excluded as the correct answer, because these initial segments of the primary bronchi exhibit cartilage rings (not the plates that are evident in this image). The conducting ducts distal to large bronchioles (choices C, D, and E) do not have cartilage plates and glandular tissue present in their walls.
Keywords: Intrapulmonary bronchi

56 **The answer is D: Thoracic aorta.** Two vascular systems supply the lung, namely the pulmonary and the bronchial circulations. This image shows an intrapulmonary bronchus (indicated by asterisk) adjacent to a pulmonary artery (indicated by dagger). The arteriole indicated by the arrow supplies the wall of the bronchus. Bronchial arteries arise from the thoracic aorta (correct answer); they supply the walls of the bronchi and the bronchioles and interstitial tissues, excluding the alveolar septa. Anastomoses between distal branches of the bronchial arteries and the pulmonary arteries are clinically significant, because these anastomoses prevent irreversible lung injury in patients with pulmonary embolism. None of the other choices listed give rise to the bronchial arteries or provide arterial blood to the intrapulmonary bronchi.

Keywords: Bronchial artery

57 The answer is A: Alveoli and alveolar septa. Pulmonary arteries and their branches travel with corresponding segments of the conducting airways and bring deoxygenated blood from the right ventricle to capillaries in the alveolar septa for gas exchange. Oxygenated blood leaves alveoli via pulmonary venous capillaries and returns to the left atrium of the heart via the four pulmonary veins. Tributaries of the pulmonary veins travel in the connective septa, between bronchopulmonary segments, at a distance from the pulmonary arteries and conducting airways. The other structures listed receive blood from the bronchial arteries.

Keywords: Pulmonary artery, alveoli

Chapter 12

Oral Cavity and Associated Glands

QUESTIONS

Select the single best answer.

1 A 48-year-old man complains of painful ulcers in his mouth. Physical examination reveals multiple shallow ulcers covered by a fibrinopurulent exudate on the inner surface of the upper lip and cheek. The patient is subsequently diagnosed with aphthous stomatitis, an inflammation of the oral mucosa. Which of the following types of epithelium lines the oral cavity?

(A) Keratinized stratified squamous
(B) Nonkeratinized stratified squamous
(C) Simple columnar
(D) Simple squamous
(E) Stratified columnar

2 A lip biopsy is sectioned and prepared with routine H&E staining (shown in the image). Identify the structures indicated by the arrows.

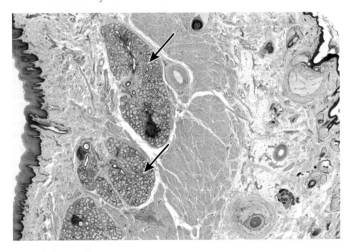

(A) Fordyce spots
(B) Minor salivary gland
(C) Sebaceous gland
(D) Sublingual gland
(E) Submandibular gland

3 A 22-year-old woman presents with a bluish, translucent cyst on her lower lip. Laboratory examination of a biopsy demonstrates a cystic cavity filled with mucus and surrounded by a layer of granulation tissue (shown in the image). Trauma to which of the following oral structures most likely resulted in the formation of this patient's mucus-filled cystic lesion?

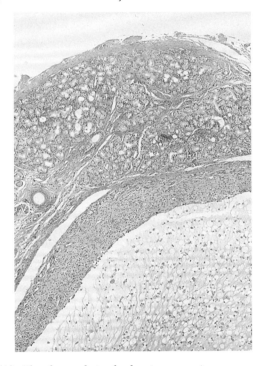

(A) Blood vessels in the lamina propria
(B) Large blood vessels in submucosa
(C) Lymphatic vessels
(D) Minor salivary glands
(E) Sublingual gland

4 A 19-year-old woman presents with painful cold sores on her lower lip. Physical examination reveals several vesicles and ulcers in the lesion area. Infection with which of the following pathogens is the common cause of cold sores?

(A) *Borrelia vincentii*
(B) Epstein-Barr virus
(C) Herpes simplex virus type 1
(D) Human herpes virus 8
(E) *Streptococcus pyogenes*

5 A 2-year-old boy suffers severe throat pain and high fever. Physical examination reveals swollen tissue masses in the posterior part of the oral cavity. Biopsy of the tissue mass is examined with routine histologic preparation (shown in the image). Identify the organ.

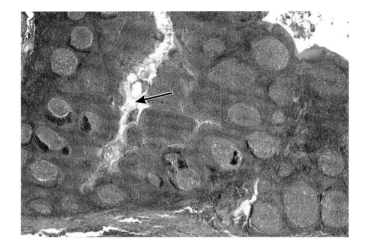

(A) Lingual tonsil
(B) Palatine tonsil
(C) Parotid gland
(D) Pharyngeal tonsil
(E) Sublingual gland

6 A tongue is examined at autopsy (shown in the image). Identify the tissue indicated by the arrows.

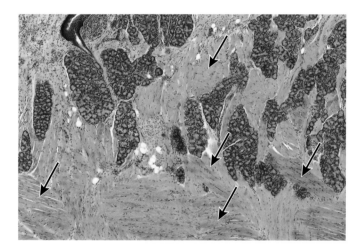

(A) Dense irregular connective tissue
(B) Dense regular connective tissue
(C) Peripheral nerve
(D) Skeletal muscle
(E) Smooth muscle

7 The epithelium overlying the dorsal surface of the tongue described in Question 6 is examined further (shown in the image). Identify the structure indicated by the arrow.

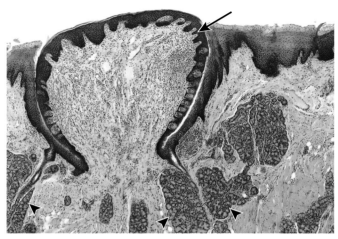

(A) Circumvallate papilla
(B) Filiform papilla
(C) Foliate papilla
(D) Fungiform papilla
(E) Lymphatic nodule

8 First-year medical students are reviewing histologic features of the tongue using a thin, plastic section obtained from a monkey. The sides of a circumvallate papilla are examined at high magnification (shown in the image). Identify the oval pale-stained structure indicated by the arrow.

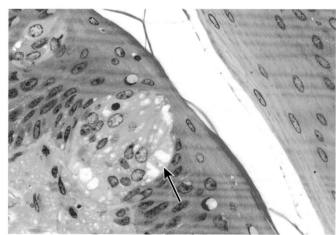

(A) Circumvallate papilla
(B) Fungiform papilla
(C) Mucous gland
(D) Serous salivary gland
(E) Taste bud

9 Taste buds in the anterior two-thirds of the dorsal surface of the tongue make synapses with special sensory axons carried by which of the following nerves?
(A) Facial nerve
(B) Glossopharyngeal nerve
(C) Hypoglossal nerve
(D) Trigeminal nerve
(E) Vagus nerve

10 The dorsal surface of a tongue specimen is examined at high magnification (shown in the image). Which of the following describes the most likely function of the structure indicated by the arrow?

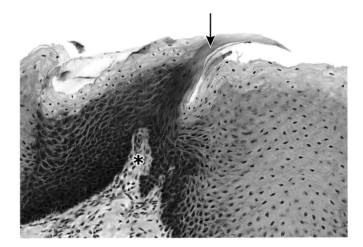

(A) Pain receptor
(B) Response to bitter taste
(C) Response to umami taste
(D) Surface for food movement
(E) Temperature receptor

11 The root of the tongue is examined at low magnification (shown in the image). Identify the structure indicated by the arrows.

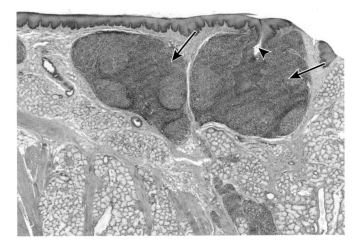

(A) Lingual tonsil
(B) Mucus lingual gland
(C) Palatine tonsil
(D) Pharyngeal tonsil
(E) Serous lingual gland

12 A 47-year-old man presents with a painless, moveable firm mass near the angle of his left mandible. Needle biopsy reveals a pleomorphic adenoma of the parotid gland, and the tumor is surgically excised. Normal glandular tissue at the margin of the surgical specimen is examined in the pathology department (shown in the image). Identify the area/structure indicated by the arrow.

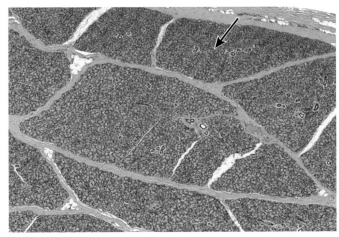

(A) Acinus
(B) Alveolus
(C) Islet
(D) Lobe
(E) Lobule

13 Two days after surgery, the patient described in Question 12 complains that he is unable to move the left side of his mouth. Physical examination reveals that the left side of his mouth is drooping. Which of the following nerves was most likely damaged during the patient's surgery?
(A) Facial
(B) Glossopharyngeal
(C) Hypoglossal
(D) Lingual
(E) Vagus

14 The parotid gland described in Question 12 is examined at high magnification (shown in the image). Identify the structure indicated by the arrow.

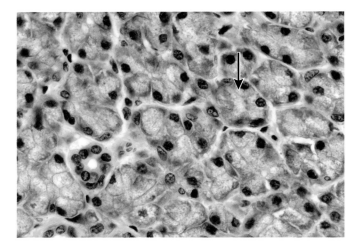

(A) Intercalated duct
(B) Mixed acinus
(C) Mucous acinus
(D) Serous acinus
(E) Serous demilune

15 Another microscopic field of the parotid gland described in Question 12 is shown in the image. Identify the structure indicated by the arrow.

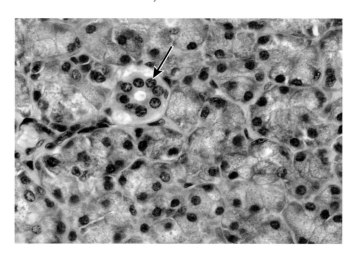

(A) Excretory duct
(B) Intercalated duct
(C) Mucous acinus
(D) Serous acinus
(E) Striated duct

16 The pleomorphic adenoma removed from the patient described in Question 12 is examined by light microscopy (shown in the image). The major cellular component of this benign tumor is identified as which of the following mesenchymal cells?

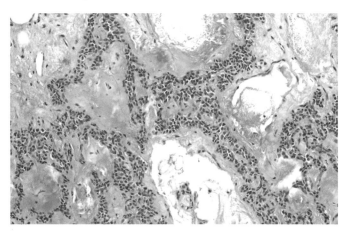

(A) Fibroblast
(B) Mucous cell
(C) Myoepithelial cell
(D) Plasma cell
(E) Serous cell

17 A submandibular gland is examined at autopsy (shown in the image). Identify the structure within the circle.

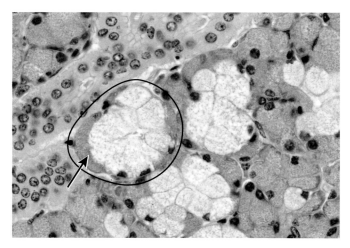

(A) Intercalated duct
(B) Mixed acinus
(C) Mucous acinus
(D) Serous acinus
(E) Striated duct

18 Another region of the submandibular gland described in Question 17 is examined at high magnification (shown in the image). Identify the structure indicated by the arrow.

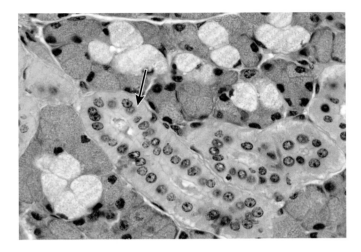

(A) Excretory duct
(B) Intercalated duct
(C) Mucous tubuloacinus
(D) Serous acinus
(E) Striated duct

19 The submandibular gland described in Questions 17 and 18 is examined further (shown in the image). The epithelium indicated by the arrows lines which of the following structures?

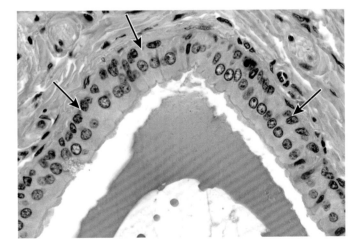

(A) Excretory duct
(B) Intercalated duct
(C) Small artery
(D) Small vein
(E) Striated duct

20 Laboratory studies demonstrate the presence of immunoglobulin A (IgA) in saliva obtained from healthy individuals. This antibody is synthesized and secreted by which of the following cells?
(A) Fibroblasts in surrounding connective tissue
(B) Mucous cells in acini
(C) Myoepithelial cells in acini
(D) Plasma cells in surrounding connective tissue
(E) Serous cells in acini

21 You are asked to lead a small group seminar on tooth development and oral hygiene. Which of the following cells produces a protective coating found on teeth referred to as pellicle?
(A) Ameloblasts
(B) Cementoblasts
(C) Mucous cells in the salivary glands
(D) Odontoblasts
(E) Serous cells in the salivary glands

22 A 7-year-old boy visits the dentist for a routine oral examination. Several microcavities (chalky white spots) are noticed on the left first molar. According to the parents, their son has not complained about any tooth pain. At this point in the development of dental caries, which of the following structures is principally affected in this patient's first molar?
(A) Cementum
(B) Dental pulp
(C) Dentin
(D) Enamel
(E) Gingiva

ANSWERS

1 **The answer is B: Nonkeratinized stratified squamous epithelium.** Oral mucosa lining the oral surfaces of the lip and cheeks, as well as the inferior surfaces of the tongue, floor of the mouth, and soft palate, is composed of a nonkeratinized stratified squamous epithelium, with associated lamina propria and a distinctive submucosa. It is referred to as lining mucosa in contrast to the mastication mucosa (keratinized stratified squamous epithelium) lining the gingiva and the hard palate. The mucosa lining the superior surface of the tongue is referred to as specialized mucosa since it is associated with the special sensation of taste. Aphthous stomatitis, also referred to as canker sores, is a common disease of the oral mucosa characterized by painful, recurrent, solitary, or multiple ulcers of the oral mucosa. Other listed epithelial types do not describe the lining mucosa of the oral cavity.
Keywords: Aphthous stomatitis, oral cavity

2 **The answer is B: Minor salivary gland.** Associated with the oral cavity, there are three pairs of major salivary glands (parotid, submandibular, and sublingual), as well as minor salivary glands. Minor salivary glands are located in the submucosa of different portions of the oral cavity, such as the inner surfaces of the lip and cheeks and inferior aspect of the tongue. They are named according to their location, that is, buccal, labial, lingual, and palatine glands. Short ducts directly convey secretions of the minor salivary glands into the oral cavity. Sublingual and submandibular glands (choices D and E) are major salivary glands and not located within the lip. Sebaceous glands (choice C) are seen in the skin below the lip, and they are associated with hair follicles. Sebaceous glands are occasionally found in the submucosa immediately lateral to the corners of the mouth; these locations are referred to as Fordyce spots (choice A).
Keywords: Minor salivary glands, lip

3 **The answer is D: Minor salivary glands.** Mucocele, also known as mucous cyst of the oral mucosa, is a mucus-filled cystic lesion associated with the minor salivary glands. Trauma to localized minor salivary glands causes escape and accumulation of mucus in the surrounding connective tissue. A fibrous wall and layer of inflammatory granulation tissue surround the mucus. Numerous macrophages and segmented neutrophils may be seen within the lumen due to concurrent acute inflammation. None of the other structures are associated with the pathogenesis of mucocele of the lip.
Keywords: Mucocele, minor salivary glands

4 **The answer is C: Herpes simplex virus type I.** Cold sores, also known as fever blisters or herpes labialis, are the most common viral infection of the lip and oral mucosa. They are caused by infection with herpes simplex virus type 1. The cold sores start with painful inflammation in the affected area. The epithelial cells undergo "ballooning degeneration" followed by the formation of vesicles. The vesicles eventually rupture, forming painful ulcers. The ulcers heal spontaneously without scar formation. Bacteria, spirochetes, viruses, and fungi are all normally present in the oral cavity and form a harmless microbial flora. The oral mucosa with its epithelial lining forms an important barrier between pathogens in the external environment and internal body tissue. Factors such as immunodeficiency, antibiotic therapy, stress, and trauma can disrupt the protective mechanisms, resulting in oral infections.
Keywords: Cold sores, herpes labialis

5 **The answer is B: Palatine tonsil.** Palatine tonsils are organized aggregations of lymphatic nodules and diffuse lymphatic tissue. They are situated between the palatopharyngeal and palatoglossal arches on either side of the pharynx. The overlying stratified squamous epithelium, continuous with the lining epithelium of the oral cavity, invaginates into the lymphatic tissue, forming deep pits referred to as tonsillar crypts (indicated by the arrow). Numerous secondary lymphatic nodules are seen with lighter stained germinal centers. In addition to palatine tonsils, there are pharyngeal tonsils (located on the roof of the pharynx, choice D), lingual tonsils (at the base of the tongue, choice A), and tubal tonsils (posterior to the opening of the auditory duct), forming a tonsillar ring around the entrance to the oropharynx. As an organ of immunity, bacterial invasion secondary to viral infection may cause acute tonsillitis characterized by sore throat, fever, and difficulty swallowing. It is the most common tonsillar disease. The parotid and sublingual glands (choices C and E) are major salivary glands and do not exhibit the lymphatic tissue seen in this biopsy.
Keywords: Tonsils

6 **The answer is D: Skeletal muscle.** The tongue is a mobile, muscular organ projecting from the oropharynx into the oral cavity. Both extrinsic and intrinsic lingual muscles are striated (skeletal) muscles that are arrayed in three dimensions. Thus, in any particular section through the tongue, muscle fibers can appear as cross-sections or as vertically- and horizontally-oriented longitudinal sections. This organization of lingual muscle fibers enables the tongue to move precisely, with enormous flexibility, which provides the structural basis for articulation. Articulation is one of the major functions of the tongue. None of the other tissues display the histologic features of skeletal muscle.
Keywords: Tongue, lingual muscles

7 **The answer is A: Circumvallate papilla.** Sulcus terminalis is a V-shaped depression on the dorsal surface of the tongue that separates the anterior two-thirds from the posterior one-third of the tongue. The surface of the tongue that is anterior to the sulcus terminalis is covered by a specialized epithelium consisting of numerous projections of the mucous membrane referred to as lingual papillae. Four types of lingual papillae are identified in humans based on shape: (1) filiform, (2) fungiform, (3) circumvallate, and (4) foliate. Circumvallate papillae are the largest dome-shaped papillae, situated just anterior to the sulcus terminalis. There are 8 to 12 circumvallate papillae arranged into a V-shaped line. Each papilla is surrounded by a deep circular invagination that is lined with stratified squamous epithelium. The epithelium lining the papilla contains numerous pale-stained taste buds. Numerous serous glands (von Ebner glands, indicated by arrowheads) are located in the underlying connective tissue and open into the circular furrow. The serous secretion of the von Ebner glands forms a continuous fluid flow that flushes material from the taste buds, so that taste buds can respond rapidly to new gustatory stimuli. None of the other structures demonstrate the characteristic histologic features of circumvallate papillae.

Keywords: Circumvallate papilla, von Ebner glands

8 The answer is E: Taste bud. Situated in the stratified squamous epithelium covering the oral cavity, taste buds appear as light-stained oval structures with a small opening, termed the taste pore, that opens at the epithelial surface. Taste buds are most numerous on the lower sides of the circumvallate papillae. They are also found in fungiform and foliate papillae and in other parts of the oral cavity. Three cell types have been identified in taste buds: (1) sensory (taste receptor) cells; (2) supporting cells, also described as immature taste cells; and (3) basal cells or precursor cells. The taste cell, the most numerous cell type, extends from the basal lamina to the taste pore, with microvilli projecting from its apical cell surface. The life spans of taste cells and supporting cells are about 10 days. Basal cells give rise to supporting cells that, in turn, develop into mature taste receptor cells. The bases of the taste receptor cells synapse with special sensory nerves. None of the other tissues exhibit histologic features of taste buds in the oral cavity.

Keywords: Taste buds

9 The answer is A: Facial nerve. Special afferent fibers carried by the facial nerve innervate the anterior two-thirds of the tongue and hard/soft palates and mediate taste sensation. Facial nerve endings synapse with taste receptor cells in taste buds located on the anterior two-thirds of the tongue. The posterior one-third of the tongue is supplied by special afferent fibers by the glossopharyngeal nerve (choice B). Vagus nerve (choice E) is believed to convey general somatic sensation from the posterior tongue and the pharyngeal area. The trigeminal nerve (choice D), through its lingual branch, innervates the anterior two-thirds of the tongue for general somatic sensation (i.e., pain, touch, and temperature) but does not convey

the sensation of taste. The hypoglossal nerve (choice C) provides somatic motor innervation to striated lingual muscles.

Keywords: Facial nerve, taste buds

10 The answer is D: Surface for food movement. The indicated structure is a filiform papilla. Filiform papillae are the smallest and most numerous type of papilla. They are found throughout the entire human tongue. Filiform papillae contain a vascular connective tissue core (indicated by the asterisk), covered by a heavily keratinized, stratified squamous epithelium. They appear as narrow cones with filamentous processes projecting posteriorly. Filiform papillae are believed to provide a rough surface on the tongue that facilitates food movement during mastication. Filiform papillae do not contain taste buds (choices B and C). Neither do they contain receptors for pain or temperature (choices A and E).

Keywords: Filiform papillae

11 The answer is A: Lingual tonsil. The lingual tonsil represents aggregates of lymphatic tissue located in the lamina propria at the base of the tongue, posterior to the sulcus terminalis. As shown in the image, the lingual tonsil is composed of diffuse and nodular lymphatic tissue (note primary and secondary nodules). The overlying stratified squamous epithelium invaginates into the tonsil forming a crypt (indicated by the arrowhead). Serous and mucous lingual salivary glands (choices B and E) are seen around and deep to the lingual tonsil and extending deep into striated lingual muscles. Palatine and pharyngeal tonsils (choices C and D) are not located at the root of the tongue.

Keywords: Lingual tonsils

12 The answer is E: Lobule. Parotid glands are the largest of the three pairs of major salivary glands. Secretomotor fibers to the parotid glands are provided by the glossopharyngeal nerve. Parotid gland secretions initiate digestion and help lubricate food. The tough dense connective tissue capsule of the parotid glands continues as connective tissue septa that penetrate and separate the parenchyma of the gland into lobes and lobules. Multiple lobules comprise a lobe (choice D). Connective tissue septa provide support to the glandular tissue and convey blood vessels, lymphatic channels, and nerves to and from secretory acini (choice A). None of the other structures exhibit histologic features of a parotid gland lobule.

Keywords: Parotid glands

13 The answer is A: Facial. After exiting the skull through the stylomastoid foramen, the facial nerve travels within the connective tissue sheath of the parotid gland to reach surrounding muscles of facial expression (e.g., orbicularis oris and zygomaticus major). Surgical resection of a pleomorphic adenoma of the parotid gland may cause injury to the facial nerve, resulting in facial nerve dysfunction. This condition is referred to as Bell palsy.

Another clinical sign of Bell palsy is ectropion (drooping of the lower eyelid), which is caused by paralysis of the orbicularis oculi muscle.

Keywords: Bell palsy, facial nerve dysfunction

14 **The answer is D: Serous acinus.** Secretory epithelial cells, especially serous cells, are often arranged into small spherical masses with very small lumens. These structures form a secretory unit that is referred to as an acinus. Parotid gland acini are composed almost entirely of serous cells that produce fluid, along with specific digestive enzymes and other proteins. Serous cells are usually pyramidal in shape, with a broad base on the basal lamina and a narrow apical surface facing the lumen. In H&E preparations, the basal domains of serous cells stain more deeply with hematoxylin, owing to an abundance of rough endoplasmic reticulum and free ribosomes. Secretory granules that stain with eosin are located in the apical cytoplasmic domain of these cells. Contractile myoepithelial cells are found between the serous cells and the basal lamina. None of the other structures exhibit histological features of a serous acinus.

Keywords: Parotid gland, serous acini

15 **The answer is B: Intercalated duct.** An extensive duct/channel system conveys salivary gland secretions to the oral cavity. Ducts draining the serous acini increase in diameter and wall thickness as they continuously merge together. The first, small segment of this extensive ductal system is the intercalated duct. Intercalated ducts drain secretory acini. They are typically lined by a squamous to low cuboidal epithelium, and the diameter of these ducts is smaller or equal in size to the size of the acini. Intercalated ducts are located within a lobule and are most well developed in the parotid glands. Several intercalated ducts join together to form a larger striated duct (choice E). None of the other choices exhibit histologic features of intercalated ducts.

Keywords: Parotid glands, intercalated ducts

16 **The answer is C: Myoepithelial cell.** Pleomorphic adenoma is the most common benign tumor of the parotid glands. It forms a slow-growing, painless, movable mass. Histologically, pleomorphic adenoma is composed of epithelial tissue intermingled with areas resembling cartilaginous, myxoid, or mucoid material. Ductal and myoepithelial cells compose the epithelial tissue component of the tumor; myoepithelial cells are the principal cellular component. Myoepithelial cells are organized into well-defined sheaths, cords, or nests with the myxoid or mucoid areas scattered between them. The other cell types do not form the major cellular component of pleomorphic adenoma.

Keywords: Pleomorphic adenoma, myoepithelial cells

17 **The answer is B: Mixed acinus.** Submandibular glands exhibit mixed serous and mucous tubuloacinar glands, although the serous acini predominant. Pure mucous

acini are rarely observed in submandibular glands. Mixed seromucous acini are scattered among the serous acini. In an H&E-stained paraffin section, the mucous cells appear empty, because their stores of mucus are removed during tissue processing. In mixed acini, serous cells form a cap on the basal aspect of the mucous cells; such caps are referred as serous demilunes (indicated by the arrow). Recent studies have shown that serous demilunes are, in fact, artifacts of conventional fixation. With improved methods, mucous and serous cells are found to be aligned in the same row facing the lumen of the acinus. Using traditional methods of tissue preparation, mucous cells swell, and the cytoplasm of serous cells is pushed to the periphery, forming a typical serous demilune. None of the other structures exhibit histologic features of mixed seromucous acini.

Keywords: Submandibular glands, serous demilune, mixed acinus

18 **The answer is E: Striated duct.** Striated ducts refer to segments of the exocrine ductal system that provide conduits between intercalated ducts and excretory ducts. Simple cuboidal to columnar epithelial cells line striated ducts as they grow in diameter and approach excretory ducts. They are so-named because of the "striations" along the basal domain of these cells. The basal plasma membrane of these duct cells forms numerous infoldings that contain longitudinally oriented mitochondria. These infoldings give the cells a striated appearance on histologic examination. They provide a mechanism for fluid reabsorption in the epithelial cells lining the striated ducts. Striated ducts are most extensive in submandibular glands and are least developed in sublingual glands. These epithelial cells reabsorb Na^+ from the primary secretion and secrete K^+ and HCO_3^-. Striated ducts located within the parenchyma of the glands are referred as intralobular ducts. They have diameters that are usually larger than that of acini. Larger striated ducts may be accompanied by small blood vessels within small amounts of connective tissue. None of the other structures exhibit the characteristic features of striated ducts.

Keywords: Submandibular glands, striated ducts

19 **The answer is A: Excretory duct.** The intralobular striated ducts join to form larger excretory ducts that travel within the interlobular and interlobar connective tissue septa. The excretory ducts eventually unite to form parotid ducts (draining the parotid glands) and submandibular ducts (draining both the submandibular and sublingual glands) that open into the oral cavity. As the diameters of the excretory ducts gradually increase, the lining epithelium changes from simple cuboidal (small excretory ducts) to stratified columnar (large excretory ducts, as shown in the image). None of the other structures exhibit histologic features of excretory ducts.

Keywords: Submandibular glands, excretory ducts

20 **The answer is D: Plasma cells in surrounding connective tissue.**   The plasma cells in the loose connective tissue surrounding the secretory acini synthesize dimeric IgA antibodies and secrete them into the surrounding extracellular matrix. Here, secretory IgA binds to a receptor protein on the basal surface of acinar cells and is carried to the apical plasma membrane where it is released into the lumen of the acinus. Salivary IgA, as well as other protein components secreted by serous cells (e.g., lysozyme and lactoferrin), provide natural immunity against bacterial and viral infections. Dysfunction of the salivary glands may result in inflammation of the oral mucosa. None of the other listed cells secrete IgA.
Keywords: Salivary IgA

21 **The answer is C: Mucous cells in the salivary glands.**   Mucous cells in the salivary glands secrete highly glycosylated mucins that lubricate the oral mucosa and form a thin protective film covering the teeth, called pellicle. Pellicle provides a barrier against acids and modulates the attachment/colonization of bacteria to the teeth and the oral cavity. Numerous proteins (e.g., lactoferrin, cystatins, histatin) and enzymes secreted by serous cells in the salivary glands (choice E) also serve to inhibit the growth of bacteria in the oral cavity. Dysfunction of the salivary glands may result in tooth decay and inflammation of the oral mucosa. Ameloblasts (choice A) produce enamel, the highly calcified superficial layer of the teeth. Cementoblasts (choice B) secrete cementum, a bone-like tissue covering the outer surface of the roots of the teeth.

Dentin, the calcified bony tissue forming the bulk of the teeth, is produced by odontoblasts (choice D).
Keywords: Pellicle

22 **The answer is D: Enamel.**   Each tooth consists of a crown (exposed portion of the tooth above the gingiva), a neck (constricted segment at the gum), and one or more roots (embedded in bony alveoli). Enamel is the extremely hard tissue layer covering the crown. A bone-like tissue layer called cementum (choice A) covers the outer surface of the root. Beneath the enamel and cementum, dentin (choice C) forms the calcified bulk of the tooth. In the center of the tooth, the pulp cavity is filled with loose connective tissue that also contains blood vessels and nerves. The narrow part of the pulp cavity in the root is referred as the root canal. Enamel is the hardest tissue in the human body. It consists almost exclusively of calcium hydroxyapatite crystals (98%), with very little organic material added. It is derived from epithelium and is not replaceable once it is formed. Despite their strength and hardness, enamel, cementum, and dentin can be decalcified and destroyed by bacteria. Bacterial colonies thriving on remnants of food on the enamel surface produce an acid environment that can demineralize the enamel and cause carious lesions (dental caries). As the caries progress, and enamel destruction continues, the dentin is exposed. At this point, the patient will experience pain that worsens when the affected tooth is exposed to heat, cold, sweet foods, or sweet drinks.
Keywords: Dental caries, tooth enamel

Chapter 13

Gastrointestinal Tract

QUESTIONS

Select the single best answer.

1 The gastrointestinal (GI) tract is compartmentalized into organs that are specialized for digestion of food and absorption of nutrients. Most variation and specialization along the length of the GI tract occur in which of the following tissue layers?
(A) Epithelium of mucosa
(B) Lamina propria
(C) Muscularis externa
(D) Muscularis mucosae
(E) Submucosa

2 During a small group discussion, you are asked to explain structural and functional differences between rugae, villi, microvilli, plicae circulares, teniae coli, and haustra. Rugae are found in which of the following segments of the GI tract?
(A) Esophagus
(B) Large intestine
(C) Rectum/anal canal
(D) Small intestine
(E) Stomach

3 A 70-year-old man undergoes chemotherapy for liver cancer, develops sepsis, and dies of multiorgan system failure. The patient's visceral organs are examined at autopsy. The plastic-embedded section shown in the image was obtained from what segment of the GI tract?

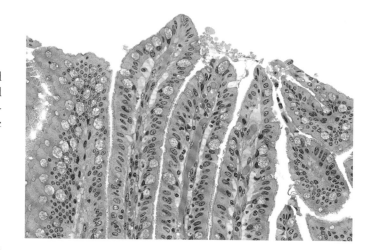

(A) Appendix
(B) Esophagus
(C) Large intestine
(D) Small intestine
(E) Stomach

4 Examination of the lamina propria of the organ identified in Question 3 reveals which of the following key histologic features of the GI tract?
(A) Brunner glands
(B) Lacteals
(C) Meissner plexuses
(D) Myenteric plexuses
(E) Pyloric glands

5 A 69-year-old man with a history of gastroesophageal reflux develops a pulmonary saddle embolus and expires. The patient's esophagus is examined at autopsy (shown in the image). Which of the following types of epithelium lines the proximal portion of this autopsy specimen?

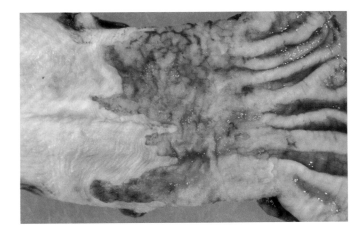

(A) Pseudostratified columnar with cilia and goblet cells
(B) Pseudostratified columnar with goblet cells
(C) Simple columnar with goblet cells
(D) Stratified squamous, keratinized
(E) Stratified squamous, nonkeratinized

6 Microscopic examination of the distal portion of the autopsy specimen provided for Question 5 reveals intestine-like glandular epithelium with goblet cells. These histopathologic findings are associated with which of following adaptations to chronic persistent cell injury?

(A) Atrophy
(B) Dysplasia
(C) Hyperplasia
(D) Hypertrophy
(E) Metaplasia

7 A section of a normal distal esophagus is examined in the histology laboratory. Identify the layer of the GI tract indicated by the arrows (shown in the image).

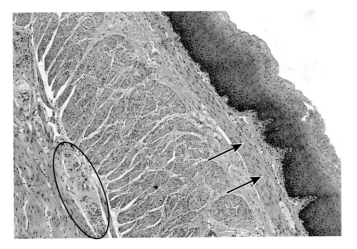

(A) Lamina propria
(B) Mucosa
(C) Muscularis externa
(D) Muscularis mucosae
(E) Submucosa

8 A 45-year-old man complains of difficulty swallowing and a tendency to regurgitate his food. Further studies demonstrate a complete absence of peristalsis and failure of the lower esophageal sphincter to relax upon swallowing. These clinicopathologic findings are explained as a deficiency (or absence) of which of the following structures in the distal esophagus?

(A) Ganglion cells in the Auerbach plexus
(B) Ganglion cells in the Meissner plexus
(C) Presynaptic parasympathetic nerves
(D) Presynaptic sympathetic nerves
(E) Smooth muscle in the muscularis externa

9 Digital slides illustrating various organs of the GI tract are examined in the histology laboratory. The specimen shown in the image was obtained from which of the following anatomic locations?

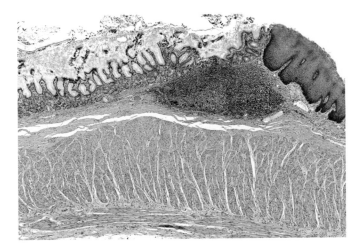

(A) Esophagogastric junction
(B) Fundus of the stomach
(C) Gastroduodenal junction
(D) Ileocecal junction
(E) Pylorus of the stomach

10 The organs identified in Question 9 are examined at higher magnification. Identify the structures indicated by the arrows (shown in the image).

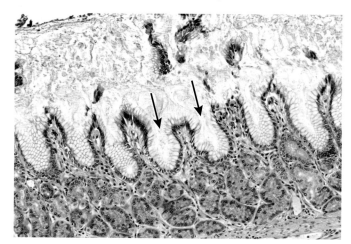

(A) Brunner glands
(B) Cardiac glands
(C) Gastric pits
(D) Intestinal glands
(E) Pyloric glands

11 The visible mucus identified in Question 10 contains a high concentration of which of the following biomolecules?
(A) Bicarbonate and potassium
(B) Hydrochloric acid
(C) Lysozyme
(D) Polypeptide hormones
(E) Proteases

12 A 58-year-old woman with a history of indigestion after meals and "heartburn" presents with upper abdominal pain. She is currently being treated with proton pump inhibitors for gastroesophageal reflux disease (GERD). Which of the following types of epithelial cells has proton pumps and generates hydrochloric acid (HCl) within the lumen of the stomach?
(A) Chief cells
(B) Enterocytes
(C) Goblet cells
(D) Paneth cells
(E) Parietal cells

13 During a clinical conference, you are asked to discuss physiological mechanisms that protect the stomach from the acidity of gastric juice and from mechanical abrasion. Which of the following small molecules plays an important role in maintaining bicarbonate secretion by surface mucous cells and increasing the thickness of the surface mucus layer in the stomach?
(A) Histamine
(B) Kinins
(C) Nitric oxide
(D) Prostaglandins
(E) Serotonin

14 You are analyzing patterns of stem cell renewal and terminal differentiation in the GI tract. As part of your research, you generate monoclonal antibodies that identify specific populations of gastric epithelial cells. One of your antibodies recognizes a protease found in zymogen granules. Which of the following cells is characterized by the presence of zymogen secretory granules?
(A) Chief cells
(B) Enteroendocrine cells
(C) Mucous cells
(D) Parietal cells
(E) Plasma cells

15 Another of your monoclonal antibodies identifies proliferating stem cells in the gastric mucosa. You hope to use this antibody to isolate these progenitor cells using fluorescence-activated cell sorting (FACS). Which of the following locations in the mucosa provides a niche for multipotent gastric stem cells?
(A) Fundus of glandular epithelium
(B) Gastric pit
(C) Isthmus of glandular epithelium
(D) Lamina propria
(E) Neck of glandular epithelium

16 A 25-year-old woman suffers massive trauma and internal bleeding in a motorcycle accident and expires. The patient's visceral organs are examined at autopsy. Identify the segment of the GI tract shown in the image.

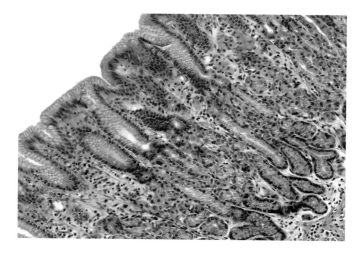

(A) Cardia of the stomach
(B) Esophagogastric junction
(C) Fundus of the stomach
(D) Gastroduodenal junction
(E) Ileocecal junction

17 The organ identified in Question 16 is examined at higher magnification (shown in the image). Name the round eosinophilic cells in these mucosal glands.

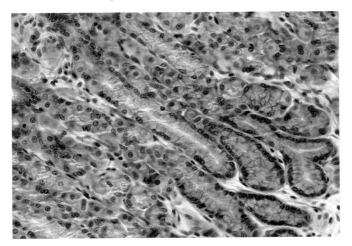

(A) Chief cells
(B) Enteroendocrine cells
(C) Mucous cells
(D) Paneth cells
(E) Parietal cells

18 For the autopsy specimen provided for Question 17, identify the basophilic cells clustered at the base of the gastric glands (lower right corner, shown in the image).
(A) Chief cells
(B) Enteroendocrine cells
(C) Mucous cells
(D) Paneth cells
(E) Parietal cells

19 A 34-year-old man presents with a 5-month history of weakness and fatigue. A peripheral blood smear shows megaloblastic anemia. Further laboratory studies demonstrate vitamin B_{12} deficiency. This patient's anemia is most likely caused by autoantibodies directed against which of the following GI cells?
(A) Chief cells
(B) Enteroendocrine cells
(C) Microfold cells
(D) Paneth cells
(E) Parietal cells

20 A 74-year-old woman complains of weakness and fatigue. She states that her stools have recently become black after taking a new nonsteroidal anti-inflammatory drug (NSAID). Gastroscopy reveals superficial, bleeding mucosal defects. What is the most likely mechanism for the development of acute erosive gastritis in this patient?
(A) Activation of Hageman factor
(B) Activation of serum kallikrein
(C) Generation of membrane attack complex
(D) Inhibition of cyclooxygenase
(E) Mast cell degranulation

21 A silver stain is used to identify enteroendocrine cells in the pyloric region of the stomach (small dark-stained cells, shown in the image). These argentaffin cells are classified as "open" or "closed" depending on whether or not their apical membranes reach the lumen of the gut. What is the primary function of "open" enteroendocrine cells in the GI tract?

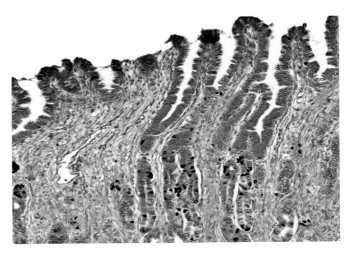

(A) Antibody secretion
(B) Antigen uptake
(C) Chemoreception
(D) Gastrin secretion
(E) Histamine release

22 You are investigating the activation of smooth muscle in the muscularis mucosae of the stomach and its role in assisting outflow from gastric glands. The cell bodies for visceral motor fibers that innervate the muscularis mucosae are present in which of the following anatomic locations?
(A) Auerbach plexus
(B) Celiac ganglion
(C) Meissner plexus
(D) Nucleus ambiguous of the CNS
(E) Sympathetic trunk

23 A 44-year-old woman presents with burning epigastric pain that usually occurs between meals. The pain can be relieved with antacids. The patient also reports a recent history of tarry stools. Gastroscopy reveals a bleeding mucosal defect in the antrum measuring 1.5 cm in diameter. Which of the following is the most likely underlying cause of peptic ulcer disease in this patient?
(A) Alcohol abuse
(B) Aspirin use
(C) Emotional stress
(D) Infection
(E) Tumor

24 A 76-year-old woman with a history of chronic infectious gastritis suffers a ruptured abdominal aortic aneurysm and expires. At autopsy, a silver stain of the patient's gastric mucosa reveals *Helicobacter pylori* (small curved rods, shown in the image). What bacterial enzyme allows these pathogens to survive in the acidic environment of the gastric lumen?

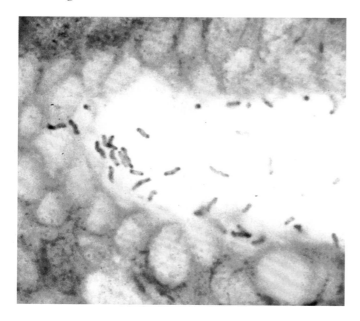

(A) Chymotrypsin
(B) Pepsin
(C) Secretase
(D) Streptokinase
(E) Urease

25 A 3-week-old boy is brought to the physician by his parents who report that he vomits forcefully immediately after nursing. Imaging studies reveal concentric enlargement of the pyloric canal. Which of the following best explains the pathogenesis of congenital pyloric stenosis in this infant?
(A) Deviation of the septum transversum
(B) Hypertrophy of smooth muscle
(C) Incomplete canalization of the primitive gut tube
(D) Malrotation of the primitive gut tube
(E) Persistence of the vitelline duct

26 Various GI organs are examined at a multiheaded microscope in the pathology department. The pathology resident asks you to comment on the glandular tissue located within the lines (shown in the image). These mucosal glands empty into which of the following segments of the GI tract?

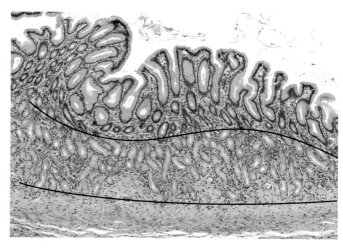

(A) Colon
(B) Duodenum
(C) Ileum
(D) Jejunum
(E) Stomach

27 Various organs of the GI tract are examined in the histology laboratory. Identify the glandular structures located between the double arrows (shown in the image).

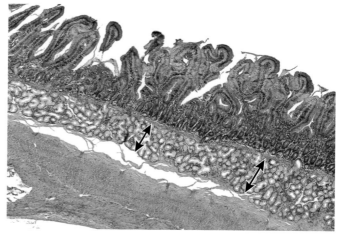

(A) Brunner glands
(B) Cardiac glands
(C) Fundic glands
(D) Intestinal glands
(E) Pyloric glands

28 Which of the following is an essential secretory product of the submucosal glands identified in Question 27?
(A) Amylase
(B) Bicarbonate ions
(C) Hydrochloric acid
(D) Lipase
(E) Pepsinogen

29 A 68-year-old man undergoes surgery to remove a gastric adenocarcinoma. A portion of the proximal duodenum at the tumor margin is examined for evidence of malignant cells. Identify the structure within the oval (shown in the image).

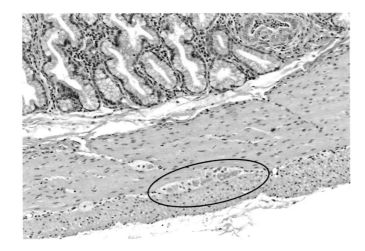

(A) Meissner plexus
(B) Myenteric plexus
(C) Peyer patch
(D) Primary lymphoid nodule
(E) Secondary lymphoid nodule

30 A 45-year-old man describes burning epigastric pain 2 to 3 hours after eating. Foods, antacids, and over-the-counter medications provide no relief, and prescribed inhibitors of acid secretion are only moderately effective. Endoscopy reveals multiple gastric and duodenal peptic ulcers. An abdominal CT scan reveals a pancreatic tumor. What polypeptide hormone is most likely secreted by this pancreatic islet cell neoplasm?
(A) Cholecystokinin
(B) Gastrin
(C) Ghrelin
(D) Motilin
(E) Secretin

31 A 68-year-old man with a history of intestinal malabsorption suffers a stroke and expires. Portions of the patient's small intestine are collected at autopsy, stained with H&E, and examined at low magnification. Identify the distinctive submucosal folds indicated by the arrows (shown in the image).

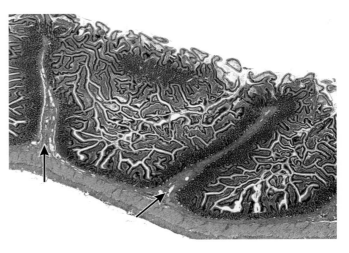

(A) Haustra
(B) Plicae circulares
(C) Rugae
(D) Teniae coli
(E) Villi

32 The autopsy specimen described in Question 31 is examined at high magnification. Identify the delicate apical membrane feature indicated by the arrows (shown in the image).

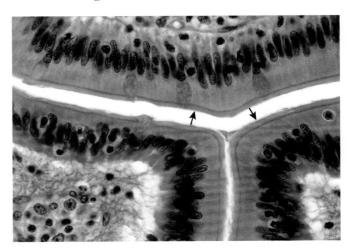

(A) Basal lamina
(B) Glycocalyx
(C) Lamina densa
(D) Lamina propria
(E) Striated brush border

33 A section of the jejunum described in Questions 31 and 32 is stained for carbohydrate using periodic acid–Schiff (PAS). Parallel arrays of intestinal villi are examined at high magnification (shown in the image). Identify the PAS-positive cells revealed in this tissue section.

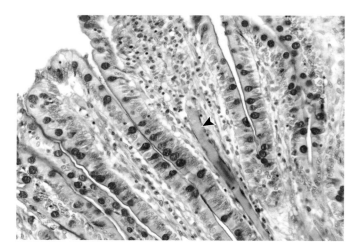

(A) Chief cells
(B) Goblet cells
(C) Histiocytes
(D) Paneth cells
(E) Parietal cells

34 You are invited to give a lecture on the pathobiology of enteroendocrine cells at a national conference on "childhood obesity" organized by First Lady Michelle Obama. During your lecture, you mention that enteroendocrine cells secrete a wide variety of polypeptide hormones. Which hormone produced in the stomach stimulates the perception of hunger?
(A) Cholecystokinin
(B) Gastrin
(C) Ghrelin
(D) Leptin
(E) Secretin

35 After your lecture, a colleague asks you to comment on recent drug discovery efforts to regulate nutrient uptake in the small intestine. What hormone stimulates gallbladder contraction and pancreatic enzyme secretion?
(A) Cholecystokinin
(B) Gastrin
(C) Ghrelin
(D) Leptin
(E) Secretin

36 A 55-year-old man undergoes abdominal surgery to remove a neuroendocrine tumor (carcinoid) of the small intestine. Normal intestinal mucosa at the margin of the tumor is embedded in plastic, sectioned at 1.5 μm, and examined at high magnification. Identify the secretory cells within the box (shown in the image).

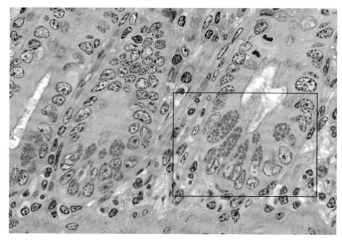

(A) Enterocytes
(B) Goblet cells
(C) Macrophages
(D) Paneth cells
(E) Plasma cells

37 The internal organs of a 78-year-old woman who died of metastatic cancer are examined at low magnification. Identify the segment of the GI tract that is shown in the image.

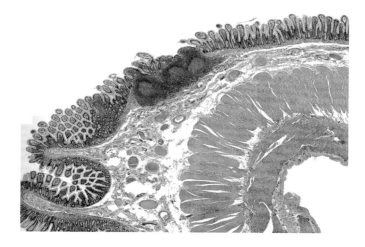

(A) Cecum
(B) Duodenum
(C) Ileum
(D) Jejunum
(E) Rectum

38 During your examination of the specimen described in Question 37, you are asked to discuss microfold (M) cells and mucosa-associated lymphoid tissue. What is the principal function of M cells in the distal ileum?
(A) Antigen uptake
(B) Fluid transport
(C) Gastrin secretion
(D) Histamine release
(E) Chemoreception

39 What cell surface glycoprotein found on M cells suggests that these phagocytic cells present antigens to lymphocytes in the GI tract?
(A) CD4
(B) CD8
(C) IgM
(D) MHC class I
(E) MHC class II

40 The autopsy specimen described in Question 37 is examined at higher magnification. Identify the glandular structures located between the lines (shown in the image).

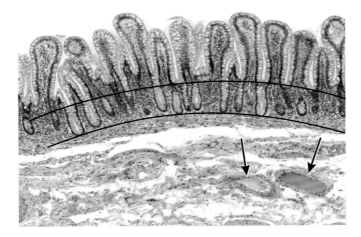

(A) Brunner glands
(B) Cardiac glands
(C) Crypts of Lieberkühn
(D) Fundic glands
(E) Pyloric glands

41 Further examination of the specimen provided for Question 40 reveals arterioles and venules (arrows, shown in the image). These blood vessels are located within which of the following layers of the GI tract?
(A) Adventitia
(B) Lamina propria
(C) Mucosa
(D) Muscularis externa
(E) Submucosa

42 An intestinal villus is examined at high magnification. Goblet cells appear to be secreting mucus into the lumen of the gut (arrows, shown in the image). Macrophages and lymphocytes visible in this slide specimen are located primarily within which of the following layers of the GI tract?

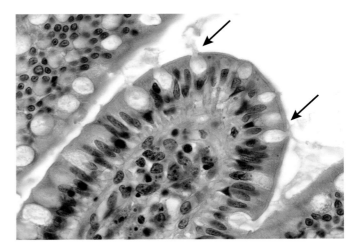

(A) Epithelium of mucosa
(B) Lamina propria
(C) Muscularis externa
(D) Muscularis mucosae
(E) Submucosa

43 A 2-year-old boy is brought to the emergency room with a 48-hour history of nausea and abdominal discomfort. Physical examination reveals right lower quadrant guarding. Ultrasound examination of the abdomen reveals a 2-cm mass near the ileocecal junction. The child is discovered to have an obstruction caused by abnormal intestinal peristalsis. What is the appropriate pathologic diagnosis?
(A) Intussusception
(B) Meconium ileus
(C) Stricture
(D) Torsion
(E) Volvulus

44 During a small group seminar, you are asked to discuss humeral immunity in the GI tract. Plasma cells in the lamina propria secrete primarily which of the following classes of immunoglobulin?
(A) IgA
(B) IgD
(C) IgE
(D) IgG
(E) IgM

45 During the seminar, you are asked to discuss the cellular mechanisms that mediate antibody transport across the epithelial barrier of the GI tract. Which of the following cells transports IgA from the lamina propria of the mucosa to the lumen of the gut?

(A) Enterocytes
(B) Goblet cells
(C) Microfold cells
(D) Paneth cells
(E) Plasma cells

46 Various organs of the GI tract are examined at low magnification in the histology laboratory. Identify the structure indicated by the arrow (shown in the image).

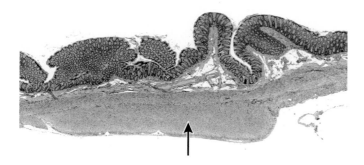

(A) Adventitia
(B) Haustra coli
(C) Omental appendices
(D) Plicae circulares
(E) Teniae coli

47 A 2-year-old girl with a history of chronic constipation since birth is brought to the emergency room because of nausea and vomiting. Physical examination shows marked abdominal distension. Abdominal radiography reveals distended bowel loops. Which of the following developmental defects explains the pathogenesis of congenital megacolon in this patient?

(A) Failure of neural crest migration
(B) Hypertrophy of smooth muscle
(C) Incomplete canalization of the primitive gut tube
(D) Malrotation of the primitive gut tube
(E) Persistence of the vitelline duct

48 Digital slides of the GI tract are examined in the histology laboratory. The double arrow (shown in the image) indicates which of the following layers of the large intestine?

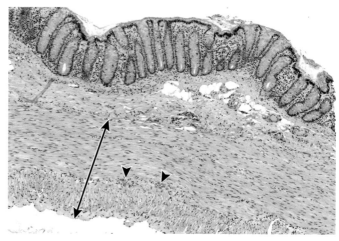

(A) Lamina propria
(B) Muscularis mucosae
(C) Mucosa
(D) Muscularis externa
(E) Submucosa

49 Your classmate opens a new digital slide and you study it together on the computer monitor. Identify the segment of the GI tract that is shown in the image.

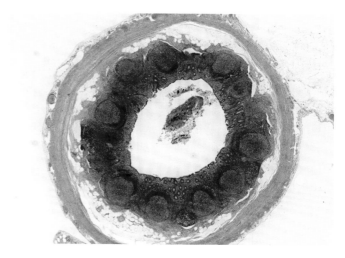

(A) Appendix
(B) Duodenum
(C) Ileum
(D) Jejunum
(E) Rectum

50 A 69-year-old woman undergoes a routine colonoscopy. During the procedure, a 2-cm mass is identified and resected. Microscopic examination shows irregular crypts lined by a pseudostratified epithelium. Normal tissue is evident at the tumor margin (shown in the image). In addition to mucin-producing goblet cells, these normal colonic glands are composed of which of the following epithelial cells?

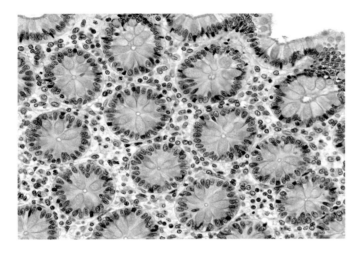

(A) Chief cells
(B) Enterocytes
(C) Enteroendocrine cells
(D) Paneth cells
(E) Parietal cells

51 You are invited to shadow a GI pathologist. A surgical specimen is examined using a double-headed microscope. This normal tissue was obtained from which of the following locations in the GI tract?

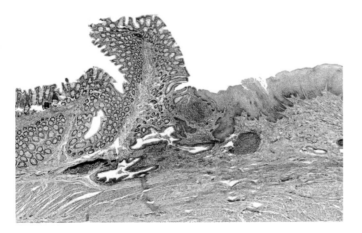

(A) Colorectal junction
(B) Esophagogastric junction
(C) Gastroduodenal junction
(D) Ileocecal junction
(E) Rectoanal junction

52 A 61-year-old man undergoes routine colonoscopy. A small, raised, mucosal nodule measuring 0.4 cm in diameter is identified and resected. The surgical specimen is shown in the image. Microscopic examination reveals goblet cells and absorptive cells with exaggerated crypt architecture but no signs of nuclear atypia. This hyperplastic polyp was most likely removed from what region of the GI tract?

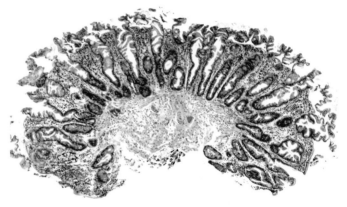

(A) Ascending colon
(B) Cecum
(C) Descending colon
(D) Rectum
(E) Transverse colon

ANSWERS

1 **The answer is A: Epithelium of mucosa.** The GI tract is composed of four tissue layers: mucosa, submucosa, muscularis externa, and serosa/adventitia (depending on whether the organ is attached to other structures). The mucosa is subdivided into lining epithelium and underlying connective tissue (lamina propria and muscularis mucosae). Lining epithelial cells regulate specific functions of the GI tract, including (1) barrier to the entry of pathogens, (2) secretion of enzymes and hormones, and (3) absorption of nutrients, electrolytes, and water. The esophagus delivers food to the stomach, where it is formed into a semiliquid mass (chyme) and transported to the small intestine. Lipases and proteases degrade proteins and complex carbohydrates to amino acids and simple sugars, respectively. Bile salts stored in the gallbladder are added to emulsify lipids. Within the jejunum and ileum, nutrients and vitamins are transported across the lining epithelium, where they enter vascular and lymphatic vessels. The other layers of the GI tract exhibit regional variation, but epithelial cells of the mucosa exhibit the greatest range of differentiation.
Keywords: Gastrointestinal tract, mucosa

2 **The answer is E: Stomach.** Rugae are characteristic features of the stomach. These longitudinal folds (or ridges) enable the stomach to distend as it fills with food. Ménétrier disease (hyperplastic hypersecretory gastropathy) is an uncommon disorder of the stomach that is characterized by enlarged rugae. Plicae circulares, villi, and microvilli are elaborations of the mucosa or submucosa in the small intestine that increase the surface area for nutrient absorption. Teniae coli are longitudinal bands of smooth muscle in the colon that regulate segmentation and peristalsis. Haustra are large sacculations of the large intestine. None of the other segments of the GI tract exhibit rugae.
Keywords: Stomach, rugae

3 **The answer is D: Small intestine.** This autopsy specimen was obtained from the small intestine (jejunum). Histologic features of intestinal mucosa include villi, enterocytes with microvilli, and mucus-secreting goblet cells. The small intestine is the principal site for nutrient absorption in the GI tract. The absorptive cells are referred to as enterocytes. These tall, columnar epithelial cells, with basal nuclei, express a variety of cell surface hydrolytic enzymes and transport proteins for uptake of amino acids, sugars, and lipids. Microvilli along the apical membrane domain of enterocytes increase the surface area of the small intestine by 600-fold. Intestinal glands in the appendix and large intestine (choices A and C) lack villi and microvilli. Gastric mucosa (choice E) features surface mucous cells and gastric pits. The

esophagus (choice B) is lined by a nonkeratinized, stratified squamous epithelium.
Keywords: Small intestine, villi

4 **The answer is B: Lacteals.** The lamina propria of the mucosa is a loose connective tissue that supports the overlying epithelium. In the GI tract, the lamina propria provides adhesion molecules for attachment and migration of epithelial cells. It also provides space for vascular and lymphatic channels. In some regions of the GI tract, the lamina propria includes mucosal glands and lymphatic tissue. The lamina propria of the small intestine is characterized by the presence of large lymphatic channels, termed "lacteals." An example of a lacteal is evident in the image. These dilated lymphatic channels transport dietary lipids from the small intestine to the circulatory system, via the thoracic duct. Free fatty acids from the diet are taken up by enterocytes and converted to triglycerides. Triglycerides are combined with cholesterol and a carrier protein (apolipoprotein B48) to form chylomicrons. These macromolecules are secreted by enterocytes into the lamina propria, where they enter the lacteals for transport. Brunner glands (choice A) are submucosal glands in the proximal duodenum. None of the other structures are found in the lamina propria of the small intestine.
Keywords: Small intestine, lacteals

5 **The answer is E: Stratified squamous, nonkeratinized.** The esophagus is a 25-cm tube that passes through the superior and inferior mediastinum. It enters the abdominal cavity at vertebral level T10 and delivers food to the stomach for mechanical and enzymatic digestion. This autopsy specimen was obtained from a patient with a history of chronic gastroesophageal (acid) reflux. It shows evidence of both normal (upper) and abnormal (lower) esophageal mucosa. The normal mucosa that lines the proximal portion of this esophagus (on the left) exhibits a nonkeratinized stratified squamous epithelium. Rugae are noted in the cardia of the stomach (on the right). None of the other types of lining epithelium describe histologic features of the esophagus.
Keywords: Barrett esophagus, gastroesophageal reflux disease

6 **The answer is E: Metaplasia.** Adaptive responses to sublethal cell injury include atrophy, hypertrophy, hyperplasia, metaplasia, and dysplasia. Metaplasia is the conversion of one cell differentiation pathway to another. In this autopsy specimen, the normal stratified squamous epithelium of the esophagus (on the left) has been replaced by columnar epithelium with goblet cells (on the right) as a result of chronic injury. The distal esophagus is said to exhibit "intestinal metaplasia." This disorder (Barrett esophagus) typically occurs in the lower third of the esophagus. Complete intestinal metaplasia with Paneth cells

and absorptive cells may also occur. Barrett esophagus is more resistant to peptic juice than normal squamous epithelium and appears to be an adaptive mechanism that serves to limit the harmful effects of acid reflux. None of the other cellular adaptations describe histopathologic findings in patients with Barrett esophagus.
Keywords: Barrett esophagus, intestinal metaplasia

7 | **The correct answer is D: Muscularis mucosae.** Several layers of the GI tract are visible in this section of the esophagus, including lining epithelium, lamina propria, muscularis mucosae, submucosa, and muscularis externa. A myenteric nerve plexus is observed between inner circular and outer longitudinal layers of the muscularis externa (oval, shown in the image). The arrows shown in the image identify the muscularis mucosae. These smooth muscle fibers run in a longitudinal direction that is parallel to the overlying epithelium. Contraction of the muscularis mucosae generates ripples in the mucosa that facilitate the movement of food during swallowing. Mucosa (choice B) is the layer that includes surface epithelium, lamina propria, and muscularis mucosae. Submucosa (choice E) is the layer of dense irregular connective tissue that is located between the muscularis mucosae and the muscularis externa. None of the other layers of the GI tract exhibit the distinctive histologic features of the muscularis mucosae.
Keywords: Esophagus, muscularis mucosae

8 | **The answer is A: Ganglion cells in the Auerbach plexus.** Absence of peristalsis and failure of the lower esophageal sphincter to relax upon swallowing are referred to as achalasia. Achalasia is associated with depletion or absence of ganglion cells in the myenteric (Auerbach) plexus. Lack of parasympathetic innervation prevents relaxation of smooth muscle in the lower esophageal sphincter during swallowing. A myenteric plexus is shown in the image provided for Question 7 (oval, shown in the image). These structures are composed of peripheral nerves and ganglion cells of postsynaptic parasympathetic neurons. Meissner plexus (choice B) is found in the submucosa of the GI tract. None of the other structures are deficient or absent in patients with achalasia.
Keywords: Achalasia, myenteric plexus

9 | **The answer is A: Esophagogastric junction.** This slide specimen was obtained from the esophagogastric junction. Examination of the image reveals an abrupt transition from a nonkeratinized stratified squamous epithelium (on the right) to a mucinous columnar epithelium with gastric pits (on the left). Diffuse lymphatic tissue is noted in the submucosa at this junction. These lymphocytes are strategically located to detect and eliminate pathogens (immune surveillance). Fundus and pylorus of the stomach (choices B and E) feature gastric glands, but they do not reveal stratified squamous epithelium. The gastroduodenal junction (choice C) is characterized by the presence of submucosal Brunner glands. The ileocecal junction (choice D) does not exhibit a stratified squamous epithelium. The muscularis externa in this distal portion of the esophagus is composed of smooth muscle; however, the muscularis externa in the upper third of the esophagus is composed of striated skeletal muscle.
Keywords: Stomach, esophagus, lymphatic tissue

10 | **The answer is C: Gastric pits.** This image shows a thick layer of visible mucus (amorphous white debris) that is secreted by the surface mucous cells. These columnar epithelial cells are filled with mucinous granules that occupy most of the apical cytoplasm. The mucinous epithelium is interrupted by deep depressions, termed gastric pits (arrows, shown in the image). Visible mucus forms a gel-like coating that protects surface epithelial cells from the harmful effects of acidic gastric juice and mechanical abrasion. Cardiac glands (choice B) are present in the lamina propria. These glands produce a neutral pH mucus that is released into the bottom of the gastric pits. A small portion of the muscularis mucosae is visible on the lower right side of the image. None of the other glands are present at the esophagogastric junction.
Keywords: Stomach, cardiac glands

11 | **The answer is A: Bicarbonate and potassium.** The visible mucus that coats the gastric lumen is composed of heavily glycosylated proteins (mucins). In addition to mucins, surface mucous cells secrete bicarbonate ions and potassium. These molecules/minerals provide the mucus with an alkaline pH that serves to neutralize stomach acid near the lining epithelium. The other biomolecules are important components of gastric juice, but mucous cells do not produce them.
Keywords: Stomach, cardiac glands

12 | **The answer is E: Parietal cells.** Gastric juice is produced primarily in the fundus and body of the stomach. It is composed of water and electrolytes, enzymes (e.g., pepsin), hormones (e.g., gastrin), intrinsic factor (essential for vitamin B_{12} absorption), mucus, and hydrochloric acid. Hydrochloric acid is generated by parietal cells in the fundic glands. Under the influence of gastrin, parietal cells produce hydrogen ions that are pumped into a complex set of membrane folds (intracellular canaliculi) by an H/K ATPase. Here, the hydrogen ions form HCl. None of the other cells produce HCl.
Keywords: Stomach, parietal cells

13 | **The answer is D: Prostaglandins.** The physiologic gastric mucosal barrier is regulated by prostaglandins (e.g., PGE_2). These hydrophobic signaling molecules are synthesized in the gastric mucosa. They play an important role in maintaining bicarbonate secretion by surface mucous cells and increasing the thickness of the surface mucus layer. Pharmacologic agents (nonsteroidal antiinflammatory drugs) that inhibit the formation of prostaglandins can compromise the gastric mucosal barrier,

leading to acute erosive gastritis. Loss of the protective alkaline mucus layer enables acidic gastric juice to injure the mucosa, leading to necrosis and hemorrhage. None of the other small molecules regulates the physiologic gastric mucosal barrier.
Keywords: Stomach, prostaglandins

14 **The answer is A: Chief cells.** Fundic glands (also called gastric glands) are composed of parietal cells, chief cells, mucous neck cells, enteroendocrine cells, and stem cells. Except for the cardiac and pyloric regions, these gastric glands are found throughout the stomach. Chief cells are typical protein-producing cells that feature an abundance of rough endoplasmic reticulum. These "protein factories" store pepsinogen (precursor enzyme) within intracellular zymogen secretory granules. Upon contact with gastric juice, pepsinogen is converted to pepsin—an aspartate protease. Pepsin was the first enzyme to be discovered in 1929 by John Northrup. Chief cells are located in deeper parts of the fundic glands. None of the other gastric cells store enzyme precursors in cytoplasmic zymogen granules.
Keywords: Stomach, chief cells

15 **The answer is C: Isthmus of glandular epithelium.** Gastric glands are branched tubular glands that extend from the bottom of the gastric pit down to the muscularis mucosae. They are connected to gastric pits via a short segment that is referred to as the isthmus. A longer neck region (choice E) connects the isthmus to the fundus of the gland (choice A). Stem cell proliferation takes place in the isthmus. Cells destined to become mucous cells migrate up toward the gastric pits (choice B), whereas the other secretory cells (e.g., parietal and chief cells) move down toward the fundus (base) of the gland. Epithelial stem cells are not found in the lamina propria of the gastric mucosa (choice D). Fluorescence-activated cell sorting (FACS) provides a valuable tool for counting and sorting dissociated single cells based on the presence or absence of cell surface markers for which probes are available.
Keywords: Stomach, stem cells

16 **The answer is C: Fundus of the stomach.** This image shows gastric glands emptying into the bottom of gastric pits. These fundic glands are populated largely by parietal cells in the neck of the gland and chief cells at the base of the gland. Parietal and chief cells are not present in cardiac and pyloric glands. Secretory cells of the gastric mucosa produce nearly 2 L of gastric juice per day. None of the other segments of the GI tract exhibit the distinctive histologic features of the fundus of the stomach.
Keywords: Stomach, fundus

17 **The answer is E: Parietal cells.** Parietal cells are large, round eosinophilic cells with central nuclei. They have extensive intracellular membrane folds (canaliculi) that provide increased surface area for the hydrogen ion

pumps (ATPases) that generate HCl. They also have an abundance of mitochondria, which provide ATP to fuel the pumps. Parietal cells are located primarily in the middle neck region of the fundic glands. Chief cells (choice A) are basophilic (not eosinophilic). Enteroendocrine cells (choice B) are present at every level of the gastric glands, but they would be difficult to identify without the use of special stains. Mucous cells (choice C) are characterized by the presence of secretory granules filled with white-appearing mucins. Paneth cells (choice D) are found in the small intestine.
Keywords: Stomach, parietal cells

18 **The answer is A: Chief cells.** Pepsinogen-secreting chief cells are located at the base of the gastric glands. Pepsin (the active enzyme) cleaves proteins within the lumen of the stomach into peptides that are further degraded to amino acids in the small intestine. Pepsinogen (the pepsin precursor enzyme) is stored within zymogen granules in the apical cytoplasm of chief cells. As mentioned above, enteroendocrine cells would be difficult to identify without the use of special stains. None of the other cells are found in the fundus of branched tubular gastric glands.
Keywords: Stomach, chief cells

19 **The answer is E: Parietal cells.** Pernicious anemia is an autoimmune disorder in which patients develop auto-antibodies against parietal cells and intrinsic factor. Parietal cell antibodies lead to atrophic gastritis. Intrinsic factor is a glycoprotein that complexes with vitamin B_{12} in the stomach and facilitates its absorption in the small intestine (ileum). Deficiency of vitamin B_{12} results in megaloblastic anemia, a hematologic condition in which the peripheral blood smear shows macrocytosis of erythrocytes and hypersegmentation of neutrophils. Megaloblastic maturation (cellular enlargement with asynchronous maturation between the nucleus and cytoplasm) is noted in bone marrow precursors from all lineages. Paneth cells (choice D) are intestinal cells that secrete antibacterial proteins. None of the other cells secrete intrinsic factor.
Keywords: Megaloblastic anemia, pernicious anemia

20 **The answer is D: Inhibition of cyclooxygenase.** Acute hemorrhagic gastritis is characterized by necrosis of the mucosa and is commonly associated with the intake of aspirin, other NSAIDs, or alcohol. Even small doses of aspirin or other NSAIDs can inhibit the production of regulatory prostaglandins in the stomach mucosa. Most NSAIDs work by inhibiting cyclooxygenase, an enzyme that generates prostaglandins from arachidonic acid precursor molecules. The factor common to all forms of acute hemorrhagic gastritis is breakdown of the mucosal barrier, which permits acid-induced injury. Mucosal injury causes bleeding from superficial erosions. Defects in the mucosa may extend into deeper tissues to form an

ulcer. None of the other mechanisms of disease is associated with pathogenesis of acute erosive gastritis.
Keywords: Gastritis, cyclooxygenase

21 **The answer is C: Chemoreception.** Enteroendocrine cells account for approximately 1% of epithelial cells in the GI tract. They develop from common enteric stem cells. Because of their similarity to secretory cells of the central nervous system, enteroendocrine cells are described as components of the diffuse neuroendocrine system. Most of these cells rest on the basal lamina, and their cytoplasm does not reach the lumen of the gut. These "closed" cells release hormones from their basal membranes into the underlying connective tissue. By contrast, "open" enteroendocrine cells have cytoplasmic extensions that reach the lumen of the gut. These cells express G protein–coupled chemoreceptors that continuously sample the contents of the gut and signal the release of hormones based on this chemical information.
Keywords: Enteroendocrine cells, diffuse neuroendocrine system

22 **The answer is C: Meissner plexus.** Visceral motor fibers that stimulate the mucosal glands and the muscularis mucosae filter through the Auerbach (myenteric) plexus (choice A) to form a secondary submucosal plexus, referred to as the Meissner plexus. This secondary plexus is difficult to identify on routine H&E-stained slides, because the ganglion cells are sparse and the nerve fibers are delicate. Postsynaptic ganglion cells and nerve fibers that innervate the muscularis mucosae are not present in the other anatomic locations.
Keywords: Meissner plexus

23 **The answer is D: Infection.** Peptic ulcer disease refers to breaks in the mucosa of the stomach and proximal duodenum that are produced by the action of acidic gastric juice. The pathogenesis of peptic ulcer disease is believed to involve an underlying chronic gastritis caused by *Helicobacter pylori*. This pathogen has been isolated from the gastric antrum of virtually all patients with duodenal ulcers and from about 75% of those with gastric ulcers. *H. pylori* gastritis is the most common type of gastritis in the United States and is characterized by chronic inflammation of the stomach. In addition to peptic ulcer disease, *H. pylori* gastritis is a risk factor for the development of gastric adenocarcinoma and gastric lymphoma. Eradication of *H. pylori* infection is curative of peptic ulcer disease in most patients. None of the other mechanisms of disease are linked to the pathogenesis of peptic ulcer disease.
Keywords: Peptic ulcer disease

24 **The answer is E: Urease.** Incidental findings are frequently encountered during an autopsy. In this case, a silver stain of the patient's gastric mucosa demonstrates *H. pylori*. These bacteria are adapted to survive in the acidic environment of the stomach. They have been shown to contain a large amount of urease. This enzyme hydrolyzes urea to generate an alkaline "ammonia cloud" that surrounds and protects the bacterium from the harmful effects of acidic gastric juice. None of the other enzymes contributes to the survival of *H. pylori* in the stomach.
Keywords: Peptic ulcer disease, chronic infectious gastritis

25 **The answer is B: Hypertrophy of smooth muscle.** Congenital pyloric stenosis is enlargement of the pyloric canal that obstructs the outlet of the stomach. This disorder is the most common indication for abdominal surgery in the first 6 months of life. Congenital pyloric stenosis has a familial tendency. The only consistent microscopic abnormality is hypertrophy of the circular muscle coat in the pyloric canal. Deviation of the septum transversum (choice A) causes congenital diaphragmatic hernia. Persistence of the embryonic vitelline duct (choice E) is known as Meckel diverticulum. None of the other congenital birth defects is associated with "projectile vomiting."
Keywords: Stomach, congenital pyloric stenosis

26 **The answer is E: Stomach.** This autopsy specimen was taken from the pylorus of the stomach. The photomicrograph shows surface mucous cells, gastric pits, and mucosal glands. These pyloric glands secrete a neutral pH mucus that drains into the bottom of the gastric pits. None of the other organs feature gastric pits and mucous glands.
Keywords: Stomach, pyloric glands

27 **The answer is A: Brunner glands.** The seromucinous glands in this slide specimen are located in submucosal connective tissue, external to the muscularis mucosae. These Brunner glands are a distinguishing feature of the proximal duodenum. Submucosal glands are also present in the esophagus (esophageal glands); however, unlike the esophagus, the mucosa shown in this image features intestinal villi lined by columnar epithelial cells (absorptive enterocytes). The open space observed between Brunner glands and the deeper muscularis externa is an artifact of paraffin embedding and sectioning. None of the other organs feature submucosal glands.
Keywords: Small intestine, Brunner glands

28 **The answer is B: Bicarbonate ions.** Brunner glands secrete a bicarbonate-rich, alkaline mucus that neutralizes the acidity of gastric juice. In addition to protecting the lining of the small intestine, these alkaline secretions establish a neutral pH that is optimum for the activity of pancreatic enzymes that enter the second part of the duodenum. Exocrine cells of the pancreas secrete amylase and lipase (choices A and D). Parietal cells of the stomach secrete HCl (choice C). Gastric chief cells secrete pepsinogen (choice E).
Keywords: Small intestine, Brunner glands

29 | **The answer is B: Myenteric plexus.** This image shows ganglion cells embedded in loose connective tissue between the inner circular and outer longitudinal layers of the muscularis externa. These structures are termed the myenteric or Auerbach plexus. They contain the ganglion cells of postsynaptic neurons that innervate the muscularis externa. The Auerbach (myenteric) plexus facilitates the movement of food along the GI tract by regulating peristalsis. The Meissner nerve plexus (choice A) is located in the submucosa. Peyer patches (choice C) are aggregates of lymphoid tissue in the mucosa and submucosa of the distal ileum. Diffuse and nodular lymphoid nodules (choices D and E) are not common in the muscularis mucosae.
Keywords: Myenteric plexus

30 | **The answer is B: Gastrin.** This patient shows evidence of Zollinger-Ellison syndrome. This syndrome is characterized by unrelenting peptic ulceration in the stomach and/or duodenum by the action of tumor-derived gastrin. Gastrin binds to receptors on parietal and chief cells to stimulate the production of gastric juice. Gastrin is secreted primarily by enteroendocrine cells in the stomach. However, for reasons that are unclear, gastrin-producing neuroendocrine tumors (gastrinomas) typically arise in pancreatic islets (microorgans composed of enteroendocrine cells). Among islet cell tumors, pancreatic gastrinomas are second in frequency only to insulinomas (insulin-producing tumors). None of the other polypeptide hormones stimulates gastric acid secretion.
Keywords: Zollinger-Ellison syndrome, gastrinoma

31 | **The answer is B: Plicae circulares.** This autopsy specimen was obtained from the jejunum. In this portion of the GI tract, the mucosa and submucosa are folded extensively to increase surface area for absorption. The submucosal folds (arrows, shown in the image) are referred to as plicae circulares. These folds/ridges extend partially around the lumen. Mucosal projections that cover the entire surface of the small intestine are referred to as villi (choice E). Intestinal villi are lined by a simple columnar epithelium with goblet cells. Haustra and teniae coli (choices A and D) are found in the large intestine. Rugae (choice C) are folds in the wall of the stomach.
Keywords: Small intestine, jejunum, plicae circulares

32 | **The answer is E: Striated brush border.** The intestinal epithelium is home to at least five different types of epithelial cells: enterocytes, goblet cells, Paneth cells, enteroendocrine cells, and microfold (M) cells. Enterocytes display thousands of delicate, apical membrane microvilli. These actin-filled membrane projections increase the surface area of the small intestine by 600-fold. They are recognized by light microscopy as a striated brush border (shown in the image). Microvilli are covered by a carbohydrate-rich glycocalyx (choice B)

that protects the lining epithelium and provides a microenvironment for the display of membrane-bound hydrolytic enzymes. The glycocalyx cannot be identified on slides stained with H&E. Basal lamina, lamina densa, and lamina propria (choices A, C, and D) are extracellular matrix structures related to the basal membrane domain of epithelial cells.
Keywords: Small intestine, striated brush border

33 | **The answer is B: Goblet cells.** PAS identifies mucin-producing goblet cells in the intestinal villi (magenta cells, shown in the image). Mucins (heavily glycosylated glycoproteins) provide a protective coating over the lining epithelial cells and help lubricate the luminal contents. This photomicrograph reveals cytologic details of the lamina propria, including a beautiful example of a lacteal (arrowhead, shown in the image). These large lymphatic channels are lined by a simple squamous epithelium (endothelium). Paneth cells (choice D) are not found in the intestinal villi.
Keywords: Small intestine, goblet cells

34 | **The answer is C: Ghrelin.** Appetite and the perception of hunger are stimulated by ghrelin, a 28-amino-acid (polypeptide) hormone that is secreted by enteroendocrine cells in the stomach and pancreas. Serum levels of ghrelin rise prior to a meal and decline following a meal. Ghrelin binds to receptors in the hypothalamus to stimulate appetite. Ghrelin receptors are found in many other organs, suggesting that this hormone has multiple functions in regulating growth and metabolism. None of the other hormones stimulate the perception of hunger.
Keywords: Enteroendocrine cells, ghrelin

35 | **The answer is A: Cholecystokinin.** Pancreatic enzymes and bile salts enter the second part of the duodenum at the ampulla of Vater. Bile salts emulsify lipids, and pancreatic enzymes degrade lipids and carbohydrates. Contraction of the gallbladder to release bile salts is stimulated by cholecystokinin. This polypeptide hormone also stimulates exocrine cells of the pancreas to synthesize and secrete amylase and lipase. Enteroendocrine cells in the duodenum and jejunum secrete cholecystokinin. None of the other hormones regulate contraction of the gallbladder and/or secretion of pancreatic enzymes.
Keywords: Enteroendocrine cells, cholecystokinin

36 | **The answer is D: Paneth cells.** These secretory cells clustered at the base of the intestinal glands are (in our opinion) among the most beautiful cells in the body. Their large secretory granules are intensely eosinophilic when stained with H&E. Paneth cells synthesize and secrete a variety of antibacterial substances, including lysozyme and defensin. Paneth cells help regulate the bacterial flora of the GI tract. None of the other cells exhibit the distinctive cytologic features of Paneth cells.
Keywords: Small intestine, Paneth cells

37 **The answer is C: Ileum.** This image reveals large aggregates of nodular lymphatic tissue that are referred to as Peyer patches. They are a characteristic feature of the ileum (particularly the distal ileum). The pale-staining regions within these lymphoid follicles represent areas of B-lymphocyte activation and proliferation. Peyer patches are located within the mucosa and the submucosa (i.e., they interrupt the muscularis mucosae). They participate in adaptive immunity and immune surveillance. Peyer patches are not present in the other segments of the GI tract.
Keywords: Peyer patches, small intestine, ileum

38 **The answer is A: Antigen uptake.** The lamina propria of the GI tract contains large numbers of acute and chronic inflammatory cells. These cells form a diffuse mucosa-associated lymphoid tissue (MALT) that protects the body from pathogens. Macrophages and other phagocytic cells may penetrate the basal lamina and migrate into the lining epithelium to ingest pathogens. In the distal ileum, however, the process of delivering pathogens to lymphocytes cells is mediated primarily by microfold (M) cells. These phagocytic cells are found in the epithelium that covers Peyer patches. M cells are professional antigen-uptake and presenting cells, with apical membrane domains that are folded to provide greater surface area for sampling the luminal contents. Antigens taken up by M cells via pinocytosis and phagocytosis are processed and presented to lymphoid cells residing within cellular recesses.
Keywords: Peyer patches, M cells

39 **The answer is E: MHC class II.** M cells degrade pathogens within phagolysosomes. Peptides are bound by MHC class II molecules and transported to the cell surface. Foreign peptides presented by MHC class II molecules stimulate helper T cells to become activated. Once activated, T cells secrete a variety of cytokines that stimulate B-cell proliferation and differentiation. CD4 and CD8 (choices A and B) are antigen coreceptors on helper and killer T cells, respectively. IgM (choice C) is the antigen receptor on most B cells. MHC class I molecules (choice D) are present on the surface of nearly every cell in the body. These membrane glycoproteins provide targets for cell-mediated immunity (e.g., killing of virally-infected cells).
Keywords: Peyer patches, M cells, major histocompatibility complex

40 **The answer is C: Crypts of Lieberkühn.** Histologic features of the small intestine include villi and mucosal glands. The intestinal glands are commonly referred to as "crypts of Lieberkühn." These simple tubular glands empty into the intestine at the base of the villi. Brunner glands (choice A) are submucosal glands in the proximal duodenum. Gastric glands (choices B, D, and E) are similar in appearance to intestinal glands (e.g., they are mucosal

glands). However, the small intestine does not feature surface mucous cells or gastric pits.
Keywords: Small intestine, intestinal glands

41 **The answer is E: Submucosa.** The submucosa consists of dense, irregular connective tissue, as well as nerves, blood vessels, lymphatic channels, and glands (esophagus and duodenum). The submucosa provides a bridge between the mucosa and the muscularis externa. It also provides a pathway for nerves and vessels to enter/exit the various GI organs. None of the other tissue layers exhibit histologic features of the submucosa.
Keywords: Small intestine, submucosa

42 **The answer is B: Lamina propria.** The core of each intestinal villus is lined by an extension of the lamina propria. This loose connective tissue is composed of fibroblasts, smooth muscle cells, endothelial cells, lymphocytes, macrophages, and plasma cells. Contraction of smooth muscle fibers in the core of the villus stimulates the movement of lymph fluid within the lacteals. Macrophages are phagocytic cells derived from circulating blood monocytes. They ingest pathogens and present antigens to passing lymphocytes. Monocytes/macrophages and lymphocytes exit the blood from postcapillary (high endothelial) venules. None of the other layers of the GI tract occupy the core of the intestinal villi.
Keywords: Mucosa-associated lymphoid tissue, lamina propria

43 **The answer is A: Intussusception.** Obstruction in this child was most likely caused by "telescoping" of the small intestine related to abnormal peristalsis. This condition (intussusception) is usually a disorder of infants or young children and occurs without a known cause. In adults, the leading point of an intussusception is usually a lesion in the bowel wall, such as Meckel diverticulum or a tumor. In addition to acute intestinal obstruction, intussusception compresses the blood supply to the affected portion of the intestine, which may undergo infarction. Meconium ileus (choice B) is intestinal obstruction in neonates with cystic fibrosis. Volvulus (choice E) is an example of intestinal obstruction, in which a segment of the gut twists on its mesentery, kinking the bowel and interrupting its blood supply. None of the other choices are related to abnormal intestinal peristalsis.
Keywords: Intussusception

44 **The answer is A: IgA.** The mucosal surface of the GI tract is exposed to a wide variety of pathogens, including bacteria, viruses, parasites, and toxins. Tight junctions (zonula occludins) between the lateral borders of enterocytes provide a crucial barrier to the spread of infections. The mucosa is also protected by cellular and humeral (antibody-mediated) immunity. Whereas IgG is the most abundant immunoglobulin found in the blood, plasma cells in the lamina propria of the GI tract secrete primarily IgA. Dimeric IgA antibodies pass to the lumen of the gut. Here, secretory IgA (sIgA) cross-links pathogens, masks pathogen adhesion molecules, and neutralizes toxins. Plasma cells in the respiratory and genitourinary system also secrete IgA. The other immunoglobulins (choices B, C, D, and E) mediate humoral immunity, but they are not secreted into the lumen of the GI tract.

Keywords: Immunoglobulins, IgA

45 The answer is A: Enterocytes. Plasma cells release dimeric IgA (dIgA) into the interstitial fluid of the lamina propria. The antibodies are then bound by "polymeric immunoglobulin receptors" that are displayed along the basal membrane domain of enterocytes that line the mucosa of the small intestine. The dIgA–receptor complex is internalized and transported to the apical membrane of the enterocyte. Here, transmembrane immunoglobulin receptors undergo proteolytic cleavage to release secretory IgA (sIgA). Microfold (M) cells (choice C) internalize pathogens and present antigenic peptides to lymphocytes. They are found in Peyer patches in the distal ileum. None of the other cells transport dIgA from the lamina propria to the lumen of the gut.

Keywords: Enterocytes, immunoglobulins, secretory IgA

46 The answer is E: Teniae coli. The large intestine includes the cecum, appendix, colon (ascending, transverse, descending, and sigmoid), rectum, and anal canal. This H&E-stained slide was obtained from the colon. The organ exhibits straight, tubular intestinal glands, as well as distinctive thickenings of the outer longitudinal layer of the muscularis externa. These bands of smooth muscle (three equally spaced bands) are referred to as teniae coli (arrow, shown in the image). These bands run longitudinally along the outer wall of the colon and are visible on gross inspection. Contractions of the teniae coli mediate segmentation and peristalsis, which serve to move the contents of the colon. Adventitia (choice A) is loose connective tissue associated with retroperitoneal visceral organs. Haustra coli (choice B) are sacculations on the external surface of the large intestine. Omental appendices (choice C) are fatty projections on the serosal surface of the colon. Plicae circulares (choice D) are submucosal folds in the small intestine.

Keywords: Large intestine, teniae coli

47 The answer is A: Failure of neural crest migration. Congenital megacolon (Hirschsprung disease) results from a congenital defect in the innervation of the large intestine, usually the rectum. Severe chronic constipation is typical. Marked dilation of the colon occurs proximal to the stenotic rectum, with clinical signs of intestinal obstruction. Congenital megacolon is caused by defective colorectal innervation that prevents relaxation of sphincter muscles. Biopsy of the rectum shows

deficiency or absence of ganglion cells in the myenteric plexus. Ganglion cells of the autonomic nervous system are derived from neural crest cells. None of the other developmental anomalies are linked to the pathogenesis of Hirschsprung disease.

Keywords: Hirschsprung disease, congenital megacolon

48 The answer is D: Muscularis externa. The layer of the GI tract indicated by the double arrow is the muscularis externa (also referred to as the muscularis propria). In the colon, the muscularis externa is composed of two layers: inner circular and outer longitudinal. As mentioned above, the outer longitudinal layer in the colon is condensed into three equally spaced bands referred to as teniae coli. A myenteric (Auerbach) plexus is present between the inner and outer layers of smooth muscle (arrowheads, shown in the image). Smooth muscle fibers in the GI tract are derived from the splanchnic mesoderm during development. None of the other layers of the GI tract exhibit the distinctive histologic features of the muscularis externa.

Keywords: Gastrointestinal tract, muscularis externa

49 The answer is A: Appendix. This digital slide illustrates histologic features of the vermiform appendix. The appendix is a small, blind pouch that arises as a projection from the cecum. Aside from its small size, histologic features of the appendix are similar to those of the colon. The appendix exhibits a mucosa, submucosa, muscularis externa, and serosa/adventitia. A distinguishing feature of the appendix is the large number of secondary lymphatic nodules that extend into the submucosa (shown in the image). None of the other organs exhibit the distinctive histologic features of the appendix.

Keywords: Large intestine, appendix

50 The answer is B: Enterocytes. This photomicrograph shows the distinctive morphology of colonic glands in cross-section. The straight tubular glands are lined by enterocytes and goblet cells. The principal function of enterocytes in the colon is absorption of water and electrolytes. The lumens of the colonic glands are small and difficult to visualize. The glands are surrounded by loose connective tissue of the lamina propria. Enteroendocrine and Paneth cells (choices C and D) may be present in the colon, but these secretory cells are not common. None of the other cells are present in the large intestine. Tubular adenomas constitute two-thirds of the benign colonic adenomas. Microscopically, tubular adenomas exhibit closely packed epithelial tubules, which may be uniform or irregular with excessive branching. Dysplasia and carcinoma often develop in tubular adenomas. As long as the dysplastic foci remain confined to the mucosa, the lesion is almost always cured by resection.

Keywords: Adenomatous polyp, enterocytes, goblet cells

51 **The answer is E: Rectoanal junction.** This surgical specimen was obtained from the junction of the rectum and the anal canal. The image shows stratified squamous epithelium on the right and colonic epithelium on the left. Diffuse lymphatic tissue is noted at the junction of these segments. The stratified squamous epithelium of the anal canal becomes keratinized as it blends with skin on the external surface of the body. The esophagogastric junction (choice B) exhibits stratified squamous epithelium but does not show colonic glands. None of the other junctions feature colonic glands and stratified squamous epithelium.

Keywords: Large intestine, rectum

52 **The answer is D: Rectum.** Hyperplastic polyps are small, sessile mucosal growths that display exaggerated crypt architecture. They are the most common polypoid lesions of the colon and are particularly frequent in the rectum. They increase with age. The crypts of hyperplastic polyps are elongated and may exhibit cystic dilations. The epithelium is composed of goblet cells and absorptive cells, without dysplasia. Hyperplastic polyps are less common in the other anatomic locations.

Keywords: Hyperplastic polyps

Chapter 14

Liver, Biliary System, and Pancreas

QUESTIONS

Select the single best answer.

1 You are asked to discuss the gross and microscopic anatomy of the liver during a pathology conference. Classic liver lobules are described as hexagonal prisms that surround which of the following anatomic structures?
(A) Bile duct
(B) Central vein
(C) Hepatic artery
(D) Portal triad
(E) Portal vein

2 A liver biopsy is examined at a multiheaded microscope in the pathology department. The surgical pathologist asks you questions to assess your understanding of normal liver histology. Identify the structure within the circle (shown in the image).

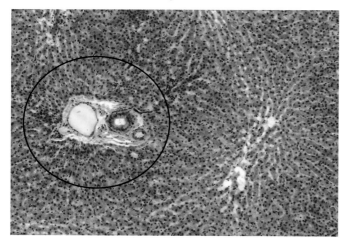

(A) Bile duct
(B) Central vein
(C) Hepatic artery
(D) Portal triad
(E) Portal vein

3 A different visual field from the slide described in Question 2 is examined at the same magnification. Identify the structures indicated by the arrows (shown in the image).

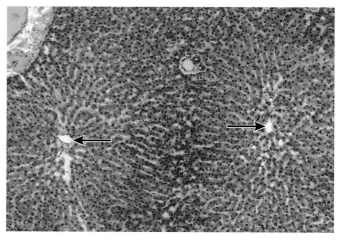

(A) Arcuate arteries
(B) Hepatic arteries
(C) Interlobular arteries
(D) Sublobular veins
(E) Terminal hepatic venules

4 A neonate born prematurely at 32-weeks' gestation develops yellow skin and sclera (physiological jaundice). Laboratory studies show elevated serum levels of bilirubin (breakdown product of heme). Inadequate bilirubin clearance by the liver in this neonate was most likely caused by organ immaturity. What liver enzyme conjugates serum bilirubin, making it water soluble, for excretion in the bile?
(A) Alanine aminotransferase
(B) Aspartate transaminase
(C) Fatty acyltransferase
(D) Galactosyltransferase
(E) Glucuronyltransferase

5 A 75-year-old man with congestive heart failure complains of increasing shortness of breath. On physical examination, the patient has an enlarged and tender liver and swollen legs. Increased venous pressure due to right-sided heart failure primarily affects which of the following regions of this patient's liver?

(A) Centrilobular hepatocytes
(B) Periportal hepatocytes
(C) Intrahepatic bile ducts
(D) Extrahepatic bile ducts
(E) Portal vein

6 Digital slides of the liver and the biliary system are examined in the histology laboratory. The sinusoids within this liver lobule (arrows, shown in the image) receive most of their blood from which of the following sources?

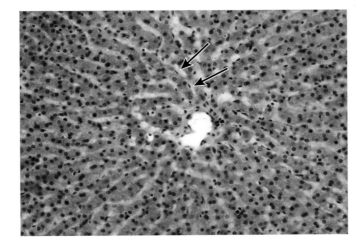

(A) Arcuate artery
(B) Hepatic artery
(C) Interlobular artery
(D) Portal vein
(E) Sublobular vein

7 The arrows on the image provided for Question 6 point to the nuclei of endothelial cells that line the hepatic sinusoids. Which of the following cytologic features best characterizes these squamous epithelial cells?

(A) Fenestrations
(B) Glycogen inclusions
(C) Secretory granules
(D) Slit-pore diaphragms
(E) Stereocilia

8 Your laboratory instructor asks you to discuss endocrine, exocrine, absorptive, and secretory functions of the liver. Secreted proteins such as albumin, clotting factors, and nonimmune globulins enter what microscopic cavity before entering the liver sinusoid?

(A) Duct of Santorini
(B) Duct of Wirsung
(C) Rokitansky-Aschoff sinus
(D) Space of Disse
(E) Space of Mall

9 During a clinical conference, you are asked to discuss iron storage disorders affecting the liver. You explain that iron overload can occur due to increased breakdown of erythrocytes (hemolysis) or increased intestinal absorption. Name the principal iron storage pigment found in hepatocytes.

(A) Bilirubin
(B) Cytochromes
(C) Hemoglobin
(D) Hemosiderin
(E) Transferrin

10 A 5-year-old girl presents with yellow skin and sclerae. The parents believe that she recently swallowed a bottle of acetaminophen tablets. A liver biopsy reveals hepatic necrosis. Which of the following enzymes metabolized acetaminophen and generated toxic metabolites in the liver of this young patient?

(A) Catalase
(B) Cytochrome P450
(C) Myeloperoxidase
(D) NADPH oxidase
(E) Superoxide dismutase

11 Phagocytic cells in the liver of an experimental animal are studied using carbon particles as a vital marker. Five hours after intravenous injection of India ink, the animal is sacrificed and the liver is processed for light microscopy. The black cells shown in the image represent Kupffer cells (macrophages) that have internalized carbon. In addition to foreign particles, Kupffer cells internalize and degrade which of the following components of portal venous blood?

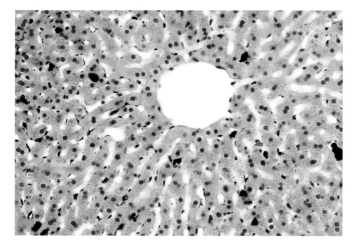

(A) Blood products from the spleen
(B) Chylomicrons and lipid micelles from the gastrointestinal tract
(C) Endocrine secretions from the pancreas
(D) Nutrients from the gastrointestinal tract
(E) Toxins from the gastrointestinal tract

12 A 40-year-old woman presents with an 8-month history of generalized itching, weight loss, fatigue, and yellow sclerae. Physical examination reveals mild jaundice. A liver biopsy discloses bile duct injury and inflammation. Which of the following cells forms the lining epithelium of the biliary tree?
(A) Cholangiocytes
(B) Endothelial cells
(C) Hepatic stellate cells
(D) Hepatocytes
(E) Kupffer cells

13 A 50-year-old malnourished man presents with a 6-month history of night blindness. Physical examination reveals corneal ulceration. The patient is subsequently diagnosed with vitamin A deficiency. Which of the following cells in the liver stores vitamin A as retinyl esters?
(A) Cholangiocytes
(B) Endothelial cells
(C) Hepatic stellate cells
(D) Hepatocytes
(E) Kupffer cells

14 Virtual microscope slides illustrating the liver and the biliary system are examined in the histology laboratory. Identify the structure indicated by the arrow (shown in the image).

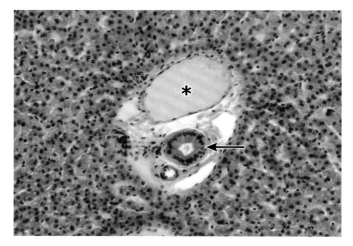

(A) Bile duct
(B) Central vein
(C) Hepatic artery
(D) Interlobular artery
(E) Portal vein

15 Injury or inflammation affecting the canal of Herring in the liver lobule is associated with which of the following pathologic changes?
(A) Fat droplets within hepatocytes
(B) Fibrosis of the common bile duct
(C) Gallstones (cholelithiasis)
(D) Hypertrophy of smooth muscle in the ampulla of Vater
(E) Intrahepatic bile lakes

16 One of your classmates casually mentions that the liver produces about 1 L of bile per day. As you attempt to confirm this surprising information through independent study, you learn that cholangiocytes continuously monitor the flow of bile. What subcellular organelle is sensitive to the directional flow of bile in the biliary tree?
(A) Cilia
(B) Flagella
(C) Hemidesmosomes
(D) Microvilli
(E) Stereocilia

17 A liver biopsy from a 62-year-old alcoholic man discloses regenerative liver nodules surrounded by fibrous scar tissue (histologic features of cirrhosis). The surgical pathologist asks you to comment on the remarkable capacity of the liver to regenerate. Hepatic stem cells that contribute to liver regeneration reside in which of the following locations?

(A) Canal of Herring
(B) Glisson capsule
(C) Hepatic sinusoid
(D) Space of Disse
(E) Space of Mall

18 A 40-year-old woman with a history of indigestion inquires about the location of her gallbladder. She also asks for information regarding risk factors for gallstones. What normal component of bile is associated with the pathogenesis of gallstones?

(A) Bicarbonate
(B) Cholesterol
(C) Cholic acid
(D) Mucin
(E) Sodium chloride

19 A 52-year-old woman presents with a 10-month history of upper abdominal pain after fatty meals. An ultrasound examination discloses multiple echogenic objects in the gallbladder (gallstones). The gallbladder is removed (cholecystectomy), and the surgical specimen is examined by light microscopy. Identify the normal epithelial structures indicated by the arrows (shown in the image).

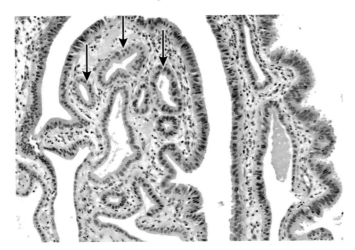

(A) Canals of Herring
(B) Hepatic ducts
(C) Mucosal folds
(D) Mucosal glands
(E) Submucosal glands

20 The surgical pathologist shows you another gallbladder for comparison (shown in the image). In contrast to other organs in the gastrointestinal system, the wall of the gallbladder lacks which of the following layers?

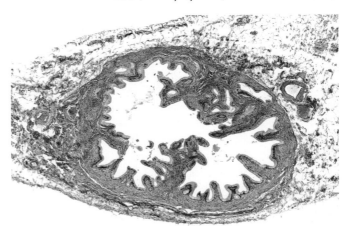

(A) Adventitia
(B) Lamina propria
(C) Muscularis externa
(D) Serosa
(E) Submucosa

21 Concentration of bile salts and pigments within the lumen of the gallbladder depends on active transport of Na^+ and HCO_3^-, as well as passive transport of H_2O. Which of the following proteins facilitates the passive transport of water across the plasma membrane of epithelial cells lining the gallbladder?

(A) Aquaporin
(B) Cadherin
(C) Occludin
(D) Perforin
(E) Porin

22 Various peritoneal and retroperitoneal organs are examined using virtual microscope slides in the histology laboratory. Identify the organ shown in the image.

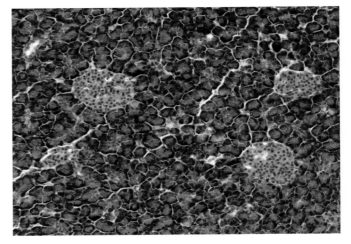

(A) Gallbladder
(B) Liver
(C) Pancreas
(D) Parotid gland
(E) Submandibular gland

23 The organ identified in Question 22 is examined at high magnification. Which of the following terms describes the glandular epithelial cells shown in the image?

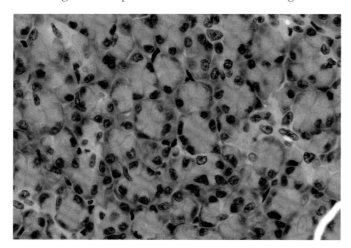

(A) Endocrine
(B) Goblet
(C) Mucous
(D) Paracrine
(E) Serous

24 The pancreas delivers an alkaline pH fluid to the duodenum that helps to neutralize the acidity of gastric juice, protect the small intestine, and provide an optimum pH for hydrolytic enzymes present in the lumen. What portion of the exocrine pancreas secretes most of this bicarbonate- and sodium-rich alkaline fluid?
(A) Intercalated ducts
(B) Interlobular ducts
(C) Intralobular ducts
(D) Pancreatic duct of Santorini
(E) Pancreatic duct of Wirsung

25 A group of medical students examine a virtual microscope slide of the pancreas at low magnification. Identify the structure indicated by the arrow (shown in the image).

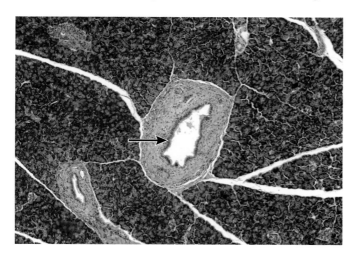

(A) Intercalated duct
(B) Interlobular duct
(C) Intralobular duct
(D) Main pancreatic duct
(E) Rokitansky-Aschoff sinus

26 During a small group seminar, you are asked to discuss pancreatic enzymes and their role in the digestion of food. Which of the following enzymes catalyzes the conversion of pancreatic proenzymes to active enzymes within the lumen of the duodenum?
(A) Alkaline phosphatase
(B) Elastase
(C) Maltase
(D) Phospholipase
(E) Trypsin

27 The virtual microscope slide described in Question 25 is examined at higher magnification. Identify the structure indicated by the arrow (shown in the image).

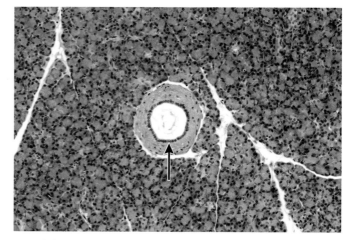

(A) Accessory pancreatic duct
(B) Intercalated duct
(C) Interlobular duct
(D) Intralobular duct
(E) Main pancreatic duct

28 A 62-year-old alcoholic presents to the emergency room with 8 hours of severe abdominal pain and vomiting. Physical examination discloses exquisite abdominal tenderness. Serum levels of amylase and lipase are elevated. These laboratory data indicate that this patient has suffered injury to which of the following internal organs?
(A) Duodenum
(B) Gallbladder
(C) Liver
(D) Pancreas
(E) Stomach

29 A 69-year-old man is brought to the emergency room in a disoriented state. Physical examination reveals an odor of alcohol, as well as jaundice and ascites. Serum levels of aspartate aminotransferase (AST), alanine aminotransferase (ALT), alkaline phosphatase, and bilirubin are all elevated. Increased serum levels of alkaline phosphatase are an indicator of injury to which of the following tissues/structures?

(A) Bile ducts
(B) Centrilobular hepatocytes
(C) Islets of Langerhans
(D) Pancreatic exocrine acini
(E) Periportal hepatocytes

30 A 44-year-old woman comes to the physician with a 6-week history of episodic hunger and fainting spells. She is currently seeing a psychiatrist because she is irritable and quarreling with her family. Laboratory studies show a serum glucose concentration of 35 mg/dL (normal = 90 mg/dL). A CT scan of the abdomen demonstrates a 1.5-cm mass in the pancreas. An EM study of the tumor reveals membrane-bound, dense-core granules. These secretory vesicles most likely contain which of the following pancreatic hormones?

(A) Glucagon
(B) Insulin
(C) Pancreatic polypeptide
(D) Secretin
(E) Somatostatin

ANSWERS

1 **The answer is B: Central vein.** The liver is the largest visceral organ in the body. It is located in the upper right quadrant of the abdominal cavity, where it is protected by the ribcage. The liver arises as a diverticulum of the embryonic foregut. It receives blood from two sources: (1) hepatic artery and (2) hepatic portal vein. The parenchymal cells of the liver, termed hepatocytes, form plates that are separated by sinusoidal capillaries. Blood filters through the sinusoids and is drained by terminal hepatic venules to the inferior vena cava. The classic liver lobule is described as a six-sided prism, with portal triads (bile duct, hepatic artery, and portal vein) located at the angles of each lobule. The terminal hepatic venule (also referred to as the central vein) is located at the center of each lobule. The liver is encapsulated with fibrous connective tissue (Glisson capsule). None of the other structures listed is found at the center of the classic liver lobule.
Keywords: Liver lobule, hepatocytes

2 **The answer is D: Portal triad.** The circle shown in the image identifies a portal triad composed of a portal vein, bile duct, and hepatic artery. The portal triad is held together by loose connective tissue. The portal vein (choice E) is thin walled, and its diameter is much larger than that of the hepatic artery (choice C). The portal vein collects blood from the superior mesenteric and splenic veins. It delivers poorly oxygenated, but nutrient-rich, blood to hepatocytes lining the sinusoids. Hepatic arteries arise from the celiac trunk—an unpaired branch of the abdominal aorta. Two or three layers of smooth muscle surround the hepatic artery/arteriole. None of the other choices exhibit histologic features of the hepatic portal triad.
Keywords: Liver, portal triad

3 **The answer is E: Terminal hepatic venules.** This image reveals the central veins (terminal hepatic venules) of two adjoining liver lobules (arrows, shown in the image). Hepatic sinusoids (open spaces) can be seen converging on the central veins. A portal triad is visible between the veins. Central veins collect blood from the hepatic sinusoids. They coalesce to form sublobular veins (choice D) that drain to hepatic veins that empty into the inferior vena cava. None of the other vessels are found at the center of a liver lobule.
Keywords: Liver, terminal hepatic venules

4 **The answer is E: Glucuronyltransferase.** Hepatocyte functions can be classified as (1) metabolic (e.g., gluconeogenesis), (2) synthetic (e.g., secretion of albumin), (3) storage (e.g., iron and triglyceride storage), and (4) excretory (e.g., secretion of bile). One of the components of bile is conjugated bilirubin (a bile pigment). Bilirubin is the end product of hemoglobin degradation. It is poorly soluble in the blood. In order to be removed from the circulation, bilirubin must be transported into hepatocytes, conjugated with glucuronic acid (to make it water soluble), and then excreted into the bile for elimination. Approximately 70% of normal newborns exhibit a transient unconjugated hyperbilirubinemia. This "physiological jaundice" is more pronounced in premature infants due to inadequate hepatic clearance of bilirubin related to organ immaturity. Fetal bilirubin levels in utero remain low because bilirubin crosses the placenta, where it is conjugated and excreted by the mother's liver. High concentrations of unconjugated bilirubin in a neonate can cause irreversible brain injury (referred to as kernicterus). The other enzymes are unrelated to bilirubin excretion by the liver.
Keywords: Neonatal jaundice

5 **The answer is A: Centrilobular hepatocytes.** Patients with right-sided heart failure have pitting edema of the lower extremities and an enlarged and tender liver. A generalized increase in venous pressure, typically from chronic right-sided heart failure, results in an increase in the volume of blood in many organs (e.g., liver, spleen, kidneys). The liver is particularly vulnerable to chronic passive congestion because the hepatic veins empty into the vena cava immediately inferior to the heart. In patients with chronic passive congestion of the liver, the central veins of the hepatic lobule become dilated. Increased venous pressure leads to dilation of the sinusoids and pressure atrophy of centrilobular hepatocytes. The other choices are less commonly affected by chronic passive congestion of the liver.
Keywords: Liver sinusoids, congestive heart failure

6 **The answer is D: Portal vein.** As mentioned above, the liver has a dual blood supply: The hepatic artery provides oxygen-rich blood, whereas the portal vein provides blood that is nutrient rich, but oxygen poor. Both sources of blood (arterial and venous) mix in the hepatic sinusoids. Approximately 75% of the blood flowing through the liver is derived from the hepatic portal vein. The other 25% of the blood supply is derived from the hepatic artery (choice B). Sublobular veins (choice E) drain to the inferior vena cava. None of the other vessels provide a major source of blood to the liver.
Keywords: Liver, portal vein

7 **The answer is A: Fenestrations.** Hepatic sinusoids are lined by a discontinuous endothelium that facilitates access of hepatocytes to the blood. The endothelial cells exhibit small windows in their cytoplasm (fenestrations). Moreover, the basal lamina of the endothelium is absent over large areas, and there are gaps between adjacent cells. Hepatic sinusoids are also lined by resident macrophages (referred to as Kupffer cells). Slit-pore diaphragms (choice D) connect podocyte foot processes in the renal glomerulus, but these structures are not found in the liver. None of the other cytologic features characterize endothelial cells lining hepatic sinusoids.

Keywords: Liver sinusoids, fenestrated capillaries

8 **The answer is D: Space of Disse.** Hepatocytes are separated from vascular endothelial cells and Kupffer cells by a perisinusoidal space (of Disse). This microscopic space provides a location for the exchange of fluid and biomolecules between hepatocytes and blood. Microvilli on the hepatocyte basal membrane fill the space of Disse and increase the surface area available for transport (endocytosis and exocytosis). Ducts of Santorini and Wirsung (choices A and B) are found in the pancreas. Rokitansky-Aschoff sinuses (choice C) are deep invaginations of the mucosa in the wall of the gallbladder. The space of Mall (choice E) is located between hepatocytes and connective tissue of the portal triads.

Keywords: Liver, hepatocytes

9 **The answer is D: Hemosiderin.** The liver stores most of the iron in the body. Iron is carried in the blood by transferrin (choice E). Receptors on hepatocytes bind transferrin and transport iron into the cell. Intracellular iron is bound by ferritin. Hemosiderin is a partially denatured form of ferritin that aggregates easily and is recognized microscopically as yellow-brown granules within the cytoplasm. Prussian blue is commonly used to identify iron storage pigments within cells. Hereditary hemochromatosis is an abnormality of iron absorption in the small intestine. In this genetic disease, iron is stored mostly in the form of hemosiderin, primarily in the liver. Bilirubin (choice A) is a product of heme catabolism that may accumulate in liver cells—but does not contain iron. Cytochromes are mitochondrial proteins that contain iron, but do not store iron within hepatocytes. Hemoglobin (choice C) is the iron-containing pigment of RBCs.

Keywords: Hemosiderosis, hemochromatosis

10 **The answer is B: Cytochrome P450.** The liver is the principal organ involved in detoxification of foreign substances, including industrial chemicals, pharmaceutical drugs, and bacterial toxins. Small doses of acetaminophen (an analgesic) are absorbed from the stomach and small intestine and conjugated in the liver to form nontoxic derivatives. In cases of overdose, the normal pathway of acetaminophen metabolism is saturated. Excess acetaminophen is then metabolized in the liver via the mixed function oxidase (cytochrome P450) system, yielding oxidative metabolites that cause predictable hepatic necrosis. These metabolites initiate lipid peroxidation, which damages the plasma membrane and leads to hepatocyte cell death. The toxic dose of acetaminophen after a single acute ingestion is in the range of 150 mg/kg in children and 7 g in adults. Drug toxicity should be suspected in all cases of acute hepatitis. None of the other enzymes metabolizes acetaminophen to generate reactive oxygen species.

Keywords: Liver, predictable necrosis

11 **The answer is A: Blood products from the spleen.** This image shows a central vein surrounded by sinusoids. The scattered black objects represent Kupffer cells that have picked up carbon particles from the circulation. Kupffer cells belong to the mononuclear phagocytic system. Their cellular processes span the hepatic sinusoids, searching for necrotic debris and foreign material to ingest. Most damaged or senescent RBCs are removed from the circulation by macrophages in the spleen; however, Kupffer cells in the liver also serve this function. Portal venous blood transports nutrients and toxins from the gastrointestinal tract (choices B, D, and E), as well as endocrine secretions from the pancreas (choice C); however, Kupffer cells do not internalize these blood components.

Keywords: Kupffer cells, hepatic sinusoids

12 **The answer is A: Cholangiocytes.** The principal excretory product of the liver is bile. Bile provides a vehicle for the elimination of cholesterol and bilirubin, and bile salts facilitate the digestion and absorption of dietary fat. Hepatocytes excrete bile into small canals (canaliculi) that drain to bile ducts within the portal triads. Intrahepatic and extrahepatic bile ducts are lined by cholangiocytes. These cuboidal to columnar epithelial cells continuously monitor the composition and flow of bile. The patient described in this clinical vignette has an autoimmune disease (primary biliary cirrhosis) that leads to chronic destruction of intrahepatic bile ducts. The bile ducts are surrounded by lymphocytes (primarily CD8+ T cells). As a result of this destructive inflammatory process, the small bile ducts all but disappear. None of the other cells provides a lining epithelium for the biliary tree.

Keywords: Primary biliary cirrhosis, cholangiocytes

13 **The answer is C: Hepatic stellate cells.** Vitamin A is essential for vision, healthy skin, and proper functioning of the immune system. Hepatic stellate cells (commonly referred to as Ito cells) store vitamin A. These mesenchymal cells are located between hepatocytes and endothelial cells in the perisinusoidal space of Disse. They store vitamin A as retinyl esters and secrete retinol bound to retinol-binding protein. Retinol is taken up by rods and cones in the retina to form the visual pigment, rhodopsin. Another derivative of vitamin A, retinoic acid, helps regulate the differentiation of squamous epithelial cells. Vitamin A deficiency causes squamous metaplasia in many tissues. In the cornea, it may progress to softening of the tissue (keratomalacia) and corneal ulceration. In response to liver injury (e.g., alcoholic hepatitis), hepatic stellate cells (Ito cells) differentiate into myofibroblasts that synthesize collagens. Collagen synthesis by Ito cells contributes to hepatic cirrhosis in patients with end-stage liver disease.

Keywords: Night blindness, vitamin A deficiency, hepatic stellate cells

14 **The answer is A: Bile duct.** This image shows a portal triad consisting of a portal vein, bile duct, and hepatic artery. The arrow points to a bile duct, and the asterisk indicates the lumen of a thin-walled, portal vein (shown in the image). The intrahepatic bile duct is lined by cholangiocytes. These columnar epithelial cells are characterized by the presence of apical membrane microvilli, tight intercellular junctions, and a complete basal lamina. Their nuclei are located in the basal cytoplasm, suggesting that their apical cytoplasm is specialized for absorption and/or secretion. None of the other structures exhibit the distinctive histologic features of intrahepatic bile ducts.

Keywords: Liver, bile ducts, portal triad

15 **The answer is E: Intrahepatic bile lakes.** Bile canaliculi join to form canals of Herring within the liver lobule. These short canals are lined by both hepatocytes and cholangiocytes. Canals of Herring deliver bile to larger ducts in the biliary tree. Intrahepatic ducts coalesce to form the hepatic duct, which joins the cystic duct to form the common bile duct. The common bile duct joins the second part of the duodenum at the ampulla of Vater. Obstruction of the canals of Herring, or the other intrahepatic bile ducts, leads to bile stasis (cholestasis). Cholestasis is characterized by the presence of bile pigment in hepatocytes and the accumulation of bile "lakes" within dilated canaliculi. None of the other pathologic changes is associated with injury to the canals of Herring.

Keywords: Cholestasis

16 **The answer is A: Cilia.** Bile contains a mixture of cholesterol, conjugated bilirubin, phospholipids, cholic acids, mucins, and electrolytes. Bile emulsifies dietary fats to facilitate enzymatic digestion and absorption. Bile excretion is stimulated by the release of polypeptide hormones (cholecystokinin, gastrin, and motilin) from enteroendocrine cells in the duodenum. Each cholangiocyte contains a primary cilium that features a basal body and a 9 + 0 arrangement of microtubules in the axoneme. These nonmotile organelles serve as molecular sensors that continuously monitor the flow of bile. Flagella (choice B) are tubulin-based organelles that provide locomotion to sperm. Cholangiocytes feature hemidesmosomes (choice C) and microvilli (choice D), but these membrane structures do not monitor the flow of bile. Stereocilia (choice E) are long microvilli found in the epididymis and inner ear.

Keywords: Biliary system, cholangiocytes, cilia

17 **The answer is A: Canal of Herring.** The liver has a remarkable ability to regenerate in response to injury. For example, in about 15% of alcoholics, hepatocellular necrosis, fibrosis, and regeneration eventually lead to the formation of fibrous septa surrounding hepatocellular nodules. These are the histopathologic features of hepatic cirrhosis. A variety of observational and experimental studies suggest that hepatic stem cells line the canals of Herring. In response to injury, these multipotent stem cells proliferate and migrate into the liver parenchyma to restore structure and function. The space of Disse (choice D) provides a location for communication between hepatocytes and blood. The space of Mall (choice E) provides a location for the accumulation and transport of lymph. None of the other locations are believed to harbor hepatic stem cells.

Keywords: Hepatic cirrhosis, alcoholic liver disease

18 **The answer is B: Cholesterol.** The gallbladder is located in the upper right quadrant of the abdominal cavity on the inferior (visceral) surface of the liver. Risk factors for cholesterol stones include female sex, diabetes, pregnancy, and estrogen therapy. Solitary, yellow, hard gallstones are associated with bile that is supersaturated with cholesterol. During their reproductive years, women are up to three times more likely to develop cholesterol gallstones than men. If the bile contains excess cholesterol, it becomes supersaturated and precipitates to form stones. In obese women, cholesterol secretion by the liver is increased. None of the other components of bile is associated with the pathogenesis of gallstones.

Keywords: Cholelithiasis, gallbladder

19 **The answer is C: Mucosal folds.** The mucosa of the gallbladder is lined by a simple columnar epithelium and a lamina propria of loose connective tissue. The mucosa of the gallbladder has numerous deep folds that may appear as glands in some tissue sections (shown in the image). The lining epithelium is characterized by the presence of tight junctions, apical membrane microvilli, and lateral membrane plications (interdigitations). Approximately 20% of men and 35% of women are found to have gallstones at autopsy. Most complications associated with cholelithiasis are related to obstruction of the biliary tree. Stones that obstruct the common bile duct lead to obstructive jaundice, cholangitis, and acute pancreatitis. Canals of Herring (choice A), hepatic ducts (choice B), and submucosal glands (choice E) are not found in the gallbladder. Mucin-secreting mucosal glands may be seen in the neck of the gallbladder; however, the epithelial structures identified in this image are not composed of mucous cells.

Keywords: Cholelithiasis, gallbladder

20 **The answer is E: Submucosa.** The wall of the gallbladder is unusual in that it does not feature a muscularis mucosae or submucosa. External to the lamina propria (choice B) is the muscularis externa (choice C). This layer is composed of randomly oriented smooth muscle fibers. Contraction of the smooth muscle forces bile through the cystic duct and down the common bile duct to the duodenum. Because the gallbladder attaches to the inferior surface of the liver, it features both an adventitia and a serosa (choices A and D).

Keywords: Gallbladder

21 **The answer is A: Aquaporin.** The concentration of bile within the lumen of the gallbladder depends on active and passive transport. Na/K ATPase in the lateral membrane domain of epithelial cells pumps sodium from the cytoplasm to the lamina propria. This energy-dependent process creates a gradient of electrolytes that draws water from the lumen of the gallbladder, through the epithelium, to the lamina propria, for removal by vascular and lymphatic channels. This active transport mechanism is supplemented by passive transport of water through special membrane pores. These water channels are composed of integral membrane proteins, termed aquaporins. Cadherins and occludins (choices B and C) are cell adhesion molecules. Perforin (choice D) is a cytotoxic protein that is secreted by killer T lymphocytes. Porins (choice E) form channels in the outer membranes of bacteria.

Keywords: Aquaporins, gallbladder

22 **The answer is C: Pancreas.** The pancreas is a retroperitoneal organ situated between the second part of the duodenum and the spleen. The pancreas is composed of both exocrine and endocrine glandular tissues. Lobules of the exocrine pancreas are separated by connective tissue septa. Endocrine cells in the pancreas are organized as compact microglands, referred to as islets of Langerhans. The image shows four spherical islets surrounded by acini of the exocrine pancreas. The pancreas contains millions of islets, primarily in the tail of the pancreas. Functional cell types in the islets of Langerhans include alpha (α), beta (β), and delta (δ) cells. Each cell type produces a different polypeptide hormone (e.g., insulin, glucagon, or somatostatin). None of the other organs feature islets of Langerhans.

Keywords: Pancreas, islets of Langerhans

23 **The answer is E: Serous.** The secretory units of the exocrine pancreas are small berry-shaped structures (acini) that are lined by a simple epithelium of enzyme-secreting serous cells. These epithelial cells store zymogen granules in their apical cytoplasm and secrete digestive enzymes that are activated within the lumen of the duodenum. The eosinophilia of pancreatic acinar cells reflects stores of zymogen granules in their apical cytoplasm. The cells are pyramidal in shape, with a broad basal membrane and a narrow apical membrane that surrounds an intercalated duct. Endocrine cells in the pancreas (choice A) are found in the islets of Langerhans. Goblet cells (choice B) are unicellular glands found in the respiratory tree and gastrointestinal tract. Mucous cells are filled with heavily glycosylated proteins that do not stain with H&E. Paracrine cells (choice D) signal to neighboring cells.

Keywords: Pancreas, exocrine glands

24 **The answer is A: Intercalated ducts.** Exocrine secretions of the pancreas drain through ducts of various sizes to reach the main pancreatic duct of Wirsung (choice E) or the accessory pancreatic duct of Santorini (choice D). The acinar cells release digestive enzymes into intercalated ducts that originate within the secretory unit. Centroacinar cells line the proximal portion of these small ducts. Intercalated ducts join to form intralobular (choice C) ducts that coalesce to form larger interlobular (choice B) ducts. Proenzymes secreted by the acinar cells are diluted with an alkaline pH fluid that is produced primarily by epithelial cells lining the intercalated ducts. Submucosal (Brunner) glands in the proximal part of the duodenum also secrete an alkaline fluid that helps to neutralize the acidity of gastric juice. The other pancreatic ducts do not contribute as much fluid as intercalated ducts.

Keywords: Pancreas, intercalated ducts

25 **The answer is B: Interlobular duct.** The arrow identifies a large pancreatic duct surrounded by dense irregular connective tissue. This duct is best described as an interlobular duct, because it is located in connective tissue septa between pancreatic lobules. Interlobular ducts are lined by low columnar epithelium, whereas intralobular ducts are lined by cuboidal epithelium. Intercalated ducts (choice A) drain pancreatic acini. Intralobular ducts (choice C) are located within pancreatic lobules. The duct indicated in the image is not large enough to be the main pancreatic duct (choice D). Rokitansky-Aschoff sinuses (choice E) are found in the wall of the gallbladder. None of the other structures exhibit the morphologic features of a pancreatic interlobular duct.

Keywords: Pancreas, exocrine ducts

26 **The answer is E: Trypsin.** The pancreas secretes about 1 L of fluid per day (about the same volume as the gallbladder). Digestive proenzymes secreted by the pancreas are activated when they reach the lumen of the duodenum. Activation is a two-step process. First, enteropeptidase in the glycocalyx of the intestinal brush border cleaves pancreatic trypsinogen to form trypsin (a serine protease). Second, trypsin cleaves other pancreatic proenzymes to yield active enzymes for the digestion of food. None of the other enzymes activates pancreatic proenzymes within the lumen of the duodenum.

Keywords: Pancreas, trypsin

27 **The answer is D: Intralobular duct.** This image shows a particularly large intralobular duct that is surrounded by dense irregular connective tissue. The duct is located entirely within a pancreatic lobule. The smallest intralobular ducts are about the same diameter as an acinus. These ducts become progressively larger as they coalesce to form interlobular ducts. None of the other pancreatic ducts exhibit the distinct histologic features of an intralobular duct.

Keywords: Pancreas, exocrine ducts

28 **The answer is D: Pancreas.**   Acute pancreatitis is defined as an inflammatory condition of the exocrine pancreas that results from injury to acinar cells. The disease presents with a spectrum of signs and symptoms. Severe forms are characterized by the sudden onset of abdominal pain, often accompanied by signs of shock (hypotension, tachypnea, and tachycardia). Amylase and lipase are digestive enzymes secreted by the pancreas. The release of these enzymes into the serum provides a sensitive marker for monitoring injury to pancreatic acinar cells. Injury to the other organs does not lead to increased serum levels of amylase and lipase.
Keywords: Pancreatitis

29 **The answer is A: Bile ducts.**   Laboratory data provide crucial information regarding the mechanisms of disease. For example, ductal epithelial cells of the pancreas express high levels of alkaline phosphatase. Injury to these ductal cells releases alkaline phosphatase into the serum. The presence of this enzyme in the blood provides a sensitive marker for monitoring injury to the biliary tree. Increased serum levels of AST, ALT, and bilirubin indicate injury to hepatocytes. Patients with end-stage liver disease often present with complications of portal hypertension, including ascites, splenomegaly, and bleeding esophageal varicose veins (varices). None of the other tissues/structures expresses high levels of alkaline phosphatase.
Keywords: Hepatic cirrhosis, alcoholic liver disease

30 **The answer is B: Insulin.**   Insulinomas are endocrine tumors that secrete insulin and cause hypoglycemia. Symptoms of hypoglycemia include hunger, sweating, irritability, epileptic seizures, and coma. Infusion of glucose alleviates these symptoms. The presence of small, membrane-bound granules with a dense core is a feature of insulinomas and other neuroendocrine tumors. These dense granules are visible by electron microscopy. Electron microscopy may aid in the diagnosis of poorly differentiated cancers, whose classification is problematic by light microscopy. None of the other hormones cause signs and symptoms of hypoglycemia.
Keywords: Insulinoma, hypoglycemia

Chapter 15

Urinary System

QUESTIONS

Select the single best answer.

1 A 46-year-old man presents with excruciating episodic (colicky) pain on the right side, radiating from the flank to his inguinal region. The episodes of pain last about 30 minutes. Imaging studies reveal a urinary stone. Based on the patient's symptoms, the stone most likely lodged in which of the following components of the urinary system?
(A) Major calyx of the kidney
(B) Renal pelvis
(C) Ureter
(D) Urethra
(E) Urinary bladder

2 A 56-year-old woman with a history of chronic renal disease complains of bone and joint pain. Laboratory studies reveal hypocalcemia and vitamin D_3 deficiency. Which of the following describes the most likely reason for vitamin D_3 deficiency in this patient?
(A) Excessive urinary loss of calcitriol (vitamin D_3)
(B) Inability to excrete serum phosphate
(C) Inadequate hydroxylation of calcidiol (vitamin D_2)
(D) Insufficient supply of vitamin D in the diet
(E) Lack of adequate exposure to sunshine

3 A 68-year-old diabetic man with chronic kidney disease complains of weakness and fatigue. Physical examination reveals marked pallor. The CBC reveals a normocytic anemia. Which of the following best describes the pathogenesis of anemia in this patient?

(A) Chronic blood loss via the urine (hematuria)
(B) Decreased serum levels of erythropoietin
(C) Inadequate supply of iron in the diet
(D) Increased destruction of circulating red blood cells
(E) Loss of erythrocyte progenitor cells from the bone marrow

4 Which of the following terms best describes the basic structural and functional unit of the kidney that filters the blood and produces urine?
(A) Cortical labyrinth
(B) Nephron
(C) Renal column
(D) Renal lobule
(E) Renal pyramid

5 You are asked to give a lecture on the development of the urinary system as part of a first-year anatomy course. The collecting ducts and major/minor calyces in the adult kidney are derived from which of the following structures during embryonic and fetal development?
(A) Mesonephric duct
(B) Mesonephric tubules
(C) Metanephric blastema
(D) Paramesonephric duct
(E) Ureteric bud

6 During your lecture, a student asks about the significance of urine production during intrauterine development. Which of the following is the most important function of the kidneys during embryonic and fetal life?
(A) Generation of amniotic fluid
(B) Maintenance of electrolyte balance
(C) Regulation of blood pH
(D) Regulation of fetal blood pressure
(E) Removal of nitrogenous waste (blood urea nitrogen)

7 A section of the kidney obtained at autopsy is examined by light microscopy (shown in the image). Identify the zone/region indicated by the double arrow.

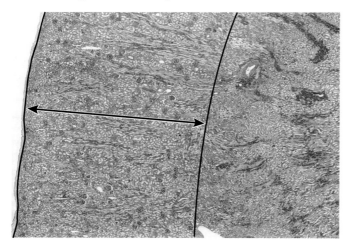

(A) Capsule
(B) Cortex
(C) Medulla
(D) Medullary ray
(E) Pyramid

8 Another section of the kidney is examined at high magnification (shown in the image). Identify the layer/region indicated by the double arrow.

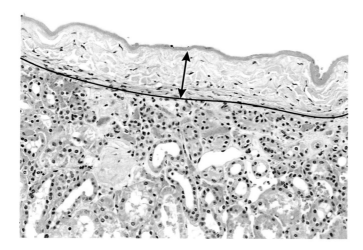

(A) Capsule
(B) Cortex
(C) Parietal peritoneum
(D) Perirenal fat
(E) Visceral peritoneum

9 A 67-year-old man is found to have blood in his urine during a routine checkup. A CT scan reveals a renal mass that is subsequently removed. Microscopic examination of the surgical specimen reveals normal tissue along the tumor margin (shown in the image). Identify the region/zone indicated by the double arrow.

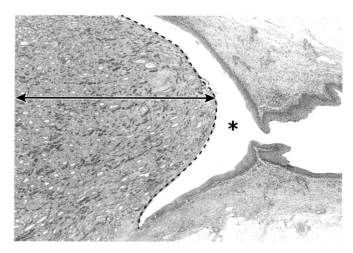

(A) Column
(B) Cortex
(C) Lobe
(D) Lobule
(E) Medulla

10 For the surgical specimen shown in Question 9, identify the open space indicated by the asterisk.
(A) Collecting duct
(B) Major calyx
(C) Minor calyx
(D) Renal pelvis
(E) Renal sinus

11 The cortical region of a kidney biopsy is examined in the pathology department. Which of the following terms best describes the regions of the cortex that are visible within the rectangular boxes (shown in the image)?

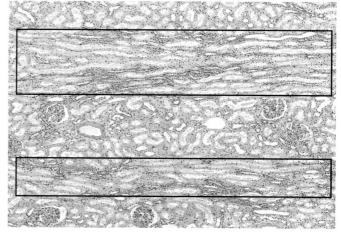

(A) Cortical labyrinths
(B) Lobes
(C) Lobules
(D) Medullary rays
(E) Renal pyramids

12 Sections of the renal biopsy described in Question 11 are prepared using the Gomori trichrome stain. Which of the following terms best describes the region of the cortex that lies between the lines (shown in the image)?

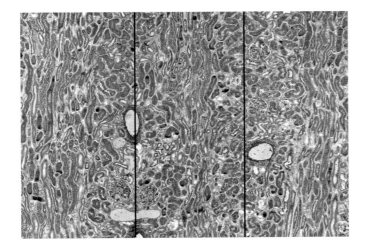

(A) Cortical labyrinth
(B) Lobe
(C) Lobule
(D) Medullary ray
(E) Renal pyramid

13 A renal biopsy is examined for pathologic changes (shown in the image). Identify the normal artery indicated by the arrow.

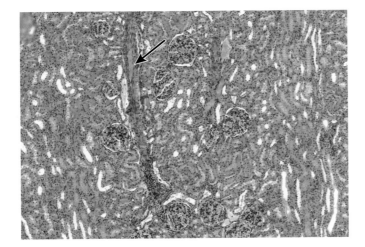

(A) Afferent arteriole
(B) Arcuate
(C) Efferent arteriole
(D) Interlobar
(E) Interlobular

14 You are asked to provide a brief overview of the anatomy and physiology of the kidney. Which of the following anatomic terms best describes the initial portion of a nephron?
(A) Collecting tubule
(B) Distal convoluted tubule
(C) Loop of Henle
(D) Proximal convoluted tubule
(E) Renal corpuscle

15 A 59-year-old woman presents with painless hematuria. A CT scan reveals a renal mass that is subsequently removed. Microscopic examination of the surgical specimen reveals normal tissue along the tumor margin (shown in the image). Identify the structure within the circle.

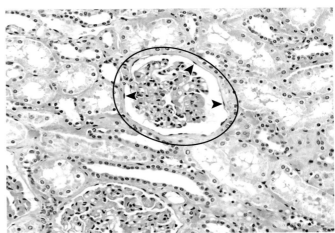

(A) Collecting duct
(B) Glomerulus
(C) Nephron
(D) Proximal convoluted tubule
(E) Renal corpuscle

16 Sections of the specimen described in Question 15 are stained with Gomori trichrome to highlight basement membrane proteins in blue and cell nuclei in red. A normal renal corpuscle is examined along with several medical students at a multiheaded microscope (shown in the image). Identify the area within the oval.

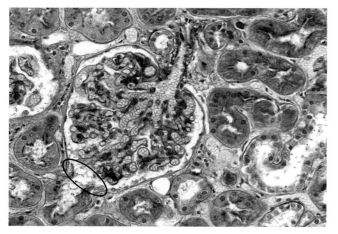

(A) Distal convoluted tubule
(B) Proximal convoluted tubule
(C) Urinary pole of the Bowman capsule
(D) Urinary space
(E) Vascular pole of the Bowman capsule

17 Another glomerulus from the section described in Question 16 is examined at higher magnification. The asterisk indicate glomerular capillary loops (shown in the image). Which of the following histologic features best characterizes these blood vessels?

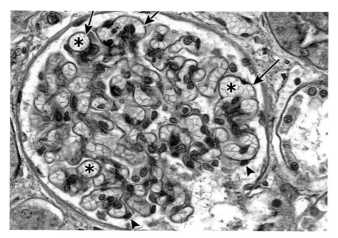

(A) Continuous capillaries lacking fenestrations
(B) Continuous capillaries with discontinuous basement membranes
(C) Discontinuous capillaries with fenestrations covered by diaphragms
(D) Discontinuous capillaries with fenestrations lacking diaphragms
(E) Sinusoidal capillaries with discontinuous basement membranes

18 For the image shown in Question 17, identify the wavy blue lines indicated by the arrows.
(A) Glomerular basement membranes
(B) Glomerular endothelial cells
(C) Mesangial cells
(D) Parietal epithelial cells
(E) Visceral epithelial cells

19 The arrowheads on the image shown for Questions 17 and 18 identify the nuclei of which of the following glomerular cells?
(A) Endothelial cells
(B) Juxtaglomerular cells
(C) Mesangial cells
(D) Parietal epithelial cells
(E) Podocytes

20 A 30-year-old woman complains of swelling of her eyelids and ankles. Urinalysis reveals proteinuria (6 g/24 h) without hematuria. A renal biopsy is obtained and examined by electron microscopy. The asterisk indicates the lumen of a single glomerular capillary loop. Identify the structures that surround the outer aspect of the glomerular basement membrane (arrow, shown in the image).

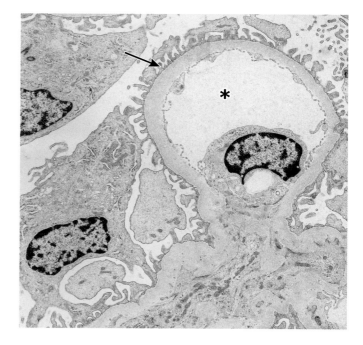

(A) Fenestrated endothelial cells
(B) Foot processes of podocytes
(C) Lamellipodia of mesangial cells
(D) Parietal epithelial cells
(E) Proliferating myofibroblasts

21 The renal biopsy described in Question 20 is examined by electron microscopy at higher magnification. Identify the delicate linear structures located between adjacent pedicles of the visceral epithelial cells (arrows, shown in the image).

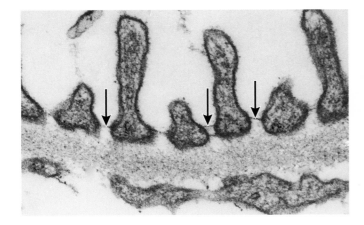

(A) Fenestrated endothelial cells
(B) Lamina rara interna of the glomerular basement membrane
(C) Parietal layer of the Bowman capsule
(D) Lamina densa of the glomerular basement membrane
(E) Slit diaphragms

22 You are involved in a translational medicine research project to identify genes that encode structural proteins associated with the glomerular filtration barrier. Which of the following is the major structural protein found in the filtration slit diaphragm?
(A) Fibrillin
(B) Fibronectin
(C) Laminin
(D) Nephrin
(E) Perlecan

23 The parents of a 2-month-old infant are concerned that their son has puffy skin and foamy urine. Physical examination confirms generalized edema. Urinalysis reveals heavy proteinuria and lipiduria (increased protein and lipid in urine). The infant is subsequently diagnosed with congenital nephrotic syndrome. This rare inherited disorder is most likely caused by mutations in the gene that encodes which of the following adhesion/matrix proteins?
(A) Fibrillin
(B) Fibronectin
(C) Laminin
(D) Nephrin
(E) Perlecan

24 A 45-year-old man presents with hematuria and bloody sputum. Over the next 3 days, he develops oliguria (decreased urine production) and renal failure. A kidney biopsy is stained with fluorescein-labeled goat anti-human IgG to reveal the distribution of autoantibodies in the patient's glomeruli. The linear pattern of staining (shown in the image) suggests that autoantibodies are bound to which of the following structures?

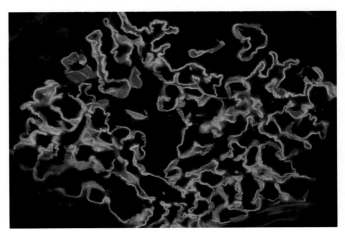

(A) Afferent and efferent arterioles
(B) Bowman capsule
(C) Glomerular basement membrane
(D) Mesangial matrix
(E) Proximal convoluted tubules

25 Laboratory analysis of serum collected from the patient described in Question 24 will reveal autoantibodies directed against which of the following basement membrane proteins?
(A) Collagen type IV
(B) Laminin B
(C) Neph-2
(D) Perlecan
(E) α-Actinin-4

26 Which of the following cells collaborates with capillary endothelial cells to synthesize the glomerular basement membrane described in Questions 24 and 25?
(A) Fibroblasts
(B) Mesangial cells
(C) Parietal epithelial cells
(D) Podocytes
(E) Smooth muscle cells

27 A 26-year-old man complains of recurrent hematuria since his youth. The hematuria typically occurs following upper respiratory tract infections. A kidney biopsy is examined by direct immunofluorescence for the presence of IgA autoantibody. The pattern of staining (shown in the image) suggests that the patient's autoantibodies are bound to which of the following structures?

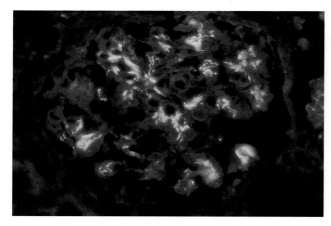

(A) Afferent arterioles
(B) Bowman capsule
(C) Efferent arterioles
(D) Glomerular basement membrane
(E) Mesangium

28 Which of the following biological processes describes the primary function of the mesangial cells described in Question 27?
(A) Hormone synthesis and secretion
(B) Maintenance of the glomerular filtration barrier
(C) Phagocytosis and endocytosis
(D) Regulation of systemic blood pressure
(E) Sodium/potassium homeostasis

29 The mesangial cells described in Questions 27 and 28 are derived from multipotential stem cells (precursors) from which of the following types of connective tissue cells?
(A) Adipocytes
(B) Fibroblasts
(C) Granulocytes
(D) Monocytes
(E) Smooth muscle cells

30 A kidney biopsy is embedded in paraffin, sectioned, stained with H&E, and examined by light microscopy (shown in the image). Identify the structure within the oval.

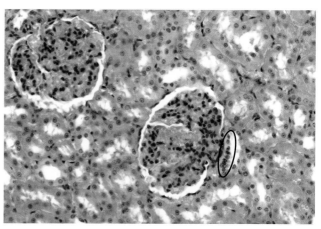

(A) Extraglomerular mesangial cells
(B) Juxtaglomerular cells
(C) Macula densa
(D) Proximal convoluted tubule
(E) Vascular pole of the Bowman capsule

31 Which of the following biological processes describes the critical function of the structure described in Question 30?
(A) Hydroxylation of vitamin D_3
(B) Monitoring Na^+ in primary urine
(C) Phagocytosis of immune complexes
(D) Reabsorption of K^+ from primary urine
(E) Secretion of aldosterone

32 During a clinical conference, you are asked to summarize the role of juxtaglomerular cells in maintaining a constant rate of glomerular filtration. Which of the following biological processes describes the function of JG cells in the kidney?
(A) Monitoring Na^+ in primary urine
(B) Reabsorption of H_2O from primary urine
(C) Reabsorption of Na^+ from primary urine
(D) Secretion of angiotensinogen
(E) Secretion of renin

33 A trichrome stain of a renal biopsy is examined in the pathology department (shown in the image). Identify the structures indicated by the asterisk.

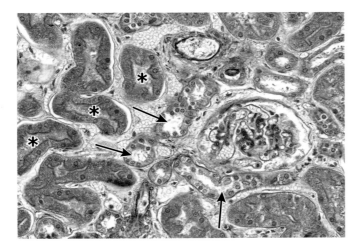

(A) Distal convoluted tubules
(B) Distal straight tubules
(C) Peritubular capillaries
(D) Proximal convoluted tubules
(E) Proximal straight tubules

34 For the biopsy described in Question 33, identify the structures indicated by the arrows.
(A) Collecting ducts
(B) Distal convoluted tubules
(C) Proximal convoluted tubules
(D) Proximal straight tubules
(E) Thin limbs of the loop of Henle

35 Another visual field from the biopsy specimen described in Questions 33 and 34 is examined in the pathology department (shown in the image). Identify the spaces/structures indicated by the arrows.

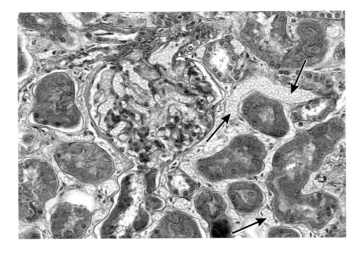

(A) Distal convoluted tubules
(B) Peritubular capillaries
(C) Thin limbs of the loop of Henle
(D) Vasa recta
(E) Vasa vasorum

36 Which of the following structures serves as the primary site for reabsorption of water, electrolytes, amino acids, sugars, and polypeptides from the glomerular ultrafiltrate?
(A) Collecting duct
(B) Distal convoluted tubule
(C) Proximal convoluted tubule
(D) Thick descending limbs of the loop of Henle
(E) Thin limbs of the long loop of Henle

37 A 48-year-old man suffers trauma in an automobile accident and expires. A kidney is harvested at autopsy and sections are stained with H&E. A medullary ray in the renal cortex is examined at high magnification. Identify the structure indicated by double arrow no. 1 (shown in the image).

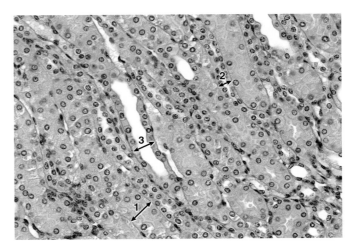

(A) Cortical collecting duct
(B) Distal convoluted tubule
(C) Proximal convoluted tubule
(D) Thick ascending limb of the loop of Henle
(E) Thick descending limb of the loop of Henle

38 For the kidney specimen described in Question 37, identify the structure in the medullary ray that is indicated by double arrow no. 2 (shown in the image).
(A) Cortical collecting duct
(B) Distal convoluted tubule
(C) Thick ascending limb of the loop of Henle
(D) Thick descending limb of the loop of Henle
(E) Thin limb of the loop of Henle

39 For the kidney specimen described in Questions 37 and 38, identify the structure in the medullary ray that is indicated by double arrow no. 3 (shown in the image).
(A) Cortical collecting duct
(B) Distal straight tubule
(C) Papillary duct
(D) Proximal straight tubule
(E) Thin limb of the loop of Henle

40 The outer medullary region of the kidney is examined in the pathology department (shown in the image). Identify the small channels indicated by the arrows.

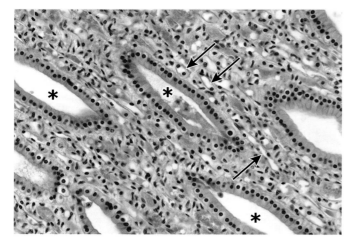

(A) Capillaries of the vasa recta
(B) Distal straight tubules
(C) Medullary collecting ducts
(D) Proximal straight tubules
(E) Thin segments of the loop of Henle

41 For the kidney specimen described in Question 40, identify the structures indicated by the asterisk.
(A) Cortical collecting tubules
(B) Distal convoluted tubules
(C) Distal straight tubules
(D) Medullary collecting ducts
(E) Proximal straight tubules

42 Examination of a transverse section through a renal pyramid reveals medullary collecting ducts, thin segments of the loop of Henle, and numerous blood vessels (red spaces, shown in the image). Which of the following describes these vascular channels?

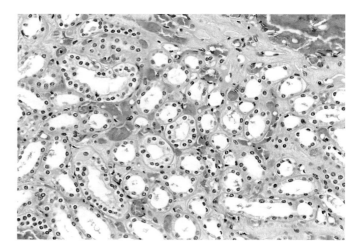

(A) Afferent arterioles
(B) Efferent arterioles
(C) Interlobular arteries
(D) Peritubular capillaries
(E) Vasa recta

43 You are asked to present a lecture on the pathophysiology of urine formation. Interstitial connective tissue is most hyperosmotic in which region of the kidney?
(A) Capsule
(B) Cortex
(C) Corticomedullary junction
(D) Medulla at apex of the pyramid
(E) Medulla at base of the pyramid

44 Which of the following best describes the physiologic mechanism responsible for the formation and excretion of hyperosmotic urine?
(A) Countercurrent multiplier system
(B) Juxtaglomerular apparatus signaling
(C) Podocyte regulation of the glomerular filtration barrier
(D) Renin–angiotensin–aldosterone system
(E) Water reabsorption in the descending limb of the loop of Henle

45 The concentration of urine in the collecting ducts is dependent on which of the following hormones?
(A) Aldosterone
(B) Angiotensin I
(C) Angiotensin II
(D) Renin
(E) Vasopressin

46 A 16-year-old boy presents with headaches and muscle weakness. His parents note that he drinks water excessively. A 24-hour urine collection shows polyuria. The fasting blood sugar is normal. This patient may have an injury affecting which of the following endocrine organs?

(A) Adrenal glands
(B) Pancreas
(C) Parathyroid glands
(D) Pituitary gland
(E) Thyroid gland

47 The apex of a medullary pyramid is examined in the histology laboratory (shown in the image). Identify the tubular structures indicated by the asterisk.

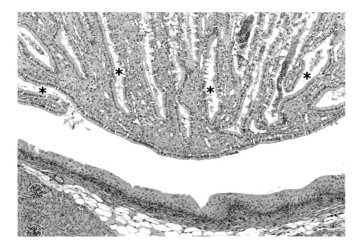

(A) Arcuate arteries
(B) Connecting tubules
(C) Cortical collecting ducts
(D) Medullary collecting ducts
(E) Papillary ducts of Bellini

48 A 55-year-old man complains of hematuria. A urinary bladder biopsy is eventually obtained and examined in the pathology department (shown in the image). Specify the type of epithelium that lines this patient's urinary bladder.

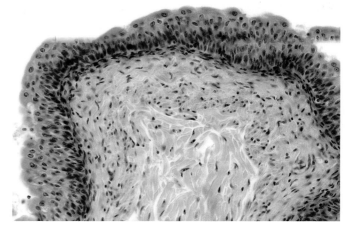

(A) Simple columnar
(B) Stratified columnar
(C) Stratified cuboidal
(D) Stratified squamous
(E) Transitional

49 First-year medical students examine the wall of the urinary bladder in the histology laboratory (shown in the image). Identify the tissue indicated by the asterisk.

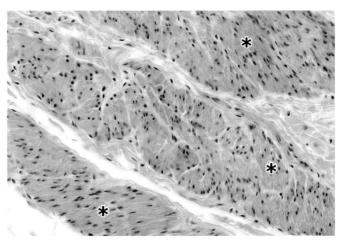

(A) Dense irregular connective tissue
(B) Dense regular connective tissue
(C) Elastic connective tissue
(D) Skeletal muscle
(E) Smooth muscle

50 Several retroperitoneal organs are examined at autopsy. One of these organs is shown in the image. The histologic features of this specimen suggest that it was obtained from which of the following anatomic locations?

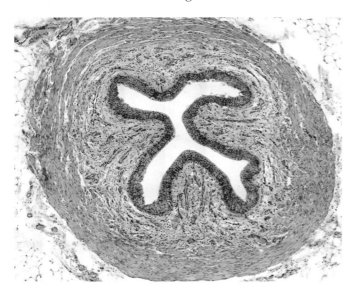

(A) Gallbladder
(B) Renal artery
(C) Ureter
(D) Urethra
(E) Urinary bladder

51 Which portion of the male urethra is surrounded by the external urethral sphincter?
(A) Distal segment of the spongy urethra
(B) Initial segment of the spongy urethra
(C) Membranous urethra
(D) Preprostatic urethra
(E) Prostatic urethra

ANSWERS

1 **The answer is C: Ureter.** The urinary system is composed of paired kidneys and ureters, as well as the urinary bladder and urethra. Urine produced in the kidneys is conveyed via the ureters to the urinary bladder. The bladder stores urine before it is released through the urethra during urination (micturition). The pelvis and calyx of the kidney are common sites for the formation and retention of calculi (stones). Renal stones can move and lodge in the ureters or urinary bladder. Large ureteric stones cause painful distention and obstruction. Patients typically complain of severe intermittent pain, caused by forceful peristaltic contractions of the ureter, as it attempts to expel the renal calculus. The pain is typically referred to the overlying cutaneous region, where it is described as passing from "loin to groin." Ureteric calculi can be removed using a nephroscope or lithotripsy—a procedure that uses shockwaves to break stones into fragments that are expelled with urine. Stones in the other anatomic locations would not typically present with flank pain radiating to the inguinal region. The presence of stones in the collecting system of the kidney is termed nephrolithiasis. The presence of stones elsewhere in the collecting system of the urinary tract is termed urolithiasis.
Keywords: Urolithiasis, renal calculi

2 **The answer is C: Inadequate hydroxylation of calcidiol (vitamin D2).** Principal functions of the kidney include removal of metabolic waste from blood and balancing serum electrolytes. The kidney also functions as an endocrine organ. For example, the kidneys synthesize the biologically active form of vitamin D (calcitriol). Calcitriol (also referred to as vitamin D_3) is required for intestinal absorption of calcium and phosphate. Inactive forms of vitamin D obtained from the diet (choice D) or from sun-exposed skin (choice E) undergo hydroxylation in the liver to form 25-OH vitamin D_2 (calcidiol). Calcidiol is converted in the kidney to 1,25-OH vitamin D_3, the biologically active form of vitamin D. In patients with chronic renal disease, hydroxylation of 25-OH vitamin D is inadequate, and patients develop signs and symptoms of vitamin D deficiency (e.g., reduced bone density). Dietary deficiency of vitamin D in children leads to developmental bone deformities and fractures. This complication of childhood malnutrition is termed rickets.
Keywords: Vitamin D, rickets

3 **The answer is B: Decreased serum levels of erythropoietin.** Erythropoietin (EPO) is a 34-kDa glycoprotein hormone that is secreted by peritubular capillary endothelial cells of the kidney. EPO binds cell surface receptors on erythrocyte progenitor cells in the bone marrow (burst-forming and colony-forming erythroid units). This interaction inhibits programmed cell death and stimulates cell survival and proliferation, leading to increased production of RBCs and increased hematocrit (relative RBC packed cell volume in the blood). Patients with end-stage kidney disease typically produce inadequate serum levels of EPO, resulting in decreased production of RBCs and decreased hematocrit. The other mechanisms of disease are unlikely causes of anemia in a patient with a history of chronic renal disease.
Keywords: Anemia, erythropoietin

4 **The answer is B: Nephron.** The kidneys filter blood to remove metabolic waste and excess water and balance concentrations of serum electrolytes. The basic functional unit of urine production is termed the nephron. The nephron consists of a (1) renal corpuscle (glomerulus and Bowman capsule), (2) proximal convoluted tubule, (3) thin and thick limbs of the nephron loop (loop of Henle), (4) distal convoluted tubule, and (5) collecting tubule. Collecting tubules from several nephrons drain into a common collecting duct. Collecting ducts transport urine to minor and then to major calyces, which drain via the ureter to the urinary bladder. Loops of Henle are straight tubules that extend deep into pyramids of the renal medulla. Cortical labyrinth (choice A) refers to regions of the cortex that contain glomeruli and convoluted tubules. Renal columns (choice C) are extensions of the cortex that lie between renal pyramids. Renal lobules (choice D) are composed of nephrons that drain to a single collecting duct. Renal pyramids (choice E) are conical structures within the medulla that provide a passage for the numerous collecting ducts that drain to the renal papillae located at the apex of the pyramid.
Keywords: Kidney, nephron

5 **The answer is E: Ureteric bud.** The metanephros (true kidney) begins to develop during the 5th and 6th weeks of development. In brief, a diverticulum (ureteric bud) of the mesonephric duct pushes its way into a mass of undifferentiated mesenchyme referred to as the metanephric blastema. These two embryonic tissues (blastema and ureteric bud) engage in complex signaling events (commonly referred to as epithelial–mesenchymal cell interactions) that establish nephrons for the production of urine and collecting ducts for the transport of urine to the urinary bladder. The collecting system of the kidney is derived entirely from the embryonic ureteric bud. The ureteric bud undergoes extensive branching morphogenesis to generate medullary collecting ducts, renal calyces, renal pelvis, and ureter. Nephrons (see Question 4) are derived from the metanephric blastema (choice C). Mesonephric ducts and tubules (choices A and B) give rise to the male genital excretory ducts. The paramesonephric duct (choice D) gives rise to the uterine tubes and uterus.
Keywords: Ureteric bud

6 **The answer is A: Generation of amniotic fluid.** The fetal kidneys (metanephroi) begin to produce urine after the 9th week of gestation. The urine leaves the urogenital sinus and enters the amniotic cavity. After 16 weeks of

gestation, urine produced by the fetal kidneys make an essential contribution to the amniotic fluid. Amniotic fluid serves many crucial functions during development, including (1) protection of the embryo and fetus; (2) regulation of fluid volume and electrolyte homeostasis; and (3) provision of space for symmetric growth of the embryo and fetus. Fetal kidneys are not essential for filtering the blood in utero, because the placenta regulates the exchange of blood gases, nutrients, electrolyte, and metabolic waste between the fetus and the mother. None of the other choices describe the primary function of the fetal kidney during gestation.
Keywords: Amniotic fluid

7 The answer is B: Cortex.   The internal architecture of the kidney consists of an outer zone (cortex) and inner zone (medulla). In living tissue, the cortex takes on a reddish brown color, since most of the blood in the renal arteries is delivered to the cortex (90% to 95%). The characteristic features of the kidney cortex are renal corpuscles and their associated tubules. Medullary rays (choice D) are portions of the cortex consisting of collecting tubules that drain to collecting ducts in the renal medulla. None of the other anatomic zones/regions exhibit key histologic features of the renal cortex.
Keywords: Kidney, renal cortex

8 The answer is A: Capsule.   A dense connective tissue capsule covers the outer surface of the kidney. Two distinct layers of the capsule are visible in this image. The outer layer features typical dense connective tissue that is composed of collagen fibers/bundles and fibroblasts. The inner layer is more cellular, with an abundance of myofibroblast cells that express nonmuscle myosin and demonstrate contractility. The fibrous capsule continues to the hilum of the kidney and coats the outer wall of the renal pelvis. Kidney cortex (choice B) is located beneath the capsule. Because the kidneys are retroperitoneal organs, they are not in contact with parietal or visceral peritoneum (choices C and E). Rather, they are surrounded by pararenal and perirenal fat. None of the other layers/regions describe a collagenous capsule for the kidney.
Keywords: Kidney, capsule

9 The answer is E: Medulla.   The renal medulla is the innermost zone of the kidney. It is composed of straight tubules, collecting ducts, and associated capillary plexuses. In humans, the renal medulla is organized into multiple cone-shaped renal pyramids. The broad base of the medullary pyramids is associated with the renal cortex. The conical apex of the pyramid faces internally and is referred to as the renal papilla (indicated by the dotted line in the image). Renal columns (choice A) are portions of the renal cortex that extend into the medulla and separate adjacent pyramids from one another. Renal cortex (choice B) is the outermost zone of the kidney. Together,

a renal pyramid and its overlying region of cortex are referred to as a lobe (choice C). Human kidneys have approximately 12 lobes. Lobules (choice D) consist of a central medullary ray surrounded by cortical labyrinth.
Keywords: Renal cell carcinoma, kidney, medulla, renal pyramid

10 The answer is C: Minor calyx.   In the medulla of the kidney, renal papillae project into small cup-like chambers, termed minor calyces (singular, calyx). Urine is excreted from the tips of renal papillae into the minor calyces, which deliver urine to the extrarenal duct system. There are many minor calices in the human kidney. Two or three minor calyces combine to form a major calyx (shown on the right side of the image). The major calyces are continuous with the renal pelvis (upper, expanded portion of the ureter) and ureter. None of the other anatomic structures describe histologic features of a minor calyx.
Keywords: Kidney, calyx

11 The answer is D: Medullary rays.   Medullary rays represent parallel striations in the renal cortex that radiate from the medulla toward the surface of the kidney. They consist of a parallel array of straight tubules and collecting ducts. Cortical labyrinths (choice A) are cortical regions that lie between adjacent medullary rays. Cortical labyrinths consist of renal corpuscles and convoluted tubules. Renal pyramids (choice E) are found in the medulla of the kidney. None of the other choices describe histologic features of cortical medullary rays.
Keywords: Kidney, medullary ray, cortical labyrinth

12 The answer is C: Lobule.   A renal lobule consists of multiple nephrons that drain to a single collecting duct. Medullary rays (choice D) form the central axis of each lobule, whereas cortical labyrinths (choice A) form the lateral borders of each lobule. Boundaries between adjacent lobules are not obvious, because intervening septa are lacking. Lobules are, however, bounded by ascending interlobular arteries (shown in the image). A renal lobe (choice B) is much larger. It consists of a single renal pyramid (with columns on either side) and an overlying region of the cortex. Interlobar arteries and veins bound renal lobes.
Keywords: Kidney, lobule, lobe

13 The answer is E: Interlobular.   Renal arteries branch to form two or three segmental arteries that enter each kidney at the hilum. Interlobar arteries (choice D) are branches of the segmental renal arteries that travel between renal pyramids. Interlobar arteries extend toward the corticomedullary junction, where they give rise to arcuate arteries (choice B). Arcuate arteries "arc" along the corticomedullary junction near the bases of the renal pyramids. Interlobular arteries (choice E) arise from the arcuate arteries at a right angle and travel through the cortex toward the surface of the kidney. Interlobular

arteries form boundaries for renal lobules. Afferent arterioles branch from interlobular arteries; they enter renal corpuscles to form a complex glomerular capillary plexus. Efferent arterioles (choice C) draining renal corpuscles in the cortex form a peritubular capillary network, whereas efferent arterioles draining juxtamedullary nephrons extend into the medulla as long, straight vessels (vasa recta). Venous blood returns to the inferior vena cava.
Keywords: Kidney, interlobular artery

14 **The answer is E: Renal corpuscle.** The nephron is the basic structural and functional unit of the kidney. There are 1 to 2 million nephrons per kidney. Each nephron begins as a spherical structure, referred to as the renal corpuscle. Renal corpuscles contain the filtration apparatus that produces primary urine (glomerular ultrafiltrate). Primary urine passes in sequence through the following additional components of the nephron: proximal convoluted tubule, proximal straight tubule (thick descending limb of the loop of Henle), descending thin limb and ascending thin limb, distal straight tubule (thick ascending limb of the loop of Henle), and distal convoluted tubule. The thin descending limb makes a hairpin turn in the medulla and is continuous with the thin ascending limb. The thin ascending limb extends toward the renal cortex and enters the cortical medullary ray as a thick ascending limb (distal straight tubule). An arched collecting tubule then connects distal convoluted tubules to collecting ducts that drain to the renal papillae.
Keywords: Kidney, renal corpuscle, nephron

15 **The answer is E: Renal corpuscle.** The renal corpuscle is the blood-filtering unit of the kidney. It consists of a double-layered cellular sac surrounding a delicate capillary tuft, referred to as the glomerulus (choice B). The cup-shaped epithelial sac is termed Bowman capsule. The visceral layer of the Bowman capsule invests capillary endothelial cells of the glomerulus. The parietal layer of the Bowman capsule (indicated by arrowheads) separates the renal corpuscle from surrounding connective tissue. The urinary space, located between the parietal and visceral layers of the Bowman capsule, receives the glomerular ultrafiltrate (primary urine). None of the other choices describe histologic features of a renal corpuscle.
Keywords: Renal cell carcinoma, renal corpuscle, glomerulus

16 **The answer is C: Urinary pole of the Bowman capsule.** The urinary space present between the layers of the Bowman capsule is continuous with the proximal convoluted tubule. The area where the proximal convoluted tubule begins is referred as the urinary pole of the Bowman capsule. The vascular pole is located on the opposite side of the renal corpuscle; here, afferent and efferent arterioles invaginate the parietal layer of the Bowman capsule to form the glomerulus. This photomicrograph clearly shows an area of open communication between the urinary space and a proximal convoluted tubule. It also provides an excellent view of an afferent arteriole (in longitudinal section), as it enters the vascular pole of the capsule and immediately branches to form the glomerulus.
Keywords: Kidney, Bowman capsule

17 **The answer is D: Discontinuous capillaries with fenestrations lacking diaphragms.** The glomerulus is a specialized capillary network (tuft) located between afferent and efferent arterioles. Glomerular capillaries are characterized by the presence of fenestrated (windowed) endothelial cells, resting on a continuous (and thick) basement membrane. Perforations through these very thin endothelial cells are approximately 60 to 100 nm in diameter. They are larger and more numerous than fenestrations observed in other tissues. Fenestrations in glomerular capillaries lack intervening extracellular diaphragms, thereby expanding the size range of molecules leaving the vascular space for the primary urine. None of the other histologic features characterize glomerular capillary endothelial cells.
Keywords: Kidney, glomerulus

18 **The answer is A: Glomerular basement membranes.** The endothelial cells of the glomerular capillaries are supported by a thick basement membrane, referred to as the glomerular basement membrane (GBM). The basement membrane is about 300 to 370 nm in thickness. When kidney tissue is prepared using special stains (e.g., PAS, trichrome), the GBM is prominently visible as is evident in this image. Capillary endothelial cells and visceral epithelial cells (podocytes) both contribute to the synthesis and deposition of the GBM. Extracellular macromolecules that make up the GBM include type IV collagen, laminin, nidogen, and proteoglycans.
Keywords: Glomerular basement membrane

19 **The answer is E: Podocytes.** Podocytes are specialized cells of the visceral layer of the Bowman capsule. Podocytes and their processes cover and are closely associated with the outer surface of the GBM. In a routine tissue preparation, the podocytes always protrude into the urinary space in the Bowman capsule, as seen in this image. Other listed choices do not exhibit features characteristic of podocytes.
Keywords: Podocytes

20 **The answer is B: Foot processes of podocytes.** The podocytes are visceral epithelial cells that rest on the outer surface of the glomerular basement membrane (GBM). They send out extensive cytoplasmic processes that wrap around the glomerular capillaries. Numerous secondary processes, termed foot processes or pedicels, arise from these cytoplasmic extensions. Adjacent pedicels (from the same podocyte or another podocyte) interdigitate and cover the outer aspect of the GBM. Podocytes and pedicels play a key role in regulating glomerular filtration. The electron micrograph shown in the image reveals numerous foot processes (pedicels) investing the outer aspect of a GBM. The nucleus of a capillary endothelial cell (choice A) protrudes into the lumen of the capillary. Mesangial matrix and a mesangial cell (choice C) are visible in the lower right corner of the image. Proteinuria, without hematuria, characterizes patients with nephrotic syndrome. None of the other cells rest on the outer aspect of the GBM.

Keywords: Nephrotic syndrome, podocytes

21 The answer is E: Slit diaphragms. The open spaces between interdigitating pedicels (foot processes) are referred to as filtration slits. These thin delicate membranes are modified adherens junctions that are referred to as slit diaphragms. The glomerular filtration barrier is composed of (1) fenestrated endothelium, (2) continuous basement membrane, and (3) podocytes and pedicels with filtration slit diaphragms. Together, these structures form a size- and charge-selective barrier that regulates glomerular ultrafiltration. Fenestrated capillary endothelial cells (choice A) are associated with the inner aspect of the GBM (lower part of the image). Components of the glomerular basement membrane (choices B and D) are visible near the center of the image. Parietal epithelial cells (choice C) do not make contact with the GBM.

Keywords: Kidney, slit diaphragm

22 The answer is D: Nephrin. The filtration slit diaphragm is a highly specialized intercellular junction. The major structural and functional protein in this junction is nephrin. Nephrin molecules are transmembrane proteins that project from the plasma membranes of adjacent pedicels. They form zipper-like sheets that interact to form a porous slit diaphragm. Pores in the slit diaphragm determine the molecular size exclusion limit for glomerular filtration; proteins with a size greater than 3.5 nm are excluded from the glomerular ultrafiltrate. Additional proteins in the slit diaphragm include podocin, α-actinin-4, Neph-1, Neph-2, and P-cadherin. Fibrillin (choice A) organizes elastic fibers in connective tissue. Fibronectin (choice B), laminin (choice C), and perlecan (choice E) are glycoprotein components of the GBM.

Keywords: Kidney, glomerulus, nephrin

23 The answer is D: Nephrin. The slit diaphragm provides a size-selective filter that normally prevents the movement of plasma proteins across the glomerular filtration barrier. The major protein component of the slit diaphragm is nephrin. Congenital nephrotic syndrome is a rare inherited disorder caused by mutations in the nephrin gene. Without nephrin, the glomerular filtration barrier fails, leading to proteinuria and lipiduria (symptoms of nephrotic syndrome). Unless the patient is given a kidney transplant, the condition is fatal within the first year of life.

Keywords: Congenital nephrotic syndrome, nephrin

24 The answer is C: Glomerular basement membrane. Anti–glomerular basement membrane antibody disease is an uncommon but aggressive form of glomerulonephritis. It may present with injury limited to the kidneys, or it may present in combination with pulmonary hemorrhage (Goodpasture syndrome). The disease is mediated by an autoimmune response against a component of the GBM. A characteristic feature of anti-GBM glomerulonephritis is diffuse linear staining for IgG. This pattern of staining indicates that autoantibodies are bound to the GBM. Autoantibodies bound to the other structures would not show a linear pattern of immunofluorescence.

Keywords: Goodpasture syndrome, glomerular basement membrane

25 The answer is A: Collagen type IV. Goodpasture syndrome is an autoimmune disorder caused by autoantibody against the NC1 domain of the α3 chain of type IV collagen. The antibody targets the GBM, causing injury and inflammation. Type IV collagen molecules form a complex network in the basement membranes of epithelial tissues throughout the body, including renal glomeruli. Like other collagen molecules, the type IV collagen monomer is a triple helix composed of three α chains. Six chains (α1 to α6) can form a type IV collagen monomer. NC1 (C-terminal) and 7S (N-terminal) domains are cross-linking sites that are required for type IV collagen monomers to form fibrillar networks within the basement membrane. The structural integrity and selective permeability of the GBM require proper assembly of type IV collagen. None of the other proteins are targets for autoantibodies in patients with Goodpasture syndrome.

Keywords: Goodpasture syndrome

26 The answer is D: Podocytes. The GBM is sandwiched between endothelium of the glomerular capillary loop and the visceral layer of the Bowman capsule. It represents a fusion of basal laminae synthesized by endothelial cells and podocytes. By electron microscopy, the GBM appears as a trilaminar structure with a central electron-dense layer (lamina densa) with two electron-lucent layers on either side. One of these electron-lucent layers faces the foot processes of the podocyte (lamina rara externa). The other electron-lucent layer faces the capillary endothelium (lamina rara interna). The GBM is a selective barrier that filters macromolecules based on their size and charge. None of the other cells contribute to the synthesis or deposition of the GBM.

Keywords: Kidney, glomerular basement membrane

27 The answer is E: Mesangium. The immunofluorescence data show focal deposits of IgA autoantibody in the mesangial areas of a glomerulus. The mesangium is composed of mesangial cells and their extracellular matrix. Mesangial areas are located between capillary loops and are most prominent near the vascular pole of the glomerulus. Mesangial cells are in direct contact with endothelial cells and are enclosed by the GBM. IgA nephropathy, also referred to as Berger disease, is the most common form of glomerulonephritis. It typically occurs following a respiratory or gastrointestinal infection that triggers an IgA immune response, leading to the deposition of secretory IgA in the mesangial areas of glomeruli. Autoantibodies bound to the other structures would not show a focal pattern of immunofluorescence.

Keywords: Berger disease, kidney, mesangium

28 The answer is C: Phagocytosis and endocytosis. Mesangial cells are phagocytic cells. They remove trapped molecules from components of the glomerular filtration barrier (i.e., GBM, slit diaphragm, and capillary endothelial cells). Mesangial cells also remove immunoglobulins and antigen–antibody (immune) complexes from glomeruli via receptor-mediated endocytosis. These phagocytic cells are essential for maintaining the structural integrity and permeability of the glomerular filtration apparatus. Mesangial cells and their mesangial matrix also provide structural support for the capillary loops. None of the other biological processes describe the principal function of mesangial cells.

Keywords: Kidney, mesangial cells

29 The answer is E: Smooth muscle cells. Although the primary function of mesangial cells is removal of debris trapped by the glomerular filtration barrier (phagocytosis), these connective tissue cells are derived from smooth muscle progenitor cells. The cytokines that regulate this stem cell differentiation pathway are largely unknown. Monocytes (choice D) are progenitor stem cells for macrophages and tissue histiocytes of the mononuclear phagocyte system. None of the other cells belong to the mesangial cell developmental lineage.

Keywords: Mesangial cells

30 The answer is C: Macula densa. The oval identifies closely packed epithelial cells in the wall of the distal convoluted tubule near the vascular pole of the Bowman capsule. These specialized cells are collectively referred as the macula densa. This tubule arises as follows: the distal part of the thick ascending limb of the loop of Henle (distal straight tubule) leaves the medullary ray and returns to the renal labyrinth. At the vascular pole of the Bowman corpuscle (where the distal straight tubule continues as the distal convoluted tubule), the tubular wall makes intimate contact with afferent and efferent arterioles. At this site, the epithelial cells of the tubular wall become closely packed and assume a low columnar morphology. None of the other structures describe histologic features of the macula densa.

Keywords: Kidney, macula densa

31 The answer is B: Monitoring Na⁺ in primary urine. The macula densa is a component of the juxtaglomerular (JG) apparatus located near the vascular pole of the Bowman capsule. Epithelial cells of the macula densa are exquisitely sensitive to changes in the concentration of Na^+ within the distal convoluted tubule. Decreased Na^+ levels in the primary glomerular ultrafiltrate stimulate cells of the macula densa to signaling other components of the juxtaglomerular apparatus (JG cells and extraglomerular mesangial cells). The macula densa controls a complex feedback loop that serves to (1) regulate blood flow through the kidney and (2) maintain a constant glomerular filtration rate. Aldosterone (choice E) is secreted by the adrenal cortex. None of the other biological processes describe the essential function of the macula densa.

Keywords: Kidney, macula densa

32 The answer is E: Secretion of renin. Modified smooth muscle cells in the wall of the afferent arteriole, near the macula densa, are termed juxtaglomerular (JG) cells. These specialized cells contain secretory granules filled with renin (a protease). In response to decreased blood volume or low sodium intake, the macula densa releases signaling molecules (e.g., adenosine) that trigger JG cells to release renin thereby activating the renin–angiotensin–aldosterone system (RAAS). Renin catalyzes the hydrolysis of serum angiotensinogen to produce angiotensin I. Angiotensin I is converted to angiotensin II in the lungs, triggering the release of aldosterone from the adrenal glands. Aldosterone stimulates distal convoluted tubules and collecting ducts in the kidney to reabsorb sodium and water, and to raise blood volume and pressure. Abnormalities associated with the RAAS may cause essential hypertension. None of the other biological processes describe the function of JG cells in the kidney.

Keywords: Juxtaglomerular apparatus, renin

33 The answer is D: Proximal convoluted tubules. As the name suggests, proximal convoluted tubules (PCTs) pursue a tortuous course through the cortical labyrinth. PCTs are longer than distal convoluted tubules (DCTs), a feature that helps explain why PCTs appear to be more numerous than DCTs in sections of the renal cortex. The PCT is lined by a simple cuboidal epithelium. The cells are large and metabolically active. Abundant microvilli extend from the apical surface of the cells, forming a prominent brush border. Brush borders are clearly visible in this photomicrograph as dark blue, fuzzy lines near the lumen of the tubules. Because the epithelial cells have extensive lateral membrane interdigitations, the boundaries between adjacent cells are not readily discernible. Numerous elongated mitochondria are oriented vertically in basal processes, forming striations that are only visible by electron microscopy. None of the other structures exhibit histologic features of PCTs.

Keywords: Kidney, convoluted tubules

34 The answer is B: Distal convoluted tubules. DCTs are shorter than PCTs (one-third as long). Cells lining the DCT are also smaller and lower in height than cells lining the PCT. Because of their smaller size, transverse sections of DCTs reveal more cells than similar sections of PCTs. Epithelial cells lining DCTs lack a brush border; hence, the lumen of these tubules appears well defined (not fuzzy). At the junction of the distal straight with the DCT, the tubule is in close proximity to the vascular pole of the renal corpuscle. The epithelial cells at this site constitute the macula densa of the JG apparatus. Thin limbs of the loop of Henle (choice E) are located in the renal medulla. Proximal straight tubules (choice D) are located in medullary rays within the renal cortex. Collecting ducts (choice A) are located in medullary rays and renal medulla. None of the other structures exhibit histologic features of DCTs.

Keywords: Kidney, convoluted tubules

35 **The answer is B: Peritubular capillaries.** The arrows identify small blood vessels that are intimately associated with both proximal and distal convoluted tubules. In brief, interlobular arteries give rise to afferent arterioles that form the glomerular capillary loops. Efferent arterioles leaving the renal corpuscle immediately branch to form a plexus of peritubular capillaries. These small vessels surround the convoluted tubules to draw electrolytes and other small molecules into the circulatory system. Vasa vasorum (choice E) refers to blood vessels within the adventitia of large elastic arteries. None of the other spaces/structures exhibit histologic features of capillaries in the kidney parenchyma.

Keywords: Kidney, peritubular capillaries

36 **The answer is C: Proximal convoluted tubule.** The kidneys produce about 180 L of primary urine every 24 hours! About 70% of this ultrafiltrate of the blood is reabsorbed into the systemic circulation by epithelial cells lining the PCTs. These cuboidal cells are specialized for the reabsorption of water and solutes. Mitochondria in the cell's basal compartment provide an abundant source of ATP to fuel Na^+/K^+ ATPase pumps that are present within lateral membrane interdigitations. These transmembrane proteins establish a transcellular osmotic gradient that provides a driving force for water uptake. PCTs also reabsorb amino acids, sugars, and polypeptides from primary urine. The other structures are involved in urine formation, but they reabsorb less of the primary urine than do PCTs.

Keywords: Kidney, convoluted tubules, urine

37 **The answer is E: Thick descending limb of the loop of Henle.** The thick descending limb of the loop of Henle is also referred to as the proximal straight tubule. It arises from the PCT and leaves the cortical labyrinth to enter the medullary ray. The thick descending limb of the loop of Henle exhibits histologic features similar to the PCT. For example, the lumens of both tubules are poorly defined, owing to the presence of a brush border membrane. Moreover, both types of tubules show indistinct

lateral membranes, owing to extensive interdigitations. Proximal and distal convoluted tubules (choices B and C) are located in the cortical labyrinth. The cortical collecting ducts (choice A) and thick ascending limb of the loop of Henle (choice E) do not exhibit histologic features of the proximal straight tubule.

Keywords: Kidney, loop of Henle

38 **The answer is C: Thick ascending limb of the loop of Henle.** The thick ascending limb (also referred to as the distal straight tubule) is continuous with the thin ascending limb after its hairpin turns in the medulla. The distal straight tubule then enters a medullary ray in the renal cortex, where its most distal portion approaches the vascular pole of its renal corpuscle of origin. At this point, the distal straight tubule becomes the distal convoluted tubule (DCT). These two types of renal tubules share similar histologic features, including low cuboidal epithelial cell morphology, lack of brush border, and lumen that is visible by light microscopy.

Keywords: Kidney, loop of Henle

39 **The answer is A: Cortical collecting duct.** Distal convoluted tubules in the labyrinth drain to collecting ducts within the medullary rays. These collecting ducts extend from the cortex to the renal medulla. The cortical portions of these ducts are referred as cortical collecting ducts. Portions within the medulla are referred to as medullary collecting ducts. Cortical collecting ducts are lined by low cuboidal cells that have distinct lateral membrane borders. The lumen of these collecting ducts is relatively large. Two populations of epithelial cells have been identified in the cortical collecting ducts using ultrastructural techniques: principal cells (light cells) and intercalated cells (dark cells). The principal cells reabsorb Na^+ and water, whereas the intercalated cells are believed to regulate acid/base chemistry (i.e., pH of urine).

Keywords: Kidney, collecting ducts

40 **The answer is E: Thin segments of the loop of Henle.** Thick descending limbs of the loop of Henle enter the outer medullary region of the kidney. Here, they continue as thin descending limbs that make a hairpin turn (loop). The arrows point to thin channels (segments) that are lined by squamous epithelial cells. The nuclei of these cells bulge into the lumens of these small channels. In contrast to vascular channels, thin segments are devoid of RBCs (the lumens are clear). The lengths of the thin segment loops vary, depending on the location of their original nephrons. Cortical nephrons have short thin segments, whereas juxtamedullary nephrons have long thin segments. Thin segments have a smaller diameter than thick segments (choices B and D). None of the other structures exhibit the histologic features of thin segments of the loop of Henle.

Keywords: Kidney, loop of Henle

41 **The answer is D: Medullary collecting ducts.** Collecting ducts that arise in the cortical medullary rays continue as medullary collecting ducts within the renal pyramids. As these collecting ducts approach the renal papilla, their lumen becomes larger and their lining epithelial cells become taller (from cuboidal to columnar). None of the other structures exhibit the distinctive morphology of medullary collecting ducts.
Keywords: Kidney, collecting ducts

42 **The answer is E: Vasa recta.** The vasa recta are straight vessels that course alongside the long loops of Henle of juxtamedullary nephrons in the medulla. After leaving the vascular pole of the renal corpuscles of the juxtamedullary nephrons, efferent arterioles branch to form numerous straight arterioles (arteriolae rectae) that extend into the inner medulla. Descending arteriolae rectae make hairpin turns and ascend as venulae rectae. Together, the straight descending arterioles and the straight ascending venules are referred to as vasa recta. These vascular channels follow the loops of Henle and help to concentrate the urine. Vasa recta can be distinguished from thin segments of the loops of Henle by the presence of RBCs within their lumen. None of the other blood vessels describe vascular channels within the renal pyramids.
Keywords: Kidney, vasa recta

43 **The answer is D: Medulla at apex of the pyramid.** Loose connective tissue surrounds the nephrons, ducts, and vascular structures. This interstitial tissue is more abundant in the medulla than in the renal cortex. The interstitium in the capsule (choice A) and cortex (choice B) are isosmotic to plasma. However, a steep osmotic gradient is established in the medulla. The interstitium that is deep in the medulla, at the apex of the renal pyramid, is hyperosmotic (approximately four times the osmolality of plasma). This osmotic gradient in the interstitial tissue of the medullary pyramids plays a key role in conserving body water and concentrating urine.
Keywords: Urine

44 **The answer is A: Countercurrent multiplier system.** Although the kidneys produce approximately 180 L of primary urine per day, all but 1 to 2 L are returned to the circulation. The PCT reabsorbs about 70% of primary urine volume. The fluid is then concentrated, and made hyperosmotic, via a countercurrent multiplier system. This system is so-named, because the filtrate flows in opposite directions in the two parallel limbs of the loop of Henle. Isosmotic fluid from the PCT enters the descending limb of the loop of Henle (which is highly permeable to water). As the descending limb descends into the hyperosmotic medulla, water and NaCl equilibrate, and the tubular fluid becomes hyperosmotic. The ascending limb of the loop of Henle is permeable to NaCl but not permeable to water; here, NaCl passively diffuses into the interstitium. Thus, as the urine reaches

the DCT, it has become hyposmotic. The fluid then drains via collecting ducts in the hyperosmotic medullary interstitium. Together, this countercurrent exchange system helps maintain an osmotic gradient and generate concentrated hyperosmotic urine.
Keywords: Countercurrent multiplier system

45 **The answer is E: Vasopressin.** Arginine vasopressin is also referred to as antidiuretic hormone (ADH). The primary action of ADH is to increase the permeability of epithelial cells lining the collecting ducts to water. The water that is reabsorbed then reenters the systemic circulation. This hormone-regulated process helps conserve body water and generate concentrated hyperosmotic urine. ADH also increases the permeability of the collecting ducts to urea in the renal medulla. Increased plasma osmolality or decreased blood volume triggers ADH secretion. Patients who become dehydrated produce an extremely hyperosmotic urine, owing to increased levels of ADH. By contrast, lack of ADH results in the formation of excessive amounts of dilute urine. None of the other hormones regulate the water permeability of epithelial cells lining collecting ducts.
Keywords: Antidiuretic hormone

46 **The answer is D: Pituitary.** ADH (arginine vasopressin) is synthesized by neurons in the hypothalamus and released from the posterior lobe of the pituitary gland. Damage to the hypothalamus or the pituitary gland can cause decreased ADH secretion, which results in polyuria and polydipsia. This condition is termed central diabetes insipidus. The patient has an increased volume of urine per day, owing to lack of water reabsorption from tubular fluid in the collecting ducts.
Keywords: Diabetes insipidus, polyuria

47 **The answer is E: Papillary ducts of Bellini.** Medullary collecting ducts descend through the medulla, toward the apex of the renal pyramids, where they merge to form large papillary ducts of Bellini. Columnar epithelial cells line the papillary ducts, which drain urine into minor calyces (visible in the image). None of the other structures exhibit morphological features of papillary ducts.
Keywords: Kidney, papillary ducts of Bellini

48 **The answer is E: Transitional.** Urine that is formed in the kidneys is transported through several excretory passages including (1) minor and major calyces, (2) renal pelvis, and (3) ureters. The urine is then stored in the bladder until it is expelled from the body through the urethra. This process of urination is also referred to as micturition. The urinary excretory passageways (from the kidney calyces to the proximal part of the urethra) are covered by a transitional epithelium (urothelium). These epithelial cells can change shape, from domed cells to flatten cells, so as to accommodate distension due to the passage of urine. Dome cells are evident in the photomicrograph. The lamina propria of the urothelium is composed of dense collagenous connective tissue (shown in the image). None of the other types of epithelium line excretory passages of the urinary system.

Keywords: Transitional epithelium, urothelium

49 **The answer is E: Smooth muscle.** The wall of the urinary bladder is composed of three layers: (1) mucosa (transitional epithelium and underlining lamina propria), (2) muscularis, and (3) adventitia. The muscularis contains abundant smooth muscle fibers that run in different directions (detrusor muscle). The detrusor muscle is innervated by parasympathetic nerve fibers that originate from spinal cord segments S2 to S4. Contraction of the detrusor muscle compresses the entire urinary bladder and expels urine into the urethra. The urethra is shorter in females than in males. Muscle fibers around the urethral opening in males form an internal urethral sphincter that is innervated by sympathetic nerve fibers. Sympathetic stimulation causes the internal urethral sphincter to contract to prevent semen reflux during sexual intercourse.

Keywords: Urinary bladder, detrusor muscle

50 **The answer is C: Ureter.** The ureters extend from the kidneys to the urinary bladder. The paired ureters are located in retroperitoneal adipose tissue that is visible in this image. The mucosa consists of a transitional epithelium and lamina propria. Two layers of smooth muscle are visible in this section: the inner longitudinal and outer circular layers. An additional longitudinal muscle layer is present in the lower portion of the ureter. Contraction of the muscularis after death causes the mucosa to fold, creating a stellate-shaped lumen. Peristaltic contractions of the smooth muscle help move urine along the ureters to the urinary bladder. The muscularis is covered by an adventitia (loose connective tissue) that fuses with the retroperitoneal adipose tissue. None of the other organs exhibit the characteristic features of the ureter.

Keywords: Ureter

51 **The answer is C: Membranous urethra.** The urethra extends from the internal urethral orifice in the bladder wall to the external urethral orifice located on the glans penis. It conveys urine from the urinary bladder to the exterior. Its length, size, and structure are different in male and female. The male urethra is about 20-cm long and is divided into four anatomic portions. The preprostatic portion (choice D) is a short segment as the bladder opens into the urethra. The prostatic urethra (choice E) travels through the prostate gland. The membranous urethra (correct answer, choice C) extends about 1 cm penetrating the deep perineal pouch. The distal and longest portion of the male urethra is the spongy urethra (choices A and B) that extends about 15 cm through the penis. Voluntary skeletal muscle fibers in the deep perineal pouch wrap around the membranous urethra to form the external urethral sphincter.

Keywords: Urethra, external urethral sphincter

Chapter 16

Male Reproductive System

QUESTIONS

Select the single best answer.

1 You are asked to give a lecture on the developmental biology of the male reproductive system. During early development, primordial germ cells (PGCs) can be unambiguously identified first in which of the following locations?
(A) Inner cell mass
(B) Lateral plate mesoderm
(C) Paraxial mesoderm
(D) Trophectoderm
(E) Yolk sac endoderm

2 During your lecture, you discuss the origin of the testes in the embryo. The urinary and genital systems both develop from which of the following types of early mesoderm?
(A) Intermediate
(B) Lateral plate somatic
(C) Lateral plate splanchnic
(D) Paraxial
(E) Somitic

3 A 30-year-old pregnant woman asks for information regarding gender determination in her unborn child. You explain that the *SRY* gene on the Y chromosome encodes a protein that determines male gonadal sex and that female reproductive organs are inhibited from developing in male embryos by müllerian-inhibiting factor (MIF). Which of the following cells in the embryo and fetus secrete this glycoprotein hormone?
(A) Follicular cells
(B) Leydig cells
(C) Mesothelial cells
(D) Primordial germ cells
(E) Sertoli cells

4 You are conducting research on mechanisms on gonadal sex determination. What is the principal effect of testis-determining factor (TDF) on the development of the male reproductive system?
(A) Arrest of PGCs in prophase of meiosis I
(B) Development of male external genitalia
(C) Differentiation of mesonephric tubules and ducts
(D) Organization and differentiation of gonadal cords
(E) Regression and loss of the uterus and uterine tubes

5 Regarding the research topic described in Question 4, testis-determining factor (TDF) belongs to which of the following families of proteins?
(A) Cytoplasmic adenylate cyclase
(B) G protein–coupled receptor
(C) Membrane tyrosine kinase
(D) Nuclear transcription factor
(E) Paracrine signaling hormone

6 A 2-month-old boy is brought to the physician because his parents cannot find one of his testicles. Physical examination confirms the parents' observation. Which of the following is the most likely medical diagnosis?
(A) Anorchia
(B) Cryptorchidism
(C) Inguinal hernia
(D) Macroorchidism
(E) Hermaphrodite

7 Beginning at puberty, under the influence of pituitary FSH and LH, the testes initiate spermatogenesis and produce sperm. Which of the following best describes the topological organization of cycles of spermatogenesis that occur in the seminiferous tubules after puberty?
(A) Lobular
(B) Patch-like
(C) Random
(D) Uniform
(E) Wave-like

8 You are asked to discuss the hormonal regulation of testicular function during a clinical conference. Which of the following cells in the postpubertal testes have receptors for both FSH and testosterone and serve as the primary regulators of spermatogenesis?
(A) Leydig cells
(B) Sertoli cells
(C) Spermatids
(D) Spermatocytes
(E) Spermatogonia

9 A thin (1.5 μm) plastic section of an adult testis is examined by light microscopy in the histology laboratory (shown in the image). Which of the following numbered arrows identifies the nucleus of a primary spermatocyte?

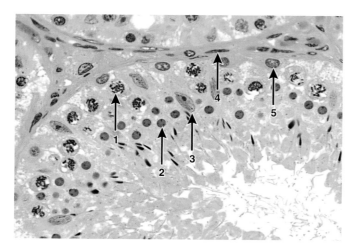

(A) Arrow 1
(B) Arrow 2
(C) Arrow 3
(D) Arrow 4
(E) Arrow 5

10 On average, when examined by light microscopy, which of the following testicular cells is most abundantly represented in the seminiferous epithelium of an adult?
(A) Leydig cells
(B) Primary spermatocytes
(C) Secondary spermatocytes
(D) Sertoli cells
(E) Spermatogonia

11 You attend a research seminar on the pathobiology of testicular cancer. Questions are raised during the talk regarding the blood–testis barrier. You explain that the seminiferous epithelium is divided into basal and adluminal compartments as a result of tight junctions between which of the following testicular cells?

(A) Leydig cells
(B) Myoid cells
(C) Primary spermatocytes
(D) Sertoli cells
(E) Spermatids

12 A lively discussion continues at the seminar described in Question 11. Which of the following germ cells would be observed within the basal compartment of the seminiferous epithelium?
(A) Primary spermatocytes
(B) Secondary spermatocytes
(C) Spermatids
(D) Spermatogonia
(E) Spermatozoa

13 A thin (1.5 μm) plastic section of an adult testis is examined at high magnification in the histology laboratory (shown in the image). Which of the following numbered arrows identifies the nucleus of a Sertoli cell?

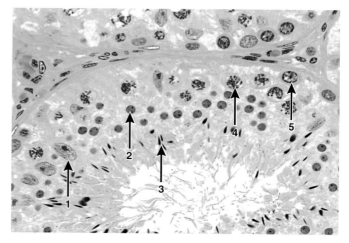

(A) Arrow 1
(B) Arrow 2
(C) Arrow 3
(D) Arrow 4
(E) Arrow 5

14 You are conducting research on the role of Sertoli cells in spermatogenesis. Which of the following cellular components permits signaling between adjacent Sertoli cells and helps coordinate the cycle of spermatogenesis within the seminiferous epithelium?
(A) Actin filament bundles
(B) Endosomes
(C) Gap junctions
(D) Hemidesmosomes
(E) Phagolysosomes

15 A 23-year-old man presents with a solid testicular mass that is removed surgically (orchiectomy). In addition to neoplastic cells, the surgical specimen shows a margin of normal testicular tissue (shown in the image). Identify the cluster of cells with rounded nuclei within the circle.

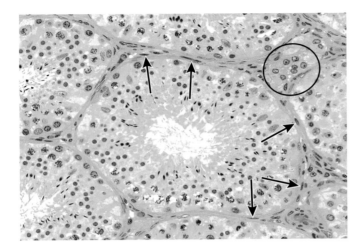

(A) Follicular cells
(B) Granulosa cells
(C) Leydig cells
(D) Oxyphil cells
(E) Parafollicular cells

16 For the surgical specimen described in Question 15, identify the peritubular cells with flattened nuclei indicated by the arrows.
(A) Endothelial cells
(B) Fibroblasts
(C) Myoid cells
(D) Plasma cells
(E) Spermatogonial stem cells

17 A 9-year-old boy is brought to the physician by his parents who are concerned about the onset of puberty in their child. Physical examination reveals facial hair and enlargement of external male genitalia. Laboratory studies show elevated serum levels of testosterone. This patient may have a testosterone-producing tumor derived from which of the following endocrine cells?
(A) Chief cells
(B) Follicular cells
(C) Granulosa cells
(D) Leydig cells
(E) Sertoli cells

18 The tumor identified in Question 17 is removed and examined by light microscopy in the pathology department. Sections of the surgical specimen are stained with

an antibody that binds to a key enzyme in the testosterone biosynthetic pathway. This enzyme is located in which of the following cellular organelles?
(A) Golgi apparatus
(B) Peroxisomes
(C) Plasma membrane
(D) Rough endoplasmic reticulum
(E) Smooth endoplasmic reticulum

19 A thin (1.5 μm) plastic section of an adult testis is examined by light microscopy in the histology laboratory (shown in the image). Which of the following numbered arrows identifies the nucleus of a late spermatid?

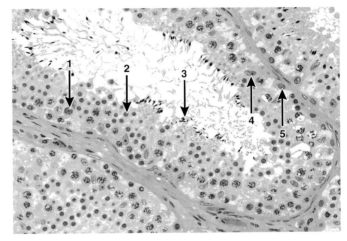

(A) Arrow 1
(B) Arrow 2
(C) Arrow 3
(D) Arrow 4
(E) Arrow 5

20 Which of the following structures helps regulate germ cell differentiation by ensuring free diffusion of signaling molecules, RNA, and proteins between daughter spermatocytes and spermatids within the seminiferous epithelium?
(A) Desmosomes
(B) Gap junctions
(C) Intercellular bridges
(D) Nuclear pores
(E) Tight junctions

21 When examined by electron microscopy, which of the following cytologic features best characterizes interstitial cells of Leydig?
(A) Apical membrane microvilli
(B) Dense core secretory granules
(C) Glycogen vacuoles
(D) Intracellular lipid droplets
(E) Segmented nuclei

22 A couple complains that they have been unable to conceive a child for the past 2 years. The man's sperm count is within the normal reference range. Electron microscopic examination of a sperm sample reveals a normal distribution of mitochondria. These intracellular organelles are located in which of the following regions of the spermatozoan?
(A) Acrosome
(B) End piece
(C) Middle piece
(D) Neck
(E) Principal piece

23 For the patient described in Question 22, electron microscopy also reveals sperm-associated microtubules and outer dense (coarse) fibers. Which of the following organelles initiates the assembly of microtubules in the axoneme of the sperm flagellum during spermiogenesis?
(A) Acrosome
(B) Centromere
(C) Centrosome
(D) Karyosome
(E) Kinetochore

24 Which of the following signaling mechanisms plays an important role in mediating "hyperactivation" of sperm motility during capacitation in the female reproductive tract?
(A) Activation of intracellular guanylate cyclase
(B) Activation of membrane Na/K ATPase
(C) Mitochondrial membrane permeability transition
(D) Opening of membrane Ca^{2+} channels
(E) Prostaglandin receptor binding

25 You are involved in a research project to investigate mechanisms of fertilization. Hydrolytic enzymes that are necessary for sperm penetration of the zona pellucida are packaged in which of the following regions of the spermatozoan?
(A) Acrosome
(B) End piece
(C) Middle piece
(D) Neck
(E) Principal piece

26 As part of your research project, you create an IgM monoclonal antibody directed to the sperm fibrous sheath protein. Indirect immunofluorescence assays using fluorescein-conjugated anti-mouse IgM demonstrate that your monoclonal antibody binds to which region of the human spermatozoan?

(A) Acrosome
(B) End piece
(C) Middle piece
(D) Neck
(E) Principal piece

27 A 55-year-old man with testicular lymphoma has his testicle removed (orchiectomy). In addition to the solid tumor, microscopic examination of the surgical specimen reveals significant thickening of peritubular tissue (tunica propria) of the seminiferous tubules. Which of the following is a complication of this incidental histopathologic finding?
(A) Hydrocele
(B) Infection
(C) Infertility
(D) Necrosis
(E) Varicocele

28 You are involved in research to identify pharmacologic compounds that inhibit the release of sperm into the lumen of the seminiferous tubule. This process of spermiation is revealed in a thin section of the hamster testis (shown in the image). Which of the following structures is removed from late spermatids prior to the release of sperm into the lumen of the seminiferous tubules?

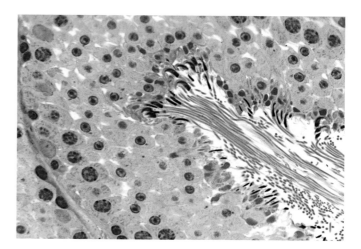

(A) Acrosomal caps
(B) Fibrous sheaths
(C) Nuclear membranes
(D) Polar bodies
(E) Residual bodies

29 During a research seminar, you are asked to discuss signaling molecules that control the development of the male reproductive system. Which of the following cells in the developing human embryo secrete a steroid hormone that stimulates the growth and differentiation of excurrent genital ducts, including the epididymis and vas deferens?
(A) Follicular cells
(B) Leydig cells
(C) Primordial germ cells
(D) Sertoli cells
(E) Spermatogonia

30 Androgen-binding protein (ABP) helps maintain a high concentration of testosterone within excurrent ducts and accessory glands of the male reproductive system. Which of the following cells in the adult testis secrete this important steroid-binding protein?
(A) Early and late spermatids
(B) Leydig cells
(C) Primary spermatocytes
(D) Principal cells of the prostate
(E) Sertoli cells

31 A section through the mediastinum of the testis is examined in the pathology department (shown in the image). Identify the structure indicated by the asterisk.

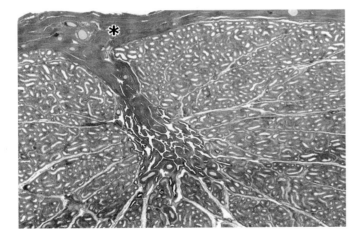

(A) Scrotal ligament
(B) Spermatic fascia
(C) Transversalis fascia
(D) Tunica albuginea
(E) Tunica vaginalis

32 The specimen described in Question 31 is examined at higher magnification (shown in the image). Identify these ducts that are lined by a simple cuboidal epithelium.

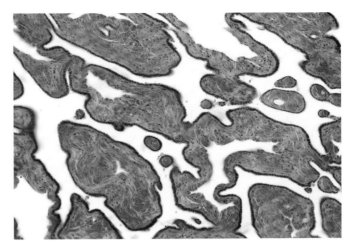

(A) Epididymis
(B) Ductuli efferentes
(C) Ductus deferens
(D) Rete testis
(E) Tubuli recti

33 Which of the following cytologic features characterizes the epithelial cells that line the efferent ductules of the testes?
(A) Cilia
(B) Dense, membrane-bound secretory granules
(C) Glycogen-rich vacuoles
(D) Intracellular lipid droplets
(E) Lamellar bodies

34 The reproductive organs of a 55-year-old man are examined at autopsy (shown in the image at low magnification). Which of the following cytologic features characterizes the epithelial cells that line this portion of the excurrent duct system?

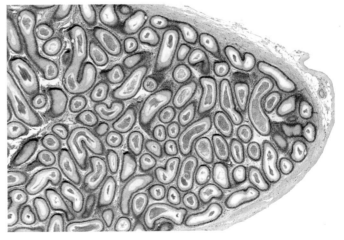

(A) Basal glycogen-rich vacuoles
(B) Dense, membrane-bound secretory granules
(C) Intracellular lipid droplets
(D) Perinuclear halos
(E) Stereocilia

35 The male reproductive organ described in Question 34 is examined at high magnification (shown in the image). What is the principal function of the cells identified by arrows in this pseudostratified epithelium?

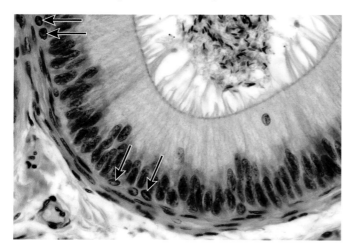

(A) Fluid uptake
(B) Reserve stem cells
(C) Secretion of sperm maturation factors
(D) Steroid hormone secretion
(E) Testosterone binding and uptake

36 Various male reproductive organs are examined at autopsy. Identify the organ shown in the image.

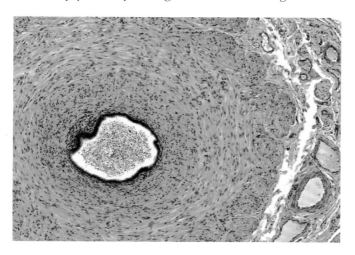

(A) Epididymis
(B) Prostate gland
(C) Seminal vesicle
(D) Testis
(E) Vas deferens

37 The excurrent genital duct identified in Question 36 was derived from which of the following structures during embryonic development?
(A) Mesonephric duct
(B) Metanephric blastema
(C) Paramesonephric duct
(D) Ureteric diverticulum
(E) Urogenital sinus

38 Which of the following organs of the male reproductive system is derived from embryonic endoderm of the urogenital sinus?
(A) Epididymis
(B) Prostate gland
(C) Seminal vesicles
(D) Seminiferous tubules
(E) Vas deferens

39 The organ described in Question 36 is examined at low magnification. Identify the structure indicated by the arrows.

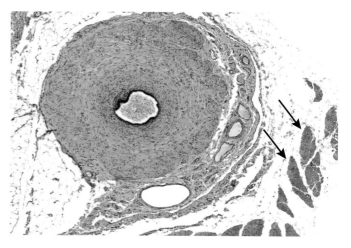

(A) Cremaster muscle
(B) Dartos fascia
(C) External oblique muscle
(D) Ampiniform venous plexus
(E) Testicular artery

40 A 65-year-old man with a history of bladder cancer develops multiple organ system failure and expires. The patient's urogenital organs are examined at autopsy for evidence of malignant disease. Identify the normal male reproductive organ shown in the image.

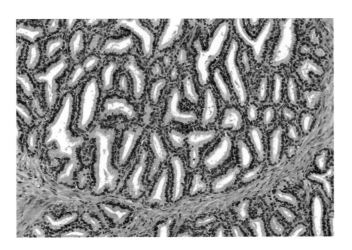

(A) Prostate gland
(B) Seminal vesicle
(C) Seminiferous tubule
(D) Urinary bladder
(E) Vas deferens

41 Which of the following best characterizes the histology of the male accessory gland identified in Question 40?
(A) Parallel cords of polygonal epithelial cells and sinusoidal capillaries
(B) Pseudostratified epithelium surrounded by a layer of smooth muscle
(C) Secretory epithelial cells lining follicles filled with glycoprotein
(D) Simple squamous epithelial cells lining open vascular spaces
(E) Small, solid clusters of epithelial cells interlaced with fenestrated capillaries

42 Microscopic examination of a seminal vesicle from a different patient shows evidence of a foamy, secretory material with the lumen of the gland (asterisk, shown in the image). Which of the following secretory products of the seminal vesicle provides the principal metabolic substrate for sperm in semen?

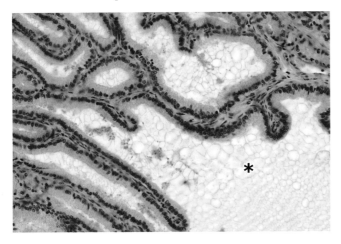

(A) Amino acids
(B) Ascorbic acid
(C) Fructose
(D) Prostaglandins
(E) Pyruvic acid

43 Digital rectal examination of a 68-year-old man reveals an enlarged prostate gland. Serum levels of prostate-specific antigen (PSA) are mildly elevated (6.8 ng/mL, normal reference range = 0 to 4 ng/mL). Enlargement of the transitional zone of the prostate in this patient would primarily affect which of the following urogenital structures?
(A) Anal canal
(B) Duct of seminal vesicles
(C) Ductus deferens
(D) Penile urethra
(E) Prostatic urethra

44 A prostate needle biopsy is obtained from a 70-year-old man with elevated serum levels of prostate-specific antigen (PSA, 10.5 ng/mL). The specimen is embedded in paraffin, stained with H&E, and examined in the pathology department (shown in the image). Identify the structure indicated by the arrow.

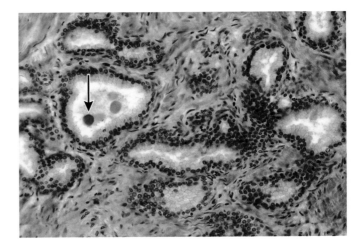

(A) Cluster of malignant cells
(B) Corpora amylacea
(C) Glassy membrane
(D) Multinucleated giant cell
(E) Residual body

45 Which of the following best describes the clinical significance of the structure identified in the image for Question 44?
(A) Chronic inflammation
(B) Circulatory disorder
(C) Neoplasia marker
(D) No clinical significance
(E) Nutritional deficiency

46 Microscopic examination of the prostate gland from a different patient is shown in the image. Which of the following is a distinctive histologic feature of this male reproductive organ?

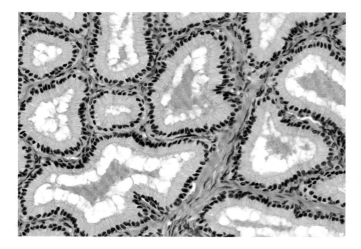

(A) Apical membrane stereocilia
(B) Colloid-filled follicles
(C) Epithelial cords and sinusoidal capillaries
(D) Fibromuscular stroma
(E) Stratified cuboidal epithelium

47 A cross-section of the penis is examined in the histology laboratory (shown in the image). Identify the structure indicated by the arrow.

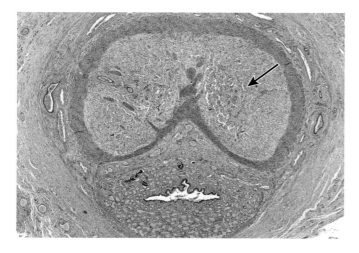

(A) Corpus cavernosum
(B) Corpus spongiosum
(C) Tunica albuginea
(D) Tunica vaginalis
(E) Tunica vascularis

48 For the specimen shown in Question 47, the erectile tissue that surrounds the spongy urethra gives rise to which of the following structures of the penis?

(A) Central vein
(B) Deep dorsal vein
(C) Glans penis
(D) Prepuce (foreskin)
(E) Urethral glands

49 The tissue specimen described in Questions 47 and 48 is examined at higher magnification (shown in the image). Which of the following types of cells lines the cavernous sinuses in this erectile tissue?

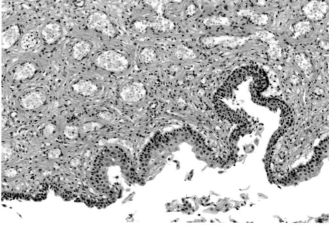

(A) Endothelial cells
(B) Mesothelial cells
(C) Myoepithelial cells
(D) Myofibroblasts
(E) Smooth muscle cells

50 A 64-year-old man with a history of hyperlipidemia and ischemic heart disease asks questions about treatment options for erectile dysfunction. Which of the following best explains the normal physiological mechanism for penile erection?
(A) Dilation of helicine arteries
(B) Dilation of spiral arteries
(C) Vasoconstriction of helicine arteries
(D) Vasoconstriction of spiral arteries
(E) Vasoconstriction of trabecular arteries

51 A 10-year-old boy is brought to the physician because his parents noticed a mass on his left testicle. Biopsy of the mass reveals a haphazard arrangement of differentiated tissues, including squamous epithelium, glandular epithelium, and cartilage. This benign tumor most likely originated from which of the following cells of the male reproductive system?
(A) Leydig cells
(B) Primordial germ cells
(C) Sertoli cells
(D) Spermatocytes
(E) Spermatogonia

ANSWERS

1 **The answer is E: Yolk sac endoderm.** Primordial germ cells (PGCs) are set aside from somatic cells during the early development. PGCs leave the epiblast during gastrulation and move in a caudal direction through the primitive streak. It has been possible to trace the origin and migration of PGCs because they express high levels of cell surface alkaline phosphatase. Using enzyme histochemistry, PGCs are identified in the yolk sac endoderm near the origin of the allantois during the 4th week of development. With subsequent folding of the embryo, PGCs are moved with the primitive gut into the intraembryonic coelom. These large, amoeboid cells migrate along the dorsal mesentery of the hindgut to reach the gonadal ridge during the 5th week of development. The inner cell mass of the blastocyst (choice A) represents a small cluster of embryonic stem cells that give rise to germ line and somatic cells of the embryo; however, PGCs cannot be identified at this stage. Lateral plate mesoderm (choice B) gives rise to the appendicular skeleton and connective tissue of the lateral body wall. Paraxial mesoderm (choice C) gives rise to the axial skeleton, skeletal muscle, and dermis. Trophectoderm of the blastocyst (choice D) is an extraembryonic epithelium that establishes contact with the maternal endometrium during implantation.
Keywords: Primordial germ cells

2 **The answer is A: Intermediate.** Mesoderm is generated through complex changes in cell adhesion and migration during gastrulation. These stem cells are organized on either side of the neural tube as blocks of tissue, referred to as paraxial, intermediate, and lateral plate mesoderm. Intermediate mesoderm gives rise to the kidneys and the gonads. The urinary and genital systems are closely associated—both anatomically and functionally. For example, the tubules and ducts of the embryonic urinary system (mesonephros) are retained in male embryos as the excurrent genital ducts. Lateral plate mesoderm (choices B and C) gives rise to the appendicular skeleton, as well as serous membranes that line body cavities and smooth muscle associated with the gut tube. Paraxial mesoderm (choice D) condenses to form somites (choice E), which give rise to the axial skeleton, skeletal (voluntary) muscle, and dermis.
Keywords: Mesoderm, testes

3 **The answer is E: Sertoli cells.** The *SRY* gene on the Y chromosome encodes testis-determining factor (TDF), which acts as a master switch to regulate the expression of several genes involved in the development of the male reproductive system (e.g., *SOX-9*, *AMH*, and *SF-1*). Female reproductive organs develop in the absence of *SRY* gene expression. Under the influence of TDF, Sertoli cells differentiate in the primitive sex cords and secrete müllerian-inhibiting factor (MIF). This large glycoprotein hormone suppresses the growth of the paramesonephric ducts that give rise to the uterus and the uterine tubes. Sertoli cells secrete MIF until the time of puberty, after which serum levels of MIF decline. Sertoli cells are the major cell population in the seminiferous tubules during embryonic and fetal development.
Keywords: Müllerian-inhibiting factor, Sertoli cells

4 **The answer is D: Organization and differentiation of gonadal cords.** During the 5th week of development, the indifferent gonads form finger-like, epithelial cords that project into the underlying mesenchyme. Male and female PGCs arriving in the indifferent gonad are incorporated into these primitive sex cords. In male embryos, testis-determining factor (TDF), encoded by the *SRY* gene, stimulates primitive sex cords to extend deeper into the medulla of the gonad. TDF also stimulates the differentiation of Sertoli cells and Leydig cells, which secrete müllerian-inhibiting factor and testosterone, respectively. The differentiation of Sertoli cells under the influence of TDF appears to be a critical step in male gonadal sex determination. Female PGCs arrest in prophase of meiosis I (choice A). Testosterone and dihydrotestosterone regulate the development of the male external genitalia (choice B), as well as differentiation of the mesonephric tubules and ducts (choice C). Regression and loss of the uterus and the uterine tubes (choice E) are regulated by müllerian-inhibiting factor.
Keywords: Gonadal cords, testis-determining factor

5 **The answer is D: Nuclear transcription factor.** Testis-determining factor (TDF) is a transcription factor that binds to a unique sequence of DNA. Binding alters the helical structure of DNA, forming a loop that permits other transcription factors to bind to DNA and modulate gene expression. None of the other choices describe TDF or its mechanism of action.
Keywords: Gonadal cords, testis-determining factor

6 **The answer is B: Cryptorchidism.** Cryptorchidism is a congenital abnormality in which one or both testes are not found in their normal position in the scrotum. It is the most common urologic condition requiring surgical treatment in infants. In 5% of male infants born at term and 30% of those born prematurely, the testes are not located in the scrotum. In the large majority of these infants, the testis will descend into the scrotum during the first year of life. The descent of the testis may be arrested at any point from the abdominal cavity to the upper scrotum. Anorchia (choice A) refers to congenital absence of testes. Inguinal hernias (choice C) represent protrusion of a portion of the small intestine through the inguinal canal. Macroorchidism (choice D) is a pathologic finding in adult patients with fragile X syndrome.
Keywords: Cryptorchidism

7 **The answer is B: Patch-like.** Spermatogenesis is the process of generating sperm from a self-renewing population of stem cells. Spermatogenesis begins at puberty and continues throughout life. Spermatogonial stem cells continuously generate spermatogonia that enter meiosis to form spermatocytes (primary and secondary), spermatids (early and late), and sperm. Extensive remodeling of spermatids to yield sperm is termed spermiogenesis. The process whereby late spermatids are released into the lumen of the seminiferous tubule is termed spermiation. The stages of spermatogenesis are not randomly distributed throughout the seminiferous tubules of the testes. Rather, groups of cells at the same stage of differentiation appear together. This grouping reflects the clonal nature of spermatogenesis, with daughter cells connected as a syncytium. In many species, spermatogenesis occurs in cycles that appear as "waves" running along the seminiferous tubules (choice E). However, recent studies indicate that spermatogenesis in humans is patch-like. Stages of spermatogenesis in humans do not extend around the circumference of the tubule, nor do they proceed sequentially along the seminiferous tubule. None of the other choices describe cycles of spermatogenesis in humans.

Keywords: Spermatogenesis seminiferous tubules

8 The answer is B: Sertoli cells.   FSH and LH are glycoprotein hormones secreted by the anterior lobe of the pituitary gland. They regulate the ovarian cycle in females and spermatogenesis in males. Sertoli cells have cell surface receptors for both FSH and testosterone and serve as the primary regulators of spermatogenesis. Interstitial cells of Leydig (choice A) have receptors for LH and produce testosterone. Germ cells (choices C, D, and E) do not express cell surface receptors for FSH and LH.

Keywords: Testes, Sertoli cells

9 The answer is A: Arrow 1.   The image shows a cross-section through a seminiferous tubule. The seminiferous epithelium is complex and stratified. Examination of the image reveals germ cells at various stages of spermatogenesis, including primary spermatocytes (arrow 1), early spermatids (arrow 2), and spermatogonia (arrow 5). The image also reveals Sertoli cells (arrow 3) and myoid cells of the tunica propria (arrow 4). Primary spermatocytes are arrested in prophase of meiosis I. Their chromosomes are duplicated and highly condensed, making primary spermatocytes easy to recognize by light microscopy. Homologous chromosomes in primary spermatocytes are paired. These tetrads undergo homologous recombination (crossing over) to enhance genetic diversity. None of the other testicular cells exhibit the distinctive nuclear morphology of primary spermatocytes.

Keywords: Spermatogenesis, primary spermatocytes

10 The answer is B: Primary spermatocytes.   The seminiferous epithelium is filled with meiotic and postmeiotic cells in the process of making sperm. Some of the stages in spermatogenesis last longer than others. For example, primary spermatocytes in humans are arrested in prophase of meiosis I for about 22 days. This pause in the cycle of spermatogenesis provides time for homologous

chromosomes to undergo crossing-over without DNA insertions or deletions. By contrast, secondary spermatocytes are very short-lived cells that rapidly complete the second meiotic division (meiosis II) to form haploid spermatids. Spermatogonial stem cells are very rare cells that have only recently been identified and cultured. Spermatogonia and Sertoli cells are less abundant than are meiotic cells in seminiferous tubules.

Keywords: Spermatogenesis, primary spermatocytes

11 The answer is D: Sertoli cells.   The blood–testis barrier separates meiotic and postmeiotic cells in the seminiferous epithelium from antibodies, pathogens, and toxins in the blood. This permeability barrier is established by the presence of tight junctions (zonula occludens) between adjacent Sertoli cells. Meiotic and haploid germ cells are located within the adluminal compartment of the seminiferous epithelium. This immunologically privileged environment is believed to protect developing germ cells from recognition and destruction by B and T lymphocytes that might otherwise become activated by "sperm-specific antigens." The blood–testis barrier also serves to concentrate secretions of Sertoli cells (e.g., testosterone and dihydrotestosterone) toward the lumen of the tubule. None of the other cells contribute to the blood–testis barrier.

Keywords: Testes, Sertoli cells

12 The answer is D: Spermatogonia.   The blood–testis barrier separates premeiotic germ cells from postmeiotic germ cells. Spermatogonial stem cells and spermatogonia are adherent to the basement membrane (tunica propria) of the seminiferous epithelium and are located in the basal compartment of the seminiferous tubule. Early spermatocytes must move past Sertoli tight junctions to enter the adluminal compartment. It is believed that Sertoli cells control this process by forming new tight junctions below primary spermatocytes and simultaneously degrading tight junctions above these cells. The other germ cells listed are located within the adluminal compartment of the seminiferous epithelium.

Keywords: Spermatogenesis, spermatogonia

13 The answer is A: Arrow 1.   This image shows a cross-section through a seminiferous tubule. Sertoli cells are tall, columnar, epithelial cells with basal membranes attached to the tunica propria and apical membranes facing the lumen of the tubule. The lateral and apical membranes of Sertoli cells envelop and nourish 30 to 50 germ cells at various stages of spermatogenesis and spermiogenesis. Sertoli cell nuclei are distinctly oval or triangular in shape. These supporting (sustentacular) cells have receptors for FSH and testosterone and serve as the principal regulator of spermatogenesis. Sertoli cells secrete many proteins, including androgen-binding protein (ABP). ABP concentrates testosterone and dihydrotestosterone within the seminiferous tubules and excurrent genital ducts. Sertoli cells also secrete inhibin—a glycoprotein

hormone that inhibits pituitary secretion of FSH. None of the other cells exhibit the distinctive nuclear morphology of Sertoli cells. These cells include early spermatids (arrow 2), late spermatids (arrow 3), primary spermatocytes (arrow 4), and spermatogonia (arrow 5).
Keywords: Spermatogenesis, Sertoli cells

14 The answer is C: Gap junctions. Junctional specializations of Sertoli cells in the seminiferous epithelium include tight junctions, gap junctions, desmosomes, and hemidesmosomes. Tight junctions create a permeability barrier between basal and adluminal compartments of the seminiferous tubules. Numerous gap junctions are also present between adjacent Sertoli cells. These junctions provide ionic coupling in the seminiferous epithelium and help coordinate the cycle of spermatogenesis. Hemidesmosomes connect the basal membranes of Sertoli cells to their underlying basal lamina. None of the other choices mediate signaling between adjacent Sertoli cells.
Keywords: Testes, Sertoli cells

15 The answer is C: Leydig cells. The circle encloses a cluster of polygonal cells in the connective tissue between adjacent seminiferous tubules. These interstitial cells of Leydig express cell surface receptors for LH and secrete testosterone. Leydig cells are the major source of androgens in males. Granulosa cells (choice B) nourish developing oocytes in the ovaries and secrete estrogen. None of the other cells are found within the testes.
Keywords: Testes, Leydig cells

16 The answer is C: Myoid cells. The tunica propria of the seminiferous epithelium is composed of multiple layers of collagen fibrils and myoid cells. These contractile cells create peristaltic waves that propel sperm and fluid through the seminiferous tubules toward the excurrent genital duct system. In addition to their contractile property, peritubular myoid cells play a role in collagen biosynthesis. The nuclei of fibroblasts (choice B) appear nearly identical to those of myoid cells; however, myoid cells are much more abundant than fibroblasts in the tunica propria. Endothelial cells (choice A), fibroblasts (choice B), and plasma cells (choice D) are present within interstitial tissue of the testes. Spermatogonial stem cells are small, nondescript cells present within the basal compartment of the seminiferous epithelium.
Keywords: Spermatogenesis, seminiferous tubules, myoid cells

17 The answer is D: Leydig cells. Leydig cell tumors are rare gonadal stromal/sex cord tumors composed of cells resembling interstitial (Leydig) cells of the testis. They can be hormonally active and secrete androgens, estrogens, or both. The androgenic effects of testicular Leydig cell tumors in prepubertal boys lead to precocious physical and sexual development. By contrast, feminization and gynecomastia are observed in some adults with this tumor. The other choices do not induce precocious puberty.
Keywords: Leydig cells, Leydig cell tumor

18 The answer is E: Smooth endoplasmic reticulum. Enzymes involved in the synthesis of steroid hormones such as testosterone and estrogen are associated with membranes of the smooth endoplasmic reticulum. Elaborate smooth endoplasmic reticula are a characteristic ultrastructural finding in steroid-secreting cells. None of the other organelles organizes enzymes involved in testosterone biosynthesis.
Keywords: Leydig cells, testosterone

19 The answer is C: Arrow 3. Spermatids are postmeiotic cells with a haploid (23n) karyotype. Spermatids undergo extensive nuclear and cytoplasmic remodeling as they differentiate into sperm. This process is termed spermiogenesis. The release of sperm into the lumen of the seminiferous tubule is termed spermiation. Early and late spermatids are distinguished by their small size, condensed chromatin, and proximity to the lumen of the seminiferous tubule. The nuclear morphology of early and late spermatids is notably different. Late spermatids have highly condensed chromatin, in which nuclear histones are replaced by small peptides termed protamines. Once late spermatids are released into the lumen of the seminiferous tubule, they are appropriately referred to as spermatozoa. None of the other cells exhibit the distinctive nuclear morphology of late spermatids.
Keywords: Spermatogenesis, testes, spermatids

20 The answer is C: Intercellular bridges. Spermatogenesis is characterized by clonal cell divisions within the seminiferous epithelium. Daughter cells arising from a single type A (dark) spermatogonial stem cell remain intimately connected to one another through intercellular bridges. These open connections are the result of incomplete cytokinesis during mitotic and meiotic cell divisions. Intercellular bridges permit haploid nuclei to share molecular resources, including RNA, proteins, and various signaling molecules. Sharing resources helps coordinate the progression of germ cells through the stages of spermatogenesis and spermiogenesis. Intercellular bridges are lost prior to the release of spermatozoa into the lumen of the seminiferous tubule.
Keywords: Spermatogenesis, spermiogenesis

21 The answer is D: Intracellular lipid droplets. Like other steroid-secreting endocrine cells, Leydig cells are characterized by the presence of innumerable intracellular lipid droplets. As a result, Leydig cells appear to have a foamy cytoplasm when examined by light microscopy. Cells with a similar, vacuolated appearance are observed in the adrenal cortex (foam cells). Membrane-bound, dense core secretory granules (choice B) are a characteristic feature of neuroendocrine cells (e.g., chromaffin cells of the adrenal

medulla). None of the other cellular organelles are ultra-structural features of Leydig cells.
Keywords: Testes, Leydig cells

22 **The answer is C: Middle piece.** The human spermatozoan has a flat, pointed head and a long tail (flagellum). The tail is divided into a short neck, middle piece, principal piece, and end piece. The middle piece of the spermatozoan contains mitochondria arranged in a helical fashion around outer dense fibers of the axonemal complex. These mitochondria provide ATP to generate whip-like motion of the flagellum (sperm motility). Of clinical significance, is the observation that sperm-associated mitochondria do not survive fertilization. As a result, the mitochondria of the embryo and adult are derived from the ovum at fertilization (i.e., maternal mitochondrial inheritance).
Keywords: Spermiogenesis, spermatozoa

23 **The answer is C: Centrosome.** The neck of the spermatozoan contains a pair of centrioles that organize the 9 + 2 arrangement of microtubules in the sperm flagellum during spermiogenesis. This microtubule-organizing center is referred to as the sperm centrosome. Acrosome (choice A) is a membrane-bound vesicle in the head region of the spermatozoan. Centromere (choice B) is a region of chromosomal DNA that organizes and links sister chromatids together and organizes the kinetochore protein complex (choice E) during cell division. Karyosome (choice D) is a discrete region of heterochromatin that may be visible by electron microscopy in the nuclei of some cells.
Keywords: Spermiogenesis, spermatozoa

24 **The answer is D: Opening of membrane Ca²⁺ channels.** Following posttesticular maturation in the epididymis, sperm must undergo capacitation in the female reproductive tract before they are competent to undergo fertilization. Capacitation results in hyperactivation of sperm motility and an increased ability of sperm to bind receptors on the zona pellucida. Biochemical changes associated with sperm capacitation include increased activity of adenylate cyclase, increased tyrosine phosphorylation, activation of membrane Ca^{2+} channels (correct answer), and other modifications of the sperm plasma membrane and glycocalyx. None of the other choices is associated with hyperactivation of sperm motility.
Keywords: Fertilization, capacitation

25 **The answer is A: Acrosome.** During spermiogenesis, small vesicles of the Golgi apparatus coalesce to form a large membrane-bound vesicle adjacent to the nucleus. In mature spermatozoa, this acrosomal cap covers the anterior two-thirds of the nucleus. It contains a variety of glycoprotein enzymes, including hyaluronidase, neuraminidase, acid phosphatase, and protease (acrosin). Binding of spermatozoa to receptors on the zona pellucida triggers the acrosome reaction. During this reaction,

the sperm plasma membrane fuses with the membrane of the acrosomal cap, thereby liberating acrosomal enzymes. These hydrolytic enzymes allow sperm to penetrate the corona radiata and zona pellucida and reach the plasma membrane of the secondary oocyte during fertilization. None of the other choices describe the location of the acrosomal cap in human sperm.
Keywords: Spermiogenesis, fertilization, spermatozoa

26 **The answer is E: Principal piece.** The principal piece of the sperm flagellum is approximately 40-µm long. It is composed of microtubules and associated molecular motor proteins (e.g., dynein). Sliding of these microtubules generates sperm motility (flagellar beat). In addition to the axoneme (9 + 2 arrangement of microtubules), the principal piece of the sperm flagellum contains outer dense fibers and a fibrous sheath. These structural proteins surround the axoneme and play an essential role in sperm motility. They influence (1) the degree of flexion of the flagellum, (2) the plane of motion of the flagellum, and (3) the curvilinear shape of the flagellar beat. Mutations in the genes for the outer dense fiber and fibrous sheath proteins lead to abnormal sperm morphology and infertility. None of the other choices describe the location of the fibrous sheath in human sperm.
Keywords: Spermiogenesis, spermatozoa

27 **The answer is C: Infertility.** Blood and lymph vessels in the testes are located outside the seminiferous tubules in the interstitial tissue. The delivery of nutrients and oxygen to spermatogenic cells requires diffusion through peritubular fascia (tunica propria). Age-related thickening of the tunica propria leads to chronic hypoxia and tissue atrophy and reduced rates of spermatogenesis. Thickening of the tunica propria earlier in life would be associated with male infertility. Hydrocele (choice A) refers to a collection of serous fluid in the scrotal sac between the two layers of the tunica vaginalis. It is the most common cause of scrotal swelling in infants and is often associated with inguinal hernia. Infection (choice B) and necrosis (choice D) are unlikely consequences of thickening of the tunica propria. Varicocele (choice E) represents a local dilation of testicular veins and presents as nodularity on the lateral side of the scrotum.
Keywords: Spermatogenesis, infertility

28 **The answer is E: Residual bodies.** The image shows late spermatids at the time of their release from the seminiferous epithelium. Acrosomal caps and sperm flagella are visible in this section. Prior to their release, late spermatids break intercellular bridges and shed residual cytoplasm. These residual bodies are internalized by Sertoli cells and degraded within phagolysosomes. Once this process has been completed, spermatozoa are released from Sertoli cells into the lumen of the seminiferous tubule. Contractions of myoid cells in the peritubular connective tissue help to propel the male gametes on their journey through the excurrent duct system. None of the other cellular structures are shed from late spermatids during spermiogenesis.

Keywords: Spermiogenesis, spermatozoa

29 **The answer is B: Leydig cells.** The *SRY* gene carried on the Y chromosome initiates gonadal sex determination, in part, by inducing the differentiation of Sertoli cells and Leydig cells in the embryonic testes. Testosterone secreted by interstitial cells of Leydig stimulates the growth and differentiation of male excurrent genital ducts, as well as morphogenesis of male external genitalia. Follicular cells of the ovary (choice A) secrete estrogen when activated by FSH after puberty. None of the other cells secrete androgens.

Keywords: Testes, Leydig cells

30 **The answer is E: Sertoli cells.** Sertoli cells are both exocrine and endocrine cells. For example, Sertoli cells release inhibin, a polypeptide hormone that provides negative feedback inhibition of FSH secretion from the pituitary gland. Sertoli cells also secrete fluid and proteins into the lumens of the seminiferous tubules. These proteins include plasminogen activator, transferrin (iron transport protein), and androgen-binding protein (ABP). ABP has high affinity for testosterone and dihydrotestosterone. ABP serves to maintain a high concentration of these steroid hormones within the seminiferous tubules and the excurrent duct system (epididymis and vas deferens), as well as within the male accessory glands (seminal vesicles and prostate gland). None of the other cells secrete androgen-binding protein.

Keywords: Sertoli cells, androgen-binding protein

31 **The answer is D: Tunica albuginea.** The seminiferous tubules are surrounded and protected by a dense, connective tissue capsule that is referred to as the tunica albuginea (white coat). The posterior wall of this tunic is thickened to form the mediastinum of the testis (shown in the image). Connective tissue septa leave the mediastinum and penetrate the testis, dividing it into approximately 250 lobules. Each lobule contains one to four seminiferous tubules, surrounded by interstitial connective tissue. Spermatic fascia (choice B) surrounds the spermatic cord; it arises during development as a continuation of transversalis fascia of the abdominal wall (choice C). Tunica vaginalis (choice E) is a serous sac derived from parietal peritoneum during descent of the fetal testes into the scrotum. None of the other choices contribute to the mediastinum of the testis.

Keywords: Testes, tunica albuginea

32 **The answer is D: Rete testis.** The seminiferous tubules terminate as short stubs (tubuli recti, choice E) that empty into an interconnected labyrinth of channels referred to as the rete testis. These anastomosing channels are embedded in dense connective tissue that is continuous

with that of the tunica albuginea. The rete testis is lined by a simple cuboidal epithelium. It provides a conduit for sperm and fluid to leave the testis for the epididymis, by way of efferent ductules (ductuli efferentes, choice B). The efferent ductules of the testis have an unusual scalloped appearance when examined on cross-section. None of the other ducts are surrounded by dense connective tissue within the mediastinum of the testis.

Keywords: Testes, rete testis

33 **The answer is A: Cilia.** Ductuli efferent are intratesticular ducts that transport sperm from the rete testis to the caput epididymis. These ducts (10 to 20) are lined by a simple epithelium composed of two populations of cells: (1) cuboidal cells with microvilli for water absorption and (2) tall columnar cells with cilia for generating fluid movement. This arrangement of tall ciliated cells and short absorptive cells gives the efferent ductules a distinctive scalloped appearance when examined on cross-section. Most of the fluid secreted by the seminiferous epithelium is absorbed by this epithelium. Lamellar bodies (choice E) are lipid-rich granules found in pneumocytes and keratinocytes. None of the other ultrastructural features characterize epithelial cells of the ductuli efferentes.

Keywords: Testes, efferent ductules

34 **The answer is E: Stereocilia.** This low-magnification image shows a cross-section through the epididymis. The epididymides are highly convoluted, 4-m ducts, located along the superior and posterior aspect of the testes. The epididymis can be divided into three segments (proximal to distal): caput, corpus, and cauda. During transit through the epididymis, sperm gain the ability to undergo capacitation and fertilization. This process is referred to as "posttesticular sperm maturation." Epithelial cells lining the epididymis are notable for the presence of nonmotile stereocilia. These apical membrane structures are actually long microvilli that contain actin filament cores (not tubulin, as would be expected in true cilia). Stereocilia are thought to be involved in fluid/electrolyte transport. None of the other ultrastructural features characterize the epithelial cells of the epididymis.

Keywords: Epididymis, stereocilia

35 **The answer is B: Reserve stem cells.** The arrows on this image identify basal stem cells. These nondescript cells, with rounded nuclei, undergo terminal differentiation to repopulate the surface epithelium. A thin layer of smooth muscle surrounds the ducts of the epididymis (note peritubular flat nuclei, shown in the image). Peristaltic contractions of these cells help to move sperm and fluid toward the vas deferens. This image also provides an excellent view of apical membrane stereocilia and sperm within the lumen of the tubule. Secretion of sperm maturation factors (choice C) is a reasonable choice for this question, but evidence to support this hypothesis is lacking. None of the other cellular functions characterize basal epithelial cells in the epididymis.

Keywords: Epididymis, stem cells

36 The answer is E: Vas deferens. The ductus (vas) deferens passes along the posterior wall of the testis and through the inguinal canal, before entering the abdomen to join the duct of the seminal vesicle and enter the prostate gland. Once the vas deferens enters the prostate gland, it is referred to as the ejaculatory duct. Unlike the other male reproductive organs listed, the vas deferens is characterized by the presence of a thick muscular wall. Close examination of this autopsy specimen reveals three distinct layers of smooth muscle fibers: inner longitudinal, middle circular, and outer longitudinal. This muscular wall contracts to expel sperm during ejaculation. All of the male reproductive organs listed possess smooth muscle external to the basal lamina of the lining epithelium; however, the muscle wall of the vas deferens is significantly thicker than any of the other choices.

Keywords: Vas deferens, smooth muscle

37 The answer is A: Mesonephric duct. The genital and urinary systems are structurally and functionally related in both males and females. They develop in close proximity within the intermediate mesenchyme of the urogenital ridge. The excurrent ducts of the male reproductive system (i.e., ductuli efferentes, epididymis, and vas deferens) are all derived from mesonephric tubules and ducts that contribute to the interim kidneys that produce urine during weeks 4 to 8 of development. Metanephric blastema (choice B) is a mass of undifferentiated nephrogenic mesenchyme that forms the nephrons within the permanent kidneys. Paramesonephric duct (choice C) forms the uterus and uterine tubes in females. Ureteric diverticulum (choice D) is a branch of the mesonephric duct that gives rise to the ureter, renal pelves, major and minor calyces, and collecting tubules/ducts of the permanent kidney. Urogenital sinus (choice E) forms the bladder, as well as various male and female reproductive organs.

Keywords: Vas deferens, mesonephric ducts

38 The answer is B: Prostate gland. During embryonic development, the urorectal septum grows and divides the primitive hindgut (cloaca) into a urogenital sinus and a rectum. The primitive hindgut and its derivatives are lined by embryonic endoderm. The urogenital sinus is further divided into three parts: the cranial (vesicle) portion forms the urinary bladder; the middle (pelvic) portion forms the urethra and prostate in males and the entire urethra in females; and the caudal (phallic) part grows toward the genital tubercle to form the penis or clitoris. The other male reproductive organs are derived from mesoderm (mesenchyme) of the urogenital ridge.

Keywords: Prostate gland, urogenital sinus

39 The answer is A: Cremaster muscle. This image shows a cross-section through the spermatic cord. The spermatic cord carries nerves and blood/lymph vessels from the posterior abdominal wall to the scrotum, and it carries the vas deferens from the scrotum to the prostate gland. The arrows on this image identify the cremaster muscle. These skeletal muscle fibers cover the spermatic cord. They represent a portion of the internal oblique muscle that extends through the inguinal canal. The cremasteric reflex serves to raise the testicles, toward the abdominal wall, in response to low temperature to safeguard spermatogenesis. Dartos fascia (choice B) is the superficial fascia of the penis and scrotum. The aponeurosis of the external oblique muscle (choice C) forms the anterior wall of the inguinal canal. The pampiniform venous plexus (choice D, shown in the image) consists of anastomosing branches of the spermatic vein. This plexus serves as a heat exchanger to lower the temperature of arterial blood entering the testes. Paired testicular arteries (choice E) arise from the abdominal aorta.

Keywords: Spermatic cord, cremaster muscle

40 The answer is B: Seminal vesicle. Examination of this image reveals a highly folded secretory epithelium, surrounded by a thin layer of smooth muscle. None of the other male reproductive organs exhibit this distinctive morphology. The paired seminal vesicles are tortuous tubes, measuring approximately 15 cm in length. They arise as outgrowths from the mesonephric ducts during embryonic development. Bladder cancer accounts for 3% to 5% of all cancer-related deaths. Urothelial (transitional) cell carcinoma of the bladder typically manifests as sudden hematuria and, less frequently, manifests as dysuria.

Keywords: Seminal vesicles, bladder cancer

41 The answer is B: Pseudostratified epithelium surrounded by layer of smooth muscle. The seminal vesicles consist of a secretory epithelium (nonciliated columnar cells), a thin layer of smooth muscle, and a fibrous coat. Parallel cords of polygonal cells (choice A) are seen in the adrenal cortex. Secretory epithelial cells lining follicles (choice C) are seen in the thyroid gland. Simple squamous cells lining open vascular spaces (choice D) are seen in sinusoid capillaries throughout the body. Solid clusters of epithelial cells (choice E) describe nests of endocrine cells that are found in many locations, including the pituitary and parathyroid glands.

Keywords: Seminal vesicles

42 The answer is C: Fructose. The accessory glands of the male reproductive tract include paired seminal vesicles, the prostate gland, and several bulbourethral glands. These organs produce secretions that mix with sperm to form semen during ejaculation. Most (70%) of the fluid in

semen is contributed by the seminal vesicles. Evidence of this viscous fluid is evident in the image. This foamy liquid contains an abundance of amino acids, simple sugars, prostaglandins (arachidonic acid derivatives), enzymes, and other proteins. Fructose is a six-carbon monosaccharide that serves as the principal metabolic substrate for sperm motility. Pyruvic acid (choice E) is a product of glycolysis and an energy source for the Krebs cycle; however, this three-carbon ketone is not secreted by the seminal vesicles. None of the other choices provide a significant source of energy for oxidative phosphorylation in sperm.
Keywords: Seminal vesicle

43 The answer is E: Prostatic urethra.   The prostate is the largest of the male accessory glands. It is located in the pelvis, below the urinary bladder. The prostate gland is divided into three zones: central, transitional, and peripheral. The transitional zone surrounds the prostatic urethra, and the central zone surrounds the paired ejaculatory ducts. Nodular hyperplasia of the prostate is a common disorder characterized clinically by enlargement of the gland and obstruction to the flow of urine through the bladder outlet, and pathologically by the proliferation of glands and stroma. Nodular prostatic hyperplasia results in the retention of urine in the bladder and predisposes to recurrent urinary tract infections. Enlargement of the prostate does not affect the other structures listed.
Keywords: Prostate gland, benign prostatic hyperplasia

44 The answer is B: Corpora amylacea.   The arrow on this image identifies secretory material of the prostate gland that has precipitated within the lumen of an alveolus. These calcified proteinaceous concretions are termed corpora amylacea (amyloid bodies). The structure revealed in this image lacks evidence of cell nuclei and is, therefore, unlikely to represent a cluster of malignant cells (choice A) or a multinucleated giant cell (choice D). Glassy membranes (choice C) represent the basement membranes of atretic ovarian follicles. Residual bodies (choice E) are large vesicles that contain shed organelles and cytoplasm of spermatids undergoing spermiogenesis.
Keywords: Prostate gland, corpora amylacea

45 The answer is D: No clinical significance.   Corpora amylacea are commonly observed in the prostate glands of elderly men. Their number increases with age. This incidental histopathologic finding does not seem to carry clinical significance. None of the other mechanisms of disease are linked to the formation of corpora amylacea in the prostate glands of elderly men.
Keywords: Nodular prostatic hyperplasia, corpora amylacea

46 The answer is D: Fibromuscular stroma.   The prostate gland contains 30 to 50 branched tubuloalveolar glands, surrounded by a fibromuscular stroma. The ducts of these glands drain to the prostatic urethra. The stroma is composed of dense, irregular connective tissue, with an abundance of smooth muscle fibers that help to expel fluid during ejaculation. Epithelial cells of the prostate gland secrete an alkaline fluid that combines with sperm and secretions of the seminal vesicles to form semen. Secretions of the prostate gland contain prostatic acid phosphatase and proteolytic enzymes that are important for the process of fertilization. None of the other choices are histologic features of the prostate gland.
Keywords: Prostate gland

47 The answer is A: Corpus cavernosum.   The erectile tissues of the penis include paired corpora cavernosa and a ventral corpus spongiosum (choice B). These cavernous spaces become engorged with blood in response to parasympathetic stimulation during penile erection. Tunica albuginea (choice C) is a dense fibroelastic layer that holds the cylindrical erectile masses together. This structure is visible in the image as a reddish band surrounding the paired corpora cavernosa. Tunica vaginalis (choice D) and tunica vascularis (choice E) are investing layers of the testes.
Keywords: Penis, corpus cavernosum

48 The answer is C: Glans penis.   The corpus spongiosum surrounds the spongy urethra along the ventral surface of the penis. The corpus spongiosum expands distally to form the glans penis. The cylindrical erectile masses of the penis contain cavernous sinuses separated by trabeculae that are composed of interstitial connective tissue, as well as blood/lymphatic vessels and smooth muscle fibers. The overlaying skin of the penis is thin and loose. Blood is supplied to the penis by the dorsal and deep arteries of the penis—branches from the internal pudendal artery. The penis is innervated by both somatic and autonomic nerve fibers. None of the other anatomic structures are derived from the corpus spongiosum of the penis.
Keywords: Penis, corpus spongiosum

49 The answer is A: Endothelial cells.   This image shows a portion of the corpus spongiosum adjacent to the spongy urethra. The cavernous spaces are components of the vascular system and lined by vascular endothelial cells. The spongy urethra is, for the most part, lined by a pseudostratified epithelium; however, the epithelium in this specimen appears stratified. Mesothelial cells (choice B) are simple squamous epithelial cells that line the body cavities (e.g., pericardium and peritoneum). Myoepithelial cells (choice C) are contractile cells that surround excretory ducts. Myofibroblasts (choice D) are contractile cells that differentiate from mesenchymal stem cells within granulation tissue to promote wound healing by primary intention. Smooth muscle cells (choice E) do not line vascular channels.
Keywords: Penis, endothelial cells

50 The answer is A: Dilation of helicine arteries.   Penile erection is a complex neurophysiological process in which erectile masses of the penis become engorged with blood. In brief, parasympathetic stimulation initiates erection by causing relaxation of trabecular smooth muscle cells surrounding the helicine arteries. Dilation of these arteries causes the cavernous sinuses to fill with blood. Expansion of erectile masses leads to compression of veins and venules against the (nondistensible) tunica albuginea, resulting in rigidity of the penis. Acetylcholine and nitric oxide stimulate relaxation of smooth muscle during erection. Sympathetic stimulation terminates erection by causing contraction of trabecular smooth muscle cells. Erectile dysfunction represents an inability to achieve and maintain an erection that is sufficient for normal intercourse. Cardiovascular disease and diabetes are linked to the pathogenesis of erectile dysfunction.
Keywords: Erectile dysfunction, helicine arteries

51 The answer is B: Primordial germ cells.   Teratomas are the most common testicular tumor in the age group between 4 and 12 years. They are derived from primordial germ cells that have become activated to initiate embryonic development. Benign teratomas in the prepubertal testes are composed of mature somatic tissues representing all three embryonic germ layers (ectoderm, mesoderm, and endoderm). Spermatogonia (choice E) give rise to monomorphic germ cell tumors, termed seminomas. None of the other testicular cells gives rise to male germ cell tumors.
Keywords: Mature teratoma, primordial germ cells

Chapter 17

Female Reproductive System and Breast

QUESTIONS

Select the single best answer.

1 You are involved in a research project to identify receptors that mediate implantation of the embryo. A section of the mouse uterus on day 4.5 postcoitum is stained with periodic acid–Schiff (PAS) reagent and counterstained with methylene blue (shown in the image). What is the appropriate name for the embryo at this stage of early development?

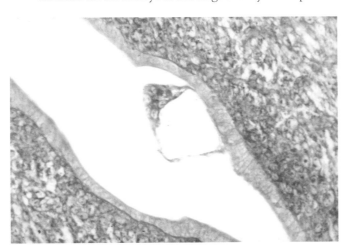

(A) Blastocyst
(B) Gastrula
(C) Morula
(D) Neurula
(E) Zygote

2 For the embryo shown in Question 1, what is the appropriate name for the epithelial cells that are adherent to the apical surface of the uterine endometrium?
(A) Amnioblast
(B) Embryoblast
(C) Inner cell mass
(D) Primitive endoderm
(E) Trophoblast

3 Which of the following maternal endocrine tissues/ organs secretes a hormone that controls the secretory phase of the uterine cycle and helps establishes a "window" for implantation of the blastocyst?
(A) Adrenal cortex
(B) Anterior pituitary
(C) Corpus luteum
(D) Graafian follicle
(E) Posterior pituitary

4 Which of the following biological processes best characterizes germ cells that have been incorporated into ovarian follicles during fetal development?
(A) Active meiosis
(B) Active mitosis
(C) Arrest in meiosis I
(D) Arrest in meiosis II
(E) Mitotic arrest

5 Microscopic examination of an ovary from a woman of reproductive age reveals follicles in various stages of maturation (shown in the image). Which of the following types of follicles is most abundant in this patient's ovary?

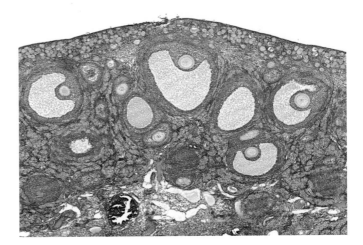

(A) Antral
(B) Graafian
(C) Multilaminar
(D) Primary
(E) Primordial

6 The cortical region of the ovary described in Question 5 is examined at higher magnification (shown in the image). Which of the following patterns of epithelial cell morphology best describes follicular cells that nourish oocytes within the oval?

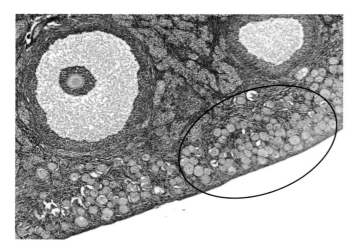

(A) Simple columnar
(B) Simple cuboidal
(C) Simple squamous
(D) Stratified cuboidal
(E) Stratified squamous

7 This high magnification view of an ovarian follicle shows cuboidal cells dividing to form a stratified epithelium (arrows, shown in the image). Identify these activated cells that surround and nourish this oocyte.

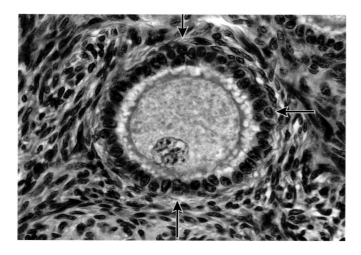

(A) Chief cells
(B) Granulosa cells
(C) Parafollicular cells
(D) Sertoli cells
(E) Theca interna cells

8 A 45-year-old woman with a family history of ovarian cancer undergoes an elective hysterectomy and oophorectomy. The patient's ovaries are sectioned and examined for pathologic changes (shown in the image). Which of the following terms describes this normal ovarian follicle?

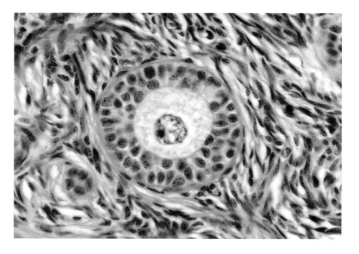

(A) Antral
(B) Atretic
(C) Graafian
(D) Primary
(E) Primordial

9 An ovary obtained at surgery is examined by light microscopy in the pathology department (shown in the image). Which of the following terms best describes this normal ovarian follicle?

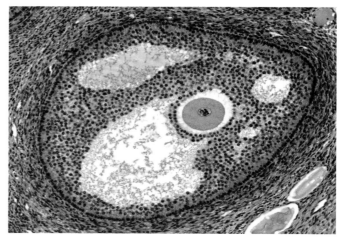

(A) Antral
(B) Atretic
(C) Graafian
(D) Primary
(E) Primordial

10 Which of the following biological processes accounts for the transformation of a primary to a secondary ovarian follicle?
(A) Deposition of the extracellular matrix
(B) Extracellular fluid accumulation
(C) Formation of a second polar body
(D) Maturation of the zona pellucida
(E) Proliferation of tissue macrophages

11 A section of ovary is stained with H&E and examined in the histology laboratory (shown in the image). Which of the numbered arrows identifies the corona radiata of this maturing follicle?

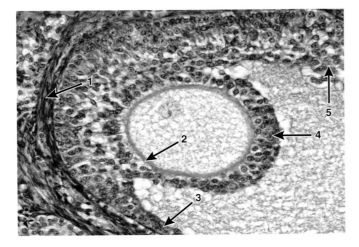

(A) Arrow 1
(B) Arrow 2
(C) Arrow 3
(D) Arrow 4
(E) Arrow 5

12 For the section of the ovary shown in Question 11, which of the numbered arrows identifies the developing zona pellucida?
(A) Arrow 1
(B) Arrow 2
(C) Arrow 3
(D) Arrow 4
(E) Arrow 5

13 Which of the following best describes the biological function of the structure identified in Question 12?
(A) Estrogen secretion
(B) Hormone secretion
(C) Selective protein uptake
(D) Sperm adhesion
(E) Sperm capacitation

14 A section of an ovary is examined by light microscopy (shown in the image). Which of the numbered regions identifies the theca interna of this preovulatory ovarian follicle?

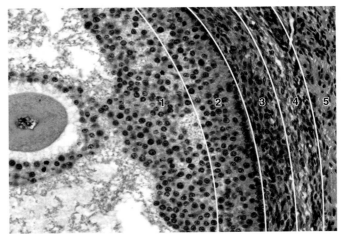

(A) Zone 1
(B) Zone 2
(C) Zone 3
(D) Zone 4
(E) Zone 5

15 The first polar body that forms near the time of ovulation is located between the germ cell plasma membrane and which of the following investing layers of the mature (graafian) follicle?
(A) Corona radiata
(B) Cumulus oophorus
(C) Theca externa
(D) Theca interna
(E) Zona pellucida

16 Which of the following ovarian cells secretes a steroid hormone that stimulates the growth of uterine glands during the proliferative phase of the menstrual cycle?
(A) Granulosa cells
(B) Granulosa lutein cells
(C) Theca externa cells
(D) Theca interna cells
(E) Theca lutein cells

17 Which of the following terms describes the female germ cell that is released into the uterine tube at the time of ovulation?
(A) Morula
(B) Oogonium
(C) Primary oocyte
(D) Secondary oocyte
(E) Zygote

18 You are asked to give a lecture on the mechanisms of ovulation, fertilization, and early development. During oogenesis, which of the following biological events/processes provides a signal for oocytes to complete the second meiotic division (meiosis II)?

(A) Fertilization
(B) First polar body formation
(C) Ovulation
(D) Second polar body formation
(E) Surge of FSH and LH

19 A couple presents with a 2-year history of infertility. Oocytes and sperm are subsequently collected for in vitro fertilization. Which of the following cytologic findings provides unambiguous evidence of fertilization?

(A) Dispersal of the corona radiata
(B) Formation of the second polar body
(C) Movement of the female pronucleus
(D) Sperm acrosome reaction
(E) Thinning of the zona pellucida

20 During an in vitro fertilization procedure in the clinic, you observe hundreds of sperm binding to the zona pellucida of an oocyte. Which of the following cellular processes in the donor oocyte provides a physiological block to polyspermy?

(A) Activation of phagolysosomes
(B) Assembly of the nuclear membrane
(C) Exocytosis of cortical granules
(D) Hydrolysis of membrane glycolipids
(E) Mitochondrial membrane permeability transition

21 Ovarian tissue from an oophorectomy specimen is examined by light microscopy (shown in the image). Which of the following terms best describes the structure within the circle?

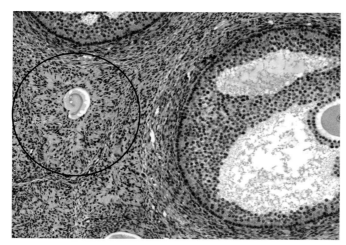

(A) Atretic follicle
(B) Corpus albicans
(C) Corpus luteum
(D) Primary follicle
(E) Primordial follicle

22 A structure similar to that identified in Question 21 is examined at high magnification (shown in the image). The folded eosinophilic band in the center of this atretic follicle represents a degradation product of which of the following follicular components?

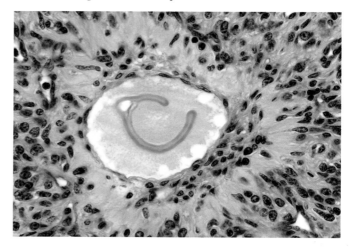

(A) Basal lamina of the stratum granulosum
(B) Cumulus oophorus
(C) Oocyte plasma membrane
(D) Theca interna
(E) Zona pellucida

23 A section through the wall of an ovarian follicle undergoing atresia reveals scattered cellular debris and chronic inflammatory cells (shown in the image). This degenerative process is mediated by activation of apoptosis in which of the following ovarian cells?

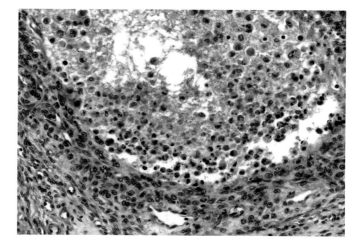

(A) Granulosa cells
(B) Primary oocytes
(C) Stromal fibroblasts
(D) Theca externa cells
(E) Theca interna cells

24 Which of the following findings is expected on gross and microscopic examination of an ovary obtained from a woman during her reproductive life?

(A) Benign germ cell tumors

(B) Collagen scar tissue

(C) Implants of endometrial tissue

(D) Neoplasia of the germinal epithelium

(E) Secondary lymphoid nodules

25 A 42-year-old woman with a family history of ovarian cancer undergoes an elective bilateral oophorectomy. A section of the patient's ovary reveals glandular epithelial tissue (shown in the image). This endocrine tissue normally develops after ovulation by morphological and functional changes in which of the following cells?

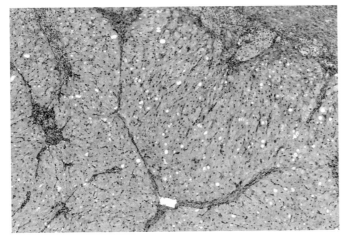

(A) Granulosa cells

(B) Leydig cells

(C) Mesothelial stem cells

(D) Stromal fibroblasts

(E) Tissue macrophages

26 The glandular tissue described in Question 25 is examined at higher magnification (shown in the image). Identify the cluster of cells indicated by the oval.

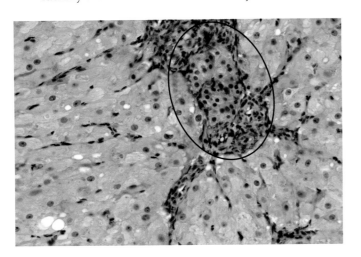

(A) Granulosa lutein cells

(B) Leydig cells

(C) Neutrophils

(D) Plasma cells

(E) Theca lutein cells

27 Examination of the contralateral ovary obtained from the patient described in Question 25 at lower magnification reveals a large pale area. Identify the structure indicated by the asterisk (shown in the image).

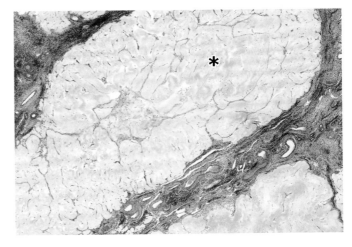

(A) Corpus albicans

(B) Corpus luteum

(C) Graafian follicle

(D) Tunica albuginea

(E) Tunica vaginalis

28 A 24-year-old pregnant woman visits her obstetrician for a routine checkup. Which of the following tissues/organs secretes a hormone that maintains the endocrine function of the corpus luteum during the first 5 months of pregnancy?

(A) Adrenal cortex

(B) Anterior pituitary

(C) Corpus luteum

(D) Cytotrophoblast

(E) Syncytiotrophoblast

29 Which of the following cells is responsible for removing tissue debris and remodeling the corpus luteum of menstruation to form the corpus albicans?

(A) Endothelial cells

(B) Lymphocytes

(C) Macrophages

(D) Mast cells

(E) Mesothelial stem cells

30 A 48-year-old woman with atypical endometrial hyperplasia undergoes an elective hysterectomy and salpingo-oophorectomy. Sections of the patient's reproductive organs are examined for pathologic changes. Identify the female reproductive organ shown in the image.

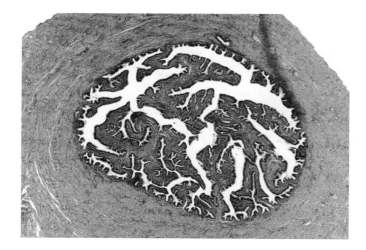

(A) Cervix
(B) Endocervix
(C) Ovary
(D) Uterine tube
(E) Vagina

31 Further examination of the organ described in Question 30 reveals a mucosa lined by ciliated epithelial cells and nonciliated "peg" cells. Proteins secreted by the peg cells are believed to mediate which of the following biological functions related to fertilization?
(A) Block to polyspermy
(B) Capacitation of sperm
(C) Formation of an endocervical plug
(D) Lysis of the zona pellucida
(E) Sperm acrosome reaction

32 A 19-year-old woman presents with a 24-hour history of intense abdominal pain. She states that she has missed two menstrual periods. Imaging studies reveal an ectopic pregnancy. Which of the following is the most likely anatomic site of embryo implantation in this patient?
(A) Ampulla of the uterine tube
(B) Endocervical canal
(C) Internal os of the uterine cervix
(D) Mesothelium of the ovary
(E) Rectouterine pouch (of Douglas)

33 The internal organs of a 34-year-old woman who died of septic shock are examined at autopsy. Identify the female reproductive organ shown in the image.

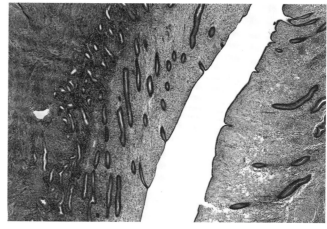

(A) Ectocervix
(B) Placenta
(C) Uterine tube
(D) Uterus
(E) Vagina

34 A 23-year-old woman complains of infertility. Pelvic examination suggests an abnormality of the patient's pelvic organs. Imaging studies reveal a double uterus (uterus bicornis). This congenital birth defect was most likely caused by failure of which of the following developmental processes?
(A) Expansion of the urorectal septum
(B) Fusion of paramesonephric ducts
(C) Involution of mesonephric ducts
(D) Migration of neural crest cells
(E) Somitogenesis in the lumbar region

35 A section of the early secretory-phase endometrium is examined by light microscopy (shown in the image). The lumen of the uterus is on the right. Which of the following arteries supplies blood to the stratum indicated by the asterisk?

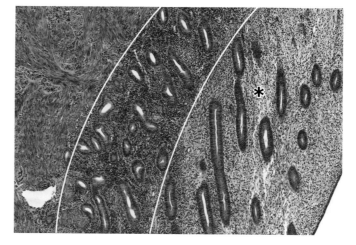

(A) Arcuate
(B) Perforating
(C) Radial
(D) Spiral
(E) Straight

36 An endometrial biopsy from a 42-year-old woman is examined in the pathology department (shown in the image). Based on the morphology of the endometrial glands, you determine that this biopsy was obtained at which phase of the patient's uterine cycle?

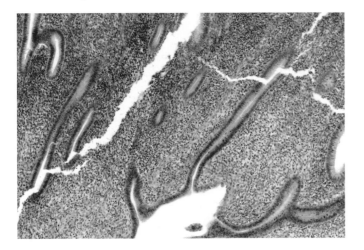

(A) Menstrual
(B) Postmenopausal
(C) Pregnancy
(D) Proliferative
(E) Secretory

37 An endometrial biopsy from a 40-year-old woman is examined in the pathology department (shown in the image). Based on the morphology of the endometrial glands, you determine that this biopsy was obtained at which phase of the patient's uterine cycle?

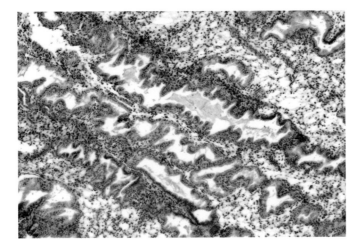

(A) Menstrual
(B) Postmenopausal
(C) Pregnancy
(D) Proliferative
(E) Secretory

38 Increased thickness of the uterine endometrium during the secretory phase of the uterine cycle is due, in part, to the accumulation of which of the following biological materials in the stratum functionalis?
(A) Adipocytes
(B) Epithelioid cells
(C) Extravascular fluid
(D) Intracellular fat droplets
(E) Intracellular glycogen vacuoles

39 A section of the early secretory-phase endometrium is examined in the pathology department (shown in the image). What is the principal function of glandular epithelial cells located in the stratum indicated by the asterisk?

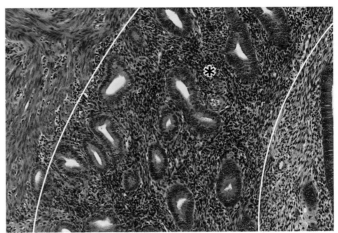

(A) Barrier to trophoblast invasion
(B) Glycogen storage and secretion
(C) Regulation of decidual reaction
(D) Reserve cells for tissue regeneration
(E) Secretion of sperm motility factors

40 The common laboratory test for pregnancy is based on the detection of a hormone that is synthesized and secreted by which of the following tissues/organs?
(A) Corpus luteum of the maternal ovary
(B) Epiblast of the developing embryo
(C) Hypoblast of the developing embryo
(D) Maternal pituitary (anterior lobe)
(E) Trophoblast of the conceptus

41 A 32-year-old woman suffers massive trauma in a motor-cycle accident. The patient's internal organs are examined at autopsy. A section of endometrial stromal tissue is examined at high magnification (shown in the image). What is the significance of these histologic findings?

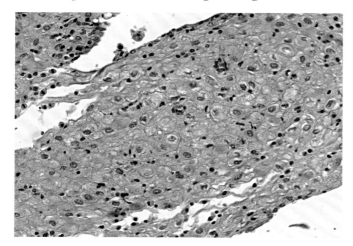

(A) Menstrual phase of the uterine cycle
(B) Pregnancy
(C) Proliferative phase of the uterine cycle
(D) Secretory phase of the uterine cycle
(E) Uterine fibroid

42 A 28-year-old woman who believes she is pregnant complains of vaginal bleeding. Ultrasound examination of the lower abdomen reveals an enlarged uterus filled with chorionic villi, but no evidence of an embryo. This patient's false pregnancy is associated with abnormal growth (hyperplasia) of which of the following cells/tissues?

(A) Amnioblast
(B) Endoderm
(C) Epiblast
(D) Hypoblast
(E) Trophoblast

43 What is the most important function of trophoblastic lacunae that form at the site of implantation during the 2nd and 3rd weeks of human development?

(A) Blood cell formation (hemopoiesis)
(B) Decidual cell formation
(C) Nutrient and gas exchange
(D) Polypeptide hormone secretion
(E) Proliferation of primordial germ cells

44 Which of the following cells is found within tertiary chorionic villi of the placenta?

(A) Amnioblasts
(B) Capillary endothelial cells
(C) Decidual cells
(D) IgA-secreting plasma cells
(E) Maternal red blood cells

45 The umbilical arteries form in close association with which of the following embryonic structures?

(A) Allantois
(B) Amnion
(C) Extraembryonic coelom
(D) Pharyngeal pouch mesenchyme
(E) Secondary yolk sac

46 Which of the following embryonic structures creates a protective fluid-filled sac that allows free movement of the embryo and fetus during pregnancy?

(A) Allantois
(B) Amnion
(C) Chorion
(D) Exocoelom
(E) Yolk sac

47 Which of the following fetal organs synthesizes steroid hormone precursors that are further metabolized to estrogen and progesterone in the placenta during the third trimester of pregnancy?

(A) Adrenal cortex
(B) Adrenal medulla
(C) Anterior pituitary
(D) Ovarian cortex
(E) Ovarian medulla

48 An ectocervical biopsy is obtained from a 25-year-old woman who presented with dysfunctional vaginal bleeding (shown in the image). This patient's biopsy shows which of the following patterns of epithelial cell differentiation?

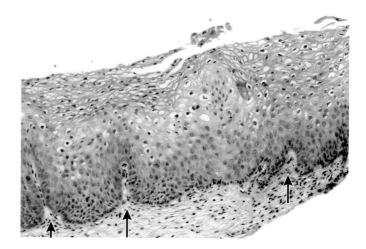

(A) Keratinized stratified squamous
(B) Nonkeratinized stratified squamous
(C) Pseudostratified columnar
(D) Pseudostratified cuboidal
(E) Simple squamous

49 The secretory epithelium lining the endocervical canal in a woman of reproductive age would most likely exhibit which of the following patterns of differentiation?
(A) Simple columnar
(B) Simple squamous
(C) Stratified columnar
(D) Stratified squamous
(E) Transitional

50 A cervical biopsy is obtained from a 36-year-old woman with a history of abnormal Pap smears. The patient's cervical biopsy is tested for human papillomavirus (HPV) by in situ hybridization using specific cDNA probes. The results are shown in the image. The dark blue viral genome is identified in which of the following subcellular locations?

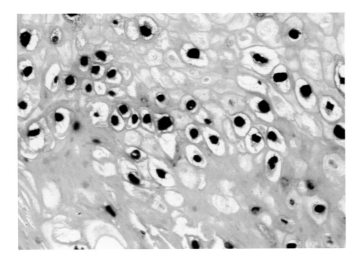

(A) Endoplasmic reticulum
(B) Golgi apparatus
(C) Nucleus
(D) Pericellular matrix
(E) Plasma membrane

51 The patient described in Question 50 is told that she is at increased risk for cervical cancer. Which of the following mechanisms of disease best explains the role of HPV in the pathogenesis of cervical neoplasia?
(A) Activation of cellular oncogenes
(B) Enhanced transcription of the telomerase gene
(C) Episomal viral replication
(D) Inactivation of tumor suppressor proteins
(E) Insertional mutagenesis

52 A vaginal smear is obtained from a 32-year-old woman who is undergoing in vitro fertilization. Which of the following cytologic features characterizes vaginal epithelial cells that are stimulated by estrogen during the menstrual cycle?
(A) Apical membrane microvilli
(B) Dense secretory granules
(C) Glycogen-filled vacuoles
(D) Intracellular lipid droplets
(E) Lamellar bodies

53 Which of the following describes the biological function of glycogen accumulation in vaginal epithelial cells during the menstrual cycle?
(A) Activation of sperm motility
(B) Enhanced bacterial growth
(C) Immune surveillance
(D) Lubrication of the mucous membrane
(E) Sperm capacitation

54 The terminal duct lobular units of an inactive mammary gland from a 34-year-old woman are examined in the pathology department (shown in the image). Which of the following types of connective tissue best describes interlobular and interlobar stromal tissue present in this breast biopsy?

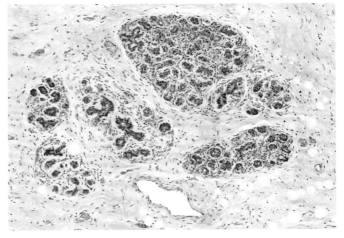

(A) Dense irregular
(B) Dense regular
(C) Elastic
(D) Loose areolar
(E) Reticular

55 A section of an active mammary gland is examined at the same magnification as was shown for the image described in Question 54. Identify the structure indicated by the arrow (shown in the image).

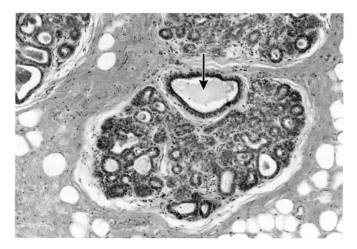

(A) Interlobular duct
(B) Intralobular duct
(C) Lactiferous duct
(D) Lactiferous sinus
(E) Sebaceous gland

56 A 32-year-old woman who recently gave birth to her first child asks for information on the physiology of nursing. The patient's milk ejection reflex is regulated by a peptide hormone that is secreted by neuroendocrine cells in which of the following anatomic locations?

(A) Adrenal cortex
(B) Adrenal medulla
(C) Hypothalamus
(D) Ovary
(E) Pituitary

57 This section of an active mammary gland shows alveolar cells with large spherical lipid droplets (shown in the image). Which of the following types of secretion best describes the manner in which these lipid droplets are released into milk during lactation?

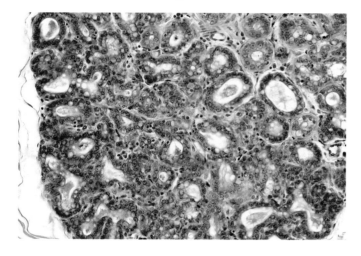

(A) Apocrine
(B) Eccrine
(C) Endocrine
(D) Holocrine
(E) Merocrine

58 A 25-year-old woman gives birth to a healthy neonate at 38-weeks' gestation and begins nursing her newborn child. The mother complains that her milk appears thick and yellow. You explain this is normal, and mention that her first milk is particularly rich in which of the following important biological molecules?

(A) Antibodies
(B) Coagulation factors
(C) Complement proteins
(D) Lipases
(E) Proteases

59 A 60-year-old woman discovers a lump in her breast on self-examination. Physical examination confirms a mass in the lower, outer quadrant of the left breast. A lumpectomy is performed, and the surgical specimen is examined in the pathology department. Based on the location of the neoplastic cells (arrows, shown in the image), this tumor most likely originated from which of the following cells within the patient's mammary gland?

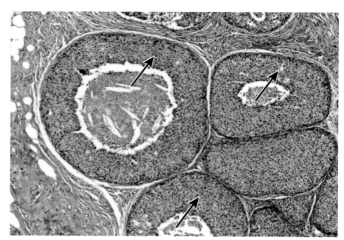

(A) Ductal epithelial cells
(B) Mesenchymal stem cells
(C) Smooth muscle cells
(D) Stromal adipocytes
(E) Stromal fibroblasts

ANSWERS

1 **The answer is A: Blastocyst.** Preimplantation embryos undergo cleavage division to form an 8- to 16-cell morula (choice C). Accumulation of fluid within this compact ball of cells transforms the morula into a fluid-filled structure referred to as the blastocyst. As shown in the image, the blastocyst is composed of two populations of cells: an inner cell mass (ICM) and an outer epithelium. Gastrula (choice B) refers to bilaminar embryos composed of epiblast and hypoblast. Neurula (choice D) refers to postimplantation embryos undergoing neurulation (folding of the neural tube). Zygote (choice E) refers to the embryo, shortly after fertilization, prior to the onset of the first cleavage division.
Keywords: Implantation, blastocyst

2 **The answer is E: Trophoblast.** As the blastocyst develops within the uterus, outer cells establish tight junctions and flatten to form a simple squamous epithelium. This outer layer of cells is referred to as trophoblast (trophectoderm). Prior to implantation, the blastocyst escapes ("hatches") from the zona pellucida. Once free of the zona pellucida, the 6-day embryo makes contact with epithelial cells lining the uterine endometrium to initiate implantation. Trophoblastic cells actively invade the maternal endometrium to establish a substrate for further development. They form two populations of cells that contribute to extraembryonic tissues of the placenta: (1) proliferative stem cells (cytotrophoblast) and (2) multinucleated giant cells (syncytiotrophoblast). The human conceptus becomes fully embedded within the maternal endometrium by day 11.
Keywords: Implantation, trophoblast

3 **The answer is C: Corpus luteum.** Implantation of the blastocyst within the endometrium is only possible during a short period of time, referred to as the "implantation window." This window of uterine receptivity is regulated by estrogen and progesterone. These steroid hormones are produced by the corpus luteum—an endocrine organ that forms in the ovary after ovulation. The anterior pituitary (choice B) secretes FSH and LH. None of the other endocrine organs secrete estrogen and progesterone.
Keywords: Ovaries, corpus luteum

4 **The answer is C: Arrest in meiosis I.** Primordial germ cells (PGCs) leave the yolk sac during the 4th and 5th weeks of development and migrate along the dorsal mesentery of the primitive gut to enter the developing gonads. Female PGCs undergo repeated mitotic cell divisions to generate millions of oogonia. Each oogonium becomes enveloped by a monolayer of follicular cells that are derived from the surface epithelium. Within these primordial follicles, female germ cells enter meiosis and arrest in prophase of meiosis I. By the 7th month of development, most oogonia have transformed into primordial oocytes. By contrast, male germ cells are incorporated into seminiferous cords and undergo mitotic arrest (choice E). Spermatogonia cells do not initiate meiosis until after puberty. None of the other types of cell division describe the behavior of germ cells within ovarian follicles during fetal development.
Keywords: Ovaries, primordial follicles

5 **The answer is E: Primordial.** Although several stages of follicular maturation are evident in this image, a majority of the follicles are primordial. Primordial follicles are located in the outer cortical region of the ovaries near the tunica albuginea. Primordial follicles are composed of a primary oocyte surrounded by a monolayer of follicular epithelial cells. Beginning at puberty, under the influence of FSH, small groups of primordial follicles are recruited to undergo maturation. Maturing follicles are less abundant than resting (primordial) follicles throughout a woman's reproductive years.
Keywords: Ovaries, primordial follicles

6 **The answer is C: Simple squamous.** The oval on this image identifies primordial follicles clustered near the periphery of the ovary. Each follicle is surrounded and nourished by follicular cells that exhibit a simple squamous epithelial morphology. Follicular cells have receptors for pituitary FSH and serve as the primary regulators of ovarian follicle development. None of the other choices describe the morphology of follicular cells associated with primordial ovarian follicles.
Keywords: Ovaries, follicular cells

7 **The answer is B: Granulosa cells.** Once activated by FSH, follicular cells differentiate into granulosa cells with altered patterns of cell behavior and metabolism. One indication of this differentiation process is a change in epithelial cell morphology from squamous to cuboidal (shown in the image). The eosinophilic material surrounding the oocyte plasma membrane represents glycoproteins forming the zona pellucida. Chief cells (choice A) are the principal cells of the parathyroid glands. Parafollicular cells (choice C) are calcitonin-secreting cells of the thyroid gland. Sertoli cells (choice D) nourish male germ cells within the seminiferous tubules. Theca interna cells (choice E) are endocrine cells that are derived from multipotential stem cells in the ovarian stroma.
Keywords: Ovaries, granulosa cells

8 **The answer is D: Primary.** This image shows a multilaminar primary follicle surrounded by spindle-shaped, connective tissue cells of the ovarian stroma. The granulosa cells have proliferated under the influence of pituitary FSH to form a stratified cuboidal epithelium. The basal lamina of the stratum granulosum appears as a thin eosinophilic ring (shown in the image). The nucleus of the primary oocyte exhibits heterochromatin and a

prominent nucleolus. None of the other choices describe the morphology of primary ovarian follicles.
Keywords: Ovaries, primary follicles

9 **The answer is A: Antral.** This image shows a developing secondary (antral) follicle. When the stratum granulosum reaches a thickness of between 6- and 12-cell layers, cystic spaces appear between the granulosa cells. These fluid-filled cavities coalesce to form a single crescent-shaped antrum. Atretic follicles (choice B) show evidence of programmed cell death (pyknosis and karyolysis). Graafian follicles (choice C) are large preovulatory follicles that reach sizes up to 10 mm in diameter. It is important to remember that germ cells within secondary (antral) ovarian follicles are primary oocytes, arrested in prophase of meiosis I. None of the other ovarian follicles describe the morphology of secondary (antral) follicles.
Keywords: Ovaries, antral follicles

10 **The answer is B: Extracellular fluid accumulation.** Secondary follicles are distinguished from primary follicles by the presence of one or more fluid-filled cavities. Granulosa cells secrete a hyaluronan-rich fluid (liquor folliculi) that creates open spaces within the stratum granulosum. Hyaluronan is a high molecular weight polysaccharide that retains extracellular (interstitial) water. None of the other biological processes are involved in the maturation of secondary (antral) follicles.
Keywords: Ovaries, antral follicles

11 **The answer is D: Arrow 4.** As the secondary follicle enlarges, granulosa cells near the oocyte form a hillock referred to as the cumulus oophorus. This mound of cells supports and protects the developing oocyte. The granulosa cells that encircle the oocyte form a crown-like structure that is referred to as the corona radiata. These cells send microvilli through openings in the zona pellucida to establish gap junction communication with the oocyte. The corona radiata remains attached to the oocyte after ovulation and may not disperse until fertilization. The eosinophilic debris within the antrum of this secondary follicle represents proteins in the liquor folliculi that precipitated during tissue fixation. None of the other structures identify the corona radiata.
Keywords: Ovaries, corona radiata

12 **The answer is B: Arrow 2.** The zona pellucida is an extracellular layer that is secreted by the oocyte during oogenesis. In this section, the zona pellucida appears as a thin, eosinophilic ring between the oocyte and the corona radiata. The zona pellucida is composed of three glycoproteins: ZP-1, ZP-2, and ZP-3. These glycoproteins form a transparent fibrous matrix that envelops the oocyte and early cleavage-stage embryo. The zona pellucida is degraded prior to implantation by proteolytic enzymes that are secreted by the blastocyst.
Keywords: Zona pellucida

13 **The answer is D: Sperm adhesion.** The zona pellucida that surrounds the oocyte provides a multivalent array of receptors for sperm adhesion and activation of the sperm acrosome reaction. These biological functions both are mediated by ZP-3. The sperm receptor for ZP-3 is, however, poorly characterized. Sperm capacitation (choice E) takes place in the uterine tube. None of the other choices describe biological functions of the zona pellucida.
Keywords: Zona pellucida, fertilization

14 **The answer is C: Zone 3.** As granulosa cells proliferate under the influence of FSH, mesenchymal stem cells surrounding the follicle form two distinct cellular layers: theca interna and theca externa. Theca interna cells express receptors for pituitary LH. They secrete a steroid hormone precursor (androstenedione) that is converted to estrogen by granulosa cells. Theca externa cells (zone 4) include fibroblasts and smooth muscle cells (fibromuscular connective tissue). Zone 1 (choice A) identifies a portion of the cumulus oophorus. Zone 2 (choice B) identifies the stratum granulosum. Zone 5 (choice E) identifies connective tissue of the ovarian stroma.
Keywords: Ovaries, theca interna

15 **The answer is E: Zona pellucida.** Primary oocytes complete the first meiotic cell division a few hours before ovulation. In response to a mid-cycle surge of FSH and LH, paired chromosomes (tetrads) separate. One set of chromosomes is retained by the secondary oocyte, while the other set is discarded, along with a small amount of cytoplasm, as the first polar body. This large vesicle forms in the perivitelline space, between the germ cell plasma membrane and the zona pellucida. Failure of homologous chromosomes to separate is termed non-disjunction. Down syndrome (trisomy 21) and Turner syndrome (45,XO) are chromosomal numerical abnormalities associated with nondisjunction. None of the other structures immediately surround the polar bodies generated during meiosis I and meiosis II.
Keywords: Oogenesis, polar bodies

16 **The answer is A: Granulosa cells.** The proliferative phase of the uterine cycle is regulated by estrogen. This steroid hormone is secreted by the stratum granulosum of maturing follicles. Granulosa cells synthesize aromatase, an intracellular enzyme that converts androstenedione into estradiol. Androstenedione is an estrogen precursor that is secreted by theca interna cells (choice D). Granulosa lutein and theca lutein cells (choices B and E) synthesize estrogen and progesterone during the secretory phase of the menstrual cycle, after formation of the corpus luteum. None of the other cells secrete estrogen.
Keywords: Ovaries, granulosa cells

17 **The answer is D: Secondary oocyte.** The first meiotic division (meiosis I) is completed prior to ovulation in response to a mid-cycle surge in levels of FSH and LH. The resulting secondary oocyte is characterized by the presence of a single (first) polar body. During ovulation, the secondary oocyte is released from the surface of the ovary and enters the ampulla of the uterine tube. Morula (choice A) is a descriptive term for mulberry-shaped 8- to 16-cell embryos. Zygote (choice E) describes the post-fertilization embryo, prior to the first cleavage division.
Keywords: Ovaries, secondary oocytes, ovulation

18 **The answer is A: Fertilization.** Whereas the completion of meiosis I is controlled by hormonal signals, the completion of meiosis II is triggered by fertilization. Sperm entry into the secondary oocyte stimulates the completion of meiosis II (the so-called reduction division) with formation of a female pronucleus and a second polar body. The biochemical mechanisms that regulate this complex process are poorly understood. None of the other cellular or physiological processes regulate the second meiotic division.
Keywords: Fertilization, meiosis

19 **The answer is B: Formation of the second polar body.** Fertilization is a complex developmental process that brings together haploid gametes, restores a diploid genome, and sets in motion early development. Binding of sperm to the zona pellucida triggers the sperm acrosome reaction (choice D). The acrosome reaction liberates hydrolytic enzymes that disperse the corona radiata (choice A) and create openings in the zona pellucida that facilitate the entry of hypermotile sperm into the perivitelline space. Movements of male and female pronuclei (choice C) would be difficult to monitor by light microscopy. On the other hand, the formation of a second polar body can be monitored easily using an inverted phase microscope. Formation of the second polar body provides unambiguous evidence of fertilization. It signifies completion of the second meiotic division and heralds the initiation of early development.
Keywords: Fertilization

20 **The answer is C: Exocytosis of cortical granules.** The postfusion oocyte undergoes a rapid sequence of changes that block the entry of more than one spermatozoan. Three postfusion blocks to polyspermy have been described: (1) membrane depolarization (fast block), (2) Ca^{2+}—mediated cortical granule release (cortical reaction), and (3) enzyme-mediated modification of the zona pellucida (zona reaction). Exocytosis of cortical granules liberates proteases that degrade sperm receptors on the oocyte plasma membrane and on the zona pellucida. Mitochondrial membrane permeability transition (choice E) regulates programmed cell death. None of the other cellular processes provide a physiological block to polyspermy. On rare occasions, two or more sperm enter an egg leading to a false pregnancy.

These partial hydatidiform moles (masses) typically exhibit a triploid karyotype (69 XXY) and present with intrauterine hyperplasia of the placental trophoblast.
Keywords: Fertilization, polyspermy

21 **The answer is A: Atretic follicle.** Although several million oocytes are present at birth, only 300,000 remain by the time of puberty, and only 400 to 500 oocytes are ovulated during a woman's reproductive years. This continuous loss of germ cells is referred to as follicular atresia. This degenerative process may take place at any stage of follicle maturation. Atretic follicles undergo degenerative changes associated with programmed cell death (apoptosis). Macrophages enter atretic follicles to remove cellular debris, and fibroblasts produce collagen scar tissue that may resorb over time. The circle shown on this image reveals a small cystic cavity surrounded by pink collagen scar tissue. This section also shows stratification of the theca folliculi that surrounds a secondary (antral) follicle.
Keywords: Ovaries, atretic follicles

22 **The answer is E: Zona pellucida.** This image shows the remains of an atretic follicle that has been invaded by stromal connective tissue. Most of the cellular debris have been removed by macrophages; however, the glycoproteins that comprise the zona pellucida are resistant to degradation. The remnant of a zona pellucida is visible in this image as an eosinophilic loop that resembles a folded rubber band. This fibrous structure is located in a cystic space that was occupied by the primary oocyte. The basal lamina of the stratum granulosum (choice A) swells during follicular atresia, forming a "glassy membrane" that is shown in this image.
Keywords: Ovaries, atretic follicles

23 **The answer is A: Granulosa cells.** Recent studies indicate that follicular atresia is triggered by down-regulation of an apoptosis-inhibitory protein in granulosa cells. Without this inhibitory protein, granulosa cells exit the cell cycle and activate hydrolytic enzymes (e.g., caspase enzymes) that degrade nuclear chromatin. Death of the oocyte ensues, and the follicle is infiltrated by macrophages that remove apoptotic bodies and necrotic tissue debris. Condensation of chromatin (pyknosis), degradation of chromatin (karyolysis), and eosinophilic apoptotic bodies provide evidence of irreversible cell injury. None of the other cells regulates ovarian follicular atresia.
Keywords: Ovaries, atretic follicles

24 **The answer is B: Collagen scar tissue.** During a woman's reproductive years, her ovaries are subjected to monthly cycles of injury associated with ovulation and follicular atresia, as well as involution of the corpus luteum. Examination of the ovaries in the pathology department would therefore reveal evidence of necrosis and apoptosis, as well as evidence of healing (collagen scar tissue). Atrophy of the ovaries occurs in postmenopausal woman, owing to the loss of hormonal stimulation. Germ cell tumors (choice A), endometriosis (choice C), ovarian cancer (choice D), and secondary lymphoid nodules (choice E) may affect the ovaries; however, these pathologic conditions are less common than normal patterns of scar tissue.

Keywords: Ovaries, ovulation

25 **The answer is A: Granulosa cells.** After ovulation, the stratum granulosum collapses and forms a temporary endocrine organ that secretes progesterone and estrogen. These steroid hormones prepare the uterus for implantation and pregnancy. This steroid hormone factory is referred to as the corpus luteum (L: yellow body). Pituitary LH programs the corpus luteum to produce steroid hormones for about 10 to 12 days. With conception, the corpus luteum of pregnancy produces steroid hormones for 4 to 5 months. Most of the cells comprising the corpus luteum are derived from the stratum granulosum of the mature (graafian) follicle. None of the other cells contribute to the corpus luteum.

Keywords: Ovaries, corpus luteum

26 **The answer is E: Theca lutein cells.** The oval highlights a cluster of theca lutein cells. After ovulation, theca interna cells acquire the ability to synthesize progesterone. These endocrine cells are smaller and less abundant than granulosa lutein cells. They are typically found as small aggregates in folds of the wall of the corpus luteum. None of the other cells exhibit the distinctive morphology of theca lutein cells.

Keywords: Ovaries, corpus luteum

27 **The answer is A: Corpus albicans.** In the absence of pregnancy, the corpus luteum of menstruation begins to degenerate about 10 to 12 days after ovulation. The degenerating glandular tissue is infiltrated by stromal fibroblasts. These cells deposit large amounts of dense collagen scar tissue to form a corpus albicans (white body). Tunica albuginea (choice D) is a collagenous tunic that surrounds the testes and ovaries. None of the other choices exhibit the distinctive (hypocellular) morphology of the corpus albicans.

Keywords: Ovaries, corpus albicans

28 **The answer is E: Syncytiotrophoblast.** Shortly after implantation, syncytiotrophoblast cells of the conceptus begin to secrete human chorionic gonadotropin (hCG). This glycoprotein hormone has LH-like activity and maintains the corpus luteum during the first and second trimesters of pregnancy. The anterior pituitary (choice B) secretes LH for only 10 to 12 days following ovulation. Pituitary LH maintains the corpus luteum of menstruation, but hCG secreted by syncytiotrophoblast cells maintains the corpus luteum of pregnancy. None of the other tissues/organs secrete hCG.

Keywords: Ovaries, corpus luteum, syncytiotrophoblast

29 **The answer is C: Macrophages.** Apoptotic bodies and necrotic debris from the degenerating corpus luteum are removed by tissue macrophages. These phagocytic cells degrade cellular debris within phagolysosomes. None of the other cells are phagocytes.

Keywords: Ovaries, corpus albicans

30 **The answer is D: Uterine tube.** The paired uterine tubes (commonly referred to as fallopian tubes) extend 10 to 12 cm from the body of the uterus toward the ovaries. Their primary function is gamete/embryo transport. The mucosa of the uterine tubes is characterized by extensive folding (folia, shown in the image). None of the other reproductive organs exhibit such extensive mucosal folding.

Keywords: Uterine tubes

31 **The answer is B: Capacitation of sperm.** Peg cells are so named because they resemble tiny pegs pounded into the epithelium lining the uterine tubes. Peg cells secrete carbohydrates and proteins that nourish and protect the oocyte, sperm, and embryo. These secretions also promote sperm capacitation—a poorly understood process whereby sperm acquire the ability to bind the zona pellucida and undergo the sperm acrosome reaction. Removal of cholesterol from the sperm plasma membrane is believed to be an essential feature of capacitation. Sperm capacitation is confirmed by documenting hyperactivation of sperm motility (i.e., whiplash motion of the sperm tail). None of the other biological functions are linked to secretions of peg cells in the uterine tubes.

Keywords: Uterine tubes, capacitation, peg cells

32 **The answer is A: Ampulla of the uterine tube.** The uterine tubes are divided into four anatomic segments: infundibulum, ampulla, isthmus, and intramural uterine portion. After ovulation, the oocyte remains viable for about 24 hours. Fertilization typically takes place in the ampulla of the uterine tube. Ciliary motion and contractions of smooth muscle normally transport the cleavage-stage embryo toward the uterus. However, the embryo may implant in a nonuterine, ectopic location (approximately 1/100 pregnancies). Most ectopic pregnancies occur in the uterine tubes, typically within the ampulla. The other choices describe possible, albeit less common, sites for ectopic pregnancy.

Keywords: Ectopic pregnancy, uterine tubes

33 **The answer is D: Uterus.** This section of the uterus shows smooth muscle (myometrium), surrounding a mucosa (endometrium) filled with tubular glands. The uterus is a highly muscular organ that provides a substrate for embryonic and fetal development. Major layers of the uterus include endometrium (glands and stroma), myometrium (smooth muscle), and perimetrium (adventitia or serosa). None of the other reproductive organs are characterized by the presence of mucosal glands.

Keywords: Uterus, endometrium

34 The answer is B: Fusion of paramesonephric ducts. The uterus and uterine tubes originate from embryonic paramesonephric ducts. The uterine tubes represent unfused cranial portions of the ducts. The uterus arises by fusion of these tubes, caudally, to form an uterovaginal primordium. Fusion of the embryonic paramesonephric ducts also brings together lateral folds of the peritoneum to form the broad ligament of the uterus. Arrest in the development of the uterovaginal primordium is associated with various types of uterine anomalies, including uterus unicornis and bicornis. None of the other developmental processes regulate morphogenesis of the uterus.

Keywords: Uterus, paramesonephric ducts

35 The answer is D: Spiral. The endometrium can be divided into two zones: stratum basalis and stratum functionalis. These zones receive blood from different arteries. Arcuate arteries branch to form (1) straight arteries that supply the stratum basalis and (2) spiral arteries that supply the stratum functionalis. The spiral arteries are uniquely sensitive to progesterone. During the secretory phase of the menstrual cycle, progesterone stimulates the growth of spiral arteries within the stratum functionalis. Decreasing serum levels of progesterone toward the end of the uterine cycle cause contractions (spasms) of the muscular wall of the spiral arteries, leading to ischemic necrosis of the stratum functionalis (menses, menstruation). None of the other arteries supplies blood to the stratum functionalis of the uterine endometrium.

Keywords: Uterus, endometrium

36 The answer is D: Proliferative. Following menstruation, the stratum functionalis is reconstituted under the influence of the estrogen secreted by granulosa cells. During this proliferative phase of the uterine cycle, the stoma appears more cellular, and the mucosal glands appear straight and empty (shown in the image). None of the other phases of the uterine cycle show this pattern of glandular epithelial morphology.

Keywords: Uterus, endometrium

37 The answer is E: Secretory. Whereas estrogen regulates the proliferative phase of the uterine cycle, progesterone secreted by the corpus luteum regulates the secretory phase of the uterine cycle. In response to progesterone, uterine glands become enlarged and coiled (tortuous). On histologic examination, the glands acquire a zigzag appearance (shown in the image). During this phase of the uterine cycle, the glandular epithelial cells secrete a glycogen- and glycoprotein-rich fluid that provides an essential growth medium for the early embryo. None of the other phases/stages of the uterine cycle show this

distinctive "sawtooth" pattern of glandular epithelial morphology.

Keywords: Uterus, endometrium, uterine endometrium

38 The answer is C: Extravascular fluid. Increased thickness of the uterine endometrium during the secretory phase of the uterine cycle is due to (1) growth of uterine glands and (2) accumulation of extravascular fluid in the stroma (i.e., lamina propria of the mucosa). Accumulation of extravascular fluid is referred to as edema. Local edema is typically caused by increased vascular permeability. The endometrial biopsy shown for Question 37 shows evidence of interstitial edema (edematous stroma). The spaces between stromal cells reflect the accumulation of extravascular edema fluid. None of the other biological materials cause increased thickness of the endometrium during the secretory phase of the uterine cycle.

Keywords: Uterus, endometrium

39 The answer is D: Reserve cells for tissue regeneration. The stratum basalis of the uterine endometrium is not shed during menstruation. During the proliferative phase of the uterine cycle, the stratum basalis provides a source of epithelial and stromal stem cells that regrow the stratum functionalis. This remarkable cyclic process of tissue regeneration and repair is regulated by estrogen. None of the other choices describe the principal function of the stratum basalis of the uterine endometrium.

Keywords: Uterus, endometrium

40 The answer is E: Trophoblast of the conceptus. Shortly after implantation, syncytiotrophoblast cells of the conceptus begin to secrete a hormone (human chorionic gonadotropin) that maintains the endocrine function of the corpus luteum during the first 4 to 5 months of pregnancy. This glycoprotein hormone (hCG) can be detected in maternal urine and blood as early as 2 weeks following conception. Most home pregnancy kits are designed to detect the beta subunit of hCG. None of the other cells are known to secrete hormones that serve as markers of pregnancy. It is also noteworthy that hCG provides a useful serum marker for men with trophoblastic tumors of the testis (choriocarcinomas).

Keywords: Pregnancy, trophoblast

41 The answer is B: Pregnancy. During early pregnancy, stromal cells surrounding the site of implantation change size, shape, and metabolic function. These connective tissue cells enlarge, store glycogen and lipid, and assume a compact epithelioid morphology (shown in the image). This transformation process is referred to as the decidual reaction. The presence of decidual cells/tissue in an endometrial biopsy provides histologic evidence of pregnancy. None of the other choices are associated with decidualization of the endometrial stroma.

Keywords: Pregnancy, decidual reaction

42 **The answer is E: Trophoblast.** Gestational trophoblastic disease is characterized by abnormal proliferation of the trophoblast. The patient described in this clinical vignette has a hydatidiform mole (L: water droplet–like mass). Complete hydatidiform mole is a placenta that has swollen and empty chorionic villi, resembling bunches of grapes. Complete mole results from the fertilization of an empty ovum that lacks functional DNA. The haploid (23,X) set of paternal chromosomes duplicates. Hence, most complete moles are homozygous 46,XX, and all chromosomes are of paternal origin. Differential methylation (imprinting) of the male genome permits the growth of trophoblast but does not support the growth and differentiation of embryonic tissues. As a result, fetal parts are absent. Malignant transformation (choriocarcinoma) develops in about 2% of cases. None of the other cells/tissues are associated with the development of a false pregnancy.
Keywords: Hydatidiform mole, trophoblast

43 **The answer is C: Nutrient and gas exchange.** Spiral arteries in the stratum functionalis of the endometrium supply blood to sinusoidal capillaries located near the lumen of the uterus. During implantation, trophoblastic giant cells organize these sinusoids into large lacunae (L: lakes) that fill with maternal blood and secretions from eroded endometrial glands. This mixture is referred to as embryotroph, because it provides essential nutrients and oxygen to the embryo during implantation. Trophoblastic lacunae establish the primordial uteroplacental circulation. None of the other biological processes describe the principal function of trophoblastic lacunae.
Keywords: Implantation, trophoblast

44 **The answer is B: Capillary endothelial cells.** Chorionic villi are finger-like projections of the chorionic sac that bring the embryonic circulatory system into close proximity with maternal blood. This intimate relationship of two circulatory systems provides the structural basis for nutrient and gas exchange between the mother and fetus during pregnancy. Tertiary chorionic villi project into pools of maternal blood (choice E). Tertiary chorionic villi contain an embryonic/fetal capillary loop surrounded by a protective layer of cytotrophoblast and syncytiotrophoblast. None of the other cells are found within the tertiary chorionic villi of the human placenta.
Keywords: Chorionic villi, endothelial cells

45 **The answer is A: Allantois.** The allantois is an endodermal outpouching from the caudal wall of the umbilical vesicle (yolk sac) that projects into the connecting stalk of the conceptus. It arises on about day 16 of development. Because of its location, blood vessels that develop in this location become the umbilical arteries. After transit through the placenta, the unpaired umbilical vein returns oxygenated, nutrient-rich blood to the embryo. None of the other embryonic structures are related to the development of paired arteries in the umbilical cord.
Keywords: Allantois, umbilical cord

46 **The answer is B: Amnion.** Shortly after implantation, the bilaminar embryo forms a protective cavity (amniotic cavity) that enlarges to surround the embryo and fetus during pregnancy. The membrane that forms this fluid-filled sac is referred to as the amnion. Amniotic fluid serves many crucial functions during development, including: (1) protection of the embryo and fetus; (2) regulation of fluid volume and electrolyte homeostasis; and (3) provision of space for symmetric growth of the embryo and fetus. The chorion (choice C) also surrounds the embryo; however, the chorionic cavity is soon obliterated by expansion of the amnion. None of the other embryonic structures envelop and protect the developing embryo and fetus.
Keywords: Amnion

47 **The answer is A: Adrenal cortex.** After the 5th month of gestation, the corpus luteum atrophies, and the placenta takes over the role of secreting steroid hormones that maintain the uterus during the last trimester of pregnancy. At this time, the cortex of the fetal adrenal glands enlarges and produces large amounts of androstenedione, which are converted to estrogens in the placenta. Thus, the fetal adrenal cortex forms part of a fetoplacental endocrine unit. Theca lutein cells associated with maturing ovarian follicles (choice D) also synthesize androstenedione; however, these endocrine cells are not metabolically active during pregnancy. None of the other endocrine organs synthesize estrogen precursors.
Keywords: Adrenal glands, pregnancy

48 **The answer is B: Nonkeratinized stratified squamous.** The image shows a nonkeratinized, stratified squamous epithelium. This epithelium is continuous with the vagina. Several connective tissue papillae are observed to penetrate the overlying stratified epithelium (arrows, shown in the image). The bulk of the cervix is composed of dense irregular connective tissue. Softening of the cervix and dilation of the birth canal during labor (cervical effacement) are caused by local degradation of collagen (collagenolysis). Possible causes of dysfunctional vaginal bleeding described in this clinical vignette include pregnancy, pelvic inflammatory disease, cervical cancer, endometrial cancer, and anovulatory uterine cycles. None of the other types of epithelium describe histologic features of the ectocervix.
Keywords: Cervix, Pap smear

49 **The answer is A: Simple columnar.** In contrast to the ectocervix, the endocervical canal is lined by a mucus-secreting columnar epithelium. The junction between these two types of epithelium is appropriately referred

to as the squamocolumnar junction. The mucosa of the endocervix contains numerous branched cervical glands. Retention of mucus within a dilated cervical gland is referred to as a nabothian cyst. None of the other types of epithelium describe histologic features of the endocervix.
Keywords: Cervix

50 **The answer is C: Nucleus.** Human papillomavirus (HPV) is a DNA virus that infects a variety of skin and mucosal surfaces to produce wart-like lesions (verrucae and condylomata, respectively). In the female reproductive tract, HPV infections are linked to the pathogenesis of cervical squamous cell carcinoma. The morphologic hallmark of HPV infection is koilocytotic atypia. This term denotes the presence of prominent perinuclear vacuoles, combined with alterations in the chromatin pattern of squamous epithelial cells. In this clinical specimen, perinuclear vacuoles are clearly visible as sharply demarcated, clear zones surrounding the nuclei of HPV-infected cells. These vacuoles are filled with actively replicating virus particles (virions). None of the other organelles provide a subcellular location for integration and transcription of the HPV genome.
Keywords: Human papillomavirus, cervical cancer

51 **The answer is D: Inactivation of tumor suppressor proteins.** Unlike RNA tumor viruses, whose oncogenes have normal cellular counterparts, the transforming genes of DNA viruses are not homologous with any cellular genes. This conundrum was resolved with the discovery that the gene products of oncogenic DNA viruses inactivate tumor suppressor proteins. For example, proteins encoded by the *E6* and *E7* genes of HPV16 bind p53 and pRb. The other choices are involved in the pathogenesis of neoplasia, but they are not specific for HPV.
Keywords: Cervical cancer, human papillomavirus

52 **The answer is C: Glycogen-filled vacuoles.** In response to estrogen, vaginal epithelial cells synthesize and store large quantities of glycogen (a large polysaccharide). As a result of glycogen accumulation, the cytoplasm of these cells typically appears empty or clear when stained with H&E. The glycogen content of vaginal cell smears can be assessed qualitatively using appropriate stains and light microscopy. Lamellar bodies (choice E) are secretory vesicles found in pneumocytes (lung) and keratinocytes (skin). None of the other cytologic features characterize the response of vaginal epithelial cells to estrogen.
Keywords: Vagina

53 **The answer is B: Enhanced bacterial growth.** As vaginal epithelial cells naturally exfoliate (desquamate), their stores of glycogen provide a source of energy for bacteria that thrive in the film of fluid that coats the vaginal mucosa. Lactic acid produced by these "healthy" bacteria lowers the pH of the vaginal mucosa (normal pH = 3.8 to 4.5), which serves to protect against the growth of

pathogenic microorganisms. None of the other biological processes describe the function of glycogen accumulation in vaginal epithelial cells during the menstrual cycle.
Keywords: Vagina, menstrual cycle

54 **The answer is A: Dense irregular.** The mammary glands consist of 15 to 25 lobes separated by dense, irregular connective tissue. This section of inactive mammary gland shows several lobules (also referred to as terminal duct lobular units). These lobules are separated by bundles of densely packed type I collagen fibers. Collagen fibers are visible in this image as wavy, extracellular pink material. By contrast, the connective tissue present within terminal duct lobular units is best described as loose areolar connective tissue (choice D). Dense regular connective tissue (choice B) is present in tendons and ligaments. None of the other types of connective tissue describe the interlobar and interlobular stromal tissue of the mammary glands.
Keywords: Mammary glands

55 **The answer is B: Intralobular duct.** The mammary glands undergo extensive branching morphogenesis both during and after pregnancy. Secretory alveoli develop at the ends of the intralobular ducts and produce milk. Growth of the mammary glands is regulated by several hormones, including estrogen, progesterone, prolactin, and human placental lactogen. The arrow on this image identifies a large intralobular duct at the margin of a lobule. This excretory duct drains milk to interlobular ducts, which drain to a lactiferous duct and sinus located near the nipple. Interlobular ducts (choice A) and lactiferous ducts (choice D) are embedded in dense irregular connective tissue (not shown). None of the other ducts/glands exhibit the distinctive histologic features of intralobular ducts of the mammary gland.
Keywords: Mammary glands

56 **The answer is E: Pituitary.** Suckling during breastfeeding initiates a sequence of neurological and hormonal changes that ensure delivery of milk to the neonate. Sensory impulses from tactile receptors in the nipple are conveyed to the hypothalamus, resulting in the release of oxytocin from the Herring bodies of terminal axons within the posterior pituitary (neurohypophysis). Oxytocin is a 9-amino-acid polypeptide hormone. It triggers contraction of smooth muscle cells surrounding lactiferous ducts and lactiferous sinuses, as well as contraction of myoepithelial cells surrounding alveoli. This hormonally mediated process of milk delivery to the neonate is referred to as the "milk ejection reflex." None of the other endocrine organs secrete oxytocin.
Keywords: Mammary glands, oxytoxin

57 **The answer is A: Apocrine.** Breast milk provides the neonate with a rich mixture of essential fluids, electrolytes, vitamins, antibodies, sugars, lipids, and proteins. The section of an active mammary gland shown in the image reveals large spherical lipid droplets within alveolar epithelial cells. Release of these stored lipids involves an apocrine secretion mechanism in which lipid droplets are shed along with a small portion of the apical cell membrane and cytoplasm. By contrast, milk proteins are released through a merocrine mechanism (choice E) in which small membrane-bound vesicles release their contents by fusing with the overlying plasma membrane. During holocrine secretion (choice D), the plasma membrane of the secretory cell ruptures and the cell dies. Holocrine secretion characterizes the release of oily/waxy materials from the sebaceous glands of the skin. None of the other types of glandular secretion describe the release of lipid droplets from alveolar cells into milk during lactation.

Keywords: Mammary glands, lactation

58 **The answer is A: Antibodies.**   The thick and yellow milk that is produced a few days after parturition is referred to as colostrum. Compared to milk that is produced over the ensuing weeks and months, colostrum is particularly rich in IgA immunoglobulins. These antibodies provide the neonate with passive humeral immunity. They are produced by mature B lymphocytes (plasma cells) that infiltrate the loose connective tissue of the breast and secrete immunoglobulins that are transported across the alveolar epithelium into breast milk. None of the other choices represent a characteristic feature of colostrum.

Keywords: Lactation, colostrum

59 **The answer is A: Ductal epithelial cells.**   Breast cancer is the most common malignancy of women in the United States, and the mortality from this disease among women is second only to that of lung cancer. This breast biopsy reveals an early stage of breast cancer termed ductal carcinoma in situ (DCIS). The neoplastic cells are derived from ductal epithelium. Although they are proliferating and enlarging the duct, the neoplastic cells are confined by the basement membrane. This cancer may extend within the duct system of the mammary gland. None of the other cells gives rise to ductal carcinoma of the breast.

Keywords: Mammary glands, breast cancer

Chapter 18

Endocrine System

QUESTIONS

Select the single best answer.

1 A 34-year-old woman with a multiple endocrine neoplasia syndrome dies of malignant thyroid cancer. The patient's organs are examined at autopsy for evidence of additional endocrine neoplasms. Identify the normal epithelial tissue in the center of the field (shown in the image).

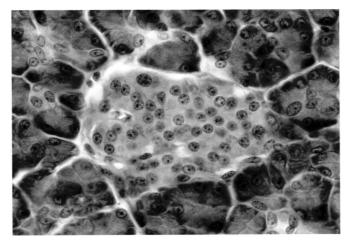

(A) Adrenal medulla
(B) Pancreatic islet
(C) Parathyroid gland
(D) Pituitary pars intermedia
(E) Thyroid follicle

2 Which of the following cytologic features is most useful for distinguishing between alpha, beta, and delta cells in the endocrine tissue identified in Question 1?
(A) Cell size and shape
(B) Differential reactivity with eosin
(C) DNA content (ploidy)
(D) Immunostaining property
(E) Size of secretory granules

3 The parents of an 8-year-old boy are concerned about his weight loss following a flu-like illness. Urinalysis reveals glucosuria (glucose in the urine). His fasting blood glucose is 220 mg/dL (normal = 50 to 100 mg/dL). The child is diagnosed with diabetes mellitus type 1. Which of the following cells in the endocrine pancreas produces insulin?
(A) Alpha cells
(B) Beta cells
(C) Delta cells
(D) F cells
(E) PP cells

4 A 24-year-old woman experiences severe bleeding during delivery of a preterm infant due to abnormal separation of the placenta. Five months later, she presents with profound lethargy, pallor, muscle weakness, failure of lactation, and amenorrhea. You suspect that the multiple hormone deficiencies in this patient were caused by postpartum injury to which of the following endocrine organs?
(A) Adrenal glands
(B) Ovaries
(C) Parathyroid glands
(D) Pituitary gland
(E) Thyroid gland

5 You are asked to give a lecture on the cellular and molecular mechanisms of hormone secretion. The cytoplasm of which of the following endocrine cells is expected to show an abundance of dense core, membrane-bound secretory granules when examined by electron microscopy?
(A) Follicular cells of the ovary
(B) Granulosa lutein cells of the ovary
(C) Interstitial cells of the testis
(D) Parafollicular cells of the thyroid
(E) Spongiocytes of the adrenal cortex

6 The parents of an 8-week-old girl complain that their child is apathetic and sluggish. Further testing reveals mental and physical retardation. The child is diagnosed with cretinism. Hormone replacement therapy is initiated. Agenesis during development of which of the following organs would explain the pathogenesis of physical and mental retardation in this infant?
(A) Adrenal glands
(B) Parathyroid glands
(C) Pineal gland
(D) Pituitary gland
(E) Thyroid gland

7 A 50-year-old man suffers massive head trauma in a motor vehicle accident and expires. Sections of the patient's hypothalamus and pituitary gland are examined at autopsy. Identify the region indicated by the asterisk (shown in the image).

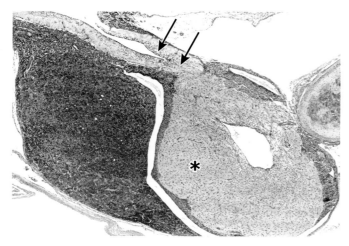

(A) Median eminence of the infundibulum
(B) Paraventricular nucleus of the hypothalamus
(C) Pars distalis of the adenohypophysis
(D) Pars nervosa of the neurohypophysis
(E) Pars tuberalis of the adenohypophysis

8 For the autopsy specimen examined in Question 7, the arrows shown in the image identify which of the following anatomic structures?
(A) Median eminence of the infundibulum
(B) Paraventricular nucleus of the hypothalamus
(C) Pars distalis of the adenohypophysis
(D) Pars nervosa of the neurohypophysis
(E) Pars tuberalis of the adenohypophysis

9 The endocrine organ identified in Questions 7 and 8 is examined at higher magnification (shown in the image). The arrows identify the nuclei of which of the following types of cells?

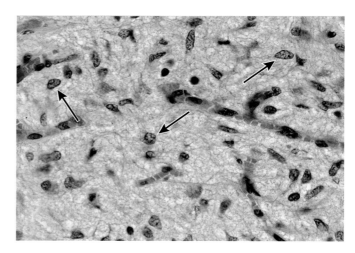

(A) Microglial cells
(B) Neurons
(C) Oligodendrocytes
(D) Pituicytes
(E) Schwann cells

10 Electron microscopic examination of the neuroendocrine tissue described in Question 9 reveals dilated terminal axons containing dense core, membrane-bound secretory vesicles. What is the appropriate term for the dilated portions of terminal axons in the posterior lobe of the pituitary?
(A) Corpora amylacea
(B) Herring bodies
(C) Neurokeratin vacuoles
(D) Neurophysin droplets
(E) Nissl substance

11 A 16-year-old boy presents with lethargy and headaches. His parents note that he drinks water excessively. A 24-hour urine collection shows polyuria. His fasting blood sugar is normal. Laboratory studies reveal decreased serum levels of antidiuretic hormone (ADH). This polypeptide hormone is synthesized in which of the following organs/glands?
(A) Adrenal cortex
(B) Adrenal medulla
(C) Hypothalamus
(D) Kidney
(E) Posterior pituitary

12 For the patient described in Question 11, ADH (arginine vasopressin) enters the systemic circulation through fenestrated capillaries that are present in which of the following anatomic locations?
(A) Median eminence of the infundibulum
(B) Paraventricular nucleus of the hypothalamus
(C) Pars distalis of the anterior pituitary
(D) Pars nervosa of the posterior pituitary
(E) Pars tuberalis of the anterior pituitary

13 Immunohistochemical methods are used to identify a subset of axons in the posterior pituitary that contain oxytocin and its intracellular-binding protein (neurophysin). Following release from these terminal axons, oxytocin travels through the circulation and binds to G protein–coupled receptors on the surface of which of the following types of cells?
(A) Clara cells
(B) Granulosa cells
(C) Parietal cells
(D) Primary oocytes
(E) Smooth muscle cells

14 A section through the pituitary gland is examined at autopsy. The cystic, epithelial structures observed between the pars nervosa and the pars distalis (indicated by arrows in the image) are most likely remnants of which of the following embryonic cells or tissues?

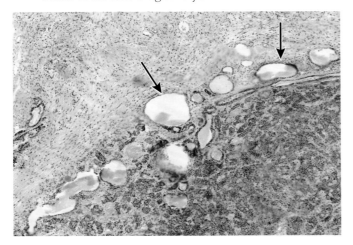

(A) Coelomic epithelium
(B) Neural crest cells
(C) Oral (pharyngeal) ectoderm
(D) Pharyngeal pouch mesenchyme
(E) Primitive gut endoderm

15 The hypothalamo–hypophyseal portal system conveys releasing hormones (neuropeptides) from the median eminence of the hypothalamus directly to which of the following anatomic locations?
(A) Infundibular nucleus of the hypothalamus
(B) Paraventricular nucleus of the hypothalamus
(C) Pars distalis of the anterior pituitary
(D) Pars nervosa of the posterior pituitary
(E) Supraoptic nucleus of the hypothalamus

16 At autopsy, a section of the hypothalamus and pituitary is stained by H&E and examined at high magnification (shown in the image). Based on the diversity of cellular morphology and the variable staining patterns (acidophils, basophils, and chromophobes), you believe that

this image was most likely obtained from which of the following locations?

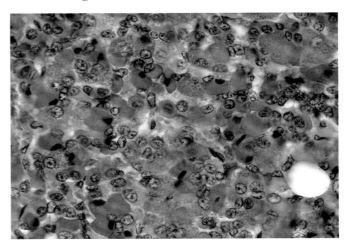

(A) Infundibular nucleus of the hypothalamus
(B) Paraventricular nucleus of the hypothalamus
(C) Pars distalis of the adenohypophysis
(D) Pars nervosa of the neurohypophysis
(E) Supraoptic nucleus of the hypothalamus

17 A subset of the cells described in Question 16 synthesize and secrete timed pulses of FSH and LH that regulate the ovarian cycle and ovulation. These gonadotropins enter the systemic circulation through which of the following vascular beds?
(A) Primary plexus of the median eminence
(B) Primary plexus of the pars distalis
(C) Primary plexus of the pars nervosa
(D) Secondary plexus of the median eminence
(E) Secondary plexus of the pars distalis

18 Binding of FSH to the plasma membranes of follicular epithelial cells in the ovary is known to activate G protein–coupled receptors that regulate the maturation of ovarian follicles. FSH receptor binding stimulates the production of which of the following second messenger molecules in ovarian follicular cells?
(A) Arachidonic acid
(B) Calcium
(C) cAMP
(D) Diacylglycerol
(E) Inositol triphosphate

19 A 33-year-old woman who is not pregnant complains of headaches and irregular menses. On physical examination, the breasts are firm and producing milk. MRI of the patient's head shows a tumor of the anterior pituitary (arrow shown on the radiograph). Which of the following pituitary tumors is the most likely cause of these clinical and pathologic findings?

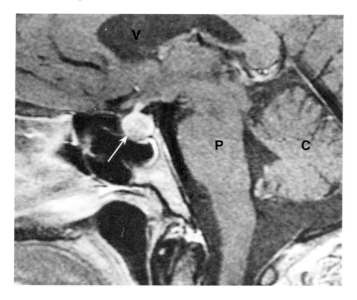

(A) Corticotroph adenoma
(B) Gonadotroph adenoma
(C) Lactotroph adenoma
(D) Somatotroph adenoma
(E) Thyrotroph adenoma

20 Which of the following cells helps to organize clusters of glandular epithelial cells in the pars distalis of the anterior pituitary?
(A) Fibrous astrocytes
(B) Folliculostellate cells
(C) Pituicytes
(D) Reticuloepithelial cells
(E) Satellite cells

21 A 52-year-old woman complains of swelling in the anterior portion of her neck that she first noticed 6 months ago. Except for some discomfort during swallowing, the patient does not report any significant symptoms. Laboratory studies show elevated serum levels of thyroid hormones (T_3 and T_4). These tyrosine-based polypeptide hormones are synthesized and secreted by which of the following endocrine cells?
(A) Chief cells
(B) Follicular cells
(C) Leydig cells
(D) Oxyphil cells
(E) Parafollicular cells

22 Physical examination of the patient described in Question 21 reveals a symmetrically enlarged thyroid gland (goiter). A portion of the goitrous thyroid is removed for cosmetic reasons. Which of the following terms best describes the material filling the lumens of the follicles shown in the image?

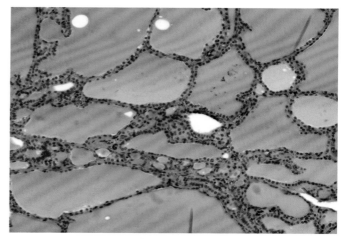

(A) Amyloid
(B) Colloid
(C) Fibrin
(D) Hyaline
(E) Mucin

23 For the patient described in Questions 21 and 22, which of the following terms best describes the biochemical composition of the material stored within the thyroid follicles?
(A) Complex carbohydrate
(B) Glycoprotein
(C) Pentapeptide
(D) Proteoglycan
(E) Steroid

24 You are asked to present a seminar on the pharmacogenetics of thyroid hormone secretion. Which of the following types of enzymes is required for the conversion of iodinated thyroglobulin to active thyroid hormones (T_3 and T_4) in the cytoplasm of follicular epithelial cells?
(A) Glycosyltransferase
(B) Lysosomal protease
(C) Myeloperoxidase
(D) Serine phosphatase
(E) Tyrosine kinase

25 A 48-year-old woman presents with flank pain. Laboratory studies show elevated serum levels of parathyroid hormone (PTH) and calcium. Imaging studies reveal stones in the patient's right renal pelvis and ureter. Which of the following endocrine cells secretes a polypeptide hormone that opposes the action of PTH and decreases serum calcium levels in this patient?
(A) Chief cells
(B) Follicular cells
(C) Leydig cells
(D) Oxyphil cells
(E) Parafollicular cells

26 A sample of the thyroid gland is collected at autopsy and embedded in plastic for computer-based morphometric analysis. Thin (1.5 μm) sections are stained with H&E and examined by light microscopy (shown in the image). Identify the clear cells within the circle.

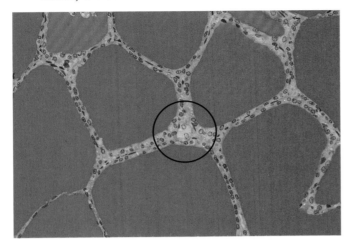

(A) Chief cells
(B) Follicular cells
(C) Macrophages
(D) Oxyphil cells
(E) Parafollicular cells

27 The cells identified in Question 26 are derived from which of the following cells/tissues during embryonic development?
(A) Coelomic epithelium
(B) Neural crest
(C) Oral (pharyngeal) ectoderm
(D) Paraxial mesoderm
(E) Primitive gut endoderm

28 A thyroid biopsy is obtained from a 46-year-old woman with an enlarged thyroid gland (shown in the image). The pathologist notes clear vacuoles (arrows shown in the image) in the colloid, next to the apical surface of the follicular epithelium. What is the biological significance of this histologic finding?

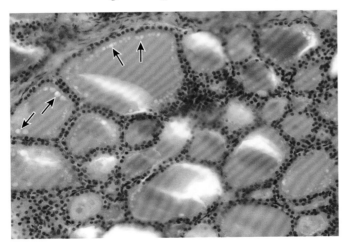

(A) Accumulation of procalcitonin
(B) Decreased section of triglycerides
(C) Decreased thyroglobulin synthesis
(D) Increased secretion of triglycerides
(E) Increased thyroglobulin uptake

29 Which of the following best describes the average epithelial morphology of a hypoactive thyroid gland?
(A) Pseudostratified columnar
(B) Simple columnar
(C) Simple squamous
(D) Stratified cuboidal
(E) Stratified squamous

30 As part of your research on mechanisms of thyroid hormone secretion, you develop a monoclonal antibody directed against the sodium/iodide cotransporter (symporter). Using indirect immunofluorescence assays, you demonstrate that this antibody specifically binds (labels) which of the following cells and membranes within the thyroid gland?
(A) Apical membranes of capillary endothelial cells
(B) Apical membranes of follicular epithelial cells
(C) Basolateral membranes of capillary endothelial cells
(D) Basolateral membranes of follicular epithelial cells
(E) Plasma membranes of parafollicular cells

31 A 36-year-old woman undergoes surgery to remove a follicular carcinoma of the thyroid. Normal tissue (shown in the image) along the margin of the surgical specimen is examined by light microscopy in the hospital. Identify the tissue/structure indicated by the arrow.

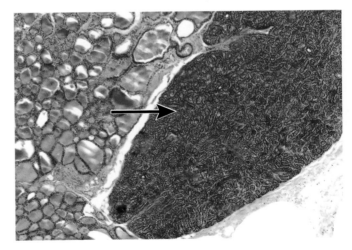

(A) Cervical ganglion
(B) Diffuse lymphatic tissue
(C) Parathyroid gland
(D) Thyroid gland
(E) Vagus nerve

32 A parathyroid gland collected at autopsy is stained with H&E and examined by light microscopy (shown in the image). Which of the following best describes the organization of principal cells in this specimen?

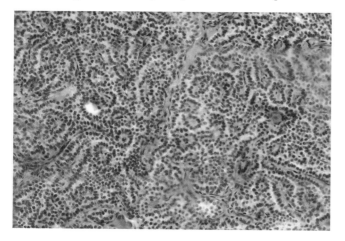

(A) Cords of epithelial cells separated by fenestrated capillaries
(B) Epithelial follicles filled with gelatinous glycoprotein
(C) Isolated polygonal cells embedded in a pseudostratified epithelium
(D) Pyramidal-shaped acinar cells lining a central lumen
(E) Simple squamous epithelial cells lining open vascular spaces

33 A 72-year-old man complains of abdominal discomfort. Physical examination reveals neuromuscular weakness. Laboratory studies show markedly elevated levels of serum calcium and parathyroid hormone (PTH). This polypeptide hormone is synthesized and secreted by which of the following endocrine cells?

(A) Chief cells
(B) Follicular cells
(C) Oxyphil cells
(D) Parafollicular cells
(E) Parietal cells

34 The parathyroid glands (shown in the image) are examined at the autopsy of an 84-year-old woman. Identify the large eosinophilic cells indicated by the arrows.

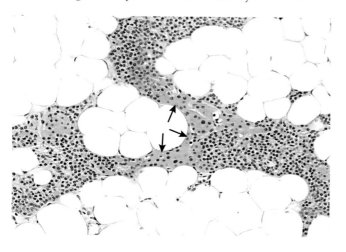

(A) Chief cells
(B) Follicular cells
(C) Oxyphil cells
(D) Parafollicular
(E) Parietal cells

35 You are asked to discuss your research on parathyroid gland pathophysiology at a national conference on "aging and the endocrine system." Which of the following cells is expected to be relatively more abundant in the parathyroid glands of an elderly patient, compared to a younger patient?

(A) Adipocytes
(B) Chief cells
(C) Endothelial cells
(D) Fibroblasts
(E) Macrophages

36 The internal organs of a 54-year-old woman who died of breast cancer are examined at autopsy. An H&E-stained section of a retroperitoneal organ is shown in the image. The pale-staining parenchymal cells that surround the central vein (indicated by the arrow) are identified as which of the following types of cells?

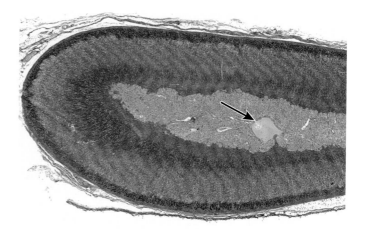

(A) Chromaffin cells
(B) Clara cells
(C) Merkel cells
(D) Parietal cells
(E) Schwann cells

37 Imaging studies demonstrate a suprarenal mass in a 50-year-old woman with a history of hypertension (indicated by the arrow on the radiograph). Histologic examination of the surgical specimen reveals a chromaffin cell neoplasm. Chromaffin cells are derived from which of the following cells/tissues during embryonic development?

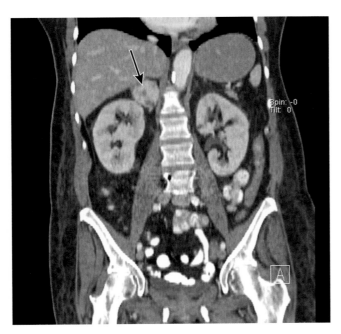

(A) Coelomic epithelium
(B) Endoderm of primitive gut
(C) Neural crest
(D) Oral (pharyngeal) ectoderm
(E) Pharyngeal pouch mesenchyme

38 A 24-year-old skydiver asks you about the physiology of the "adrenaline rush" that she experiences when jumping from airplanes. Which of the following neurotransmitters stimulates the release of adrenalins from chromaffin cells in the adrenal medulla?
(A) Acetylcholine
(B) Dopamine
(C) Glutamate
(D) Norepinephrine
(E) Serotonin

39 A high-magnification view of the adrenal gland and central vein is shown in the image. Which of the following proteins provides a useful marker for dense core, secretory granules in the cytoplasm of these neuroendocrine cells?

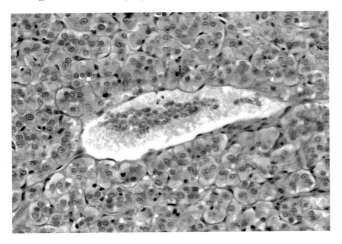

(A) Chromogranin
(B) Connexin
(C) Eumelanin
(D) Netrin
(E) Neurophysin

40 A section of the adrenal gland collected at autopsy is stained with H&E and examined by light microscopy. Name the region of the gland indicated by the rectangular box shown in the image.

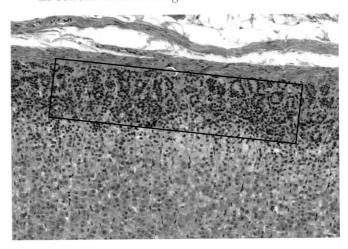

(A) Capsule
(B) Medulla
(C) Zona fasciculata
(D) Zona glomerulosa
(E) Zona reticularis

41 A 40-year-old woman complains of recent changes in her bodily appearance, including upper truncal weight gain and moon facies. Endocrine studies reveal elevated serum levels of cortisol and corticotropin (ACTH). The patient is subsequently diagnosed with Cushing disease. ACTH is synthesized primarily by endocrine cells in which of the following anatomic locations?
(A) Adrenal cortex, zona fasciculata
(B) Adrenal cortex, zona glomerulosa
(C) Adrenal cortex, zona reticularis
(D) Anterior pituitary
(E) Neurohypophysis

42 A 53-year-old man complains of muscle weakness and dizziness of 3 months' duration. His blood pressure is elevated (185/100 mm Hg). Endocrine studies reveal elevated serum levels of aldosterone. Cells in which of the following anatomic locations secrete this mineralocorticoid?
(A) Adrenal cortex, zona fasciculata
(B) Adrenal cortex, zona glomerulosa
(C) Adrenal cortex, zona reticularis
(D) Adrenal medulla
(E) Anterior pituitary

43 Another section of the adrenal gland (shown in the image) collected at autopsy shows long, parallel cords of epithelial cells separated by sinusoidal capillaries. These histologic features are characteristic of which of the following zones or regions?

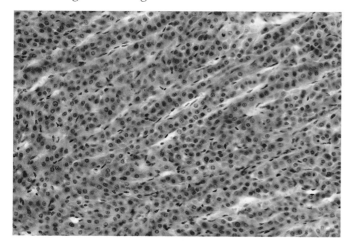

(A) Capsule
(B) Medulla
(C) Zona fasciculata
(D) Zona glomerulosa
(E) Zona reticularis

44 A high-magnification view of the adrenal cortex is examined by light microscopy (shown in the image). Which of the following cytologic features best characterizes the glandular epithelial cells in this specimen?

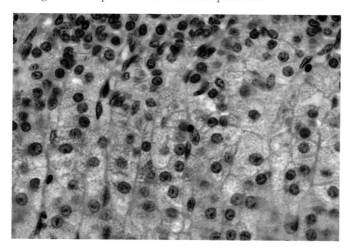

(A) Apical membrane microvilli
(B) Dense, membrane-bound secretory granules
(C) Glycogen-filled vacuoles
(D) Intracellular lipid droplets
(E) Segmented nuclei

45 A 44-year-old woman suffers from long-standing peptic ulcer disease that is largely unresponsive to pharmacologic therapy. Laboratory studies reveal high serum levels of gastrin. If this patient has a gastrin-secreting tumor, then imaging studies would most likely reveal a mass in which of the following organs/glands?

(A) Adrenals
(B) Pancreas
(C) Parathyroids
(D) Pituitary
(E) Thyroid

46 You are asked to discuss the neuropharmacology of the pineal gland at a conference on "advances in psychobiology." What is the principal hormone produced by the pineal gland located in the posterior wall of the third ventricle of the brain?

(A) Dopamine
(B) β-Endorphin
(C) Melatonin
(D) Proopiomelanocortin
(E) Serotonin

47 A newborn is discovered to have ambiguous genitalia (shown in the image). Virilization of female genitalia in this neonate was most likely caused by increased production of androgens by fetal cells located in which of the following endocrine organs?

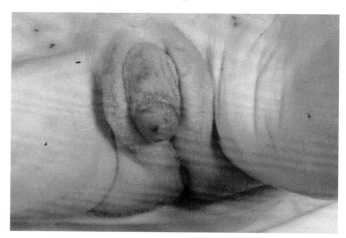

(A) Adrenal glands
(B) Ovaries
(C) Pancreas
(D) Pituitary gland
(E) Thyroid gland

48 What is the major source of cholesterol present in the foamy cytoplasm of spongiocytes in the zona fasciculata of the adrenal cortex?

(A) Chylomicrons
(B) De novo biosynthesis
(C) High-density lipoproteins
(D) Low-density lipoproteins
(E) Very low-density lipoproteins

ANSWERS

1 **The answer is B: Pancreatic islet.** This autopsy specimen shows an islet of Langerhans in the pancreas, surrounded by exocrine acini. The pancreas contains millions of islets, primarily in the tail of the pancreas. These microglands regulate blood glucose levels. The functional cell types in the islets of Langerhans include alpha (α), beta (β), and delta (δ) cells. Each cell type produces a different polypeptide hormone (e.g., insulin, glucagon, or somatostatin). Patients with multiple endocrine neoplasia (MEN) syndromes have gene mutations that make them susceptible to neoplasia or hyperplasia of multiple organs. For example, patients with MEN 2A (Sipple syndrome) develop medullary carcinoma of the thyroid and pheochromocytoma of the adrenal medulla. One-third of these patients also exhibit hyperparathyroidism as a result of parathyroid hyperplasia or parathyroid adenoma. None of the other choices feature the distinctive morphology of pancreatic islets.
Keywords: Pancreas, islets of Langerhans, multiple endocrine neoplasia

2 **The answer is D: Immunostaining property.** Pancreatic islets contain a variable number of cells, ranging from only a few cells, to many hundreds of cells. Each endocrine cell typically secretes one polypeptide hormone. Monospecific antibodies directed to unique polypeptide chains can be used to identify specific hormone-producing cells (e.g., insulin- or glucagon-producing cells). None of the other choices provide a reliable basis for distinguishing between types of functional cells in the endocrine pancreas.
Keywords: Pancreas, islets of Langerhans

3 **The answer is B: Beta cells.** Type 1 diabetes mellitus (T1DM) is a lifelong disorder of glucose homeostasis that results from the autoimmune destruction of the beta (β) cells in the islets of Langerhans. The clinical onset of T1DM often coincides with another acute illness, such as a febrile viral or bacterial infection. The disease is characterized by few (if any) functional beta cells in the islets of Langerhans and limited or absent insulin secretion. Alpha cells (choice A) secrete glucagon. Delta cells (choice C) secrete somatostatin. F cells (also termed PP cells) (choices D and E) secrete pancreatic polypeptide, which stimulates gastric chief cells and inhibits intestinal motility.
Keywords: Pancreas, islets of Langerhans, diabetes mellitus

4 **The answer is D: Pituitary gland.** This patient experienced postpartum ischemic necrosis of the pituitary gland (Sheehan syndrome). This rare complication of labor and delivery may occur following a severe drop in blood pressure (hypotension) induced by postpartum hemorrhage. The pituitary is particularly susceptible at this time, because its enlargement during pregnancy renders it vulnerable to a reduction in blood flow. The varied clinical manifestations of Sheehan syndrome are related to panhypopituitarism. These clinical manifestations include pallor (decreased MSH), hypothyroidism (decreased TSH), failure of lactation (decreased prolactin), adrenal insufficiency (decreased ACTH), and ovarian failure (decreased FSH and LH). Injury to the other endocrine organs would not lead to the constellation of hormonal insufficiencies observed in this patient.
Keywords: Pituitary, Sheehan syndrome

5 **The answer is D: Parafollicular cells of the thyroid.** Hormones are molecules that "set in motion" the metabolic activities of cells, tissues, and organs. These regulatory molecules (hundreds of unique molecules) are typically released into the circulatory system for distribution throughout the body (endocrine signaling). Hormones may also travel through hydrated interstitial space (tissue compartments). Hormones are classified chemically as steroids, polypeptides, or amino acids. They exhibit target specificity, because nuclear and cell surface receptors display restricted patterns of developmental expression. Neuroendocrine cells, such as parafollicular cells of the thyroid, typically store hormones within membrane-bound dense core granules. These secretory granules provide a useful EM marker for the diagnosis of certain poorly differentiated tumors. The other endocrine cells synthesize steroid hormones and do not contain dense core, membrane-bound secretory granules.
Keywords: Thyroid gland, parafollicular cells

6 **The answer is E: Thyroid gland.** Cretinism denotes physical and mental insufficiency that is secondary to congenital hypothyroidism. Iodination of salt has reduced the incidence of cretinism in the United States and other countries. The most common cause of neonatal hypothyroidism today is agenesis of the thyroid, which occurs at a rate of 1 in 4,000 newborns. Hypothyroidism in pregnant women also has grave neurologic consequences for the fetus, expressed after birth as cretinism. Symptoms of congenital hypothyroidism appear in the early weeks of life and include sluggishness, low body temperature, and anemia. Mental retardation, stunted growth, and characteristic facies become evident. If thyroid hormone replacement therapy is not promptly provided, congenital hypothyroidism results in mentally retarded dwarfs. None of the other choices produce the signs and symptoms of cretinism.
Keywords: Thyroid gland, cretinism

7 **The answer is D: Pars nervosa of the neurohypophysis.** The pituitary gland (hypophysis) is located at the base of the brain within the sella turcica (L: Turkish saddle). This "master gland" has two components: the posterior lobe (neurohypophysis) and the anterior lobe (adenohypophysis).

The posterior lobe of the pituitary shown in the image is composed of lipid-rich (pale staining) nonmyelinated axons, supporting glial cells, and capillary endothelial cells. The hypothalamus (choice B) is not visible in the image but is located superior to the pituitary in the brain. Hormonal secretions of the hypothalamus regulate pituitary function. The anterior lobe of the pituitary (choice C) is visible on the left side of the image. This lobe features small cords of glandular epithelial cells. None of the other choices exhibit the distinctive morphologic features of the neurohypophysis.

Keywords: Pituitary, neurohypophysis

8 The answer is A: Median eminence of the infundibulum. The pituitary is derived from two different tissues during embryogenesis. The anterior lobe is derived from an evagination from the roof of the oropharynx (oral ectoderm). By contrast, the posterior pituitary is derived from a downgrowth of neuroectoderm from the diencephalon of the developing forebrain. This funnel-shaped downgrowth is referred to as the infundibulum (pituitary stalk). The portion of the infundibulum that is continuous with the hypothalamus is referred to as the median eminence. The arrows in the image indicate a portion of the infundibulum that contains neurosecretory axons emanating from the hypothalamus. These nerve axons form the hypothalamo–hypophyseal tract. The pars tuberalis of the adenohypophysis (choice E) is visible in the image as glandular tissue along the margins of the pars nervosa. None of the other choices exhibit the distinctive morphologic features of the infundibulum.

Keywords: Pituitary, infundibulum

9 The answer is D: Pituicytes. Pituicytes are specialized glial cells present in the pars nervosa of the posterior pituitary. They support and nourish the terminal axons that originate in specific hypothalamic nuclei. They display an intricate stellate morphology, similar to astroglial cells of the CNS. Microglial cells (choice A) are phagocytic cells of the CNS. Although axons are present in the pars nervosa, the nucleated nerve cell bodies (choice B) are located in supraoptic and paraventricular nuclei of the hypothalamus. Oligodendrocytes (choice C) provide myelin sheaths to axons in the CNS; however, the axons in the posterior pituitary are nonmyelinated nerve fibers. Schwann cells (choice E) provide myelin to peripheral nerve fibers.

Keywords: Pituitary, pituicytes

10 The answer is B: Herring bodies. Axon terminals in the posterior pituitary are dilated, owing to an abundance of membrane-bound neurosecretory vesicles. These dilated portions of terminal axons are termed Herring bodies, after Percy Theodore Herring, who first described them in 1908. Corpora amylacea (choice A) are protein concretions found in the prostate glands of elderly

men. Neurokeratin vacuoles and neurophysin droplets (choices C and D) do not contain dense core secretory vesicles. Nissl substance (choice E) refers to a basophilic region of the neuronal cell body (soma) that features an abundance of rough endoplasmic reticulum and ribosomes.

Keywords: Pituitary, Herring bodies

11 The answer is C: Hypothalamus. Herring bodies in the posterior pituitary store oxytocin and antidiuretic hormone (ADH). These powerful nonapeptide hormones are synthesized in supraoptic and paraventricular hypothalamic nuclei, respectively. They are liberated from high molecular weight prohormones (neurophysins) via proteolytic cleavage during axonal transport. The patient described in this clinical vignette has diabetes insipidus. Diabetes insipidus is characterized by an inability to concentrate the urine, with consequent chronic water diuresis, thirst, and polydipsia. The disease reflects a deficiency of ADH (arginine vasopressin), which is secreted from the posterior pituitary under the influence of the hypothalamus. ADH signals epithelial cells of the renal collecting ducts to reabsorb water to help maintain blood volume and regulate the osmolarity of body fluids. None of the other endocrine tissues synthesize or secrete ADH.

Keywords: Diabetes insipidus, antidiuretic hormone

12 The answer is D: Pars nervosa of the posterior pituitary. Following exocytosis from terminal axons, ADH enters fenestrated (windowed) capillaries within the pars nervosa of the posterior pituitary. These capillaries represent terminal branches of paired inferior hypophyseal arteries that arise from the paired internal carotid arteries. ADH is not released via the hypophyseal portal circulation (choices A, C, and E), nor is it released to the systemic circulation in the hypothalamus (choice B).

Keywords: Pituitary, arginine vasopressin

13 The answer is E: Smooth muscle cells. Oxytocin stimulates the contraction of (1) smooth muscle cells in the myometrium of the uterus during orgasm, menstruation, and parturition and (2) myoepithelial cells associated with breast ducts and alveoli during breast-feeding and milk ejection. Synthetic analogs of oxytocin are used clinically to initiate or accelerate the pace of labor and delivery. Oxytocin has been suggested to play a role in pair bonding and has been described recently as the "cuddle hormone." None of the other cells express receptors for oxytocin.

Keywords: Pituitary, oxytocin

14 The answer is C: Oral (pharyngeal) ectoderm. The anterior pituitary is derived from an evagination of the oropharynx during embryonic development that is referred to as Rathke pouch. It is named after Martin Rathke, who first described it in 1839. Rathke pouch makes contact with

a downgrowth from the diencephalon to form the pituitary gland. Remnants of Rathke pouch are preserved as cystic epithelial structures located between the pars nervosa and the pars distalis. These cystic structures can give rise to epithelial tumors that invade and compress adjacent tissues. Destruction of the posterior lobe of the pituitary, the source of ADH, causes diabetes insipidus (see Question 11). One-fourth of the cases of diabetes insipidus are associated with brain tumors, particularly craniopharyngiomas. This tumor arises above the sella turcica from remnants of Rathke pouch. None of the other choices contribute to the formation of the pituitary gland during embryonic development.
Keywords: Pituitary, Rathke pouch

15 The answer is C: Pars distalis of the anterior pituitary. Neuropeptides that regulate the metabolic and secretory functions of the anterior pituitary are synthesized by neurons in the hypothalamus and conveyed to the median eminence of the infundibulum via nerve axons that run along the hypothalamo–hypophyseal tract. After their release in the median eminence, these neuropeptides enter a primary capillary plexus and are distributed via portal veins of the hypothalamus–hypophyseal portal system to the pars distalis of the anterior pituitary. The hypothalamo–hypophyseal portal system does not convey hypothalamic hormones by a direct route to the other choices listed.
Keywords: Pituitary, portal circulation

16 The answer is C: Pars distalis of the adenohypophysis. The anterior lobe of the pituitary is composed of small cords of glandular epithelial cells separated by sinusoidal capillaries. These cells respond to hormonal signals from the hypothalamus and secrete many polypeptide hormones, including FSH, LH, ACTH, TSH, MSH, PRL, and GH (somatotropin). Each cell typically secretes one or a limited number of protein hormones. Immunohistochemical assays are useful for identifying cells that produce a particular polypeptide hormone. Based on their H&E staining properties, glandular epithelial cells of the anterior pituitary are classified as acidophils, basophils, or chromophobes. None of the other tissues exhibit the distinctive histologic features of the pars distalis of the anterior pituitary.
Keywords: Pituitary, adenohypophysis

17 The answer is E: Secondary plexus of the pars distalis. Polypeptide hormones released from endocrine cells in the anterior pituitary enter sinusoidal capillaries for distribution to the systemic circulation. The vascular bed within the pars distalis of the anterior pituitary is referred to as the secondary capillary plexus. Most of the venous blood from the pituitary gland drains to the cavernous sinus. The primary capillary plexus (choice A) is located upstream of the pituitary portal system in the median eminence of the infundibulum.

None of the other choices describe the process of gonadotropin release from the anterior pituitary.
Keywords: Pituitary, portal circulation

18 The answer is C: cAMP. Binding of FSH to its G protein–coupled receptor leads to the activation of adenylate cyclase and the production of cAMP. Most polypeptide hormone signaling pathways involve membrane-associated G proteins that activate the cyclic adenosine monophosphate (cAMP) system. This second messenger system serves to amplify the primary hormonal signal and initiate (1) complex changes in cellular physiology and (2) altered patterns of gene expression. None of the other second messenger molecules plays a primary role in FSH-mediated signal transduction in the ovary.
Keywords: Ovary, follicular cells

19 The answer is C: Lactotroph adenoma. Pituitary adenomas are benign neoplasms of glandular epithelial cells of the anterior lobe of the pituitary. They may be associated with excess secretion of specific pituitary hormones (endocrine hyperfunction). They occur in both sexes at almost any age but are more common in men between the ages of 20 and 50 years. Hyperprolactinemia is the most common endocrinopathy associated with pituitary adenoma. Almost half of all pituitary adenomas synthesize prolactin (PRL). Functional lactotroph adenomas lead to amenorrhea, galactorrhea, and infertility in women and erectile dysfunction in men. The set of answer choices for this question represents tumors arising from the five functional types of cells in the pars distalis of the anterior pituitary. None of the other tumors secrete PRL or lead to galactorrhea.
Keywords: Pituitary adenoma, galactorrhea

20 The answer is B: Folliculostellate cells. In addition to hormone-producing cells (gonadotropes, thyrotropes, and corticotropes), the anterior pituitary is home to folliculostellate cells that organize the secretory cells. These large, stellate cells communicate with one another through gap junctions. Their long, star-shaped cytoplasmic processes encircle the clusters of hormone-producing cells. Fibrous astrocytes (choice A) and satellite cells (choice E) provide support for neurons in the CNS and autonomic ganglia, respectively. Pituicytes (choice C) are found in the posterior pituitary, where they support terminal nerve fibers. Reticuloepithelial cells (choice D) are found in the thymus, where they coordinate positive and negative selection of immature thymocytes.
Keywords: Pituitary, folliculostellate cells

21 The answer is B: Follicular cells. The thyroid gland is composed of numerous hollow, spherical structures (follicles) lined by a simple epithelium. The apical surface of these cells faces the follicular lumen, whereas the basal surface of these cells rests on an extracellular basal lamina. Follicular epithelial cells respond to TSH,

which is secreted by the anterior pituitary. Follicular cells synthesize, store, and secrete thyroid hormones (T_3 and T_4). These iodinated, tyrosine-based hormones regulate growth and development, as well as general body metabolism and heat production. Chief cells (choice A) secrete gastric enzymes (e.g., pepsin). Leydig interstitial cells (choice C) secrete testosterone. Oxyphil cells (choice D) are present in the parathyroid gland. Parafollicular cells (choice E) represent a minor endocrine cell population in the thyroid gland.
Keywords: Thyroid gland, follicular cells

22 The answer is B: Colloid. The gelatinous material stored within thyroid follicles is referred to as colloid. This distinguishing feature of the thyroid gland represents a large store of the thyroid hormone precursor (3-month supply). Enlarged thyroid glands are referred to as goiters. They range from double the size of a normal gland (40 g) to massive thyroid glands weighing hundreds of grams. Microscopically, the epithelial cells of nontoxic goiters exhibit hypertrophy and hyperplasia. Amyloid (choice A) represents extracellular deposits of abnormal fibrillar proteins. Fibrin (choice C) is the insoluble end product of the coagulation cascade. Hyaline (choice D) is a descriptive term for eosinophilic inclusions and deposits that are associated with various normal and pathologic conditions. Mucins (choice E) are hydrophilic polysaccharide chains that protect and lubricate delicate mucous membranes.
Keywords: Thyroid gland, colloid, goiter

23 The answer is B: Glycoprotein. The principal biochemical component of colloid is thyroglobulin, a large (660 kDa) glycoprotein. This prohormone undergoes sequential oxidation (via thyroid peroxidase) and iodination of specific tyrosine residues. Glycogen and starch are examples of complex carbohydrates (choice A). Proteoglycans (choice D) are composed of a core protein and specific glycosaminoglycan side chains. None of the other choices describe the chemical nature of thyroglobulin.
Keywords: Thyroid gland, colloid, thyroglobulin

24 The answer is B: Lysosomal protease. When stimulated with TSH, follicular epithelial cells absorb thyroglobulin from colloid by receptor-mediated endocytosis. Endosomes containing thyroglobulin are referred to as "colloidal resorption droplets." These endosomes fuse with existing lysosomes. Proteases within lysosomes degrade high molecular weight thyroglobulin and release the low molecular weight active hormones: triiodothyronine (T_3) and thyroxine (T_4). T_4 is more abundant than T_3 in the circulation (20:1). It is converted to T_3 (the more potent hormone) within target organs such as the kidney, liver, and heart. Iodine deficiency causes hypertrophy and hyperplasia of follicular epithelial cells (goiter), because the feedback loop that turns off TSH secretion from the anterior pituitary cannot take place without iodinated thyroid hormones. None of the other

enzymes participate in the intracellular processing of thyroglobulin to generate thyroid hormones.
Keywords: Thyroglobulin, thyroid gland, follicular cells

25 The answer is E: Parafollicular cells. The action of PTH to increase serum calcium levels is opposed by the action of calcitonin. Calcitonin is a 32-amino-acid polypeptide that is secreted by parafollicular cells (C cells) of the thyroid gland. Calcitonin rapidly decreases serum calcium levels and opposes the action of PTH to maintain calcium homeostasis. Levels of blood calcium regulate the secretion of calcitonin by parafollicular cells. Chief cells (choice A) secrete PTH. Follicular cells (choice B) secrete thyroid hormone. Leydig cells (choice C) secrete testosterone. Oxyphil cells (choice D) are nonsecretory cells of the parathyroid glands.
Keywords: Thyroid gland, parafollicular cells

26 The answer is E: Parafollicular cells. The circle in the image identifies large clear cells (C cells) in the connective tissue between adjacent thyroid follicles. These parafollicular cells are scattered throughout the thyroid gland. They are present within the basal lamina of follicles and as isolated clusters between follicles. EM studies of parafollicular cells reveal an abundance of membrane-bound, dense core secretory granules. Follicular cells (choice B) are not found outside the basal lamina. None of the other cells are found in the thyroid gland.
Keywords: Thyroid gland, parafollicular cells

27 The answer is B: Neural crest. The thyroid gland forms during early development as an endodermal outpouching (thyroglossal duct) of the foregut (choice E). Parafollicular cells, however, arise from neural crest cells that are set aside as "ultimobranchial bodies" within paired branchial pouches. These ultimobranchial bodies eventually fuse with the primordium of the thyroid gland, and the neural crest cells are dispersed among the developing thyroid follicles. Oral ectoderm (choice C) gives rise to the anterior lobe of the pituitary. Paraxial mesoderm (choice D) arises during gastrulation and gives rise to the paired somites. None of the other choices describe the embryonic origin of parafollicular cells of the thyroid gland.
Keywords: Neural crest, parafollicular cells

28 The answer is E: Increased thyroglobulin uptake. The clear vacuoles observed in this image are visual evidence of thyroglobulin uptake by activated epithelial cells. When stimulated by TSH, activated follicular epithelial cells "drink" colloid for the processing of thyroglobulin and the export of active thyroid hormones T_3 and T_4. Procalcitonin (choice A) is the precursor polypeptide for calcitonin. It is not stored within the lumens of the thyroid follicles. None of the other choices describe the process of thyroglobulin uptake by follicular epithelial cells.
Keywords: Goiter, thyroid gland, colloid

29 **The answer is C: Simple squamous.** Morphology of cells and tissues provides important clues to understanding biological function. For example, active thyroid glands have follicles lined by columnar cells (choice B), whereas hypoactive glands have follicles lined by squamous or low cuboidal epithelial cells (correct answer, choice C). Stratified or pseudostratified epithelia (choices A, D, and E) are not found in the thyroid gland.
Keywords: Thyroid gland, follicular cells

30 **The answer is D: Basolateral membranes of follicular epithelial cells.** Follicular cells of the thyroid sequester iodide from the circulation using an ATPase-dependent sodium/iodide cotransporter (symporter). This transmembrane protein localizes to the basolateral membranes of epithelial cells and is therefore in close proximity to the blood supply. Once within the cytoplasm of the epithelial cells, iodide is pumped into the lumens of thyroid follicles by an iodide/chloride transporter termed pendrin. Here, iodide undergoes oxidation to form iodine—the active chemical element that forms covalent bonds with tyrosine residues of thyroglobulin. The sodium/iodide symporter does not distribute or localize to the other membrane domains.
Keywords: Thyroid gland, colloid, thyroid hormone

31 **The answer is C: Parathyroid gland.** The tissue identified in this surgical specimen is a normal parathyroid gland. These small, oval-shaped glands are typically located in the connective tissue along the posterior wall of the thyroid gland, but they may be found in various ectopic locations. Most individuals have four parathyroid glands (two superior and two inferior). None of the other anatomic structures describe the distinctive morphologic features of the parathyroid glands.
Keywords: Parathyroid glands

32 **The answer is A: Cords of epithelial cells separated by fenestrated capillaries.** The parathyroid glands are composed of small nests or cords of densely packed glandular epithelial cells, separated by discontinuous fenestrated capillaries. Epithelial follicles (choice B) are found in the thyroid gland. Pyramidal-shaped acinar cells (choice D) are a characteristic feature of many exocrine glands. Simple squamous epithelial cells lining open vascular spaces (choice E) describes endothelial cells of the circulatory system.
Keywords: Parathyroid glands, chief cells

33 **The answer is A: Chief cells.** Parenchymal cells of the parathyroid glands include chief cells and oxyphil cells. Chief cells are more numerous than oxyphil cells. They secrete parathyroid hormone (PTH) in response to decreased levels of serum calcium. Elevated serum levels of PTH in this patient may be due to increased mass of parathyroid tissue (hyperplasia or neoplasia).

This syndrome is referred to as primary hyperparathyroidism. Excessive PTH secretion leads to excessive loss of calcium from the bones and enhanced calcium resorption by the renal tubules. The clinical manifestations of hyperparathyroidism range from asymptomatic hypercalcemia to major constitutional symptoms related to renal stones, bone loss, mental status changes, and abdominal pain. This constellation of clinical features is summarized (memorably) as "stones, bones, moans, and groans." None of the other cells secrete PTH.
Keywords: Parathyroid glands, chief cells, hyperparathyroidism

34 **The answer is C: Oxyphil cells.** The large eosinophilic cells indicated by the arrows in the image are oxyphil cells. These epithelial cells represent a minor cell population in parathyroid glands. They are nonsecretory cells, and their function (if any) remains to be determined. Chief cells (choice A) are the principal cells of the parathyroid glands. They are visible in this image as densely packed polygonal cells with basophilic central nuclei. The large vacuolated cells with peripheral nuclei are adipocytes. Follicular and parafollicular cells (choices B and D) are found in the thyroid gland. Parietal cells (choice E) are gastrin-secreting cells found in the stomach.
Keywords: Parathyroid glands, oxyphil cells

35 **The answer is A: Adipocytes.** The abundance of oxyphil cells and adipocytes in the parathyroid glands increases with advancing age. For example, oxyphil cells do not appear in the parathyroid glands until after the time of puberty, and adipocytes populate the parathyroid glands of the elderly. None of the other cells have been reported to undergo age-related changes in the endocrine organs.
Keywords: Parathyroid glands, adipocytes

36 **The answer is A: Chromaffin cells.** The adrenal (suprarenal) glands are small, flat organs, embedded in fat near the superior poles of the kidneys. This photomicrograph of the adrenal gland shows a pink-stained cortical region surrounding a pale-stained central (medullary) region. The parenchymal cells of the adrenal medulla are termed chromaffin cells. These large epithelioid cells secrete catecholamines—commonly referred to as the "flight-or-fight" hormones. The adrenal medulla has a dual blood supply that arises from (1) medullary arterioles that bypass the adrenal cortex and (2) capillary sinusoids that perfuse the adrenal cortex (adrenocortical sinusoids). The central adrenomedullary vein indicated by the arrow on this image drains to the inferior vena cava. None of the other choices describe the parenchymal cell of the adrenal medulla.
Keywords: Adrenal medulla, chromaffin cells

37 **The answer is C: Neural crest.** Chromaffin cells of the adrenal medulla arise from the neural crest lineage during embryonic development. They represent postganglionic cells of the sympathetic nervous system that populate the adrenal glands. Neoplasms of chromaffin cells in the adult are termed pheochromocytomas. These tumors secrete catecholamines, which cause episodic, malignant hypertension. Mesothelial cells of the coelomic epithelium (choice A) contribute to the development of male and female gonads. Endoderm of the primitive gut (choice B) forms many internal organs, including the liver, gallbladder, and pancreas. Oral ectoderm (choice D) gives rise to Rathke pouch that forms the anterior pituitary. Pharyngeal pouch mesenchyme (choice E) gives rise to many structures in the head and neck, including the thyroid and parathyroid glands.
Keywords: Neural crest, adrenal medulla

38 **The answer is A: Acetylcholine.** The release of adrenalins (epinephrine and norepinephrine) from secretory granules stored in chromaffin cells is stimulated by acetylcholine. This neurotransmitter is released by sympathetic axons (i.e., preganglionic sympathetic nerve endings) that synapse with individual chromaffin cells in the adrenal medulla. Release of epinephrine and norepinephrine to the circulation increases blood pressure, as well as heart rate and respiration rate. None of the other neurotransmitters trigger the release of catecholamines from the adrenal medulla.
Keywords: Adrenal medulla, acetylcholine

39 **The answer is A: Chromogranin.** Epinephrine and norepinephrine are stored in dense core granules within chromaffin cells of the adrenal medulla. These secretory granules also contain binding proteins, termed chromogranins. Antibodies to chromogranins are used routinely to identify neuroendocrine neoplasms, such as neuroblastoma and pheochromocytoma. Eumelanin (choice C) is a pigment protein synthesized by melanocytes of the skin that is derived from the amino acid tyrosine. Connexins (choice B) are gap junction proteins. Netrins (choice D) are involved in axonal path finding during embryonic development. Neurophysins (choice E) are binding proteins for oxytocin and antidiuretic hormone within Herring bodies in the posterior pituitary.
Keywords: Chromaffin cells, chromogranins

40 **The answer is D: Zona glomerulosa.** The adrenal cortex arises from mesoderm during development and undergoes extensive remodeling at the time of birth. Endocrine cells of the adrenal cortex secrete a variety of cholesterol-based steroid hormones. After birth, the permanent cortex is divided structurally and functionally into three discrete zones: zona glomerulosa, zona fasciculata, and zona reticularis. Although there is overlap, each zone typically secretes a characteristic set of steroid hormones. The region of the adrenal cortex indicated on this photomicrograph can be identified as the zona glomerulosa, because of its proximity to the collagenous capsule. The zona glomerulosa is composed of cords of epithelial cells that are continuous with cells of the zona fasciculata. Glomerulosa cells secrete mineralocorticoids that regulate sodium and potassium homeostasis (water balance). None of the other choices describe the distinctive histologic features of the zona glomerulosa of the adrenal cortex.
Keywords: Adrenal glands, cortex

41 **The answer is D: Anterior pituitary.** Cushing *disease* is caused by pituitary tumors that secrete corticotropin (ACTH) resulting in elevated serum levels of cortisol (adrenal hyperfunction). Tumors of the adrenal cortex are also associated with an increase in serum cortisol; however, adrenal hyperfunction in these patients with Cushing *syndrome* is not pituitary dependent. Pituitary-dependent Cushing disease is five times more frequent than Cushing syndrome associated with tumors of the adrenal cortex. Patients with Cushing disease/syndrome commonly present with diabetes mellitus (hyperglycemia) and an accumulation of subcutaneous fat on the posterior neck (buffalo hump). Tumors that arise in the other anatomic locations listed do not secrete ACTH.
Keywords: Pituitary, Cushing disease

42 **The answer is B: Adrenal cortex, zona glomerulosa.** Malignant hypertension and elevated serum levels of aldosterone suggest a diagnosis of Conn syndrome. Primary hyperaldosteronism (Conn syndrome) reflects inappropriate secretion of aldosterone by an adrenal adenoma (75% of cases) or hyperplastic adrenal glands (25% of cases). Most patients with primary aldosteronism are diagnosed after the detection of asymptomatic hypertension. Muscle weakness and fatigue are due to the effects of potassium depletion on skeletal muscle physiology. None of the other tissues secrete aldosterone.
Keywords: Adrenal glands, Conn syndrome

43 **The answer is C: Zona fasciculata.** Endocrine cells in the middle zone of the adrenal cortex are arranged in long, parallel cords separated by sinusoidal capillaries. These cells secrete glucocorticoids that regulate systemic glucose and fatty acid metabolism. None of the other zones/regions of the adrenal gland exhibit the distinctive histologic features of the zona fasciculata.
Keywords: Adrenal glands

44 **The answer is D: Intracellular lipid droplets.** Endocrine cells of the zona fasciculate contain numerous intracellular lipid droplets. Lipid extraction during tissue embedding and processing leaves these cells with a characteristic foamy appearance that can be observed by light microscopy (shown in the image). For this reason, these cells are referred to as spongiocytes. Intracellular lipid droplets provide a store of cholesterol, fatty acids, and phospholipids for the synthesis of steroid hormones. None of the other cytologic features describe the morphology of spongiocytes in the adrenal cortex.

Keywords: Adrenal glands, spongiocytes

45 **The answer is B: Pancreas.** This patient has Zollinger-Ellison syndrome, which is characterized by intractable gastric hypersecretion, severe peptic ulceration of the duodenum, and elevated serum levels of gastrin. The gastrin-secreting tumor responsible for Zollinger-Ellison syndrome is commonly a pancreatic gastrinoma. Gastrinomas are typically located in the pancreas, but they may arise in other parts of the gastrointestinal tract, most notably the duodenum. None of the other endocrine organs secrete gastrin.

Keywords: Pancreas, islets of Langerhans, Zollinger-Ellison syndrome, gastrinoma

46 **The answer is C: Melatonin.** The pineal gland is a neuroendocrine gland that helps regulate day/night (circadian) rhythms. This light-sensitive organ is located in the posterior wall of the third ventricle of the brain. It receives axonal input from the retina via sympathetic fibers that run along the retinohypothalamic tract. The principal hormone secreted by the pineal gland is melatonin (not to be confused with melanin). This tryptamine-based hormone is released primarily in the dark. It appears to regulate gonadal functions, as well as emotional responses to reduced daylight hours during winter at high latitude (seasonal affective disorder). Tumors that destroy the pineal gland are associated with the onset of precocious puberty. None of the other neurotransmitters or hormones are secretory products of the pineal gland.

Keywords: Pineal gland, melatonin, circadian rhythm

47 **The answer is A: Adrenal glands.** This photograph shows a markedly virilized and hypertrophic clitoris and partial fusion of labioscrotal folds in a genetic female. Congenital deficiency in the synthesis of corticosteroids in the adrenal cortex results in excessive secretion of ACTH by the anterior pituitary, resulting in adrenal hyperplasia. The adrenal glands become greatly enlarged, weighing as much as 30 g (normal = 4 g). Adrenal hyperfunction leads to excessive secretion of weak androgens by cells of the zona reticularis, leading to virilization of the female external genitalia that occurs during fetal development. Androgens are cholesterol-based steroid hormones that are secreted by the testes, ovaries, placenta, and the adrenal glands. Congenital deficiency of 21-hydroxylase results in virilization of the external genitalia in female infants and is referred to as adrenogenital syndrome. None of the other organs secrete androgens.

Keywords: Adrenal glands, adrenogenital syndrome

48 **The answer is D: Low-density lipoproteins.** The adrenal cortex can be thought of as a cholesterol uptake, modification, and delivery "factory." These endocrine cells take up cholesterol from the circulation and synthesize various steroid hormones, including aldosterone, cortisol, and dehydroepiandrosterone (a weak androgen). The major source of cholesterol for adrenal cortical cells is low-density lipoproteins present in the blood. Cholesterol is primarily stored within intracellular lipid droplets as cholesterol esters. Chylomicrons (choice A) deliver free fatty acids from the gut to the liver. High-density lipoproteins (choice C) return cholesterol to the liver. None of the other choices provide a major source of cholesterol for adrenal cortical cells (spongiocytes).

Keywords: Adrenal glands, low-density lipoproteins

Chapter 19

Special Sense Organs

QUESTIONS

Select the single best answer.

1 A 56-year-old woman complains of decreased vision in her left eye of 4 years' duration. White discoloration of her left pupil is noted on physical examination (shown in the image). The white appearance of the pupil in this patient represents a pathologic change affecting which of the following components of the eye?

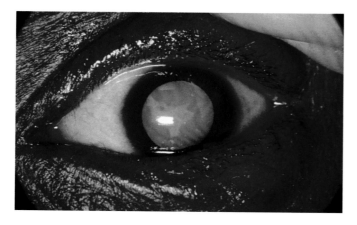

(A) Conjunctiva
(B) Cornea
(C) Iris
(D) Lens
(E) Vitreous body

2 You are looking in the mirror and examining your eye. You notice that your pupils are black. Which of the following structures gives a black appearance to the pupils?
(A) Aqueous humor
(B) Iris
(C) Lens
(D) Uvea
(E) Vitreous body

3 A cornea is obtained and examined by light microscopy (shown in the image). Identify the layer indicated by the double arrow.

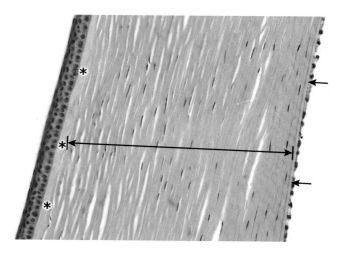

(A) Bowman membrane
(B) Corneal epithelium
(C) Descemet membrane
(D) Endothelium
(E) Stroma

4 In the image shown for Question 3, identify the zone indicated by the asterisk.
(A) Bowman membrane
(B) Corneal endothelium
(C) Corneal epithelium
(D) Descemet membrane
(E) Stroma

5 A 23-year-old man who wears contact lenses complains of severe pain, foreign body sensation, and photophobia in his right eye. Physical examination reveals localized roughening of the corneal epithelium. The patient is subsequently diagnosed with recurrent corneal erosion. Separation between which of the following pairs of structures underlies this patient's condition?
(A) Bowman membrane and corneal stroma
(B) Corneal epithelium and Bowman membrane
(C) Corneal stroma and Descemet membrane
(D) Descemet membrane and corneal endothelium
(E) Neighboring epithelial cells

268

6 A 7-year-old girl complains of pain, excessive tearing, and decreased vision in her left eye. She was diagnosed with a herpes simplex virus infection 6 months ago. Physical examination reveals multiple, minute corneal ulcers. Which of the following structures is primarily affected in this superficial punctate keratopathy?

(A) Corneal endothelium
(B) Corneal epithelium
(C) Iris
(D) Lacrimal gland
(E) Lens

7 Corneal epithelium is composed of which of the following types of tissue?

(A) Keratinized stratified squamous epithelium
(B) Nonkeratinized stratified squamous epithelium
(C) Pseudostratified epithelium
(D) Stratified columnar epithelium
(E) Stratified cuboidal epithelium

8 A 39-year-old woman afflicted with corneal perforation receives a corneal transplant. Her vision is restored. The corneal graft is well tolerated and becomes fully integrated with the patient's other ocular tissues. Which of the following structural features provides the best explanation for why the corneal graft is not rejected by the recipient?

(A) Basal cells of the corneal epithelium are able to regenerate.
(B) The Bowman membrane protects against the spread of infections.
(C) Collagen fibers are regularly packed.
(D) Cornea is avascular and lacks lymphatic drainage.
(E) Regeneration of the Descemet membrane assists wound healing.

9 A 29-year-old man with myopia inquires about the benefits of LASIK (laser-assisted in situ keratomileusis) surgery to correct and improve vision. You explain to him that LASIK surgery reshapes which of the following components of the eye?

(A) Cornea
(B) Iris
(C) Lens
(D) Retina
(E) Vitreous body

10 A 39-year-old woman complains of double vision. During the physical examination, you notice that the patient is unable to abduct her left eye, suggesting paralysis of the lateral rectus muscle. The patient is subsequently diagnosed with abducent nerve palsy. The lateral rectus muscle inserts to which of the following components of the eye?

(A) Conjunctiva
(B) Lens
(C) Retina
(D) Sclera
(E) Uvea

11 An eyeball obtained at autopsy is sectioned and stained with H&E. The wall of the globe is shown in the image. Identify the layer indicated by the double arrow.

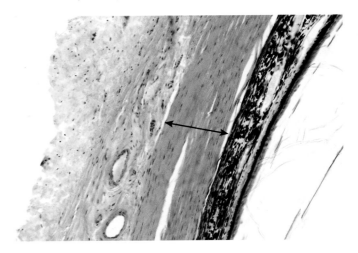

(A) Choroid
(B) Cornea
(C) Retina
(D) Sclera
(E) Uvea

12 A 28-year-old man presents with pain, tearing, and the sense of a foreign object in his left eye. A tiny dust particle is observed and carefully removed. Minor corneal abrasions caused by the dust particle are also noted. After a few days, the scratches on the cornea have completely disappeared. Stem cells that populate the basal layer of the corneal epithelium and facilitate the healing of corneal abrasions originate from which of the following locations?

(A) Blood vessels in the sclera
(B) Bowman membrane
(C) Corneal stroma
(D) Corneoscleral limbus
(E) Descemet membrane

13 The corneoscleral limbus of an enucleated globe is examined at high magnification (shown in the image). Identify the channel indicated by the arrowhead.

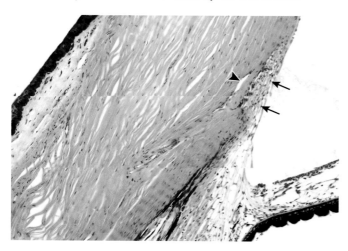

(A) Arteriole
(B) Artifact
(C) Canal of Schlemm
(D) Lymphatic vessel
(E) Trabecular meshwork

14 A 68-year-old woman complains of gradual vision loss over the past year. Ophthalmic examination reveals elevated intraocular pressure. Funduscopic examination reveals optic cupping. The patient is subsequently diagnosed with open-angle glaucoma. Which of the following mechanisms of disease is associated with this patient's medical condition?
(A) Corneal abrasion
(B) Degeneration of the choroid
(C) Degeneration of the lens
(D) Increased resistance to the outflow of the aqueous humor
(E) Retinal ischemia

15 The eye specimen described in Question 13 is examined at the junction between the cornea and sclera. Identify the structure indicated by the double arrow.

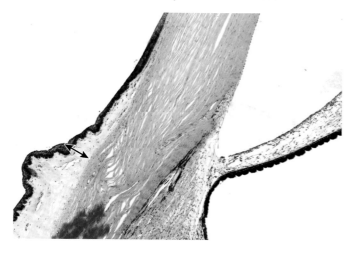

(A) Bulbar conjunctiva
(B) Choroid
(C) Cornea
(D) Palpebral conjunctiva
(E) Sclera

16 A 45-year-old Asian woman complains itching and irritation in both eyes. Physical examination reveals photophobia and fibrovascular opacity in the superior cornea (shown in the image). Histological examination of a conjunctival scraping exhibits cytoplasmic inclusion bodies. Which of the following best describes these clinicopathologic findings?

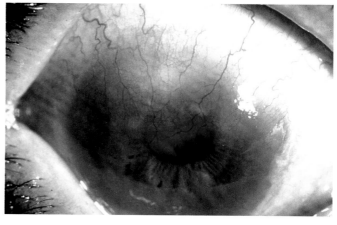

(A) Conjunctivitis
(B) Corneal ulceration
(C) Iritis
(D) Keratitis
(E) Scleritis

17 The posterior segment of an enucleated eye is examined at autopsy. Multiple layers form the posterior aspect of the globe. Identify the heavily pigmented layer indicated by the double arrow (shown in the image).

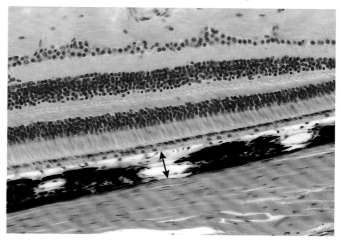

(A) Choroid
(B) Iris
(C) Neural retina
(D) Pigmented retina
(E) Sclera

18 A section of the anterior segment of the eye obtained at autopsy is prepared with routine H&E staining and examined at low magnification (shown in the image). Identify the structure indicated by the dotted line.

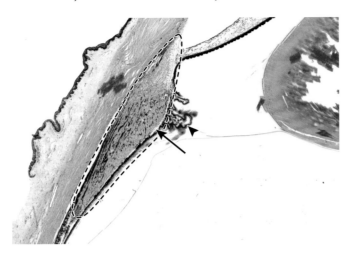

(A) Limbus
(B) Ciliary body
(C) Ciliary process
(D) Iris
(E) Zonular fibers

19 The specimen described in Question 18 is examined at high magnification and a portion of a ciliary process is shown in the image. The apical, nonpigmented epithelial cells indicated by the arrow are derived from which of the following structures?

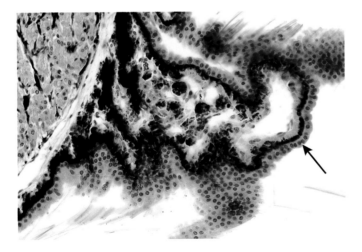

(A) Inner layer of the optic cup
(B) Lens vesicle
(C) Mesenchyme
(D) Optic stalk
(E) Outer layer of the optic cup

20 A 62-year-old man presents with persistent headaches and gradual visual field loss in his right eye. Ophthalmic examination demonstrates high intraocular pressure. The patient is subsequently diagnosed with closed-angle glaucoma, caused by inadequate drainage of aqueous humor. Which of the following structures in the eye produces aqueous humor?
(A) Choroid
(B) Corneal endothelial cells
(C) Corneal epithelial cells
(D) Nonpigmented epithelial cells of the ciliary process
(E) Pigment epithelial cells of ciliary process

21 An iris biopsy is examined in the pathology department (shown in the image). Identify the structure indicated by the arrows.

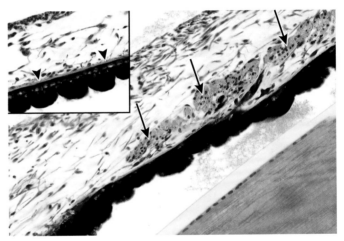

(A) Ciliary muscle
(B) Dilator pupillae
(C) Iris stroma
(D) Macrophages
(E) Sphincter pupillae

22 A 37-year-old woman complains that her right pupil is smaller than her left pupil. Physical examination confirms this observation and further reveals that the patient's right hand is atrophic, warm, and dry. A subsequent neurological examination demonstrates an interruption of the patient's right cervical sympathetic trunk. Which of the following mechanisms of disease explains constriction of the patient's right pupil?
(A) Increased tension of the zonular fibers
(B) Paralysis of the ciliary muscle
(C) Paralysis of the dilator pupillae
(D) Tonic contraction of the ciliary muscle
(E) Tonic contraction of the sphincter pupillae

23 A group of first-year medical students examine a histologic section of the anterior segment of an eyeball (shown in the image). Identify the cellular layer indicated by the arrow.

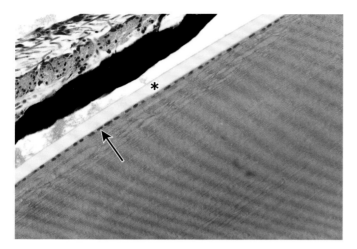

(A) Developing lens fibers
(B) Iris epithelium
(C) Lens capsule
(D) Lens epithelium
(E) Mature lens fibers

24 A 54-year-old woman complains blurry vision when reading. Her vision of distant objects is fine. Which of the following age-related changes underlies presbyopia in this patient?
(A) Dilated pupil
(B) Flattened lens
(C) Opacity of the lens
(D) Relaxed zonular fibers
(E) Rounded lens

25 A 14-year-old girl with a 4-year history of type 1 diabetes presents with blurred vision. Ophthalmic examination reveals "snowflake" cataracts. Which of the following abnormalities accounts for the pathogenesis of cataracts in this patient?
(A) Accumulation of sorbitol in the lens
(B) Increased anteroposterior diameter of the eye
(C) Increased intraocular pressure
(D) Macular degeneration
(E) Retinitis pigmentosa

26 A 48-year-old man loses vision in his right eye after an automobile accident. Funduscopy reveals intraocular hemorrhage and detachment of the retina. Retinal detachment occurs between which of the following paired tissue layers?
(A) Bipolar cell layer and ganglion cell layer
(B) Bruch membrane and retinal pigmented epithelium
(C) Choroid and Bruch membrane
(D) Outer nuclear layer and inner nuclear layer
(E) Retinal pigmented epithelium and retinal photoreceptor layer

27 During a small group seminar, you are asked to explain how neural impulses originating from an image on the retina are conducted to the brain via the optic nerve. Which of the labeled arrows shown in the image identifies the location of cell bodies of the optic nerve?

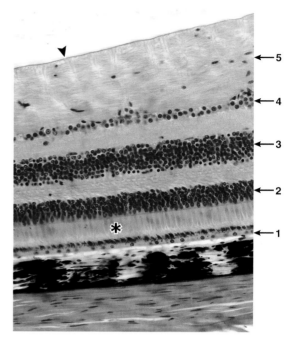

(A) Arrow 1
(B) Arrow 2
(C) Arrow 3
(D) Arrow 4
(E) Arrow 5

28 In the image described in Question 27, the layer indicated by the asterisk contains which of the following cellular structures?
(A) Dendrites of bipolar neurons
(B) Inner rod and cone fibers
(C) Outer segments of rods and cones
(D) Synapse between photoreceptor cells and bipolar cells
(E) Synapse between rods and cones

29 In the image described in Questions 27 and 28, the inner limiting membrane indicated by the arrowhead is produced by which of the following cells?
(A) Amacrine
(B) Bipolar
(C) Cone and rod
(D) Ganglion
(E) Müller

30 An 18-year-old man is color-blind and fails his physical examination for military pilot training. Deficiency in which of the following cells accounts for his color blindness?
(A) Bipolar
(B) Cone
(C) Ganglion
(D) Müller
(E) Rod

31 When reading, detailed patterns of letters on the printed page are detected primarily in which of the following areas of the retina?
(A) Fovea
(B) Lamina cribrosa
(C) Macula lutea
(D) Optic disc
(E) Optic papilla

32 A 72-year-old man complains that he has had poor vision for 3 years. Ophthalmic examination reveals a loss of central vision, although the patient's peripheral vision remains unaffected. Which of the following structures is most likely affected?
(A) Cornea
(B) Iris
(C) Lens
(D) Macula lutea
(E) Optic nerve

33 An enucleated eye obtained at autopsy is sectioned and stained with H&E. The posterior portion of the globe is examined in the histology laboratory (shown in the image). Identify the region indicated within the oval line.

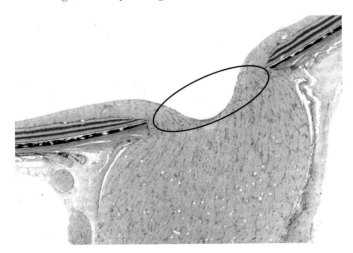

(A) Fovea
(B) Lamina cribrosa
(C) Macula lutea
(D) Optic disc
(E) Sclera

34 The primary visual cortex that processes and interprets the visual image captured by the retina is located in which of the following parts of the central nervous system?
(A) Frontal lobe
(B) Occipital lobe
(C) Parietal lobe
(D) Temporal lobe
(E) Thalamus

35 A 72-year-old woman with a history of coronary heart disease complains of blurred vision in her left eye. Funduscopic examination reveals a cherry-red spot. Which of the following abnormalities underlies this pathologic finding?
(A) Cataract
(B) Central retinal artery occlusion
(C) Central retinal vein occlusion
(D) Melanoma
(E) Retinal detachment

36 The mother of a 2-year-old boy complains about her son's eye. Physical examination reveals two small red bumps and localized swelling on the outside of the patient's top right eyelid. Acute inflammation of which of the following structures most likely caused the stye observed in this patient?
(A) Conjunctiva
(B) Dermis
(C) Lacrimal gland
(D) Sebaceous gland of Zeis
(E) Tarsus

37 A 6-year-old boy who does not respond when his mother calls him is brought in for evaluation. Large earwax masses are found to be plugging both of his ears. The major component of earwax, cerumen, is produced by which of the following structures in the external acoustic meatus?
(A) Cartilage tissue
(B) Eccrine sweat gland
(C) Modified apocrine sweat gland
(D) Hair follicle
(E) Tympanic membrane

38 The mother of an 18-month-old girl complains that her daughter has a fever, cough, and nasal discharge. Physical examination reveals an upper respiratory tract infection and a bulging tympanic membrane. The patient is subsequently diagnosed with otitis media secondary to an upper respiratory tract infection. The infection and inflammation in this patient affect which of the following areas of the ear?
(A) Cochlear labyrinth
(B) External acoustic meatus
(C) Semicircular canal
(D) Tympanic cavity
(E) Vestibular labyrinth

39 The auditory tube described in Question 38 is lined by which of the following types of epithelium?
(A) Ciliated pseudostratified columnar
(B) Simple cuboidal
(C) Simple squamous
(D) Stratified columnar
(E) Stratified squamous

40 A 36-year-old woman complains about progressive hearing loss in the last year and is diagnosed with otosclerosis. Otosclerosis primarily affects which of the following structures of the ear, leading to impaired hearing?
(A) Auditory ossicles
(B) Auditory tube
(C) Cochlear labyrinth
(D) Tympanic membrane
(E) Vestibular labyrinth

41 A section of the internal ear obtained from a guinea pig is examined in the histology laboratory (shown in the image). The space indicated by the asterisk represents which of the following structures?

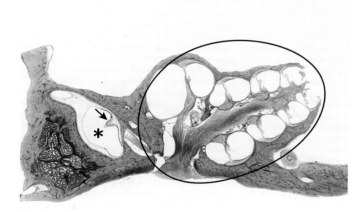

(A) Ampulla of a bony semicircular canal
(B) Cochlea
(C) Internal acoustic meatus
(D) Membranous ampulla of a semicircular duct
(E) Tympanic cavity

42 The ampulla of the semicircular duct described in Question 41 is examined at high magnification (shown in the image). Identify the cells indicated by the arrows.

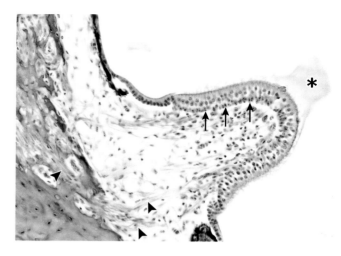

(A) Afferent neurons
(B) Schwann cells
(C) Supporting cells
(D) Type I hair cells
(E) Type II hair cells

43 An epithelial thickening is found in another region of the membranous labyrinth (indicated in the rectangular box, shown in the image). Which of the following terms describes histological features of this epithelial receptor?

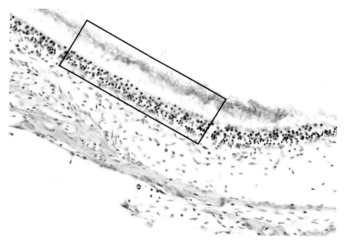

(A) Crista ampullaris
(B) Macula
(C) Organ of Corti
(D) Saccule
(E) Utricle

44 An 18-year-old man experiences seasickness while on a deep-sea fishing excursion. Overstimulation of which of the following structures causes vertigo in this patient?
(A) Cochlear labyrinth
(B) Crista ampullaris
(C) Macula
(D) Organ of Corti
(E) Semicircular ducts

45 A first-year medical student is studying a cochlea specimen obtained from a guinea pig (shown in the image). Identify the structure indicated by the double arrow.

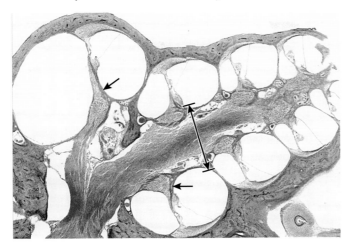

(A) Cochlear canal
(B) Cochlear duct
(C) Internal acoustic meatus
(D) Modiolus
(E) Vestibule

46 A section of the cochlear canal is examined at higher magnification (shown in the image). Identify the space indicated by the asterisk.

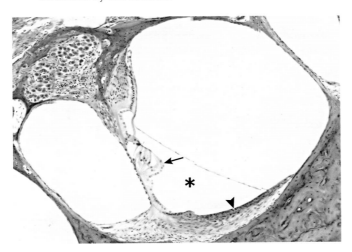

(A) Cochlear canal
(B) Internal spiral tunnel
(C) Scala media
(D) Scala tympani
(E) Scala vestibule

47 Cells in which of the following structures produce endolymph in the scala media?
(A) Basilar membrane
(B) Organ of Corti
(C) Periosteum
(D) Stria vascularis
(E) Vestibular membrane

48 The scala media at the base of the cochlea specimen described in Question 46 is examined at higher magnification (shown in the image). Identify the structure indicated by the arrow.

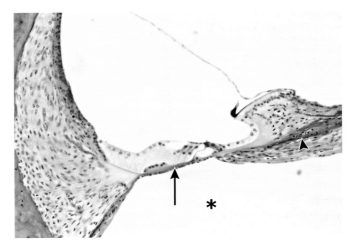

(A) Basilar membrane
(B) Osseous spiral lamina
(C) Spiral ligament
(D) Tectorial membrane
(E) Vestibular membrane

49 A section through the cochlea near the apex is examined in the histology laboratory (shown in the image). Identify the structure indicated by the arrow.

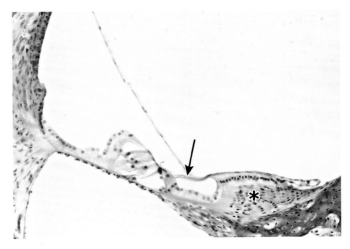

(A) Basilar membrane
(B) Osseous spiral lamina
(C) Spiral limbus
(D) Tectorial membrane
(E) Vestibular membrane

50 The cochlea is sectioned at its first spiral turn and the spiral organ of Corti is revealed at high magnification. Identify the space indicated by the asterisk.

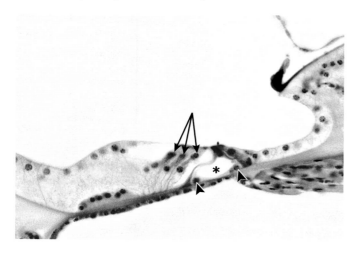

(A) Scala media
(B) Scala tympani
(C) Scala vestibuli
(D) Sulcus spiralis internus
(E) Tunnel of Corti

51 In the image shown for Question 50, identify the three cells indicated by the arrows.
(A) Hensen cells
(B) Inner hair cells
(C) Outer hair cells
(D) Phalangeal cells
(E) Pillar cells

52 Which of the following structures transforms vibrations of the ossicles into waves of fluid in the cochlea?
(A) Ampullae of semicircular ducts
(B) Oval window
(C) Round window
(D) Saccule
(E) Utricle

53 You are invited to attend an outdoor concert in the park during the summer. Your ear detects delightful changes in the frequency of sound vibrations (notes with different pitch). Which of the following structures in the internal ear encodes this frequency-based acoustic information and converts it into nerve impulses that are conveyed to the brain?
(A) Basilar membrane
(B) Crista ampullaris
(C) Macula of saccule
(D) Macula of utricle
(E) Vestibular membrane

54 Which of the following types of cells initiates neuronal transduction during sound perception?
(A) Hair cells of the crista ampullaris
(B) Hair cells of the macula of utricle
(C) Hair cells of the spiral organ of Corti
(D) Phalangeal cells
(E) Pillar cells

55 A 42-year-old woman complains of attacks of loss of balance and spinning sensation (vertigo). She states that nausea, vomiting, and hearing loss, lasting about 24 hours, accompany these intermittent attacks. She has experienced several of these episodes over the past year. The patient is subsequently diagnosed with Ménière disease. Which of the following mechanisms of disease is most likely responsible for this patient's symptoms?
(A) Degeneration of the hair cells in the crista ampullaris
(B) Dilation of the endolymphatic system
(C) Injury of cranial nerve VIII
(D) Labyrinth toxicity
(E) Viral labyrinthitis

ANSWERS

1 **The answer is D: Lens.** Cataract is a degenerative change of the crystalline lens due to biological aging. The lens is a transparent, biconvex avascular structure suspended in the anterior segment of the eye. It is a refractile component of the eye that helps focus light on the retina. Clouding (opacification) of the lens obstructs the pathway of light to photoreceptors in the back of the eye, leading to vision loss. Cataracts are the major cause of visual impairment and blindness throughout the world. Surgical removal of the cataract lens is the most convenient treatment. Conjunctiva (choice A) refers to the epithelium overlying the sclera and internal surface of the eyelid. Cornea (choice B) is the anterior one-sixth of the external layer of the eye. Iris (choice C) is a contractile diaphragm over the anterior surface of the lens. Vitreous body (choice E) refers to the transparent gelatinous substance in the vitreous chamber that is posterior to the lens. None of these structures are involved in the pathogenesis of cataract.
Keywords: Cataract

2 **The answer is D: Uvea.** Three concentric layers constitute the wall of the eye (globe). They include (from outer to inner) (1) cornea and sclera, (2) uvea, and (3) retina. There are also three distinct, but interconnected, chambers inside the eye. The lens serves as a boundary for these chambers. The anterior chamber is the space between the cornea and the iris; the posterior chamber is between the iris and the anterior aspect of the lens. The vitreous chamber is between the posterior surface of the lens and the retina. Aqueous humor, a watery fluid, circulates through anterior and posterior chambers. The transparent vitreous body occupies the vitreous chamber. The pupil is the central circular aperture of the iris. When looking at the eye, one looks through the transparent cornea, lens, and vitreous body, toward the heavily pigmented uvea at the back of the eye. The iris (choice B) is usually heavily pigmented, and the color of the iris is referred to as eye color. The other structures are transparent and do not contribute to the black appearance of the pupil.
Keywords: Eye, pupil

3 **The answer is E: Stroma.** Cornea is the transparent portion of the outer fibrous coat of the eye that covers the anterior one-sixth of the eye. The cornea is about 0.8 to 1.1 mm thick and extremely rich in free nerve endings. The cornea is composed of five layers; from anterior to posterior, they are (1) corneal epithelium, (2) Bowman membrane, (3) stroma, (4) Descemet membrane, and (5) endothelium. Corneal stroma, also referred to as substantia propria, accounts for 90% of the thickness of the cornea and is formed by highly organized collagen fibers. Collagen fibers in the corneal stroma are composed primarily of type I and type V collagen and exhibit a precise, small diameter. The fibers are parallel and arranged into thin layers or lamellae. There are about 60 lamellae in the corneal stroma. The fibers in neighboring lamellae are oriented at approximately right angles. Slender, flattened fibroblasts are situated between lamellae. The ground substance is rich in proteoglycans containing negatively charged chondroitin and keratin sulfate side chains that serve to covalently bind water. Transparency of the cornea depends on the precise arrangement of collagen lamellae and the affinity for water for extracellular matrix. Nerves reaching the corneal epithelium traverse the stroma, but the stroma itself is avascular.
Keywords: Cornea, stroma

4 **The answer is A: Bowman membrane.** Bowman membrane is the thickened basement membrane that corneal epithelial cells (choice C) rest upon. It is a transparent, homogeneous fibrillar lamina located between the corneal epithelium and stroma. It ends at the corneoscleral limbus, the junction of the cornea and the sclera. The Bowman membrane serves as a protective barrier to the spread of bacterial invasion. Descemet membrane (choice D, indicated by the arrows) is the thick basal lamina of corneal endothelial cells (choice B).
Keywords: Cornea, Bowman membrane

5 **The answer is B: Corneal epithelium and Bowman membrane.** Recurrent corneal erosion is a condition characterized by detachment of corneal epithelial cells from the underlying Bowman membrane. It is usually secondary to previous corneal injury or corneal diseases. The affected eye can be excruciatingly painful, due to the exposure of abundant sensory nerve endings in the cornea. None of the other conditions are related to recurrent corneal erosion.
Keywords: Recurrent corneal erosion

6 **The answer is B: Corneal epithelium.** Herpes simplex virus has a predilection for corneal epithelium and causes corneal lesions with corneal ulceration occurring in severe cases. Most of the lesions are asymptomatic and heal without ulceration. Corneal ulceration is associated with high serum levels of antiviral antibodies.
Keywords: Corneal ulceration

7 **The answer is B: Nonkeratinized stratified squamous epithelium.** As shown in the image for Questions 3 and 4, the corneal epithelium consists of approximately five layers of nonkeratinized stratified squamous cells. Neighboring cells adhere to one another via desmosomes. As in skin, basal columnar cells give rise to maturing squamous cells in the outer layers of the epithelium. These basal stem cells provide the cornea with a remarkable capacity for regeneration and wound healing, as evidenced in the healing of the corneal lesions described in Question 6. Numerous microvilli on the apical surface of the

superficial layer of cells retain a protective film of tears. Tears keep the corneal surface wet and lubricated; they prevent drying and ulceration of the cornea. Numerous free nerve endings penetrate the stroma and innervate the cornea. As a result, the cornea is very sensitive to touch. Even very small foreign bodies, such as dust particles, can elicit blinking, flow of tears, and acute pain.
Keywords: Corneal epithelium

8 **The answer is D: Cornea is avascular and lacks lymphatic drainage.** Corneal transplantation, also known as penetrating keratoplasty, is the most common and successful tissue transplantation. Cornea is one of the few organs that is not rejected as allografts by the recipient's immune system. Lack of immune rejection contributes to the remarkable success of this surgical procedure. The cornea does not normally contain blood and lymphatic vessels. This prevents the delivery of immunogenic materials to regional lymph nodes and further prevents the migration of activated immune cells to the allograft. In addition, recent studies have shown that major histocompatibility complex (MHC) class II molecules are not expressed in the cornea. The avascular cornea is nourished by aqueous humor in the anterior chamber of the eye. None of the other choices describe a structural basis for the lack of immune rejection of corneal transplants.
Keywords: Corneal transplantation

9 **The answer is A: Cornea.** LASIK, commonly known as laser eye surgery, is a refractive surgery to correct certain visual abnormalities involving the ability to focus. The cornea has a small radius of curvature and is the chief refractive element of the eye. Working together with the lens, the cornea refracts light rays and focuses them on photoreceptor cells of the retina. In patients with myopia, hypermetropia, or astigmatism, the refractile media (cornea and lens) do not accommodate for proper focus. LASIK has become a popular option that provides a permanent alternative to the use of eyeglasses. It reshapes the cornea, using an excimer laser, in a highly controlled manner to improve the refractive ability of the cornea and improve the patient's vision. LASIK does not affect the other structures listed.
Keywords: Cornea, LASIK

10 **The answer is D: Sclera.** The sclera is the tough, opaque part of the outer fibrous coat that covers the posterior five-sixths of the eye. Along with the cornea, the sclera forms the external fibrous skeleton for the eye, providing shape and resistance, as well as attachment sites for extraocular muscles. It is commonly referred to as "the white of the eye," and its anterior part is visible. Diseases of the central nerve system (notably the brainstem) involving the oculomotor and/or abducent nerve may paralyze one or more extraocular muscles. Conjunctiva (choice A) is the transparent mucous membrane covering the internal surface of the eyelids (palpebral conjunctiva)

and the anterior part of the sclera (bulbar conjunctiva). Bulbar conjunctiva adheres to the periphery of the cornea. None of the other choices provide attachment sites for the extraocular muscles.
Keywords: Sclera

11 **The answer is D: Sclera.** Sclera, the thick fibrous coating of the eye, is composed of dense, irregular collagenous connective tissue with bundles of collagen fibers oriented in various directions and in planes parallel to the surface of the eye. The sclera also contains a rich network of elastic fibers. Externally, the sclera is in contact with periorbital adipose tissue. Internally, the sclera faces the choroid (choice A)—a heavily pigmented layer to the right of the indicated sclera. The choroid is a richly vascular sheet within the uvea (choice E). Uvea is the middle layer of the wall of the eye containing blood vessels. A thin layer of loose connective tissue, known as suprachoroid lamina, separates the sclera from choroid. Anteriorly, the sclera is continuous with the cornea (choice B)—the anterior portion of the outer fibrous coat of the eye that exhibits dense regular connective tissue in its stroma. Posteriorly, the sclera is continuous with the dura mater covering the central nervous system. Retina (choice C) is the inner layer of the eye that contains photoreceptor cells and multiple layers of neurons. Histologic features of the retina are not evident, because the image shows only the anterior portion of the eye.
Keywords: Sclera

12 **The answer is D: Corneoscleral limbus.** The cornea and sclera are continuous. The transitional zone encircling the cornea is termed the corneoscleral limbus or corneoscleral junction. This zone is where the transparent cornea merges with the opaque sclera. Stem cells for the corneal epithelium are concentrated at the limbus. From this stem cell niche, rapidly dividing cells move centripetally into the corneal epithelium. Minor lesions of cornea can heal rapidly without treatment due to the significant regenerative capacity of the cornea. The stem cells also serve as a barrier to conjunctival epithelial cells to prevent them from migrating into the cornea. Depletion of the stem cell niche at the limbus, due to disease or injury, may result in an abnormal corneal surface and "conjunctivalization" of the cornea. Basal cells of the corneal epithelium are recruited from the stem cells and further differentiated into squamous cells moving toward the surface. Other listed choices do not provide stem cells for the corneal epithelium.
Keywords: Corneoscleral limbus

13 **The answer is C: Canal of Schlemm.** At the inner aspect of the limbus region, close to the angle between the cornea and the iris, the corneal endothelium and Descemet membrane are replaced with a plexus of irregular endothelium-lined channels, referred to as trabecular meshwork (choice E, indicated by arrows in the image).

Adjacent and deep to these channels, a larger space (the canal of Schlemm or scleral venous sinus) is situated in the stroma of the limbus. The canal of Schlemm forms a complete circle at the apex of the anterior chamber angle. The canal of Schlemm and trabecular meshwork form an apparatus for the outflow of the aqueous humor. Aqueous humor from the anterior chamber is slowly and continuously drained into the trabecular meshwork, then enters the canal of Schlemm, and eventually returns to veins of the sclera. The endothelial lining of the space indicates that it is not an artifact. None of the other choices exhibit histologic features of the canal of Schlemm.

Keywords: Canal of Schlemm, aqueous humor circulation

14 **The answer is D: Increased resistance to the outflow of the aqueous humor.** Glaucoma refers to a collection of disorders resulting from increased intraocular pressure. Glaucoma features an optic neuropathy accompanied by a characteristic excavation of the optic nerve head (cupping) and a progressive loss of visual field sensitivity. Primary glaucoma may develop with no apparent underlying eye disease and can be subdivided into open-angle and closed-angle glaucoma. In open-angle glaucoma, the anterior chamber angle is open and appears normal, but increased resistance to the outflow of the aqueous humor due to the degeneration or obstruction of the trabecular meshwork is present within the vicinity of the canal of Schlemm. Deficient aqueous humor absorption leads to increased resistance and intraocular pressure. None of the other choices cause glaucoma.

Keywords: Glaucoma

15 **The answer is A: Bulbar conjunctiva.** At the corneoscleral junction, corneal epithelium transitions to conjunctival epithelium that covers the sclera (bulbar conjunctiva). It is also reflected onto the internal surface of the eyelids (palpebral conjunctiva, choice D). Conjunctival epithelium is a nonkeratinized stratified squamous epithelium with numerous goblet cells. Melanocytes are also present as seen in the image. Beneath the epithelium is a layer of loose connective tissue (lamina propria) that contains blood vessels and lymphatic channels. Conjunctival epithelium and its underlying loose vascular connective tissue are referred to as conjunctiva. Cornea epithelium (choice C, a small portion is visible at the top of the image) is about five to seven cell layers thick and rests on the Bowman membrane. The Bowman membrane abruptly disappears under the conjunctival epithelium. Other listed structures do not describe features of the conjunctiva.

Keywords: Conjunctiva

16 **The answer is A: Conjunctivitis.** Conjunctivitis is a common infectious or allergic ocular disease. Virtually, everyone develops conjunctivitis at some point in his or her life. Chronic contagious conjunctivitis caused by *Chlamydia trachomatis* is referred to as trachoma. It is the

most common cause of blindness in the world, especially in Asia, the Middle East, and parts of Africa. It affects the upper half of the conjunctiva more than the lower half and typically involves both eyes. When inoculated into the eye, the organism reproduces within the conjunctival epithelium, inciting a mixed acute and chronic inflammatory infiltrate. As the disease progresses, blood vessels invade the cornea and fibroblasts form a trachomatous pannus. Keratitis (choice D) is inflammation of the cornea. Inflammation associated with the disruption of the corneal epithelium and/or stroma is referred to as corneal ulceration (choice B). Iritis (choice C) is inflammation of the iris. Scleritis (choice E) is an inflammatory disease of the sclera.

Keywords: Trachoma, conjunctivitis

17 **The answer is A: Choroid.** Choroid is the large posterior portion of the uvea, the middle layer of the wall of the eye. It is composed of highly vascular loose connective tissue and coats the posterior two-thirds of the eye. Abundant melanocytes are present in this layer and give it a characteristic black color (see Question 2). The choroid blocks light from entering the eye except through the pupil, and its melanin helps to limit uncontrolled light reflection to avoid perception of confusing images. The outer part of the choroid (suprachoroidal lamina) binds the sclera, and an inner, thin, hyaline sheet (Bruch membrane) adheres to the retina. Branches of posterior ciliary vessels, nerves, and lymphatic channels are present in the suprachoroidal lamina. Microvasculature supplying the outer retina constitutes a less pigmented layer, termed the choriocapillary lamina. Sclera (choice E) is seen at the bottom of the image as dense connective tissue. Iris (choice B) is the most anterior part of the uvea and is not visible in the image. Neural and pigmented retinal (choices C and D) layers are observed deep to the choroid.

Keywords: Choroid, uvea

18 **The answer is B: Ciliary body.** Ciliary body is the expansion of the choroid at the level of the lens. It forms a thickened tissue ring lying inside the anterior part of the sclera. The connective tissue stroma of the ciliary body consists of a thick, outer layer of smooth muscle (ciliary muscle) and an inner vascular layer (indicated by the arrow). Ciliary processes (choice C, indicated by the arrowhead) are radial ridges extending from the vascular layer of the ciliary body. The surfaces of ciliary processes and the ciliary body facing posterior/vitreous chambers are covered by ciliary epithelium—a double layer of low columnar epithelial cells. A circular system of zonular fibers (choice E) extends from the surface epithelial cells in grooves between ciliary processes and attaches to the lens capsule. This structure is also referred to as the suspensory ligament of the lens. Contraction of ciliary muscles decreases the diameter of the ciliary body ring and reduces tension on the zonular fibers. This enables the lens to become rounded and to focus light from nearby objects onto the

retina. Continuous contraction of ciliary muscles (e.g., prolonged reading) may result in muscle spasm, loss of visual accommodation, and myopia. None of the other structures exhibit histologic features of the ciliary body.
Keywords: Ciliary body

19 The answer is A: Inner layer of the optic cup.   The ciliary epithelium covering the ciliary body and ciliary processes consists of two layers of low columnar epithelial cells. The outer pigmented layer is the anterior projection of the pigmented retinal epithelium, while the inner nonpigmented layer is continuous with the sensory neural retina. The retina is derived from a double-layered optic cup that arises as an outpouching of the developing brain. The outer layer of the optic cup (choice E) gives rise to the pigmented retinal epithelium, while the inner layer cells proliferate to form the stratified neural retina. The neural retina extends anteriorly and becomes a monolayer of cells. The anterior projection of pigmented retinal epithelium and the single layer of neural retinal cells form the ciliary epithelium, which covers the ciliary body and ciliary processes. Lens vesicle (choice B) gives rise to the lens. The vitreous body, uvea, and sclera are derived from embryonic mesenchyme (choice C). Optic stalk (choice D) connects the optic cup to the brain.
Keywords: Ciliary epithelium, optic cup

20 The answer is D: Nonpigmented epithelial cells of the ciliary process.   The cells of the nonpigmented layer of the ciliary epithelium demonstrate characteristic features of fluid-transporting cells, namely tight junctions, extensive basal infolding, and Na–K pumps in their lateral plasma membranes. These cells transport fluid from the vascular stroma of the ciliary processes into the posterior chamber, located between the posterior surface of the iris and the anterior surface of the lens. The ionic composition of aqueous humor is similar to plasma, except for reduced protein content (0.1% in aqueous humor vs. 7% in plasma). Aqueous humor in the posterior chamber flows through the pupil into the anterior chamber of the eye, where it nourishes the lens and cornea. Aqueous humor is drained through the trabecular meshwork located at the iridocorneal angle and returned to veins through the canal of Schlemm. In closed-angle glaucoma, the iridocorneal angle is completely closed due to anterior displacement of the iris root against the cornea, thereby obstructing the outflow of aqueous humor through the trabecular meshwork. This leads to an accumulation of fluid and increased intraocular pressure. None of the other structures produce aqueous humor.
Keywords: Glaucoma, ciliary process, aqueous humor

21 The answer is E: Sphincter pupillae.   Iris is the most anterior extension of the choroid that forms a contractile diaphragm with a central aperture (pupil). The peripheral portion of the iris partially covers the lens. The uveal portion of the iris is composed of loose connective tissue,

with abundant melanocytes and fibroblasts (choice C). The number of pigmented melanocytes determines the color of the iris. Near the margin of the iris, an involuntary sphincter pupillae muscle is arranged in a circular array. The posterior aspect of the iris is lined by a double layer of cuboidal epithelial cells that represent the anterior continuation of the ciliary epithelium. The cells of both layers are pigmented, and this heavy pigmentation ensures that light enters the eye only through the pupil. The deep layer consists of myoepithelial cells that constitute the dilator pupillae (choice B, inserted image, indicated by the arrowheads). Contractions of dilator and sphincter muscles regulate the diameter of the pupil and control the amount of light entering the eye. Ciliary muscle (choice A) is smooth muscle found in the ciliary body.
Keywords: Iris, sphincter pupillae, dilator pupillae

22 The answer is C: Paralysis of the dilator pupillae.   Dilator pupillae are radially oriented, pigmented myoepithelial cells of the iris epithelium. These contractile cells are innervated by *sympathetic* fibers from the cervical sympathetic trunk. Contraction of the dilator pupillae dilates the pupil to enable more light to enter the eye. Sphincter pupillae are a circular band of smooth muscle fibers in the iris stroma around the pupil. These contractile cells are innervated by *parasympathetic* fibers carried by the oculomotor nerve. Contraction of the sphincter pupillae constricts the pupil in response to bright light. Disruption of either component of the autonomic nervous system results in the loss of pupil diameter regulation. Lesions of sympathetic fibers innervating the eye lead to Horner syndrome, which is characterized clinically as (1) ptosis (upper eyelid drooping), (2) miosis (constriction of the pupil), and (3) anhidrosis (absence of sweating). Unopposed contraction of the sphincter pupillae muscle (due to paralysis of the dilator muscle) causes miosis in Horner syndrome. Similarly, unopposed contraction of dilator pupillae in oculomotor nerve palsy results in a fully dilated pupil.
Keywords: Horner syndrome, dilator pupillae, sphincter pupillae

23 The answer is D: Lens epithelium.   The lens is a transparent, biconvex, elastic, and avascular structure situated immediately behind the iris and pupil. The bulk of the lens consists of elongated concentric lens fibers. The lens epithelium is a monolayer of cuboidal epithelial cells covering the anterior surface of the lens. They are referred to as a subcapsular epithelium, because a thick basal lamina (elastic lens capsule) covers the epithelium. The subcapsular epithelial cells near the equator of the lens proliferate and differentiate into new lens fibers (choice A), a process responsible for the growth of the lens and continuous deposition of new fibers throughout life. As the new lens fibers mature (choice E), they move toward the center of the lens. Lens capsule (choice C, indicated by the asterisk) is a thick, homogeneous membrane that provides an attachment site for zonular fibers. Iris epithelium (choice B) is seen on the image as a pigmented epithelium covering the iris.

Keywords: Eye, lens

24 **The answer is B: Flattened lens.**   Visual accommodation is mediated by changes in lens shape. A flattened lens enables distant vision, whereas a rounder lens focuses light on nearby objects. Contraction of the ciliary muscle and tension on the zonular fibers (that attach to the equatorial region of the lens capsule) contribute to the accommodation process. With age, the lens loses elasticity and accommodation for near objects becomes increasingly difficult. While distant vision is fine, the patient cannot focus on near objects. This normal aging-related process is termed presbyopia. Presbyopia can be corrected by wearing convex lens glasses. Rounded lens (choice E) is related to myopia, in which near vision is fine but far vision is deficient. Opacity of the lens (choice C) is associated with cataract, a degenerative lens disease. Relaxed zonular fibers (choice D) result in a rounded lens that is best suited for near vision.

Keywords: Presbyopia, visual accommodation

25 **The answer is A: Accumulation of sorbitol in the lens.** "Snowflake" cataracts that develop in patients with type 1 diabetes consist of numerous, white opacities in the lens immediately beneath the lens capsule. These opacities develop owing to high levels of sorbitol in patients with hyperglycemia. Sorbitol is a by-product of glucose metabolism. The major, soluble proteins found in lens fibers are filensin and crystallins. In patients with hyperglycemia (diabetes mellitus), sorbitol accumulation in the lens serves to reduce the solubility of the crystallins, resulting in the appearance of "snowflake" cataracts. None of the other abnormalities cause cataracts in patients with diabetes mellitus.

Keywords: Cataracts, diabetic retinopathy

26 **The answer is E: Retinal pigmented epithelium and retinal photoreceptor layer.**   Retina is the innermost layer of the wall of the globe. It is derived from the optic cup and is composed of two layers: (1) the inner neural retina (light sensitive photoreceptors and conducting neurons) and (2) the outer nonsensory retinal pigmented epithelium, which firmly attaches to the choroid through the Bruch membrane. A potential space is present between the pigmented epithelium and the photoreceptor cell layer of the sensory retina. Traumatic hemorrhage can cause separation between these two layers, leading to retinal detachment. This is a medical emergency that requires immediate treatment. Blindness and permanent damage may occur if retinal detachment is not repaired urgently. Retinal defects, diminished pressure on the retina, and vitreous traction can also lead to this medical emergency. None of the other tissue layers are associated with retinal detachment.

Keywords: Retinal detachment

27 **The answer is D: Arrow 4.**   The visual apparatus focuses light on the retina, which converts the image to neural impulses that are sent to the brain via the optic nerve (cranial nerve II). As seen in the image, the retina is a multilayered structure with three major cellular layers: (1) outer nuclear layer (arrow 2) containing nuclei of photoreceptor rod and cone cells; (2) inner nuclear layer (arrow 3) composed of bipolar neuron cell bodies; and (3) an internal ganglion cell layer (arrow 4). Regions containing the fibers and synapses between adjacent inner and outer nuclear layers are referred as outer plexiform layers. The inner plexiform layer contains bipolar axons and the dendrites of ganglion cells. Ganglion cells are large, multipolar neurons with their cell bodies located in the cellular ganglion cell layer. Their axons form the nerve fiber layer (arrow 5) that is internal to the ganglion cell layer. These nerve fibers converge at the optic disc to form the optic nerve. The retina also contains supporting glial cells, Müller cells, and other association neurons (horizontal neurons and amacrine neurons). Arrow 1 indicates pigmented epithelial cells of the retina.

Keywords: Retina, optic nerve

28 **The answer is C: Outer segments of rods and cones.**   Two photoreceptor neurons are found in the retina, namely rods and cones. Both are elongated cells with specialized structural and functional polarity. Their cytoplasm consists of an outer segment and an inner segment. The outer segment of the rods is cylindrical, whereas the outer segment of the cones is conical (hence their names). The outer segment is formed by stacks of flat disks (plasma membrane infoldings) that contain photopigment. The inner segment shows cytologic features of cells actively synthesizing proteins. A stalk connects both segments. Photosensitivity occurs at the outer segment; the inner segment provides support. The proximal processes of rods and cones, the inner rod fibers and inner cone fibers (choice B), are located in the outer plexiform layer of the retina and form synapses with dendrites of bipolar neurons (choices A and D).

Keywords: Photoreceptors, rod and cones

29 **The answer is E: Müller.**   The inner limiting membrane is the innermost boundary of the retina and separates the retina from the vitreous body. It represents the basal lamina of Müller cells. Müller cells are supporting glial cells with their nuclei located in the inner nuclear layer, span most of the retina, and extend from the inner to the outer limiting membrane. The outer limiting membrane, external to the outer nuclear layer, is a distinct boundary formed by junctional complexes (zonula adherens) between rods, cones, and Müller cells. None of the other cells produce the inner limiting membrane.

Keywords: Müller cells

30 **The answer is B: Cone.**   There are three types of cones, each containing a different visual pigment molecule that is sensitive to different wavelengths in the color spectrum (blue, green, and red). Normally, impulses generated by three cone photoreceptor types can be processed accurately and mixed to discriminate almost any color. When any one of the three types of color-receptive cones is missing, the individual cannot distinguish certain colors. In the case of red-green blindness (all patients are male), the red- and green-sensitive photopigments are missing, due to a defect in genes that are present on the X chromosome. None of the other cells contribute to the pathogenesis of color blindness.

Keywords: Color blindness, photosensitivity

31   **The answer is A: Fovea.**   Fovea (also known as fovea centralis) is a shallow depression in the retina on the temporal side of the optic disc. Its center is located near the posterior pole of the optical axis. This area of the retina is specialized for color vision, discrimination of details, and precise visual acuity. In the center of the fovea, the photoreceptor layer is composed entirely of cones. Cones in this region are longer and narrower than in other areas, and they are oriented at an angle around the margin of the fovea. In the region of the fovea, the other layers of the retina are greatly reduced and blood vessels are absent. Thus, the fovea exhibits histological features that allow light to freely access photoreceptors, thereby increasing visual acuity. The fovea with its high concentration of cones is responsible for sharp, acute vision, and color discrimination. Other areas of the retina (having both rods and cones) provide peripheral and night vision. Lamina cribrosa (choice B) is the portion of the sclera at the optic disc that is pierced by the optic nerve fibers leaving the eye. Macula lutea (choice C) is the area immediately surrounding the fovea. It has a characteristic yellowish appearance due to the presence of xanthophyll. Optic disc (choice D) is the exit point of the optic nerve—a location where photoreceptors are absent. For this reason, the optic disc is commonly referred to as the blind spot. Optic papilla (choice E) is the region around the optic disc where bundles of nerve fibers exit the retina.

Keywords: Fovea

32   **The answer is D: Macula lutea.**   Macula lutea surrounds the fovea and protects cone cells of the fovea. With advanced age, the retina around the macula lutea may undergo degenerative changes resulting in age-related macular degeneration (ARMD). ARMD is the most common cause of impaired visual acuity and blindness in the elderly population. Degenerative lesions in the area of macula lutea involve focal thickening of the Bruch membrane, as well as atrophy and depigmentation of the retinal pigmented epithelium and obliteration of capillaries in the choroid layer. Eventually, photoreceptor cells are affected and a blind spot is produced. None of the other structures are involved in the pathogenesis of ARMD.

Keywords: Macular degeneration

33   **The answer is D: Optic disc.**   Axons arising from ganglion cells traverse the nerve fiber layer of the retina and merge to form the optic nerve at the optic disc. The optic disc lacks the typical, layered retinal architecture and only contains unmyelinated nerve fibers. As shown in the image, there is a central depression in the optic disc. When intraocular pressure increases, the optic disc becomes concave; when intracranial pressure decreases, the disc swells (becomes convex). None of the other structures exhibit histologic features of the optic disc.

Keywords: Optic disc

34   **The answer is B: Occipital lobe.**   The optic nerves convey visual impulses into the central nervous system. The occipital lobe of the cerebrum is concerned with visual functions. The primary visual cortex is situated in and around the calcarine sulcus, a deep cerebral infolding along the medial aspect of the occipital lobe. The rest of the occipital lobe is considered a visual association cortex that is involved in higher-order processing and interpretation of visual information. Other cerebral lobes do not contain the primary visual cortex.

Keywords: Primary visual cortex

35   **The answer is B: Central retinal artery occlusion.**   The outer layers of the retina are nourished by diffusion from choriocapillaris in the choroid. Inner retinal layers are supplied by the central retinal artery, which enters the eye through the center of the optic nerve. Central retinal artery occlusion may occur following thrombosis of the artery, as may be seen in patients with atherosclerosis or giant cell arteritis. Intracellular edema and retinal pallor are prominent, especially in the macula lutea, where multilayer ganglion cells are present. By contrast, the fovea stands out as a prominent cherry-red spot because of the underlying, rich choroidal vasculature. If not treated, permanent damage and blindness may ensue. Central retinal vein occlusion (choice C) typically features flame-shaped hemorrhages. None of the other abnormalities are associated with a cherry-red spot.

Keywords: Central retinal artery

36   **The answer is D: Sebaceous gland of Zeis.**   Anteriorly, the eye is protected by the eyelids, as well as the conjunctiva and tears produced by the lacrimal gland. The eyelid is lined by skin externally and conjunctiva internally. Muscle fibers of the orbicularis oculi are situated in the dermis. The tarsal plate (tarsus) is a supportive fibroelastic tissue facing the conjunctiva. Tarsal glands (meibomian glands) are long sebaceous glands embedded in the tarsus. Eyelashes are present at the margins of the eyelids. The sebaceous glands of Zeis and sweat glands of Moll are associated with hair follicles of the eyelashes. Infections of sebaceous glands of Zeis or glands of Moll, generally caused by *Staphylococcus aureus*, lead to external styes on the outside of the eyelids. Infections near the openings of the ducts of the tarsal glands of meibomian can cause internal styes that appear as red bumps beneath the eyelid. None of the other structures are involved in localized styes.

Keywords: Stye, eyelid

37 The answer is C: Modified apocrine sweat gland. Modified apocrine glands are found in the skin lining the external acoustic meatus of the external ear. They are also referred to as ceruminous glands, because the cells secrete cerumen—a waxy, yellowish material. The ear consists of three chambers, from lateral to medial: external ear, middle ear, and internal ear. The external acoustic meatus is a skin-lined canal through the temporal bone extending from the auricle to the tympanic membrane. The skin here contains sebaceous glands and hair follicles, but lacks eccrine sweat glands (choice B). Earwax is the mixture of secretions of the ceruminous glands and sebaceous glands. It has important protective and antimicrobial functions. Excessive accumulation of cerumen can block the meatus and result in conducting hearing loss. Other listed structures do not produce cerumen.

Keywords: Ears, external acoustic meatus, ceruminous glands

38 The answer is D: Tympanic cavity. Tympanic cavity is an air-filled space within the temporal bone that is separated from the external acoustic meatus laterally by the tympanic membrane and from the internal ear medially by the bony wall. The tympanic cavity, along with three small auditory ossicles, is referred as the middle ear. The auditory tube (eustachian tube or pharyngotympanic tube) connects the middle ear to the nasopharynx. Otitis media is very common in childhood. Upper respiratory tract infections can cause swelling and obstruction of the auditory tube. Air in the middle ear cannot enter the tube and is absorbed through the mucosa, leading to negative pressure in the middle ear cavity. Accumulation of extravascular fluid results in a middle ear effusion. Semicircular canals, cochlear labyrinth, and vestibular labyrinth (choices C, A, and E) are structures located in the internal ear and are not involved in otitis media.

Keywords: Otitis media, tympanic cavity

39 The answer is A: Ciliated pseudostratified columnar. The auditory tube is continuous with the nasopharynx and is lined by respiratory epithelium. At the end of the tube near the middle ear cavity, this ciliated pseudostratified columnar epithelium is gradually replaced by a simple cuboidal epithelium (choice B) that lines the tympanic cavity. None of the other types of epithelium lines the auditory tube.

Keywords: Auditory tube

40 The answer is A: Auditory ossicles. The auditory ossicles are three small bones that are articulated with one another in the tympanic cavity. They include, from lateral to medial, the malleus, incus, and stapes. The malleus attaches to the tympanic membrane and the stapes to the membrane of the oval window (one of two membrane-covered openings of the medial bony wall of the middle ear). The incus links the malleus and the stapes. Sound waves reach the tympanic membrane through the external acoustic meatus and cause vibration of the latter. The three ossicles convert air vibration into mechanical vibration in the fluid-filled chambers of the internal year through the oval window. In the internal ear, sensory receptors convert mechanical forces into electrical impulses. Otosclerosis is an autosomal dominant hereditary defect uniquely affecting the temporal bone and the auditory ossicles. It is the most common cause of acquired conductive hearing loss in young and middle-aged adults in the United States. The most frequently affected site is the stapes, immediately anterior to the oval window. With progressive immobilization of the footplate, the stapes can no longer vibrate and transmit sound waves into the internal ear.

Keywords: Otosclerosis, auditory ossicles

41 The answer is D: Membranous ampulla of a semicircular duct. The internal ear, located within the temporal bone, consists of the bony labyrinth and the membranous labyrinth. The membranous labyrinth represents a set of continuous epithelium-lined tubes and chambers filled with endolymph. Membranous labyrinth is suspended in the perilymph of the larger bony labyrinth—a set of interconnected canals and spaces. Three semicircular ducts of the membranous labyrinth, situated, respectively, within the three semicircular canals, are oriented at approximately right angles to each other in sagittal, frontal, and horizontal planes. They open into a central oval space called the vestibule. The end of each semicircular canal and duct is dilated to form the ampulla. As seen in the image, the crista ampullaris (indicated by the arrow) is located in the membranous ampullae of the semicircular ducts; this structure provides a sensory receptor for angular movements of the head. Ampulla of a bony semicircular canal (choice A) is the space surrounding the membranous ampulla. Cochlea (choice B) refers to the cone-shaped helical space connected with and anterior to the vestibule. Internal acoustic meatus (choice C) is a channel in the temporal bone for the vestibulocochlear nerve to pass. Tympanic cavity (choice E) is not seen in this image.

Keywords: Ears, semicircular duct, bony labyrinth, membranous labyrinth

42 The answer is C: Supporting cells. The enlarged ampulla end of each semicircular duct contains a crista ampullaris, a mechanoreceptor formed by an elongated ridge-like thickening of the epithelium. The ridge is perpendicular to the long axis of the semicircular duct. Crista ampullaris consists of hair cells, supporting cells, and nerve endings associated with hair cells. Cell types can be distinguished based on the location of the cells. The supporting cells are basal, while the hair cells are more superficial. There are

two types of hair cells (choices D and E) in the epithelium, but they cannot be distinguished by light microscopy. Electric impulses generated by hair cells are transmitted by afferent nerve fibers. Afferent neuron cell bodies (choice A) and Schwann cells (choice B) are not located in the crista ampulla. Nerve fibers of the vestibular division of vestibulocochlear nerve (indicated by the arrowheads) can be seen reaching the crista ampullaris. A gelatinous proteoglycan layer known as the cupula (indicated by the asterisk) is seen covering the crista ampullaris.
Keywords: Ears, crista ampullaris

43 **The answer is B: Macula.**   Maculae represent small areas of thickened neuroepithelial cells in the saccule and the utricle that sense the position of the head and its linear movement. Three semicircular ducts and two connected sacs (the saccule and utricle) comprise the vestibular labyrinth. The saccule and utricle (choices D and E) are located within the central vestibule and are lined by a simple squamous epithelium. Two maculae are found in the walls of the saccule and utricle, and they are oriented perpendicular to each other. Histologically, they are composed of mechanosensitive hair cells, supporting cells, and associated nerve endings. A layer of gelatinous polysaccharide material (otolithic membrane) covers the surface of macula that faces the endolymph. The outer surface of the otolithic membrane contains otoliths, small crystalline bodies of calcium carbonate. Maculae respond to linear acceleration, gravity, and tilting of the head. Crista ampullaris (choice A) is located in the ampulla of the semicircular ducts. Organ of Corti (choice C) is found in the cochlea.
Keywords: Ears, macula, saccule, utricle

44 **The answer is C: Macula.**   The stereocilia of the hair cells embedded in the gelatinous otolithic membrane covering the maculae are sensitive to gravity and linear acceleration. Otoliths lie on the outer surface of the otolithic membrane and are heavier than the endolymph. When the head is not moving, the stereocilia bundles are deflected by gravity. When the individual is moving in a straight line, the otolithic membrane with the stereocilia of the hair cells is dragged by inertia, and this movement activates and depolarizes the hair cells. When one is moving by flight, train, or ship, repetitive changes in linear acceleration and direction can overstimulate the maculae in the utricles and cause motion sickness. Spinning the body and rotational movements create excessive stimulation of the crista ampullaris and semicircular ducts (choices B and E), which also cause vertigo. Organ of Corti (choice D) is situated in the cochlear labyrinth (choice A) and is responsible for hearing perception.
Keywords: Motion sickness

45 **The answer is D: Modiolus.**   Modiolus refers to the central bony core surrounded by the cone-shaped spiral cochlear canal. In humans, the cochlea makes two and one-half turns around the modiolus. The cochlea of the guinea pig makes three and one-half turns, as shown in this section through the central axis of the cochlea. The modiolus is composed of spongy bone containing blood vessels, as well as spiral ganglion and nerve fibers of the cochlear branch of the eighth cranial nerve. Bony extensions from the modiolus form the osseous spiral laminae (indicated by the arrows), which provide attachment sites to the basilar membrane of the spiral organ of Corti. Cochlear canal (choice A) is the bony space hosting the membranous cochlear duct (choice B). Vestibule (choice E) is the central compartment of the bony labyrinth containing the membranous saccule and utricle.
Keywords: Ears, cochlea, modiolus

46 **The answer is C: Scala media.**   The cochlear duct, the membranous cochlear labyrinth, is suspended in the cochlear canal (bony cochlea, choice A). The cochlear canal is divided into three parallel longitudinal channels (compartments) running from the base to the apex of the cochlea. The cochlear duct itself is the triangular middle compartment (scala media) that contains endolymph. It is bounded superiorly by the vestibular membrane and inferiorly by the basilar membrane with the organ of Corti (indicated by the arrow) resting upon it. Laterally, the scala media is bordered by a special epithelium termed stria vascularis (indicated by the arrowhead). Scala vestibule and scala tympani (choices D and E) are perilymph-containing channels flanking the scala media. The scala vestibule begins at the oval window, and the scala tympani ends at the round window membrane (second tympanic membrane). They communicate with each other at the apex of the cochlea, through a narrow slit (helicotrema). Internal spiral tunnel (choice B) is a space within the organ of Corti.
Keywords: Ears, cochlea, scala media

47 **The answer is D: Stria vascularis.**   Bordering the lateral aspect of the scala media (shown in the image for Question 46 and indicated by the arrowhead), the periosteal tissue adhering to the inner surface of the bony cochlea is thickened. This thickened periosteal connective tissue is referred as the spiral ligament. Its endolymph-facing surface is lined by a specialized secretory epithelium (stria vascularis) that contains a complex capillary network and produces most of the endolymph in the membranous labyrinth. There are three cell types in the stria vascularis, namely (1) marginal cells lining the endolymphatic space of the scala media, (2) pigment-containing cells scattered among the capillaries, and (3) basal cells separating the stria vascularis from the underlying connective tissue of the spiral ligament. Cells of periosteum (choice C) and cells lining the perilymph-facing surface of the membranous labyrinth secrete the perilymph that fills the scala vestibuli and scala tympani. Vestibular membrane (choice E), also termed the Reissner membrane, is a thin membrane composed of two layers of simple squamous epithelium separated by a basal lamina. It serves mainly as a diffusion barrier between endolymph in the scala media and perilymph in the scala vestibule. None of the other structures produce endolymph.

Keywords: Ears, endolymph, stria vascularis

48   **The answer is A: Basilar membrane.**   The basilar membrane is a thick basement membrane stretching from the spiral ligament (choice C) laterally to the osseous spiral lamina (choice B, indicated by the arrowhead) medially. It forms the floor of the scala media and separates it from the scala tympani (indicated by the asterisk). The highly specialized epithelium, the spiral organ of Corti, superimposes on the basilar membrane. A layer of cuboidal cells secreting perilymph lines its surface facing the scala tympani. The width and stiffness of the basilar membrane vary as it coils from base to apex of the cochlea. It is widest and least stiff at the apex of the cochlea and narrowest and most stiff at the base. Sound waves transmitted into the inner ear induce movement of fluid in the cochlea that causes displacement of the basilar membrane. Hair cells of the organ of Corti are subsequently stimulated and activated to convert these mechanical signals into electric nerve impulses.

Keywords: Ears, basilar membrane

49   **The answer is D: Tectorial membrane.**   The tectorial membrane is a stiff, gelatinous acellular plate that extends from the spiral limbus. The spiral limbus represents a thickened periosteum of the osseous spiral lamina on the medial aspect of the scala media (indicated by the asterisk). The lateral margin of the tectorial membrane overlies the organ of Corti. The stereocilia of the outer hair cells in the organ of Corti are embedded in the lower surface of the tectorial membrane. The tectorial membrane is composed of collagen types II, V, and IX in an amorphous ground substance containing tectorin and otogelin; these glycoproteins are unique to the inner ear and are secreted by cells in the spiral limbus. None of the other structures exhibit characteristic features of the tectorial membrane.

Keywords: Ears, tectorial membrane

50   **The answer is E: Tunnel of Corti.**   The tunnel of Corti is a small triangular tunnel-like space at the central part of the spiral organ. It appears triangular in cross-section. Two rows of cells, inner and outer pillar cells (indicated by the arrowheads), line the borders of the tunnel of Corti. The bases of the pillar cells are expanded and rest on the basilar membrane. Their cell bodies are widely separated but come in contact along the apical aspects of the cells, thereby enclosing a triangular space. Pillar cells contain bundles of keratin that make the cells stiff to outline the tunnel of Corti. Sulcus spiralis internus (choice D) represents the concavity created by the inner projection of the spiral limbus (right side of the image). The tectorial membrane hangs over this space to reach the spiral organ, thereby creating a tunnel-like space

(referred to as the internal spiral tunnel). Other named spaces do not exhibit histologic features of the tunnel of Corti.

Keywords: Ears, tunnel of Corti

51   **The answer is C: Outer hair cells.**   The spiral organ of Corti is a highly specialized epithelium resting on the basilar membrane and exposed to the endolymph in the scala media. It is composed of hair cells, phalangeal cells, pillar cells, Hensen cells, and several other cell types whose functions are not fully known. Hair cells are special auditory receptors and sensory transducers that detect the amplitude and frequency of sound waves. There are two types of hair cells in the spiral organ, namely inner and outer hair cells. The inner hair cells (choice B) form a single row of cells along the inner pillar cells. The outer hair cells are organized into three rows at the base of the cochlea (as shown in this specimen) and increase to five rows at the apex. Phalangeal cells (choice D) and pillar cells (choices E, indicated by arrowheads) provide support to the hair cells. The outer phalangeal cells can be distinguished from the outer hair cells by their location in this image (the three well-aligned nuclei immediately below the three outer hair cells). Hensen cells (choice A) are external limiting cells on the lateral aspect of the spiral organ.

Keywords: Ears, spiral organ of Corti, hair cells

52   **The answer is B: Oval window.**   The oval window and round window are two openings of the bony labyrinths within the temporal bone. The oval window is situated on the lateral wall of the vestibule of the bony labyrinth. The footplate of the stapes fits into the oval window. On the inner side, the oval window is the beginning of the scala vestibuli. The three-ossicle chain connects the tympanic membrane to the oval window. Movement of the stapes induced by the vibration of the tympanic membrane stirs up the mechanical vibration of the perilymph contained in the scala vestibuli, which in turn causes vibration of the endolymph in the scala media and, subsequently, the perilymph in the scala tympani. The round window (choice C) is located at the inferior aspect of the base of the cochlea and is covered by an elastic membrane termed secondary tympanic membrane. Pressure changes of fluid in the cochlea cause movement (bulging out or in) of this membrane. None of the other structures mediate sound wave conduction from the middle ear to the internal ear.

Keywords: Sound conduction, ears, oval window

53   **The answer is A: Basilar membrane.**   As sound vibrations are transferred to the internal ear, a pressure pulse of the perilymph of the scala vestibule causes a traveling wave of deformation along the basilar membrane. The traveling wave of sound of a specific frequency reaches its peak amplitude at a particular location along the basilar membrane. As discussed earlier, the basilar membrane is narrow and relatively stiff at the base of the cochlea but increases in width and decreases in stiffness as it coils toward the apex of the cochlea. High-frequency sounds cause maximal amplitude of the basilar membrane near the base of the cochlea. By contrast, the basilar membrane near the apex of the cochlea undergoes maximal displacement in response to low-frequency sounds. Thus, different sites along the basilar membrane are specific for sounds with particular frequencies (pitch) and provide a structural basis for frequency discrimination. The receptor cells of the organ of Corti resting on a particular site of the basilar membrane respond best to sounds at particular frequency and convert the mechanical tuning of the basilar membrane into nerve pulses. The degree of displacement of the basilar membrane, in another words, the amplitude at any particular frequency, reflects the intensity or loudness of sound. None of the other structures encode acoustic information based on sound frequency or amplitude.

Keywords: Ears, basilar membrane

54 **The answer is C: Hair cells of the spiral organ of Corti.** The receptor hair cells of the organ of Corti are supported and surrounded by phalangeal cells. At their apical surface, stereocilia of the hair cells attach to the tectorial membrane. Thus, stereocilia connect the basilar membrane to the tectorial membrane. The basilar membrane stretches from the osseous spiral lamina medially to the lateral spiral ligament, whereas the tectorial membrane hinges from the spiral limbus. Vibrations of the basilar membrane and tectorial membrane create a shearing effect that deflects and activates stereocilia of the hair cells. The activated hair cells generate action potentials that are conveyed by the cochlear nerve to the central nervous system. Hair cells of the crista ampullaris and macula (choices A and B) are receptor cells responsible for balance and equilibrium. Phalangeal and pillar cells (choices D and E) are support cells.

Keywords: Sound perception

55 **The answer is B: Dilation of the endolymphatic system.** Ménière disease is the triad of vertigo, sensorineural hearing loss, and tinnitus. Ménière disease is characterized pathologically by hydropic distention of the endolymphatic channels of the membranous labyrinth. Dilation of the cochlear duct and saccule occurs at the early stage of disease, and eventually, the entire endolymph-containing network of channels is involved. The membranous wall can be ruptured and endolymph escapes into the perilymph. Patients are afflicted with extensive vertigo and tinnitus, accompanied by nausea and vomiting. Permanent hearing loss may develop as the disease progresses. None of the other mechanisms of disease are associated with the pathogenesis of Ménière disease.

Keywords: Ménière disease

Chapter 20

Comprehensive Review

QUESTIONS

Select the single best answer.

Plate 1. Various organs and tissues are examined during the autopsy of a 70-year-old woman. The sections shown below represent five basic tissue types. Questions 1 to 5 are based on these five images.

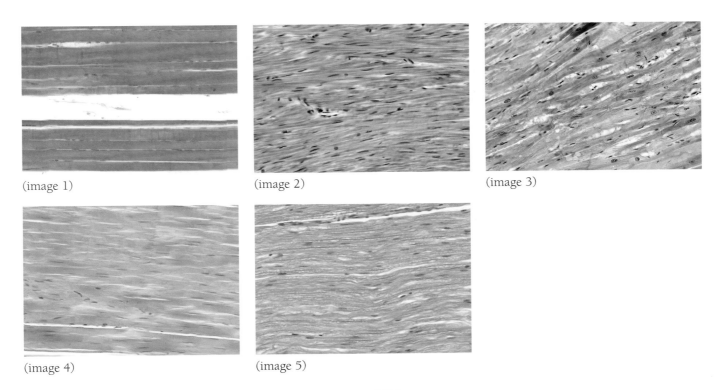

(image 1)

(image 2)

(image 3)

(image 4)

(image 5)

1 Which of the images shown above represents an example of skeletal muscle?
(A) Image 1
(B) Image 2
(C) Image 3
(D) Image 4
(E) Image 5

2 Which of the images shown above represents an example of cardiac muscle?
(A) Image 1
(B) Image 2
(C) Image 3
(D) Image 4
(E) Image 5

3 Which of the images shown above represents tissue that would be present in the muscularis externa of the small intestine?

(A) Image 1
(B) Image 2
(C) Image 3
(D) Image 4
(E) Image 5

4 Which of the images shown above represents tissue that would be expected to show pathologic changes in a patient suffering from chronic tendinitis?

(A) Image 1
(B) Image 2
(C) Image 3
(D) Image 4
(E) Image 5

5 An 8-year-old boy presents to the emergency department with a laceration on the lateral side of his index finger. The wound is cleaned and sutured; however, the boy suffers temporary loss of sensation distal to the wound. Which of the images shown above represents an example of a tissue that would be expected to show degenerative changes in the injured finger of this patient?

(A) Image 1
(B) Image 2
(C) Image 3
(D) Image 4
(E) Image 5

Plate 2. Nerve tissues collected at autopsy are examined by light microscopy. The sections shown below represent four different components of the nervous system. Questions 6 to 9 are based on these four images.

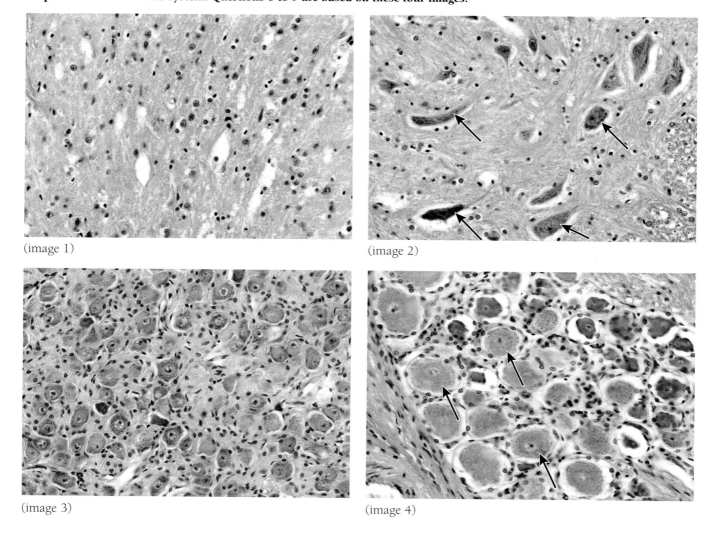

(image 1)

(image 2)

(image 3)

(image 4)

6 The tissue shown in image 1 was most likely obtained from which of the following regions/components of the nervous system?
(A) Brachial plexus
(B) Dorsal horn of the spinal cord
(C) Dorsal root ganglion
(D) Enteric ganglion
(E) Ventral horn of the spinal cord

7 Which of the following best describes the large cells indicated by the arrows shown in image 2?
(A) Glial cells
(B) Lower motor neurons
(C) Postsynaptic parasympathetic neurons
(D) Postsynaptic sympathetic neurons
(E) Sensory neurons

8 The tissue shown in image 3 was most likely obtained from which of the following regions/components of the nervous system?
(A) Dorsal horn of the spinal cord
(B) Dorsal root ganglion
(C) Periphery nerve
(D) Sympathetic ganglion
(E) Ventral horn of the spinal cord

9 Which of the following tissues or structures is most likely innervated by the neurons indicated by the arrows shown in image 4?
(A) Cardiac myocytes
(B) Skeletal muscle fibers
(C) Skin
(D) Smooth muscle fibers
(E) Sweat glands

Plate 3. Multiple organs and tissues are examined at autopsy. The five sections shown below were obtained from cell-rich glandular tissues that are organized into clusters, acini, or cords. Questions 10 to 14 are based on these five images.

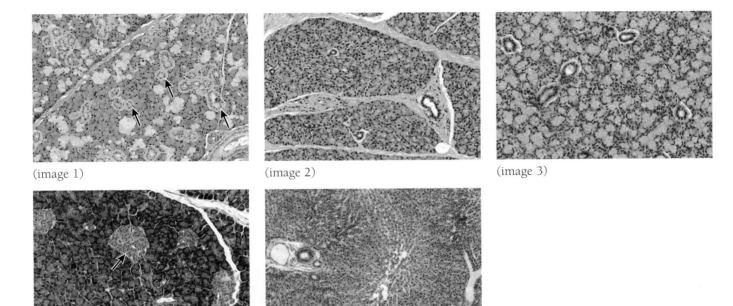

(image 1)

(image 2)

(image 3)

(image 4)

(image 5)

10 The facial nerve exits the stylomastoid foramen and penetrates the organ represented by which of the following images?
(A) Image 1
(B) Image 2
(C) Image 3
(D) Image 4
(E) Image 5

11 Image 3 represents a section through which of the following organs?
(A) Palatine tonsil
(B) Pancreas
(C) Parotid gland
(D) Sublingual salivary gland
(E) Submandibular salivary gland

12 Identify the structure indicated by the arrow shown in image 4.
(A) Langerhans islet
(B) Mucous acinus
(C) Primary lymphoid nodule
(D) Secondary lymphoid nodule
(E) Serous acinus

13 Identify the structures indicated by the arrows shown in image 1.
(A) Bile ducts
(B) Intralobular ducts
(C) Langerhans islands
(D) Mucous acini
(E) Serous acini

14 Identify the organ that is represented by image 5.
(A) Liver
(B) Lymph node
(C) Pancreas
(D) Parotid gland
(E) Spleen

Plate 4. Various lymphoid organs are examined at low magnification in the histology laboratory. Questions 15 to 18 are based on these four images.

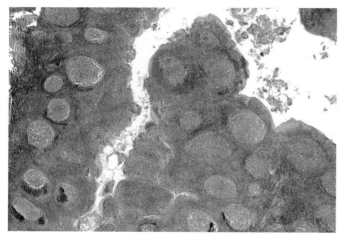

(image 1)

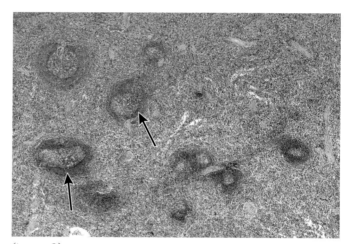

(image 2)

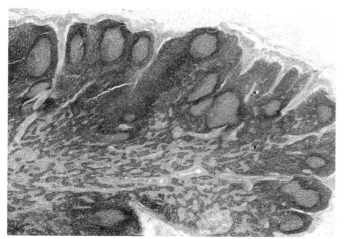

(image 3)

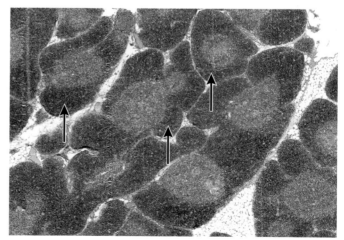

(image 4)

15 Identify the organ represented by image 1.
(A) Lingual tonsil
(B) Lymph node
(C) Palatine tonsil
(D) Spleen
(E) Thymus

16 Image 3 represents a section through which of the following organs?
(A) Appendix
(B) Lymph node
(C) Palatine tonsil
(D) Spleen
(E) Thymus

17 Identify the structures indicated by the arrows shown in image 2.
(A) Hassall corpuscles
(B) Lobules
(C) Medullary cords
(D) Red pulp
(E) White pulp

18 Identify the dark-stained areas indicated by the arrows shown in image 4.
(A) Cortex
(B) Germinal center
(C) Medulla
(D) Red pulp
(E) White pulp

Plate 5. Various segments of the gastrointestinal tract are examined at autopsy. The five images shown below were obtained at low magnification. Questions 19 to 23 are based on these five images.

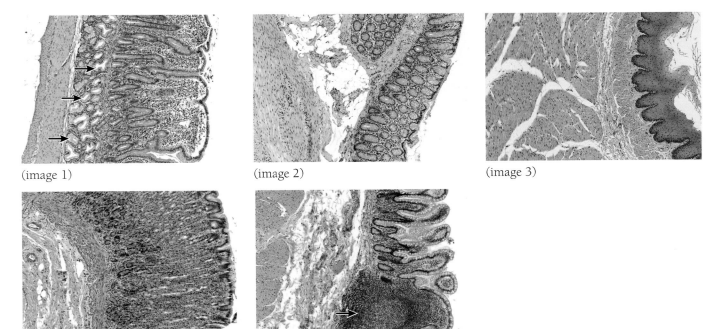

(image 1)   (image 2)   (image 3)

(image 4)   (image 5)

19 Identify the organ represented by image 2.
(A) Colon
(B) Duodenum
(C) Ileum
(D) Jejunum
(E) Stomach

20 Identify the structures indicated by the arrows shown in image 1.
(A) Brunner glands
(B) Crypts of Lieberkühn
(C) Gastric pits
(D) Myenteric ganglia
(E) Peyer patches

21 Identify the organ represented by image 4.
   (A) Appendix
   (B) Duodenum
   (C) Esophagus
   (D) Ileum
   (E) Stomach

22 Identify the structure indicated by the arrow in image 5.
   (A) Brunner gland
   (B) Diverticulum

   (C) Gastric gland
   (D) Peyer patch
   (E) Pyloric sphincter

23 Identify the segment of the gastrointestinal tract represented by image 3.
   (A) Anal canal
   (B) Lower esophagus
   (C) Rectum
   (D) Stomach
   (E) Upper esophagus

Plate 6. Various portions of the digestive tract are examined by light microscopy at low magnification. Questions 24 to 28 are based on these five images.

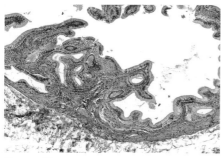

(image 1)

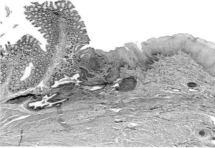

(image 2)

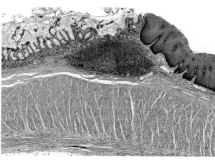

(image 3)

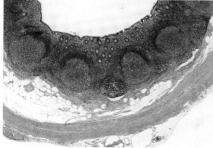

(image 4)

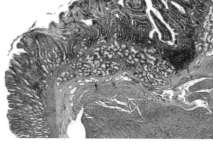

(image 5)

24 Which of the images in Plate 6 represents a section through the anorectal junction?
   (A) Image 1
   (B) Image 2
   (C) Image 3
   (D) Image 4
   (E) Image 5

25 Image 3 was obtained from what portion of the gastrointestinal tract?
   (A) Anorectal junction
   (B) Esophagogastric junction
   (C) Gastroduodenal junction
   (D) Pyloric stomach
   (E) Upper portion of the esophagus

26 Image 5 was obtained from what segment of the gastrointestinal tract?
   (A) Appendix
   (B) Gallbladder
   (C) Gastric cardia
   (D) Gastroduodenal junction
   (E) Ileocecal junction

27 Which of the images in Plate 6 represents a section through the gallbladder?
   (A) Image 1
   (B) Image 2
   (C) Image 3
   (D) Image 4
   (E) Image 5

28 Image 4 was obtained from what portion of the gastro-intestinal tract?

(A) Appendix
(B) Esophagus
(C) Gallbladder
(D) Ileum
(E) Rectum

Plate 7. Various endocrine and reproductive organs are examined at low magnification in the histology laboratory. Questions 29 to 32 are based on these five images.

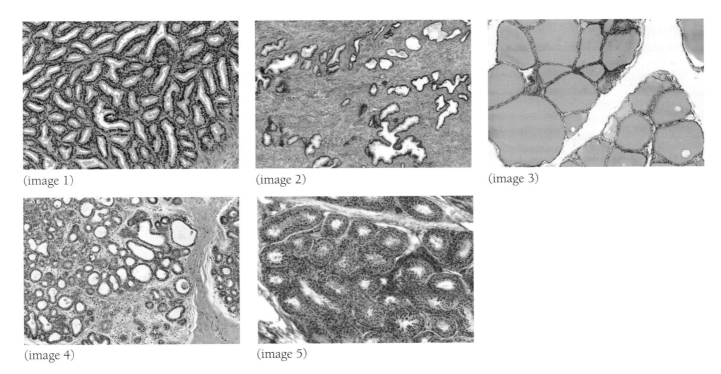

(image 1)   (image 2)   (image 3)

(image 4)   (image 5)

29 Which of the following organs depicted in Plate 7 produces milk?

(A) Image 1
(B) Image 2
(C) Image 3
(D) Image 4
(E) Image 5

30 Which of the following organs depicted in Plate 7 sequesters iodide from the blood to synthesize tyrosine-based hormones?

(A) Image 1
(B) Image 2
(C) Image 3
(D) Image 4
(E) Image 5

31 Which of the following organs depicted in Plate 7 secretes approximately 70% (v/v) of the fluid present in ejaculated semen?

(A) Image 1
(B) Image 2
(C) Image 3
(D) Image 4
(E) Image 5

32 Which of the following organs depicted in Plate 7 exhibits cells with flagella?

(A) Image 1
(B) Image 2
(C) Image 3
(D) Image 4
(E) Image 5

A 48-year-old man complains of a swollen, painful lip that he first noticed 4 months ago. Physical examination shows an ulcerated lesion of the left lower lip. Biopsy reveals a well-differentiated squamous cell carcinoma. You examine the biopsy and observe several normal structures in a region adjacent to the neoplasm (shown in the image). Questions 33 to 35 are based on this image.

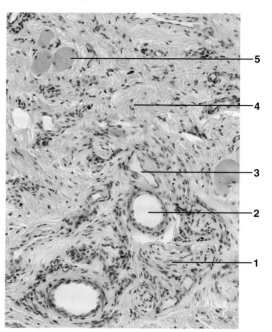

33 Which of the following numbered structures is a terminal nerve?
(A) Line 1
(B) Line 2
(C) Line 3
(D) Line 4
(E) Line 5

34 Line 2 indicates which of the following structures?
(A) Adipocyte
(B) Arteriole
(C) Hair follicle
(D) Lymphatic vessel
(E) Venule

35 Line 4 identifies which of the following types of tissue?
(A) Dense irregular connective tissue
(B) Dense regular connective tissue
(C) Loose connective tissue
(D) Periphery nerve fibers
(E) Skeletal muscle fibers

The superior part of the trachea is collected at autopsy. A transverse section through the posterior aspect of this organ is examined by light microscopy (shown in the image). Questions 36 to 39 are based on this image.

36 Identify the gland indicated by the arrow.
(A) Parathyroid
(B) Sublingual
(C) Submandible
(D) Thyroid
(E) Tracheal gland

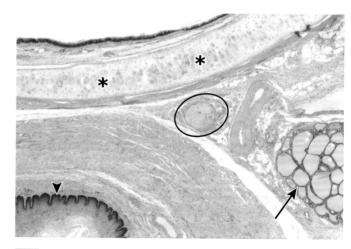

37 Identify the tissue indicated by the asterisk.
(A) Compact bone
(B) Elastic cartilage
(C) Hyaline cartilage
(D) Loose connective tissue
(E) Spongy bone

38 The arrowhead identifies an epithelial tissue that lines which of the following organs?
(A) Aorta
(B) Esophagus
(C) Inferior vena cava
(D) Sympathetic ganglion
(E) Trachea

39 The structure within the circle represents which of the following nerves?
(A) Hypoglossal
(B) Lingual
(C) Recurrent laryngeal
(D) Superior laryngeal
(E) Vagus

A biopsy of the submandibular gland is examined in the pathology department. Multiple tissue types are observed in a single visual field (shown in the image). Questions 40 to 45 are based on this image.

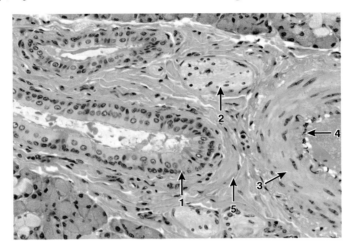

40 What type of epithelium is indicated by arrow 1?
(A) Pseudostratified columnar
(B) Simple columnar
(C) Simple cuboidal
(D) Stratified columnar
(E) Transitional

41 Identify the structure lined by the epithelium indicated by arrow 1.
(A) Artery
(B) Excretory duct
(C) Intralobular duct
(D) Secretory acinus
(E) Vein

42 Arrow 2 indicates which of the following types of tissue?
(A) Adipose tissue
(B) Elastic connective tissue
(C) Loose connective tissue
(D) Peripheral nerve
(E) Reticular connective tissue

43 Which of the arrows shown in the image identifies simple squamous epithelium?
(A) Arrow 1
(B) Arrow 2
(C) Arrow 3
(D) Arrow 4
(E) Arrow 5

44 Arrow 3 identifies which of the following types of tissue?
(A) Elastic connective tissue
(B) Loose connective tissue
(C) Periphery nerve
(D) Smooth muscle
(E) Stratified squamous epithelium

45 Arrow 5 identifies which of the following types of tissue?
(A) Dense irregular connective tissue
(B) Loose connective tissue
(C) Skeletal muscle
(D) Smooth muscle
(E) Stratified squamous epithelium

A lung biopsy is examined in the pathology department. A longitudinal section through the respiratory tree is shown in the image. Questions 46 to 48 are based on this image.

46 The space indicated by number 1 is best identified as which of the following?
(A) Alveolar duct
(B) Alveolar sac
(C) Large bronchiole
(D) Respiratory bronchiole
(E) Terminal bronchiole

47 Which of the numbered spaces shown in the image identifies an alveolar sac?
(A) Space 1
(B) Space 2
(C) Space 3
(D) Space 4
(E) Space 5

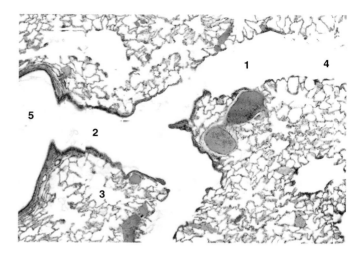

48 The space labeled 4 represents which of the following pulmonary structures?
(A) Alveolar duct
(B) Alveolar sac
(C) Alveolus
(D) Respiratory bronchiole
(E) Terminal bronchiole

49 The tissue shown in this image was obtained from which of the following anatomic locations?

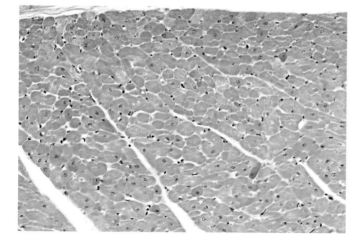

(A) Achilles tendon
(B) Heart
(C) Lower esophagus
(D) Pancreas
(E) Upper esophagus

50 The section shown below represents which of the following basic types of tissue?

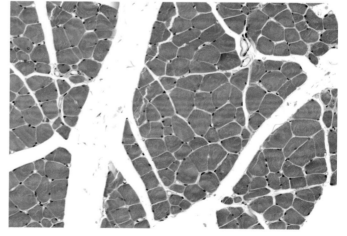

(A) Cardiac muscle
(B) Dense regular connective tissue
(C) Peripheral nerve
(D) Skeletal muscle
(E) Smooth muscle

51 The tissue shown in this image was most likely obtained from which of the following anatomic locations?

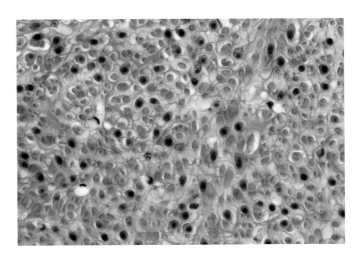

(A) Biceps brachii muscle
(B) Lateral cord of the brachial plexus
(C) Left ventricle of the heart
(D) Muscularis externa of the colon
(E) Palmaris longus tendon

52 Various organs are examined in the histology laboratory using virtual microscope slides. Identify the tissue shown in the image.

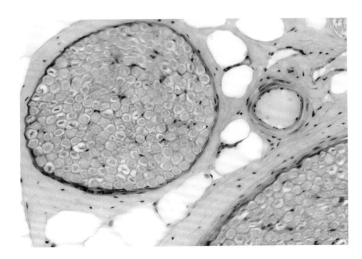

(A) Cardiac muscle
(B) Dorsal root ganglion
(C) Peripheral nerve
(D) Smooth muscle
(E) Sympathetic ganglion

53 Identify the tissue and the structures indicated by the arrows (shown in the image).

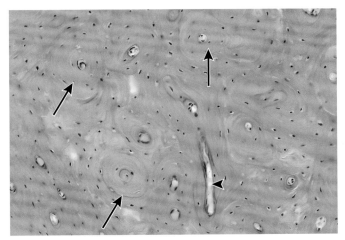

(A) Compact bone/haversian system
(B) Glandular epithelium/mucous acini
(C) Hyaline cartilage/isogenous groups
(D) Skeletal muscle/fascicles
(E) Skin/pacinian corpuscles

54 Identify the tissue and the structures indicated by the arrows (shown in the image).

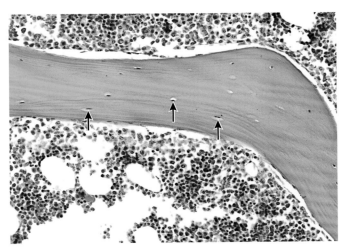

(A) Bone/osteocytes
(B) Cartilage/chondrocytes
(C) Dense regular connective tissue/fibroblasts
(D) Large artery/smooth muscle cells
(E) Peripheral nerve/Schwann cells

55 Which of the following is a feature that is common to the lamina propria of the GI tract, as well as bone, hyaline cartilage, and tendon?
(A) Abundance of macrophages
(B) Complexity of cells and extracellular matrix
(C) Connective tissue capsule
(D) Predominance of type I collagen fibers
(E) Rich arterial blood supply

56 Various organs are examined in the histology laboratory. Identify the epithelium shown in the image.

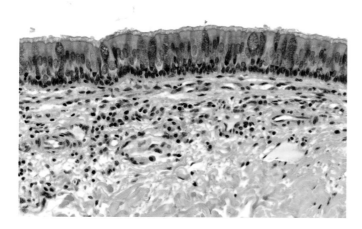

(A) Pseudostratified columnar
(B) Simple columnar
(C) Stratified columnar
(D) Stratified squamous
(E) Transitional

57 The tissue shown in the image was obtained from which of the following organs?

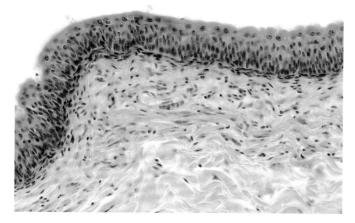

(A) Esophagus
(B) Skin
(C) Stomach
(D) Trachea
(E) Urinary bladder

58 A virtual microscope slide is examined in the histology laboratory. The instructor asks you to identify the type of epithelium that is shown in the image.

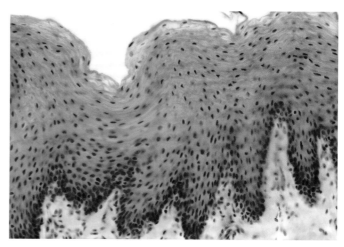

(A) Keratinized stratified squamous
(B) Simple squamous
(C) Stratified cuboidal
(D) Stratified squamous
(E) Transitional

59 Identify the tissue indicated by the arrow (shown in the image).

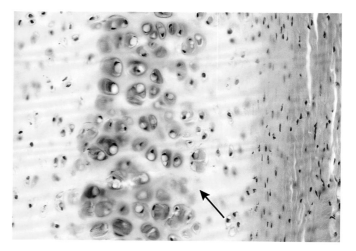

(A) Adipose tissue
(B) Compact bone
(C) Elastic cartilage
(D) Hyaline cartilage
(E) Loose connective tissue

60 The tissue indicated by the arrow (shown in the image) is most likely found in which of the following structures?

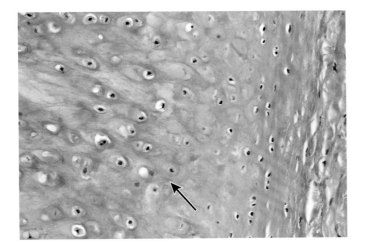

(A) External ear
(B) Head of femur
(C) Patellar ligament
(D) Primary bronchus
(E) Pubic symphysis

61 Various tissues and organs are examined at the autopsy of a 50-year-old man. Identify the organ shown in the image.

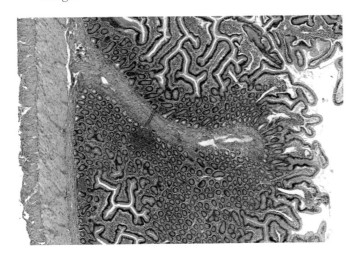

(A) Colon
(B) Duodenum
(C) Ileum
(D) Jejunum
(E) Stomach

62 This image was obtained from which of the following organs?

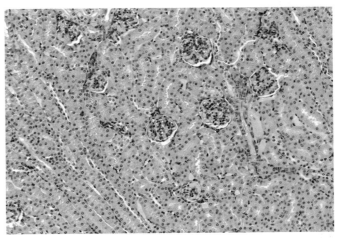

(A) Adrenal gland
(B) Kidney
(C) Liver
(D) Pancreas
(E) Pituitary gland

63 Examination of an inner ear specimen reveals a spiral ganglion (shown in the image). Which of the following best describes the neurons in this auditory ganglion?

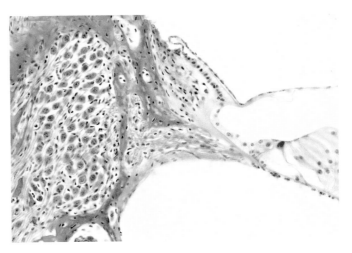

(A) Bipolar
(B) Intermediate
(C) Motor
(D) Multipolar
(E) Pseudounipolar

64 Male and female reproductive organs are examined in the histology laboratory. Identify the cells indicated by the arrow (shown in the image).

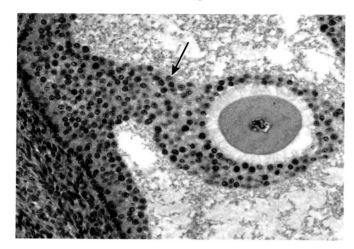

(A) Decidual cells
(B) Granulosa cells
(C) Leydig cells
(D) Parafollicular cells
(E) Theca interna cells

65 Which of the following numbered arrows (shown in the image) identifies the nucleus of a germ cell that has entered prophase of meiosis I?

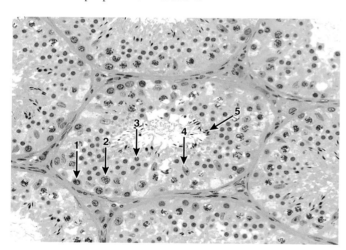

(A) Arrow 1
(B) Arrow 2
(C) Arrow 3
(D) Arrow 4
(E) Arrow 5

66 For the image provided for Question 65, which of the following numbered arrows (shown in the image) identifies the nucleus of a cell that secretes androgen-binding protein?

(A) Arrow 1
(B) Arrow 2
(C) Arrow 3
(D) Arrow 4
(E) Arrow 5

67 Your laboratory instructor asks you to identify the organ shown in the image.

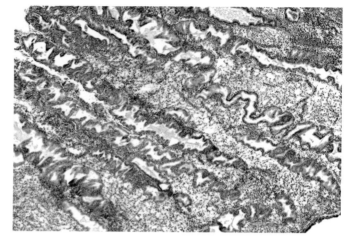

(A) Ampulla of the uterine tube
(B) Endocervical canal
(C) Fimbriae of the uterine tube
(D) Proliferative-phase endometrium
(E) Secretory-phase endometrium

68 The endocrine organ shown in the image secretes which of the following hormones?

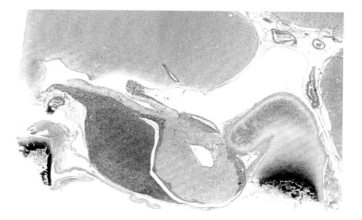

(A) Epinephrine
(B) Erythropoietin
(C) Estrogen
(D) Thyroxine
(E) Vasopressin

69 Name the parenchymal cells of the organ indicated by the arrow (shown in the image).

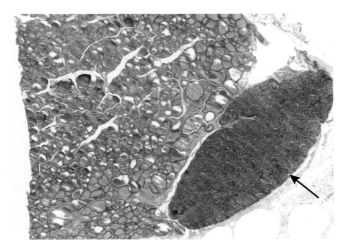

(A) Beta cells
(B) Chief cells
(C) Follicular cells
(D) Ganglion cells
(E) Lymphocytes

70 Which of the following numbered layers in this organ (shown in the image) is primarily responsible for the synthesis and secretion of cortisol?

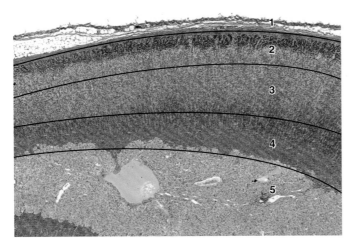

(A) Layer 1
(B) Layer 2
(C) Layer 3
(D) Layer 4
(E) Layer 5

71 A neurovascular bundle obtained at autopsy is sectioned and stained using a trichrome reagent. Identify the blood vessel shown in the image.

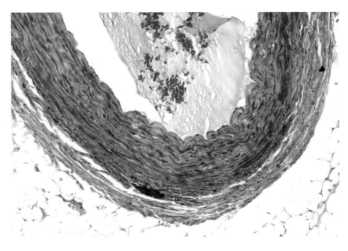

(A) Large vein
(B) Larger elastic artery
(C) Medium vein
(D) Muscular artery
(E) Small artery

72 A skin biopsy is stained with H&E and examined at high magnification. Identify the structure indicated by the arrow (shown in the image).

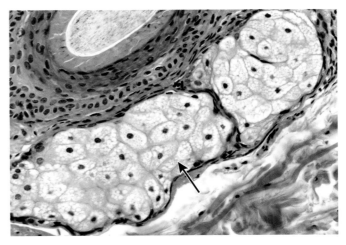

(A) Apocrine sweat gland
(B) Eccrine sweat gland
(C) Hair follicle
(D) Pacinian corpuscle
(E) Sebaceous gland

73 Various organs and tissues are examined at autopsy. Identify the tissue.

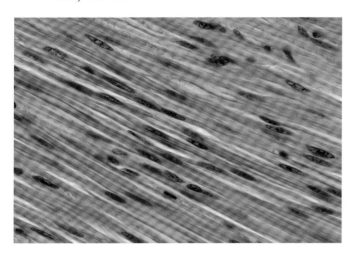

- (A) Cardiac muscle
- (B) Dense regular connective tissue
- (C) Fibrocartilage
- (D) Skeletal muscle
- (E) Smooth muscle

74 A tissue section is prepared using a special stain (hematoxylin/permanganate oxide). Identify the tissue.

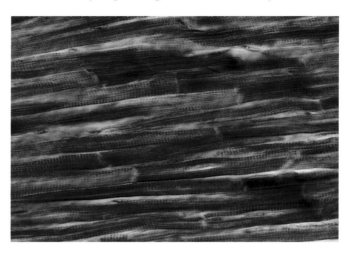

- (A) Cardiac muscle
- (B) Compact bone
- (C) Dense regular connective tissue
- (D) Skeletal muscle
- (E) Smooth muscle

ANSWERS

1 **The answer is A: Image 1.** Longitudinal sections of these basic tissue types may look similar. Skeletal muscle cells (image 1) form large-diameter fibers with peripheral nuclei. Transverse striations composed of alternating dark and light bands are visible across the fiber width. None of the other images show these histologic features.
Keywords: Skeletal muscle

2 **The answer is C: Image 3.** Like skeletal muscle, cardiac muscle fibers show transverse striations. However, cardiac myocytes can be distinguished from skeletal muscle fibers by their distinctive cellular branching patterns. Cardiac myocytes also exhibit central nuclei and intercalated disks. None of the other images show these histologic features.
Keywords: Cardiac muscle

3 **The answer is B: Image 2.** The muscularis externa in the wall of the gastrointestinal tract is composed predominantly of smooth muscle (image 2). Smooth muscle fibers are identified as short, spindle-shaped cells with single, centrally located nuclei. These fibers lack transverse striations (rules out image 1). Smooth muscle is more cellular than dense connective tissue, and smooth muscle nuclei are located in the center of each fiber (rules out image 4).
Keywords: Smooth muscle

4 **The answer is D: Image 4.** This section of tendon shows dense, regular connective tissue that is characterized by densely packed, parallel collagen fibers and bundles. The fibroblast nuclei are flat, elongated, and oriented parallel to the collagen fibers. Fibroblast nuclei display primarily heterochromatin. None of the other images shows these distinct histologic features. Tendinitis represents inflammation of a tendon. It may be caused by repetitive stress injury (e.g., tennis elbow).
Keywords: Dense regular connective tissue

5 **The correct answer is E: Image 5.** Proper palmar digital nerves travel along the medial and lateral sides of the finger and are subject to injury. In a severed nerve, the axons and myelin sheaths would be expected to undergo degeneration. Longitudinal sections of a peripheral nerve (image 5) can be discerned by finding "empty" spaces among dark-stained wavy axons and scattered Schwann cell nuclei. These unstained (empty) spaces form when lipids making up the myelin sheaths of axons are extracted during tissue preparation. None of the other images show these histologic features.
Keywords: Peripheral nerve

6 **The answer is B: Dorsal horn of the spinal cord.** Dorsal horn refers to the dorsal portion of the central grey matter in the spinal cord. The dorsal horn contains small, second-order sensory neurons and interneurons. Many of the small nuclei visible in this image represent glial cells. Nerve fibers and capillaries are distributed among the neurons and glial cells.
Keywords: Spinal cord, dorsal horn

7 **The answer is B: Lower motor neurons.** The characteristic feature of the ventral horn of the spinal cord is the presence of large, multipolar lower motor neurons. Numerous small nuclei of glial cells (choice A) are observed among the nerve fibers. Sensory neurons (choice E) are small neurons found in the dorsal horn. None of the other listed structures show the characteristic features of the ventral horn of the spinal cord.
Keywords: Spinal cord, ventral horn

8 **The answer is D: Sympathetic ganglion.** Sympathetic ganglia are composed of clusters of large, multipolar neuronal cell bodies, with eccentric nuclei. Satellite cells are present, but these glial cells do not form a complete ring around the neuronal cell bodies.
Keywords: Sympathetic ganglion

9 **The answer is C: Skin.** Image 4 shows a section through a dorsal root ganglion. These large neurons are pseudounipolar. Their nuclei are centrally located, and a complete layer of small satellite cells surrounds each neuronal cell body. Multipolar neurons in a sympathetic ganglion exhibit different histologic features (see image 3 for comparison). Dorsal root ganglia contain the cell bodies of both somatic and visceral afferent neurons. Somatic afferent neurons provide sensory innervation to the skin. The other cells/tissues listed require motor innervation for their function.
Keywords: Dorsal root ganglion

10 **The answer is B: Image 2.** Images 1 to 4 illustrate characteristic features of glandular epithelial tissue. The secretory cells are organized into clusters or acini. Image 2 shows serous acini that are enclosed by dense, irregular connective tissue septa. These are the unique histologic features of the parotid gland. The facial nerve (cranial nerve VII) exits the stylomastoid foramen and penetrates the parotid gland, before innervating muscles of facial expression.
Keywords: Parotid glands

11 **The answer is D: Sublingual salivary gland.** The sublingual gland contains primarily mucous acini with a small number of serous cells. Mucous cells appear pale in routine slide preparations, because they are filled with heavily glycosylated proteins (mucins) that are poorly stained by H&E.
Keywords: Sublingual gland

12 **The answer is A: Langerhans islet.** Image 4 shows clusters of light-stained endocrine epithelial cells scattered among

serous acini. These islets of Langerhans are a unique histologic feature of the pancreas. Their presence helps distinguish the pancreas from the parotid gland. Endocrine cells in the pancreas do not form acini. This observation helps distinguish islets of Langerhans from light-stained mucous acini that are found in the submandibular gland.
Keywords: Pancreas, islets of Langerhans

13 **The answer is B: Intralobular ducts.** Image 1 reveals glandular tissue that is composed of both serous and mucous acini. These are the characteristic features of the submandibular gland. A complex system of ducts transports watery secretions of the salivary glands to the oral cavity. Intralobular ducts are located within the lobules of these glands (arrows, shown in the image). In the submandibular gland, the most abundant intralobular duct segments are referred to as striated ducts.
Keywords: Submandibular gland

14 **The answer is A: Liver.** Hepatocytes form anastomosing plates that appear as interconnected cords of cells in tissue sections. Sinusoidal capillaries separate the hepatic plates. Classic liver lobules are described as hexagonal prisms with hepatocyte plates and sinusoids radiating from a central vein (terminal hepatic venule). Portal triads are located at the peripheral angles of the liver lobules. Portal triads are composed of branches of the portal vein, hepatic artery, and bile duct. These structures and lymphatic channels are surrounded by connective tissue that forms portal canals.
Keywords: Liver, lobules

15 **The answer is C: Palatine tonsil.** Palatine tonsils are aggregates of diffuse and nodular lymphatic tissue that are located between palatopharyngeal and palatoglossal arches in the oropharynx. Stratified squamous epithelium covers this lymphoid tissue and dives deep into the tonsils, forming tonsillar crypts.
Keywords: Tonsils, palatine

16 **The answer is B: Lymph node.** Lymph nodes are encapsulated secondary lymphoid organs. Extensions of the capsule form connective tissue trabeculae that penetrate the lymph node. Tightly packed lymphocytes form nodules in the cortex and cords in the medulla.
Keywords: Lymph nodes

17 **The answer is E: White pulp.** Image 2 shows a low-magnification section through the spleen. Examination of the specimen reveals scattered splenic lymphoid nodules (white pulp) surrounded by venous sinuses (red pulp). A dense connective tissue capsule encloses the spleen from which numerous trabeculae penetrate the parenchymal tissue. The spleen filters the blood and provides a microenvironment for generating immune responses to blood-borne antigens.
Keywords: Spleen, white pulp

18 **The answer is A: Cortex.** At low magnification, lobules of the thymus (with dark-stained cortex and light-stained medulla) may resemble secondary lymphoid follicles. However, thymic lobules are much larger than lymphoid follicles, and unlike lymphoid follicles, thymic lobules are separated by thin connective tissue septa (trabeculae). Hassall corpuscles in the medulla of the thymus also help distinguish thymic lobules from secondary lymphoid nodules.
Keywords: Thymus, cortex

19 **The answer is A: Colon.** This image shows the distinctive morphology of colonic glands in cross section. The straight tubular glands are lined by enterocytes and goblet cells. The principal function of enterocytes in the colon is absorption of water and electrolytes. The lumens of these colonic glands are small and difficult to visualize. The glands are surrounded by loose connective tissue of the lamina propria.
Keywords: Colon

20 **The answer is A: Brunner glands.** The glands indicated by the arrows are located in submucosal connective tissue, deep to the muscularis mucosae. These submucosal (Brunner) glands are a distinguishing feature of the proximal duodenum. In addition to mucus, Brunner glands secrete an alkaline pH fluid that helps neutralize the acidity of gastric juice. The lamina propria in this autopsy specimen is filled with mucosa-associated lymphoid tissue.
Keywords: Duodenum, Brunner glands

21 **The answer is E: Stomach.** This image shows gastric glands emptying into the bottom of the gastric pits. These fundic glands are populated largely by eosinophilic parietal cells in the neck of the gland and basophilic chief cells at the base of the gland. Gastric glands are branched tubular glands that extend from the bottom of the gastric pits down to the muscularis mucosae.
Keywords: Stomach, fundus

22 **The answer is D: Peyer patch.** This section of the distal ileum shows a large aggregate of diffuse and nodular lymphatic tissue that is referred to as a Peyer patch. The pale-staining region within this lymphoid tissue represents an area of B lymphocyte activation and proliferation. Peyer patches participate in adaptive immunity and immune surveillance. They are a distinguishing feature of the mucosa of the distal ileum.
Keywords: Peyer patches

23 **The answer is B: Lower esophagus.** The esophagus is lined by a nonkeratinized stratified squamous epithelium (shown in the image). Upper and lower portions of the esophagus can be distinguished on the basis of their muscularis externa. The muscularis externa in the lower (distal) esophagus is composed of smooth muscle, whereas the muscularis externa in the upper (proximal) esophagus is composed of striated skeletal muscle. We can infer that this autopsy specimen was obtained from the lower esophagus, because the muscularis externa is composed entirely of smooth muscle. The anal canal also features stratified squamous epithelium; however, this segment of the GI tract would show striated muscle of the external sphincter.

Keywords: Esophagus

24 **The answer is B: Image 2.** This specimen was obtained from the junction of the rectum and the anal canal. The image shows colonic epithelium on the left (rectum) and a nonkeratinized stratified squamous epithelium on the right (anal canal). The stratified squamous epithelium of the anal canal becomes keratinized as it blends with skin on the external surface of the body. The esophagogastric junction also exhibits stratified squamous epithelium but does not show colonic glands. None of the other images reveal colonic glands and stratified squamous epithelium.

Keywords: Anorectal junction

25 **The answer is B: Esophagogastric junction.** This specimen was obtained from the esophagogastric junction. The image shows an abrupt transition from a nonkeratinized stratified squamous epithelium (on the right) to a mucinous columnar epithelium with gastric pits (on the left). None of the other segments of the GI tract exhibit these distinct histologic features.

Keywords: Esophagogastric junction

26 **The answer is D: Gastroduodenal junction.** This image reveals gastric pyloric glands on the left and intestinal villi on the right. The junction of the stomach and duodenum is also characterized by the presence of submucosal Brunner glands (shown in the image). None of the other organs feature submucosal Brunner glands.

Keywords: Gastroduodenal junction

27 **The answer is A: Image 1.** The mucosa of the gallbladder features a simple columnar epithelium and a lamina propria of loose connective tissue. In contrast to other segments of the GI tract, the wall of the gallbladder does not exhibit a muscularis mucosae or submucosa. The muscularis externa of the gallbladder is located immediately external to the lamina propria (shown in the image). The other organs illustrated in Plate 6 all feature a muscularis mucosae and a submucosa.

Keywords: Gallbladder

28 **The answer is A: Appendix.** The appendix is a small, blind pouch that arises as a diverticulum of the cecum. Histologic features of the appendix are similar to those of the colon. The appendix exhibits a mucosa, submucosa, muscularis externa, and serosa/adventitia. A distinguishing feature of the appendix is the large number of secondary lymphatic nodules that extend into the submucosa (shown in the image).

Keywords: Appendix

29 **The answer is D: Image 4.** The mammary gland is a compound tubuloalveolar gland that produces milk to nourish the newborn. In response to pregnancy-associated hormones, the mammary gland undergoes extensive proliferation of terminal duct lobular units and branching morphogenesis. Loose areolar connective tissue present within terminal duct lobular units of the inactive gland appears sparse as the glandular tissue proliferates. Secretions of the terminal alveoli drain to large intralobular ducts (shown in the image), which drain to interlobular ducts and lactiferous ducts that drain to the nipple. None of the other organs features secretory alveoli surrounded by loose areolar connective tissue.

Keywords: Mammary gland

30 **The answer is C: Image 3.** The thyroid gland stores a large reserve of thyroid hormone precursor molecules within numerous follicles (shown in the image). The gelatinous material within these follicles is referred to as colloid. The principal component of colloid is thyroglobulin, a large glycoprotein. This thyroid prohormone undergoes iodination of tyrosine residues. As needed, this thyroglobulin is internalized through endocytosis and proteolytically cleaved to form active hormones that carry either three or four iodotyrosine residues (T_3/T_4). The thyroid gland actively absorbs iodide from the blood (iodide trapping). None of the other organs feature large follicles filled with colloid or sequester iodide.

Keywords: Thyroid gland, thyroid hormones

31 **The answer is A: Image 1.** Accessory glands of the male reproductive tract include paired seminal vesicles, the prostate gland, and several bulbourethral glands. These organs produce secretions that mix with sperm to form semen during ejaculation. Most (70%) of the fluid in semen is contributed by the seminal vesicles. This fluid contains an abundance of amino acids, simple sugars, prostaglandins, and enzymes. Histologic features of paired seminal vesicles include a highly folded secretory epithelium, surrounded by a thin layer of smooth muscle. None of the other organs exhibit the distinctive histologic features of the seminal vesicles.

Keywords: Seminal vesicles

32 **The answer is E: Image 5.** Spermatogenesis is a complex developmental process that generates haploid male gametes with flagella. Sperm motility is based on the whip-like motion of the sperm flagellum. The sperm tail is composed of microtubules and associated molecular motor proteins (e.g., dynein). Sliding of these microtubules generates a flagellar beat. The testis is the only organ in the body that produces cells with a flagellum.

Keywords: Spermatozoa, flagellum

33 **The answer is A: Line 1.** Multiple tissue types sectioned in various planes are evident in this lip biopsy. To identify these soft tissues requires a comprehensive and integrated understanding of histology. In this section, line 1 identifies a peripheral nerve with a distinct wavy appearance. The nerve is captured in cross section at an oblique angle. Dark-stained axons may be identified at higher magnification. Nerve is typically more cellular and more highly organized than connective tissue.
Keywords: Oral cancer, peripheral nerve

34 **The answer is B: Arteriole.** Arterioles are the smallest and most terminal components of arterial blood vessels. They typically contain one or two layers of smooth muscle in their tunica media and exhibit a round lumen. By contrast, venules (line 3) typically feature a very thin wall and exhibit a collapsed lumen. Cross sections of a few skeletal muscle fibers are present in this microscopic field (line 5).
Keywords: Oral cancer, arterioles

35 **The answer is A: Dense irregular connective tissue.** Dense irregular connective tissue fills the space between the structures described above. It is typically less cellular and poorly organized, with pink-stained collagen fibers running in various directions.
Keywords: Dense irregular connective tissue

36 **The answer is D: Thyroid.** The thyroid gland is an endocrine organ in the anterior neck. It neighbors the larynx, superior trachea, and esophagus. The thyroid features large follicles that are filled with a pink-stained gelatinous material (colloid). None of the other glands exhibit follicles.
Keywords: Thyroid gland, trachea

37 **The answer is C: Hyaline cartilage.** A series of C-shaped cartilaginous rings provide structural support to the trachea. The rings are composed of hyaline cartilage that features chondrocytes in lacunae and a glassy translucent matrix.
Keywords: Trachea, cartilage rings

38 **The answer is B: Esophagus.** The esophagus is situated immediately posterior to the trachea. It is lined by a stratified squamous epithelium and features a thick muscular wall that is lined by striated muscle (upper esophagus) or smooth muscle (lower esophagus). Striated muscle fibers are evident in this section of the esophagus.
Keywords: Esophagus

39 **The answer is C: Recurrent laryngeal.** This question highlights an important anatomic relationship in the anterior neck. The recurrent branch of the vagus nerve (cranial nerve X) ascends in a groove between the trachea and esophagus to innervate the larynx. None of the other nerves are found in this anatomic location.
Keywords: Recurrent laryngeal nerve

40 **The answer is D: Stratified columnar.** Arrow 1 points to a stratified epithelium composed of a basal layer of cuboidal cells and an upper layer of columnar cells. The shape of the upper layer of cells designates the type of stratified epithelium.
Keywords: Stratified columnar epithelium

41 **The answer is B: Excretory duct.** This arrow points to a section through a large excretory duct that is lined by stratified columnar epithelium. The duct is surrounded by dense connective tissue. Intralobular ducts in salivary glands are lined by cuboidal to low columnar epithelium, depending on the diameter of the duct.
Keywords: Salivary glands, excretory ducts

42 **The answer is D: Peripheral nerve.** This is an oblique section through a peripheral nerve. Note the wavy appearance of the axons and the pale-stained space where lipid-rich myelin was removed in tissue processing. These are the characteristic features of peripheral nerves in routine H&E slide preparations. The nuclei within the nerve tissue belong to neural crest–derived Schwann cells.
Keywords: Peripheral nerves

43 **The answer is D: Arrow 4.** This arrow points to the lining epithelium of a blood vessel that is filled with red blood cells. Simple squamous epithelial cells (endothelial cells) line all vascular and lymphatic channels in the body.
Keywords: Simple squamous epithelium

44 **The answer is D: Smooth muscle.** The arrow identifies smooth muscle in the tunica media of a small artery. The myocytes are spindle-shaped cells with central nuclei. The nuclei are generally aligned with the arc of the tunica media. Some of the nuclei assume a "corkscrew" appearance, due to postmortem contraction of the muscle cells. These nuclear features help distinguish smooth muscle from connective tissue (choices A and B).
Keywords: Smooth muscle

45 **The answer is A: Dense irregular connective tissue.** Large, coarse, and densely packed collagen bundles with few fibroblast cell nuclei are the characteristic features of dense connective tissue. The presence of collagen fibers running in many different directions provides evidence of irregular collagen assembly.
Keywords: Dense irregular connective tissue

46 **The answer is D: Respiratory bronchiole.** Respiratory bronchioles are distal to terminal bronchioles (the space indicated by number 2). They are transitional regions between conducting and respiratory portions of the respiratory system. They have incomplete walls that are interrupted by openings to respiratory alveoli. Smooth muscle cells are still visible in portions of the bronchiole wall located beneath the simple cuboidal epithelium.
Keywords: Respiratory system, respiratory bronchioles

47 The answer is C: Space 3.   Gas exchange occurs within pulmonary alveoli. These microscopic sac-like structures give the lungs a spongy texture. Clusters of alveoli open into a common space referred to as an alveoli sac. Alveoli sacs are continuous with alveolar ducts.
Keywords: Respiratory system, alveolar sacs

48 The answer is A: Alveolar duct.   Alveolar ducts are long, thin-walled tubules whose walls are entirely lined by openings of alveoli and alveolar sacs. Proximally, alveolar ducts are continuous with respiratory bronchioles.
Keywords: Respiratory system, alveolar ducts

49 The answer is B: Heart.   The image shows a transverse section through a group of cardiac muscle fibers. The muscle fibers demonstrate relatively large diameters with centrally located nuclei. Myofibrils can be identified at higher magnification.
Keywords: Cardiac muscle

50 The answer is D: Skeletal muscle.   The image shows a transverse section through a skeletal muscle. The muscle fibers are organized into fascicles. Their nuclei are situated at the periphery of the muscle cells.
Keywords: Skeletal muscle

51 The answer is D: Muscularis externa of the colon.   This is a cross-section through smooth muscle tissue. Smooth muscle fibers are spindle-shaped cells with single, centrally located nuclei. Thus, in a given transverse section, many cells are expected to appear without nuclei. In cells whose nuclei are visible in the section plane, the nuclei are located in the center of the cytoplasm. Smooth muscle fibers are smaller in diameter than those of skeletal and cardiac muscle.
Keywords: Smooth muscle

52 The answer is C: Peripheral nerve.   This image represents a cross section through a peripheral nerve. The axons are tightly packed and enveloped with perineurium and epineurium. The dark-stained axons are surrounded by a pale circular space that represents the lipid-rich myelin sheath that was removed during tissue processing. Endoneurium is a delicate layer of connective tissue that encloses each axon and its associated myelin sheath.
Keywords: Peripheral nerve

53 The answer is A: Compact bone/haversian system.   This section through compact bone reveals bone-forming cells in lacunae and well-organized, eosinophilic collagen lamellae. The concentric layers of collagen surround a centrally located canal (haversian canal) that forms part of the haversian system. The arrowhead indicates a Volkmann canal.
Keywords: Compact bone

54 The answer is A: Bone/osteocytes.   This image shows a bone spicule that is composed of densely packed collagen lamellae. The bone-forming cells that are located within the lacunae are osteocytes. The cellular tissue surrounding the spicule is red bone marrow.
Keywords: Bone, osteocyte

55 The answer is B: Complexity of cells and extracellular matrix.   Bone, cartilage, tendon, and lamina propria are all connective tissues composed of cells and extracellular matrix. The organization of the extracellular matrix is chiefly responsible for their specific functions. Macrophages (choice A) are abundant in the lamina propria of the GI tract, but they are not abundant in bone, cartilage, and other dense connective tissues. Connective tissue capsules (choice C) surround bone (periosteum), cartilage (perichondrium), and tendon (epitendineum), but capsules do not surround loose connective tissues such as the lamina propria. Type I collagen fibers (choice D) are the major component of bone, tendon, and lamina propria, whereas type II collage fibrils are the predominant fibrous component of cartilage. Finally, bone and lamina propria receive a rich blood supply (choice E), but tendons do not, and cartilage is avascular.
Keywords: Connective tissue

56 The answer is A: Pseudostratified columnar.   This image shows a cross section of the trachea. The respiratory epithelium exhibits numerous goblet cells with dark-stained mucus. Cilia are visible along the apical surface of the epithelial cells. The respiratory epithelium appears stratified, because the lining cells differ in height; however, all of the cells are attached to the underlying basal lamina.
Keywords: Pseudostratified columnar epithelium

57 The answer is E: Urinary bladder.   Several distinct cell layers are evident in this lining epithelium. The dome-shaped apical cells indicate this is a transitional epithelium that lines organs of the urinary system (bladder, ureters, and proximal portion of the urethra).
Keywords: Transitional epithelium, urotholium

58 The answer is D: Stratified squamous.   The epithelium contains numerous cell layers with squamous cells in the most apical layer. The apical cells are nucleated, and the epithelium is not keratinized.
Keywords: Stratified squamous epithelium

59 The answer is D: Hyaline cartilage.   Histologic features of this slide include (1) translucent extracellular matrix, (2) chondrocytes situated in lacunae, and (3) isogenous groups. These are the typical characteristics of hyaline cartilage. The eosinophilic stained connective tissue surrounding the cartilage is perichondrium.
Keywords: Hyaline cartilage

60 **The answer is A: External ear.** This image illustrates histologic features of elastic cartilage. Chondrocytes are visible in lacunae, and fibrous components are present in the extracellular matrix. Compared to coarse, eosinophilic collagen fibers in the surrounding perichondrium, elastic fibers are smaller in diameter and more basophilic. Elastic cartilage has a restricted distribution in the body. This type of cartilage is only found in the Eustachian tube, epiglottis, and external ear.
Keywords: Elastic cartilage

61 **The answer is D: Jejunum.** This autopsy specimen was obtained from the jejunum. In this portion of the GI tract, the mucosa and submucosa are folded extensively to increase surface area for absorption. These submucosal folds are referred to as plicae circulares.
Keywords: Gastrointestinal tract, plicae circulares

62 **The answer is B: Kidney.** This image shows renal corpuscles, convoluted tubules, and straight tubules. These are histologic features of the renal cortex.
Keywords: Kidney, renal cortex

63 **The answer is A: Bipolar.** The spiral ganglion cells located in the bony core of the cochlea are bipolar neurons. Their dendrites synapse with hair cells of the spiral organ, and their axons form the auditory nerve that extends into the central nervous system.
Keywords: Bipolar neuron

64 **The answer is B: Granulosa cells.** This image shows a tangential section through a secondary oocyte in the ovary. Granulosa cells surround the oocyte to form a cumulous oophorus and corona radiata. They secrete steroid hormone precursors that are converted to estrogen by a layer of theca interna cells that surrounds each follicle. Decidual cells (choice A) are found in the uterine endometrium during pregnancy. Leydig cells (choice C) are interstitial cells in the testes that secrete testosterone. Parafollicular cells (choice D) are calcitonin-producing cells in the thyroid gland. Theca interna cells (choice E) are visible in this image (lower left side), as a band of connective tissue cells in contact with the stratum granulosum.
Keywords: Granulosa cells, ovarian follicles

65 **The answer is B: Arrow 2.** This thin plastic section of a seminiferous tubule shows meiotic and haploid germ cells at various stages of spermatogenesis and spermiogenesis. Primary spermatocytes feature highly condensed chromatin that is undergoing homologous recombination and crossing-over during prophase of meiosis I. None of the other cells exhibit the distinct nuclear morphology of primary spermatocytes.
Keywords: Spermatogenesis, spermiogenesis

66 **The answer is D: Arrow 4.** Sertoli cells regulate spermatogenesis through direct interactions with germ cells. Their basal membrane is attached to the basement membrane, and their apical membrane extends to the lumen of the seminiferous tubule. Sertoli cell nuclei are typically described as having an oval or almond shape (shown in the image). Sertoli cells secrete a variety of hormones and transport proteins, including anti-müllerian hormone, inhibin, and androgen-binding protein (ABP). ABP concentrates testosterone and delivers it to the male genital ducts and glands (e.g., seminal vesicles and prostate). None of the other testicular cells secrete ABP.
Keywords: Sertoli cells

67 **The answer is E: Secretory-phase endometrium.** This shows the typical sawtooth appearance of uterine glands during the secretory phase of the uterine (menstrual) cycle. The glands become tortuous and secretory under the influence of progesterone that is secreted by the corpus luteum after ovulation. None of the other female reproductive organs exhibit the distinct histologic features of the secretory-phase uterine endometrium.
Keywords: Uterine endometrium, menstrual cycle

68 **The answer is E: Vasopressin.** This image shows two lobes of the pituitary bland connected to the hypothalamus through the infundibulum. The anterior lobe of the pituitary is composed of glandular epithelial cells that secrete a wide variety of polypeptide hormones, such as FSH and LH. The posterior pituitary is composed of terminal nerve axons with Herring bodies that secrete vasopressin and oxytocin. Vasopressin is also referred to as antidiuretic hormone (ADH). The pituitary does not secrete the other hormones listed.
Keywords: Pituitary, antidiuretic hormone

69 **The answer is B: Chief cells.** The arrow identifies a parathyroid gland along the posterior wall of the thyroid gland. The thyroid gland is filled with numerous, colloid-filled follicles. When examined at higher magnification, the parathyroid gland is observed to consist of tightly packed cords and clusters of glandular epithelial cells. Chief cells secrete parathyroid hormone (PTH). None of the other cells are found in the parathyroid gland or secrete PTH.
Keywords: Parathyroid gland, chief cells

70 **The answer is C: Layer 3.** The adrenal gland has two functional layers, namely the cortex and medulla. The cortex is further subdivided into three zones based on cell morphology and endocrine secretion. These zones include zona glomerulosa (layer 2, aldosterone secretion), zona fasciculate (layer 3, cortisol secretion), and zona reticularis (layer 4, weak androgen secretion). In this image, layer 5 identifies the adrenal medulla. The zona fasciculata is

characterized by long cords of epithelial cells separated by fenestrated capillaries. The other zones in the adrenal cortex synthesize small amounts of cortisol; however, the zona fasciculata secretes most of this steroid hormone.
Keywords: Adrenal gland, cortex

71 **The answer is D: Muscular artery.** Trichrome stains are commonly used to distinguish collagen connective tissue from smooth muscle. In this photomicrograph, many layers of red-stained smooth muscle fibers are visible in the tunica media of a muscular artery. RBCs are visible in the vascular lumen.
Keywords: Muscular artery

72 **The answer is E: Sebaceous gland.** Secretory cells in sebaceous glands are large and swollen cells, and they exhibit a central pyknotic nucleus. The cytoplasm is foamy and pale, owing to the extraction of lipids and waxes during tissue preparation. Small, dark-stained basal cells can proliferate and differentiate into secretory cells to replace mature cells that are lost as a result of programmed cell death during holocrine secretion.
Keywords: Sebaceous glands

73 **The answer is E: Smooth muscle.** This is a longitudinal section of smooth muscle through the muscularis externus of the colon. The histologic features of the different tissue types have been described in previous chapters, as well as earlier in this review chapter. This smooth muscle section is similar in appearance to dense regular connective tissue and fibrocartilage. However, dense regular connective tissue contains fewer cells, and the fibroblast nuclei are flat and display heterochromatin; abundant large collagen bundles occupy the extracellular space. In fibrocartilage, type I collagen fibers in the extracellular matrix may resemble the cytoplasm of smooth muscle cells; however, most of the cells in fibrocartilage are chondrocytes, and they are located in lacunae.
Keywords: Smooth muscle

74 **The answer is A: Cardiac muscle.** This section of cardiac muscle was stained with hematoxylin/permanganate oxide to highlight intercalated disks (vertical white lines, shown in the image). Cardiac and skeletal muscles are similar in appearance: both tissues feature large muscle fibers with transverse striations. However, cardiac muscle is uniquely characterized by the presence of intercalated disks. Special stains can be used to identify these anchoring junctions.
Keywords: Cardiac muscle, intercalated disks

Chapter 21

Introduction to Histopathology

QUESTIONS

Select the single best answer.

1 A 54-year-old woman presents with a 4-month history of increasing abdominal girth. Percussion of the patient's abdomen indicates fluid within the peritoneal cavity (ascites). Aspiration of the ascites reveals small, gland-like structures (shown in the image). These pathologic findings are consistent with which of the following mechanisms of disease?

   (A) Cell adaptation
   (B) Chronic inflammation
   (C) Hemodynamic disorder
   (D) Neoplasia
   (E) Nutritional pathology

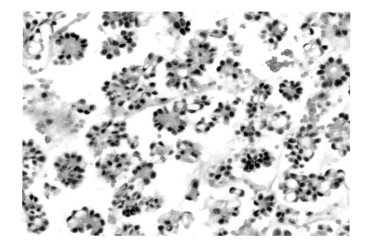

2 You examine a slide with a surgical pathologist at a double-headed microscope (shown in the image) and are asked to describe what you see. Which of the following best describes this tissue and the response to injury?

   (A) Cardiac muscle, fibrosis
   (B) Cardiac muscle, necrosis
   (C) Skeletal muscle, inflammation
   (D) Smooth muscle, fibrosis
   (E) Smooth muscle, inflammation

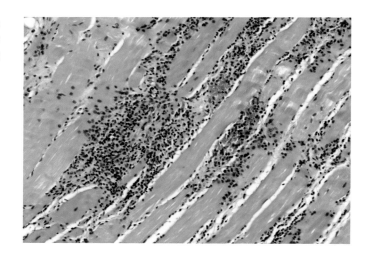

3 A 75-year-old woman with terminal cancer develops multiple organ failure and expires. The heart at autopsy is enlarged and weighs 380 g (normal = 230 to 280 g in women). A section of heart muscle is stained with H&E (shown in the image). How does the microscopic appearance of the patient's myocardium (image on right) differ from that of a normal myocardium (image on left)?

(A) There has been irreversible injury to myocytes.
(B) There is accumulation of lipid material within the myocytes.
(C) There is an inflammatory infiltrate in the myocardium.
(D) There is deposition of collagen in the myocardium.
(E) There is enlargement of individual myocytes.

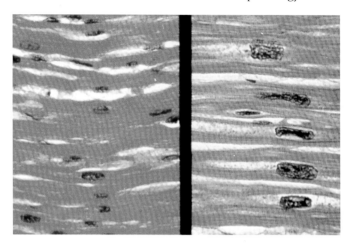

4 A 30-year-old woman suffers weakness of her right leg following an automobile accident, and a muscle biopsy is obtained (shown in the image). Compared to normal muscle fibers on the left, abnormal muscle fibers on the right side of this biopsy show which of the following histopathologic changes?

(A) Abnormal pattern of myocyte differentiation
(B) Accumulation of glycogen within myofibers
(C) Decrease in the size of myocytes
(D) Increased numbers of otherwise normal myocytes
(E) Transformation of one differentiated cell type to another

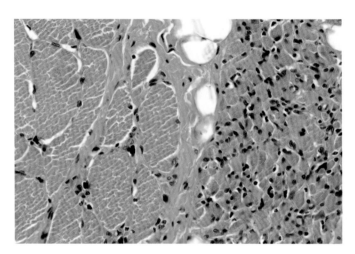

5 An endometrial biopsy is obtained from a 42-year-old woman with a history of dysfunctional uterine bleeding (shown in the image). Compared to normal endometrial tissue on the left of the indicated line, abnormal tissue on the right side of this biopsy shows which of the following histopathologic changes?

(A) Accumulation of chronic inflammatory cells
(B) Deposition of amorphous eosinophilic material
(C) Focal atrophy of the glandular epithelium.
(D) Increased cellularity of the glandular epithelium
(E) Irreversible injury (coagulative necrosis)

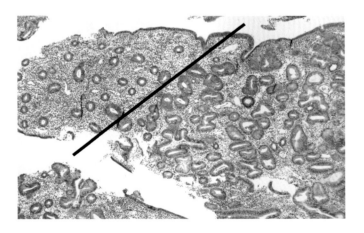

6 A 38-year-old woman complains of cold intolerance and frequent constipation. Physical examination reveals soft tissue swelling (edema) and a firm, diffusely enlarged thyroid gland. Serum levels of T_3 and T_4 are abnormally low. A thyroid biopsy is shown in the image. Which of the following describes histopathologic findings observed in this patient's thyroid gland?

(A) Calcification within the gland
(B) Enlargement and growth of follicular epithelial cells
(C) Evidence of irreversible cell injury
(D) Extensive fibrosis within the gland
(E) Infiltrate of chronic inflammatory cells

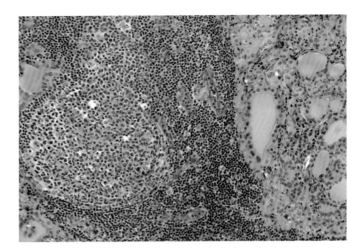

7 A 65-year-old man presents with a lesion on the dorsal aspect of a finger. A biopsy of the mass is examined by light microscopy (shown in the image). The pathologist states that the neoplastic cells resemble cells of the stratum spinosum of the epidermis. Based on your understanding of skin histology, what is the appropriate pathologic diagnosis?

(A) Adenocarcinoma
(B) Hemangioma
(C) Malignant melanoma
(D) Squamous cell carcinoma
(E) Transitional cell carcinoma

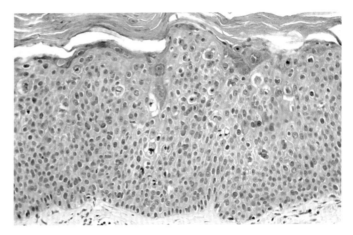

8 A 74-year-old man from a mountain region of the country develops respiratory insufficiency and expires. The patient's organs are examined at autopsy. Compared to a normal bone marrow (image on left), the patient's bone marrow (image on right) demonstrates which of the following reversible adaptive changes?

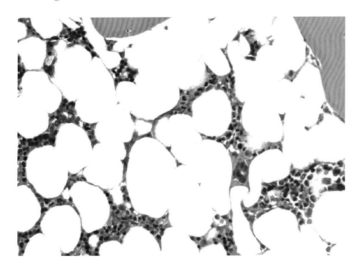

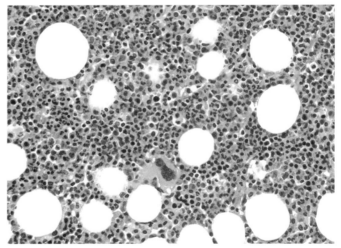

(A) Atrophy (decreased cell size/function)
(B) Dysplasia (abnormal maturation)
(C) Hyperplasia (increased numbers of cells)
(D) Hypertrophy (increased cell size/function)
(E) Metaplasia (new differentiation pathway)

9 A 34-year-old woman presents with a 3-month history of fatigue, mild fever, and skin rash. Physical examination reveals erythematous (red) plaques on the trunk and neck with silvery scales that induce bleeding when removed. Biopsy of lesional skin is obtained. Compared to normal skin (image on left), the patient's biopsy (image on right) shows which of the following histopathologic changes?

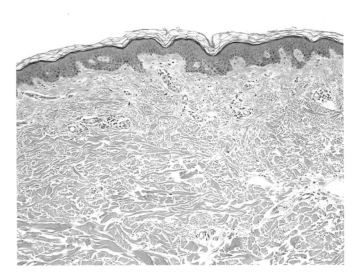
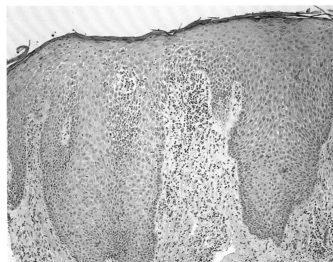

(A) Abnormal pattern of cellular maturation
(B) Increased numbers of otherwise normal cells
(C) Invasion of neoplastic cells through the basement membrane
(D) Transformation of one differentiated cell type to another
(E) Ulceration and necrosis of the epithelium

10 A 22-year-old woman complains of intense bone pain. Physical examination reveals enlargement of her spleen (splenomegaly). A percutaneous spleen biopsy is obtained. Compared to a normal spleen (image on left), the patient's spleen biopsy (image on right) shows which of the following histopathologic changes?

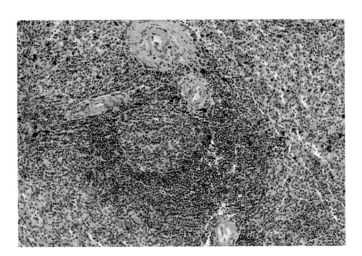
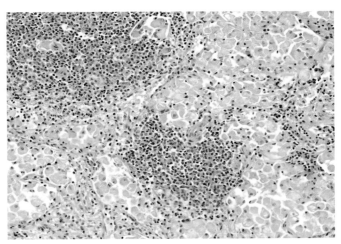

(A) Absence of lymphoid follicles
(B) Accumulation of abnormal cells
(C) Hemorrhage from trabecular arteries
(D) Presence of multinucleated giant cells
(E) Proliferation of small lymphocytes

11 A 78-year-old farmer presents with an encrusted lesion on his cheek, and a biopsy is obtained. How does the histologic appearance of the patient's skin biopsy (image on right) differ from that of normal skin (image on left)?

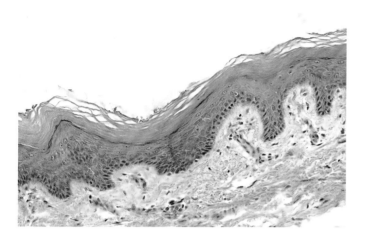
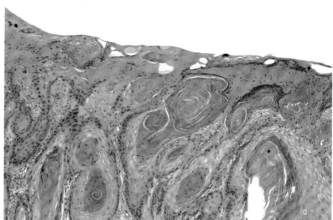

(A) There are intravascular blood clots within dermal arterioles.
(B) There is a neoplastic proliferation of keratinocytes.
(C) There is an accumulation of lipid material within dermal macrophages.
(D) There is an inflammatory infiltrate in the papillary dermis.
(E) There is deposition of collagenous scar tissue in the dermis.

12 A 70-year-old man with a history of recurrent episodes of chest pain (angina) suffers a heart attack and expires. At autopsy, a section of the patient's heart is stained for elastic tissue and examined by light microscopy. Compared to a normal muscular artery (image on left), the patient's left anterior descending artery (image on right) shows which of the following histopathologic changes?

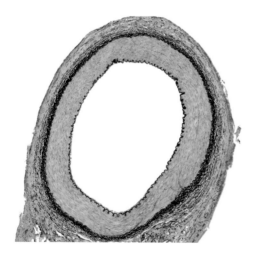
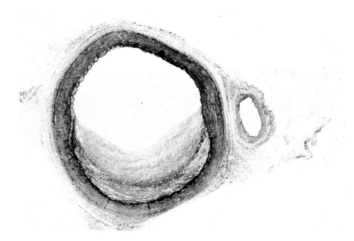

(A) Accumulation of cells and lipid material in the arterial wall
(B) Destruction of the vessel wall by inflammatory cells
(C) Dissecting aneurysm and formation of a second lumen
(D) Loss of elastic fibers and cystic medial necrosis
(E) Uncontrolled proliferation of vascular endothelial cells

13 A 74-year-old woman with a history of systemic hypertension develops heart failure and expires. At autopsy, a section of the patient's aorta is stained with aldehyde fuchsin and examined by light microscopy. Compared to a normal aortic media (image on left), the media of the patient's thoracic aorta (image on right) shows which of the following histopathologic changes?

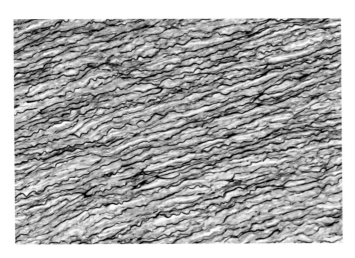 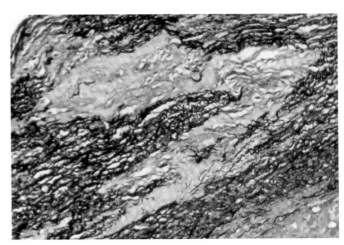

(A) Disruption of elastic fibers
(B) Excess deposition of collagen
(C) Infiltration by chronic inflammatory cells
(D) Occlusion of the vasa vasorum
(E) Proliferation of vascular endothelial cells

14 A 76-year-old woman with a history of smoking and hypertension suffers a massive heart attack and expires. The patient's coronary arteries are examined at autopsy. Compared to a normal artery (image on left), the patient's posterior interventricular artery (image on right) shows which of the following histopathologic changes?

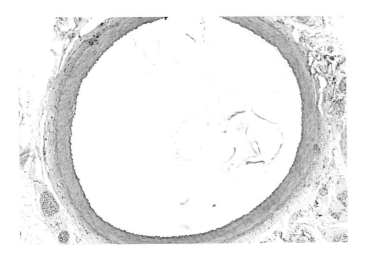 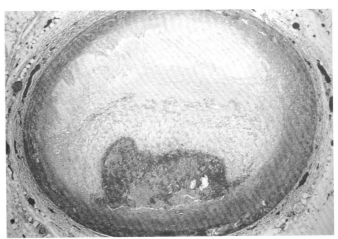

(A) Destruction of the vessel wall by inflammatory cells
(B) Dissecting aneurysm and formation of a second lumen
(C) Loss of elastic fibers and cystic medial necrosis
(D) Occlusion of the lumen by a thrombus
(E) Uncontrolled proliferation of vascular endothelial cells

15 A 68-year-old woman is admitted to the hospital in severe respiratory distress. Her temperature is 38.7°C (103°F), respirations 32/minute, and blood pressure 130/90 mm Hg. She coughs constantly and expectorates bloody sputum. The patient subsequently develops infection of the blood and expires. The lungs are examined at autopsy. How does the histologic appearance of the patient's lung (image on right) differ from that of a normal lung (image on left)?

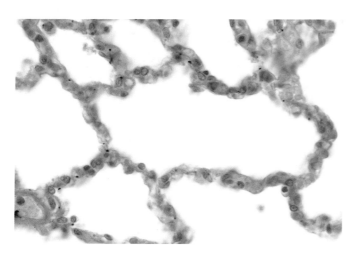 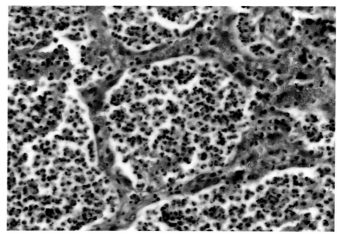

(A) The air spaces are filled with fluid.
(B) The air spaces are filled with inflammatory cells.
(C) The air spaces are overly distended.
(D) There is enlargement of type II pneumocytes.
(E) There is excess collagen in the alveolar septa.

16 A 69-year-old man with a long-standing history of systemic hypertension complains that his face and ankles appear swollen. Urinalysis reveals mild proteinuria, and a kidney biopsy is obtained. How does the histologic appearance of this patient's renal arteriole (image on right) differ from that of a normal renal arteriole (image on left)?

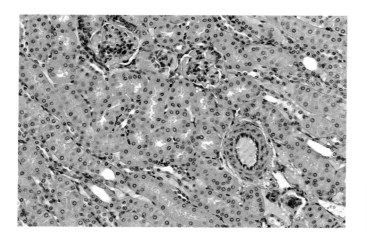 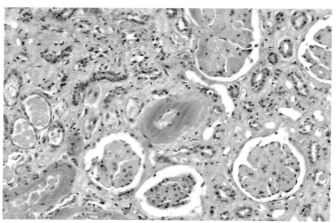

(A) The lumen of the vessel is occluded by a blood clot.
(B) The wall of the vessel has been destroyed by inflammatory cells.
(C) There is a proliferation of endothelial cells.
(D) There is an accumulation of lipid material in the vessel wall.
(E) There is thickening of the arteriole wall.

17 A 76-year-old man with congestive heart failure complains of persistent cough and shortness of breath (dyspnea) on exertion. The patient subsequently suffers a stroke and expires. The brain and internal organs are examined at autopsy. How does the histologic appearance of the patient's lung (image on right) differ from that of a normal lung (image on left)?

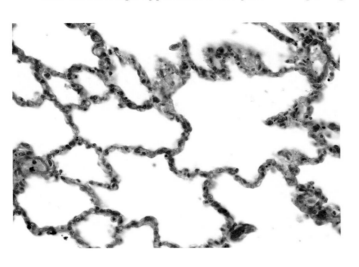
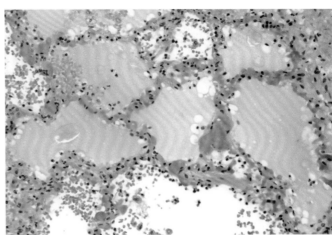

(A) The air spaces are filled with fluid.
(B) The air spaces are filled with inflammatory cells.
(C) The air spaces are overly distended.
(D) There is excess collagen in the alveolar septa.
(E) There is enlargement of type II pneumocytes.

18 A 68-year-old woman with a history of chronic hepatitis B presents with fever, weight loss, and hemorrhagic skin lesions. Four years later, the patient suffers a stroke and expires. The internal organs are examined at autopsy. Compared to normal arterioles (image on left), submucosal arterioles in this patient's gallbladder (image on right) show which of the following histopathologic changes?

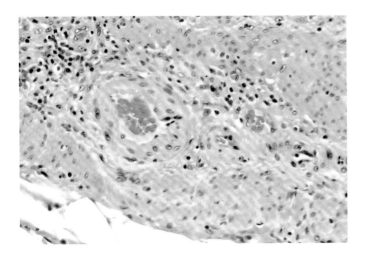
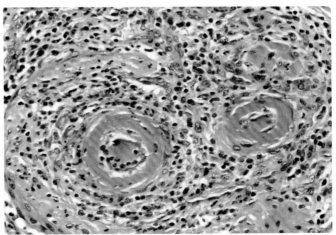

(A) Accumulation of lipid material in the arterial wall
(B) Destruction of the vessel wall by inflammatory cells
(C) Intimal tear with dissecting aneurysm and formation of a second lumen
(D) Loss of elastic fibers and cystic medial necrosis
(E) Uncontrolled proliferation of vascular endothelial cells

19 A 38-year-old man with AIDS presents with fever and a persistent dry cough. A chest x-ray shows bilateral diffuse infiltrates. A transbronchial lung biopsy is obtained. Compared to a normal lung (image on left), the patient's lung biopsy (image on right) shows which of the following histopathologic changes?

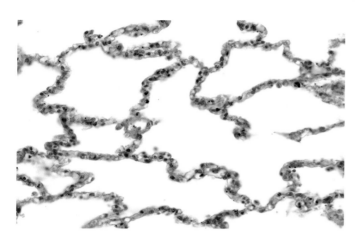
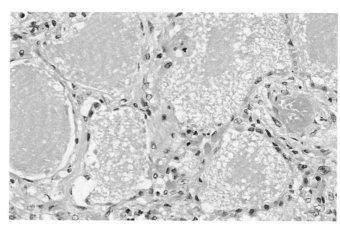

(A) Air spaces filled with inflammatory cells
(B) Enlargement of type II pneumocytes
(C) Foamy exudate within the air spaces
(D) Hemorrhage in the air spaces
(E) Neoplastic change in the respiratory epithelium

20 A 70-year-old man dies from complications of congestive heart failure. At autopsy, a section of heart muscle is stained with Masson trichrome. Compared to a normal myocardium (image on left), the patient's myocardium (image on right) shows which of the following histopathologic changes?

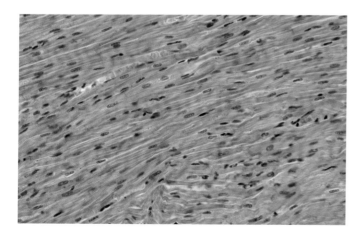
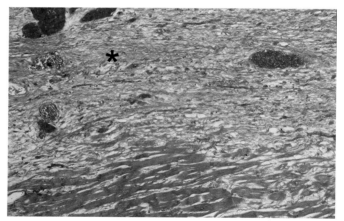

(A) Accumulation of glycogen within the myocytes
(B) Deposition of collagen in the myocardium
(C) Enlargement of individual cardiac myocytes
(D) Inflammatory infiltrate in the myocardium
(E) Neoplastic proliferation of cardiac myocytes

21 A 56-year-old man is admitted to the hospital with increasing shortness of breath and dry cough for the past 3 years. He is "gasping for air" and walks with difficulty, because he becomes breathless after only a few steps. The patient subsequently dies of cancer. A section of his lung is examined at autopsy. How does the histologic appearance of the patient's lung (image on right) differ from that of a normal lung (image on left)?

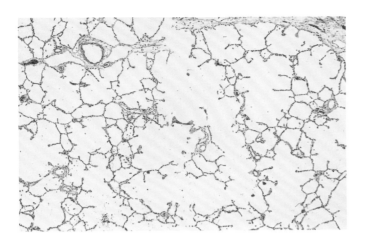 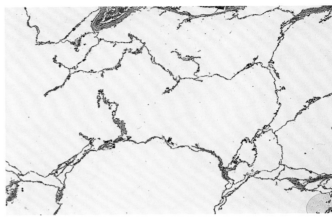

(A) The air spaces are filled with fluid.
(B) The air spaces are filled with inflammatory cells.
(C) The air spaces are overly distended.
(D) There is enlargement of type II pneumocytes.
(E) There is excess collagen in the alveolar septa.

22 A 20-year-old man dies suddenly while playing basketball, and his heart is examined at autopsy. Compared to a normal myocardium (image on left), the patient's myocardium (image on right) shows which of the following histopathologic changes?

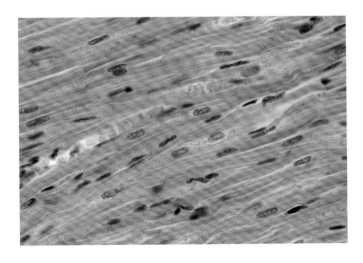 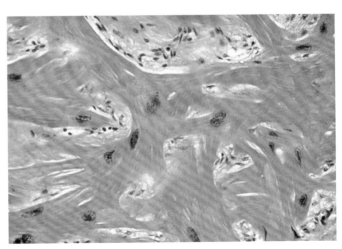

(A) Accumulation of lipid material within myocytes
(B) Disarray of the cardiac myocytes
(C) Enlargement of individual myocytes
(D) Inflammatory infiltrate in the myocardium
(E) Irreversible injury to the myocytes

23 A 75-year-old man who handled asbestos fibers in a shipyard for many years developed progressive shortness of breath and died of respiratory insufficiency. A section of his lung is examined at autopsy. How does the histologic appearance of the patient's lung (image on right) differ from that of a normal lung (image on left)?

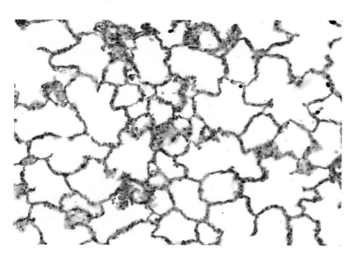 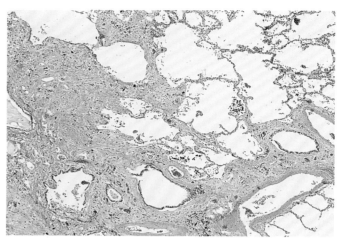

(A) The air spaces are filled with eosinophils.
(B) There are fibrin-rich membranes in the air spaces.
(C) There is a neoplastic change in the respiratory epithelium.
(D) There is enlargement of type II pneumocytes.
(E) There is excess collagen in the alveolar septa.

24 An endoscopic biopsy of the distal esophagus is obtained from a 50-year-old man with a history of chronic epigastric pain (heartburn). How does the histologic appearance of the patient's biopsy (image on right) differ from that of a normal esophagus (image on left)?

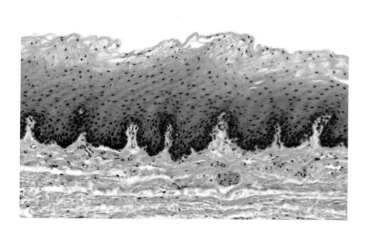 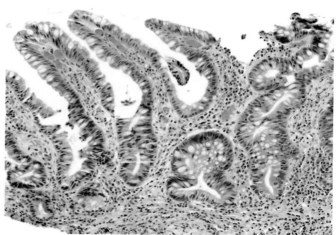

(A) The cell type of the surface epithelium has changed.
(B) The esophageal mucosa has been eroded.
(C) There has been a neoplastic change in the epithelium.
(D) There is a foreign material within the epithelium.
(E) There is an infectious process within the epithelium.

25 A 55-year-old alcoholic presents with upper gastrointestinal bleeding and expires. The distal esophagus is examined at autopsy. Compared to a normal esophagus (image on left), the patient's esophagus (image on right) shows which of the following histopathologic changes?

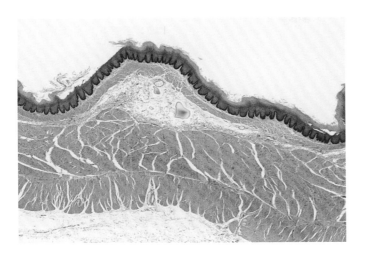 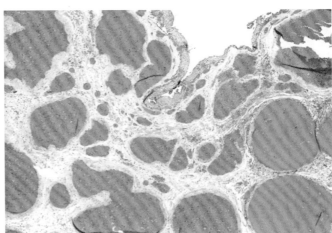

(A) Accumulation of inflammatory cells in the submucosa
(B) Alteration of the submucosal vasculature
(C) Erosion of the esophageal mucosa
(D) New uncontrolled growth of the lining epithelium
(E) Thickening of the muscular wall of the esophagus

26 A 56-year-old woman suffers major trauma in a motor vehicle accident and expires. An incidental finding is observed at autopsy. How does the histologic appearance of the patient's stomach (image on right) differ from that of the normal stomach (image on left)?

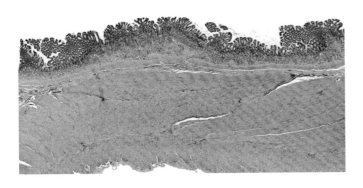 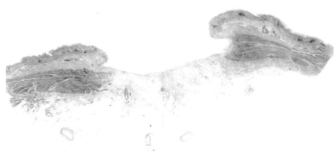

(A) The cell type of the surface epithelium has been changed.
(B) The gastric mucosa has been eroded.
(C) The muscular wall of the stomach is thickened.
(D) The submucosal vasculature has been altered.
(E) There has been a neoplastic change in the epithelium.

27 A 50-year-old woman with a history of chronic hepatitis C presents with jaundice and chronic fatigue. A liver biopsy is stained with Masson trichrome and examined by light microscopy. How does the histologic appearance of the patient's liver (image on right) differ from that of the normal liver (image on left)?

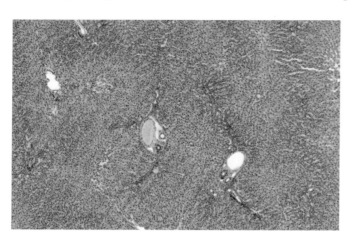
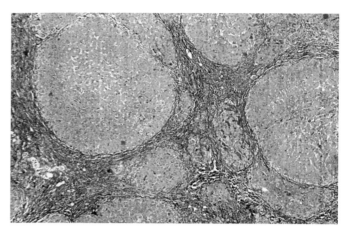

(A) The bile canaliculi are dilated by bile plugs.
(B) The hepatic architecture has been distorted by scar tissue.
(C) There is a vascular alteration within the liver.
(D) There is excess iron deposition in the hepatocytes.
(E) There is fat accumulation within the hepatocytes.

28 A 4-year-old child is brought to the family physician with parental concerns regarding diarrhea and growth retardation. Laboratory studies demonstrate intestinal malabsorption. A biopsy of the child's proximal small intestine is obtained. How does the histologic appearance of the patient's intestinal biopsy (image on right) differ from that of a normal intestine (image on left)?

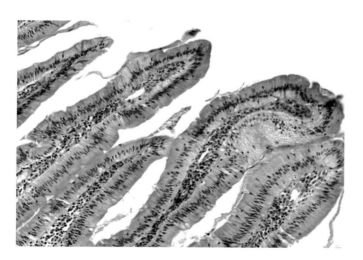
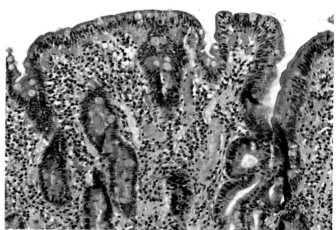

(A) The absorptive surface has been attenuated.
(B) The cell type of the surface epithelium has been changed.
(C) The submucosal vasculature has been altered.
(D) There is an infectious process within the epithelium.
(E) There is erosion of the surface epithelium.

29 A liver biopsy is obtained from a 45-year-old man with mildly elevated liver enzymes (aminotransferases). Compared to a normal liver (image on left), the patient's liver biopsy (image on right) shows which of the following histopathologic changes?

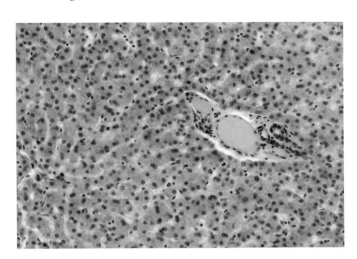 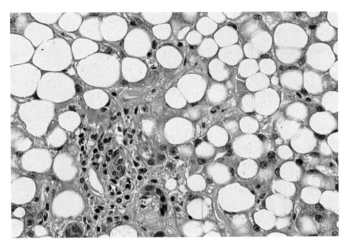

(A) Bile canaliculi dilated by bile plugs
(B) Deposition of lipofuscin in hepatocytes
(C) Excess iron deposition in hepatocytes
(D) Fat accumulation within hepatocytes
(E) Vascular alteration within the liver

30 A 68-year-old woman with varicose veins of her legs develops acute pulmonary thromboembolism. Despite treatment, the patient develops multiple organ system failure and expires. An incidental finding is discovered at autopsy. Compared to a normal colon (image on left), the patient's colon (image on right) shows which of the following histopathologic findings?

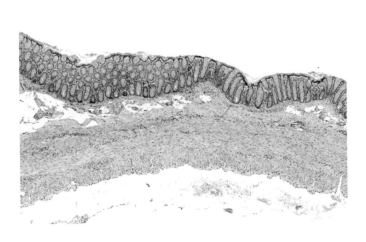 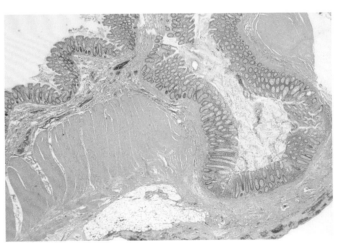

(A) Alteration of submucosal vasculature
(B) Benign neoplasm of the epithelium
(C) Defect in the wall of the colon
(D) Submucosal collagen deposition
(E) Superficial inflammatory membranes

31 A 34-year-old woman with a recent history of sore throat complains of a recent change in the color of her urine. Physical examination reveals soft tissue swelling (generalized edema). Laboratory studies demonstrate hematuria and moderate renal insufficiency (elevated serum levels of creatinine). A percutaneous renal biopsy is stained with Masson trichrome and examined by light microscopy. How does the microscopic appearance of the patient's glomerulus (image on right) differ from that of the normal control (image on left)?

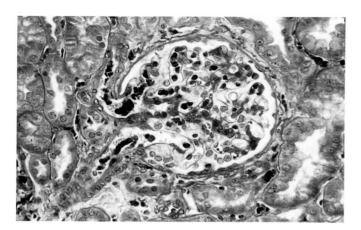 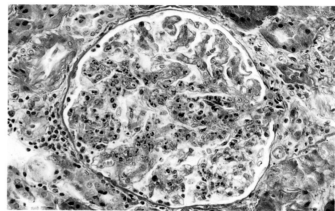

(A) The glomerulus appears normal.
(B) The glomerulus is hypercellular.
(C) The glomerulus shows marked atrophy.
(D) There is diffuse necrosis of the glomerulus.
(E) There is thickening of the glomerular capillary loops.

32 A colon biopsy is obtained from a 58-year-old man with a history of intermittent rectal bleeding. How does the histologic appearance of the patient's colon biopsy (image on right) differ from that of a normal colon (image on left)?

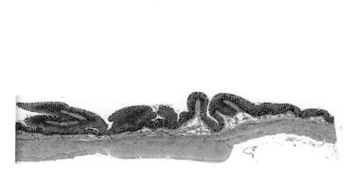 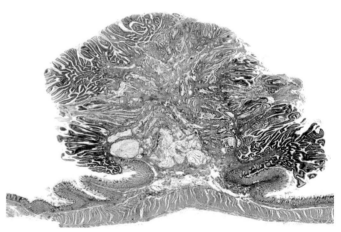

(A) The submucosal vasculature has been altered.
(B) There has been a neoplastic change in the epithelium.
(C) There is a defect in the wall of the colon.
(D) There is an increase in submucosal collagen.
(E) There is destruction of the glandular epithelium.

33 A 60-year-old obese woman (BMI = 34 kg/m^2) complains of excessive thirst and urine production (polydipsia and polyuria). Laboratory studies reveal glucosuria (sugar in urine) and proteinuria (protein in urine). A renal biopsy is obtained and stained with PAS reagent. How does the microscopic appearance of the patient's glomerulus (image on right) differ from that of the normal control (image on left)?

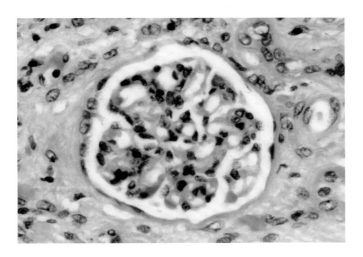 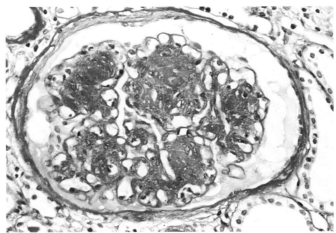

(A) There is acute inflammation of the glomerulus.
(B) There is diffuse necrosis of the glomerulus.
(C) There is expansion of the mesangium-forming nodular lesions.
(D) There is hemorrhage into the urinary space.
(E) There is marked atrophy of the glomerulus.

34 A 50-year-old man from Egypt presents with blood in his urine (hematuria). The patient's past medical history is significant for a parasitic infestation of his bladder (schistosomiasis). A biopsy of the bladder wall is obtained. How does the microscopic appearance of the patient's bladder (image on right) differ from that of normal bladder epithelium (image on left)?

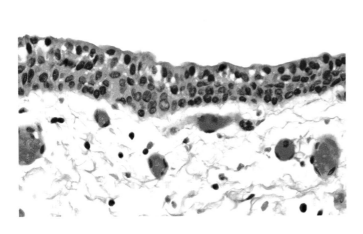 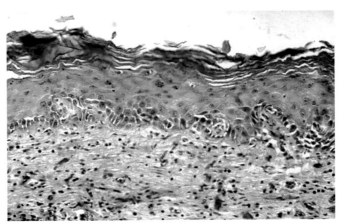

(A) The cell type of the epithelium has been changed.
(B) The epithelium shows new uncontrolled growth.
(C) The lamina propria of the mucosa is absent.
(D) There is an infectious process within the epithelium.
(E) There is erosion of the surface epithelium.

35 A testicular biopsy is obtained from a 24-year-old man who, along with his wife, is being evaluated for infertility. How does the histologic appearance of the patient's testis (image on right) differ from that of the normal testis (image on left)?

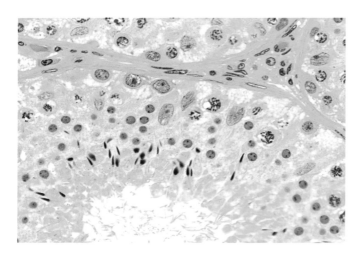
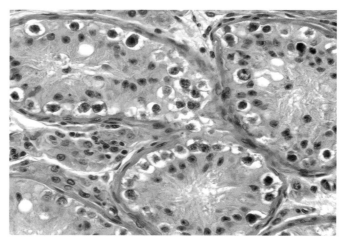

(A) Spermatogenesis appears essentially normal.
(B) There is a chronic inflammatory cell infiltrate.
(C) There is a proliferation of abnormal germ cells.
(D) There is an increase in stromal cells with tubular atrophy.
(E) There is evidence of irreversible germ cell injury.

36 A prostate biopsy is obtained from a 55-year-old man with an elevated serum level of prostate-specific antigen (PSA = 9.5 ng/mL, normal = 0 to 4 ng/mL). Compared to a normal prostate (image on left), the patient's prostate biopsy (image on right) shows which of the following histopathologic changes?

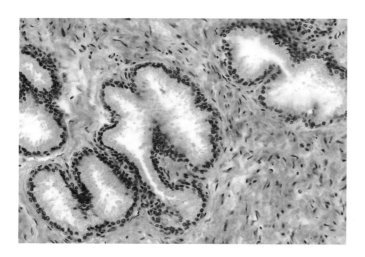
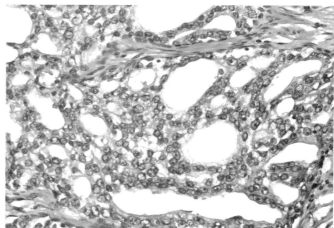

(A) Accumulation of chronic inflammatory cells
(B) Atrophy of glandular epithelium
(C) Expansion of fibromuscular stroma
(D) Irreversible cell injury
(E) Proliferation of epithelial cells

37 A cervical Pap smear is obtained from a 28-year-old woman. Compared to normal cervical epithelial cells (image on left), the patient's epithelial cells (image on right) exhibit which of the following pathologic features?

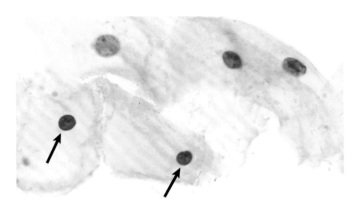 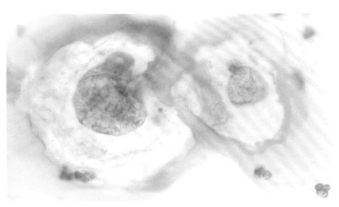

(A) Lewy bodies
(B) Nuclear pyknosis
(C) Papillary morphology
(D) Perinuclear halos
(E) Squamous metaplasia

38 A 32-year-old woman complains of heat intolerance, heart palpitations, and recent weight loss. Serum levels of T_3 and T_4 are elevated. A biopsy of the thyroid is obtained. How does the histologic appearance of the patient's thyroid gland (image on right) differ from that of a normal thyroid (image on left)?

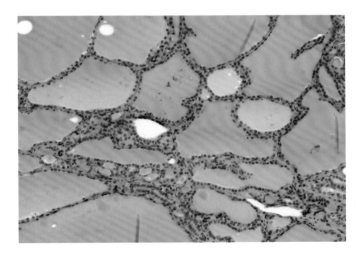 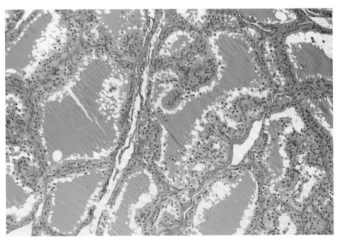

(A) There are areas of calcification within the gland.
(B) There is a chronic inflammatory cell infiltrate.
(C) There is enlargement and growth of follicular cells.
(D) There is evidence of irreversible injury.
(E) There is extensive fibrosis of the gland.

39 A 59-year-old woman discovers a lump in her breast. Mammography demonstrates a linear and punctate pattern of abnormal calcification. Compared to normal breast tissue (image on left), the patient's breast biopsy shows malignant cells confined by the gland's basement membrane (image on right). Which of the following best describes these histopathologic findings?

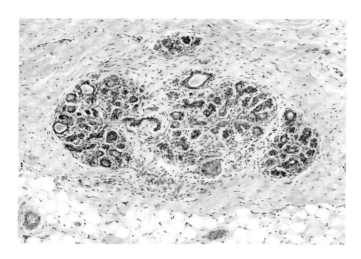 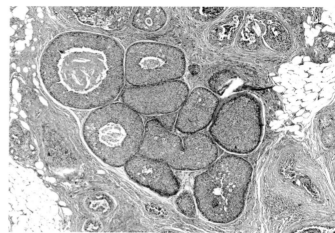

(A) Atypical ductal hyperplasia
(B) Carcinoma in situ
(C) Intraductal papilloma
(D) Metastatic carcinoma
(E) Microinvasive carcinoma

40 A 35-year-old woman presents with a swelling in her neck. Physical examination reveals a solitary nodule of the thyroid gland measuring 2 cm in diameter. Thyroid function tests are within normal limits. A biopsy of the nodule is obtained. How does the histologic appearance of the patient's thyroid biopsy (image on right) differ from that of a normal thyroid (image on left)?

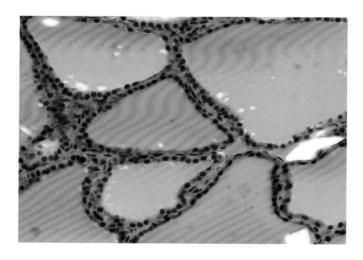 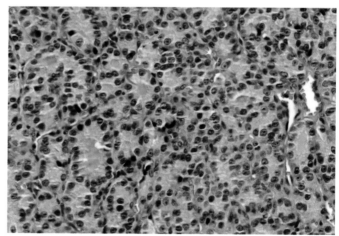

(A) There is a chronic inflammatory cell infiltrate.
(B) There is evidence of irreversible injury.
(C) There is focal atrophy of the gland.
(D) There is hemorrhage within the gland.
(E) There is increased cellularity of the gland.

ANSWERS

1 The answer is D: Neoplasia. Examination of ascites fluid in this patient demonstrates small, gland-like cellular structures (shown in the image). This histopathologic finding is consistent with a diagnosis of neoplasia (new uncontrolled cell growth). Patients with ovarian cancer typically present with a history of increasing abdominal girth, owing to an accumulation of neoplastic cells and fluid within their peritoneal cavity. Neoplasms are genetic diseases that are associated with acquired mutations in growth regulatory or DNA repair genes. The ascites fluid obtained from this patient does not show evidence of inflammatory cells (choice B). None of the other choices would explain the presence of neoplastic cells within the peritoneum.

Keywords: Ovarian cancer, metastasis, neoplasia

2 The answer is C: Skeletal muscle, inflammation. This biopsy reveals skeletal muscle myofibers with peripheral nuclei surrounded by chronic inflammatory cells (numerous basophilic nuclei). The patient may have been an elderly man recovering from the "flu" who complains of marked fatigability. He may report that he cannot climb stairs two at a time as he used to. He may also describe pain in the thighs. Inflammatory myopathies are thought to have an autoimmune origin. The most common morphologic characteristics in the inflammatory myopathies are (1) inflammatory cells, (2) necrosis and phagocytosis of muscle fibers, (3) a mixture of regenerating and atrophic fibers, and (4) fibrosis. Polymyositis is one example of an inflammatory myopathy that is related to direct muscle cell damage produced by cytotoxic T cells. Healthy muscle fibers are initially surrounded by CD8+ T lymphocytes and macrophages, after which muscle fibers degenerate. The patient's biopsy does not show cardiac or smooth muscle (choices A, B, D, and E).

Keywords: Inflammatory myopathy, polymyositis

3 The answer is E: There is enlargement of individual myocytes. These paired images contrast normal cardiac myocytes (image on left) with hypertrophic cardiac myocytes (image on right). The increased weight of the heart suggests that this patient suffered from chronic hypertension. Chronic hypertension causes compensatory left ventricular hypertrophy. The overall weight of the heart increases, exceeding 375 g in men and 350 g in women. Microscopically, hypertrophic myocardial cells exhibit an increased diameter with enlarged, hyperchromatic, rectangular (boxcar) nuclei. Myocardial hypertrophy adds to the ability of the heart to handle an increased workload. However, there is a limit beyond which hypertrophy is no longer compensatory. This upper limit may reflect an increasing diffusion distance between the interstitium and the center of each myofiber; if the distance becomes too great, the supply of oxygen to the myofiber will be deficient. Hypertension also increases the severity of atherosclerosis. The combination of increased cardiac workload and narrowed coronary arteries leads to a greater risk of myocardial ischemia, infarction, and congestive heart failure. None of the other choices feature hypertrophic cells with boxcar nuclei.

Keywords: Hypertensive heart disease, hypertrophy

4 The answer is C: Decrease in the size of myocytes. The patient's biopsy shows normal skeletal muscle fibers on the left side of the image and a cluster of smaller fibers on the right side of the image. This pathologic finding is consistent with denervation muscle atrophy (reduced cell size and function). When a skeletal muscle fiber becomes separated from contact with its motor neuron, it invariably atrophies due to the progressive loss of myofibrils. On cross section, atrophic fibers have a characteristic angular configuration, seemingly compressed by the surrounding normal muscle fibers. If a muscle fiber is not reinnervated, atrophy proceeds to complete loss of myofibrils. In the end stage, muscle fibers disappear and are replaced by adipose tissue. None of the other choices describe histopathologic features of denervation muscle atrophy.

Keywords: Skeletal muscle, atrophy, denervation injury

5 The answer is D: Increased cellularity of the glandular epithelium. This endometrial biopsy reveals normal glandular tissue on the left of the indicated line and hyperplastic or neoplastic glandular epithelium on the right (note increased cellularity). The pathologist will carefully examine the glandular architecture, to distinguish between the estrogen field effect of benign hyperplasia and a more concerning monoclonal neoplastic growth. Endometrial intraepithelial neoplasia (EIN) is a clonal, neoplastic proliferation that is prone to malignant transformation. Endometrial glands affected by EIN typically show loss of the *PTEN* tumor suppressor gene. Women with EIN have a 40% chance of developing endometrial cancer within 1 year. The biopsy does not show evidence of acute or chronic inflammatory cells (choice A). None of the other choices describe increased cellularity of the glandular epithelium.

Keywords: Endometrial intraepithelial neoplasia, hyperplasia

6 The answer is E: Infiltrate of chronic inflammatory cells. This thyroid biopsy reveals an infiltrate of chronic inflammatory cells (note the numerous small basophilic nuclei) and a prominent, secondary, lymphoid follicle. These pathologic findings are seen in patients with chronic thyroiditis (Hashimoto thyroiditis), a common cause of hypothyroidism. This autoimmune disease is characterized by circulating antibodies to thyroid antigens and cell-mediated immunity to thyroid tissue. The disorder arises commonly in the fourth and fifth decades of life, and women are six times more likely to be affected than men. On gross examination, the gland in patients with Hashimoto thyroiditis is diffusely enlarged and firm. On microscopic examination, the thyroid displays an infiltrate of chronic inflammatory cells (lymphocytes and plasma cells) and atrophy of follicles. None of the other choices describe features of chronic inflammation.

Keywords: Hashimoto thyroiditis

7 | **The answer is D: Squamous cell carcinoma.**   The epidermis in this skin biopsy is filled with atypical cells that resemble keratinocytes of the normal stratum spinosum. Mitotic and apoptotic cells are also evident. This early stage of cancer progression is referred to as "carcinoma in situ," because malignant cells have not yet penetrated the basement membrane at the dermal–epidermal junction. Squamous cell carcinoma of the skin typically arises in sun-damaged patches or plaques, referred to as actinic keratoses (from the sun's rays). Over time, patches of actinic keratoses may evolve into squamous cell carcinoma in situ and, finally, into invasive squamous cell carcinoma. However, most actinic keratosis are stable and many regress. Adenocarcinomas (choice A) are malignant neoplasms of glandular epithelium (e.g., breast and prostate cancer). Hemangiomas (choice B) are benign neoplasms of vascular endothelial cells. Melanomas (choice C) are malignant neoplasms of melanocytes. Transitional cell carcinomas (choice E) are malignant neoplasms of the urothelium (e.g., cancer of the ureters and urinary bladder).

Keywords: Squamous cell carcinoma of the skin

8 | **The answer is C: Hyperplasia (increased numbers of cells).** These paired images contrast normal bone marrow (image on left) with hyperplastic bone marrow (image on right) from a patient living at high altitude. As an adaptation to low atmospheric oxygen content, erythrocyte precursors in the patient's bone marrow undergo compensatory hyperplasia to increase the delivery of oxygen-carrying erythrocytes to the blood. Note that cellularity of the patient's bone marrow is increased and that fat content is decreased. None of the other choices describe increased numbers of hematopoietic cells in the bone marrow.

Keywords: Bone marrow, hyperplasia, polycythemia

9 | **The answer is B: Increased numbers of otherwise normal cells.** These paired images, obtained at the same magnification, contrast normal epidermis (image on left) with epidermal hyperplasia (image on right) in a patient with psoriasis. The epidermis in the patient with psoriasis is thickened, owing to an increase in the number of squamous epithelial cells. Psoriasis is a chronic disease of the dermis and epidermis that is characterized by persistent epidermal hyperplasia. It is frequently a familial disorder that features large, erythematous, scaly plaques, commonly on the dorsal extensor cutaneous surfaces of the body. Abnormal pattern of cellular maturation (choice A)

is a description of dysplasia, which is not evident in this patient's biopsy. None of the other choices describe increased numbers of normal squamous epithelial cells in the epidermis.

Keywords: Psoriasis, hyperplasia

10 | **The answer is B: Accumulation of abnormal cells.**   The patient's spleen biopsy shows an accumulation of abnormal, lipid-laden macrophages that have displaced normal cells. These abnormal macrophages have a foamy cytoplasm and an eccentrically located nucleus. They are found in patients with lysosomal storage diseases. For example, they are present in the red pulp of the spleen, liver sinusoids, lymph nodes, lungs, and bone marrow of patients with Gaucher disease—an autosomal recessive genetic disease that is characterized by the accumulation of glucosylceramide (a glycolipid) within lysosomes. The underlying abnormality in Gaucher disease is a deficiency in glucocerebrosidase, a lysosomal acid glucosidase. Lipid-laden macrophages in patients with Gaucher disease are termed Gaucher cells; they are derived from the resident macrophages in respective organs (e.g., Kupffer cells in the liver and alveolar macrophages in the lung). Gaucher cells are not multinucleated (choice D), and they are not small lymphocytes (choice E). None of the other choices describe histopathologic features of Gaucher disease.

Keywords: Gaucher disease, macrophage, lysosomal storage disease

11 | **The answer is B: There is a neoplastic proliferation of keratinocytes.**   The patient's biopsy shows a well-differentiated squamous cell carcinoma of the skin. Malignant cells have penetrated the epidermal–dermal junction and are infiltrating the dermis. The spheroidal, eosinophilic bodies observed in this specimen are referred to as "keratin pearls." These structures represent an attempt on the part of the neoplastic cells to recapitulate normal squamous epithelial cell differentiation. Keratin pearls are a useful marker for squamous cell carcinomas arising in many different location, including the esophagus, cervix, skin, and lung. None of the other choices describe histopathologic features of this skin cancer.

Keywords: Squamous cell carcinoma of the skin, keratinocyte

12 | **The answer is A: Accumulation of cells and lipid material in the arterial wall.**   These paired images contrast a normal muscular artery (image on left) with a diseased coronary artery (image on right) from a patient with advanced atherosclerosis and ischemic heart disease. The patient's artery shows a well-developed fibrofatty plaque within the intima, along the inferior vessel wall. Atherosclerosis is a chronic disease of large and medium-sized elastic and muscular arteries that results in the progressive accumulation within the intima of inflammatory cells, hyperplastic smooth muscle cells, lipids, and connective tissue. The resulting characteristic lesion, the fibrofatty plaque (atheroma), contains pools of extracellular lipid, and numerous lipid-laden macrophages (foam cells). Atherosclerosis is not an acute inflammatory or a neoplastic disease (choices B and E). Cystic medial necrosis and dissecting aneurysms are typically diseases of the aorta (choices C and D).

Keywords: Atherosclerosis, myocardial infarction

13 **The answer is A: Disruption of elastic fibers.** These paired images contrast normal elastic media (image on left) with disrupted elastic fibers (image on right) in the aorta of an elderly patient with a history of systemic hypertension. The patient's aortic media shows disruption of elastic fibers (the wavy black lines), as well as pools of metachromatic material (mostly proteoglycans). These histopathologic findings are referred to as "cystic medial necrosis." They may be observed in elderly patients with systemic hypertension and in younger patients with Marfan syndrome—an autosomal dominant genetic disease associated with diminished integrity of elastic tissue. This autopsy specimen does not reveal chronic inflammatory cells (choice C), nor does it show proliferation of endothelial cells (choice E). Occlusion of the vasa vasorum (choice D) is a feature of secondary syphilis.

Keywords: Cystic medial necrosis, hypertension

14 **The answer is D: Occlusion of the lumen by a thrombus.** This autopsy specimen shows a coronary artery with severe atherosclerosis and a recent thrombus lodged in the narrowed lumen. Intravascular thrombi are adherent to the wall of the vessel. They are composed of insoluble fibrin, various clotting factors, platelets, and other formed blood elements. A mature atheroma (fibrofatty plaque) is highly thrombogenic. A thrombus formed on an atherosclerotic plaque can abruptly occlude the lumen of medium-sized muscular arteries causing ischemic necrosis and acute myocardial infarction. None of the other choices describe the histopathology of atherosclerosis and thrombosis.

Keywords: Myocardial infarction, atherosclerosis, thrombosis

15 **The answer is B: The air spaces are filled with inflammatory cells.** The alveolar air spaces in this autopsy specimen are filled with acute inflammatory cells (primarily neutrophils), eosinophilic fibrin stands, and necrotic debris. The neutrophils recognize, internalize, and digest bacteria and cellular debris. This process is termed phagocytosis, and the effector cells are known as phagocytes. Despite the impact of antibiotic therapy, pneumonia caused by *Streptococcus pneumoniae* (pneumococcus) remains a significant problem. The onset of pneumococcal pneumonia is acute, with fever and chills. The most common outcome of bacterial pneumonia is complete resolution, particularly with appropriate antibiotic treatment. Choice A (air spaces filled with fluid)

is partially correct, because activated endothelial cells in the lung become leaky, causing an exudate to accumulate within intra-alveolar air spaces. None of the other choices describe histopathologic features of acute bacterial pneumonia.

Keywords: Pneumonia, inflammation

16 **The answer is E: There is thickening of the arteriole wall.** This renal biopsy shows arterioles that are markedly thickened by the deposition of basement membrane material and by the accumulation of plasma proteins. The glassy, pink-stained material in the wall of these injured vessels is termed "hyaline," and the disease process is referred to as "hyaline arteriolosclerosis." Thickening of the arteriolar wall reduces blood flow to the kidney, causing the renal glomeruli and tubules to undergo atrophy (reduced size and function). Arterioles exhibit concentric hyaline thickening of the wall, often with the loss of smooth muscle cells. None of the other choices describe histopathologic features of hyaline arteriosclerosis.

Keywords: Benign nephrosclerosis, arteriosclerosis

17 **The answer is A: The air spaces are filled with fluid.** Examination of the patient's lungs at autopsy reveals pink fluid within the intra-alveolar air spaces. This extravascular fluid is termed pulmonary edema. It is a characteristic finding in patients with congestive heart failure. Increased hydrostatic pressure associated with failure of the left ventricle causes fluid (transudate) to move from pulmonary capillaries into interstitial tissue and intra-alveolar air spaces of the lung. Patients in left-sided congestive heart failure complain of shortness of breath (dyspnea) on exertion and when recumbent (orthopnea). They may be awakened from sleep by sudden episodes of shortness of breath (paroxysmal nocturnal dyspnea). Patients with pulmonary edema have crackling breath sounds (rales) caused by expansion of the fluid-filled alveoli. None of the other choices describe histopathologic features of pulmonary edema.

Keywords: Pulmonary edema, congestive heart failure

18 **The answer is B: Destruction of the vessel wall by inflammatory cells.** The submucosal arterioles in the patient's gallbladder exhibit chronic inflammation (numerous basophilic nuclei), destruction of the wall, and fibrinoid necrosis. Fibrinoid necrosis is an alteration of injured blood vessels, in which the insudation and accumulation of plasma proteins causes the wall to stain intensely with eosin. These clinicopathologic findings are consistent with a diagnosis of polyarteritis nodosa—an acute necrotizing vasculitis that affects medium-sized and smaller muscular arteries. The most common pathologic feature of polyarteritis nodosa is fibrinoid necrosis, in which the medial muscle and adjacent tissue are fused into an eosinophilic mass that stains for fibrin. Approximately 15% of patients with this disease demonstrate either

HBsAg or anti-HCV antibodies. Accumulation of lipid (choice A) is a hallmark of atherosclerosis. None of the other choices describe histopathologic features of a necrotizing arteritis.

Keywords: Polyarteritis nodosa, arteritis

19 The answer is C: Foamy exudate within the air spaces. This lung biopsy reveals a foamy exudate within the alveolar air spaces. The interstitium is also thickened and contains a chronic inflammatory cell infiltrate. A bronchoalveolar lavage obtained from this patient would show clusters of *Pneumocystis* organisms and establish a diagnosis of *Pneumocystis* pneumonia. *Pneumocystis jiroveci* (formerly *P. carinii*) is the most common cause of infectious pneumonia in patients with acquired immunodeficiency syndrome (AIDS). Once considered a protozoan, the organism has been reclassified as a fungus. The classic lesions of *Pneumocystis* pneumonia are a foamy intra-alveolar exudate and an interstitial infiltrate of plasma cells and lymphocytes. None of the other choices describe the common histopathologic features of *Pneumocystis* pneumonia.

Keywords: *Pneumocystis* pneumonia, *Pneumocystis jiroveci*

20 The answer is B: Deposition of collagen in the myocardium. Examination of the patient's heart reveals a healed myocardial infarct with mature collagen-rich scar tissue (asterisk, shown in the image). Infarcts are geographic areas of necrosis caused by lack of arterial blood flow (ischemia). Soon after the heart attack, neutrophils, macrophages, fibroblasts, and capillary endothelial cells infiltrate the injured heart muscle. Over the next weeks-to-months, necrotic debris is replaced with mature scar tissue (primarily collagen type I) that is synthesized by fibroblasts. Glycogen accumulation (choice A) is seen in patients with certain inborn errors of metabolism (e.g., Hunter and Hurler syndromes). Enlargement of cardiac myocytes (choice C) is a hallmark of hypertensive heart disease. Inflammatory infiltrates (choice D) are hallmarks of infections and ischemic necrosis.

Keywords: Myocardial infarct, fibrosis

21 The answer is C: The air spaces are overly distended. Examination of the patient's lung at autopsy reveals large, irregular air spaces and a reduction in the number of alveoli (shown in the image on right). These findings are the hallmark of pulmonary emphysema. Emphysema is a chronic lung disease, characterized by enlargement of the air spaces distal to terminal bronchioles, with destruction of their walls, but without fibrosis. The major cause of emphysema is cigarette smoking; however, it is also seen in younger patients with alpha-1-antitrypsin deficiency (genetic disease). Moderate to severe emphysema is rare in nonsmokers. None of the other choices describe histopathologic features of pulmonary emphysema.

Keywords: Emphysema

22 The answer is B: Disarray of the cardiac myocytes. Examination of the patient's heart muscle at autopsy reveals myofiber disarray and hyperplasia of interstitial cells. These pathologic findings are seen in patients with hypertrophic cardiomyopathy, a condition in which cardiac hypertrophy is out of proportion to the hemodynamic load placed on the heart. This disorder is an autosomal dominant trait in about half of the patients, involving mutations in genes that encode cardiac muscle contractile proteins. The wall of the left ventricle is typically thickened (hypertrophic) and its cavity is small. The most notable histologic characteristic of this disorder is myofiber disarray, which is most extensive in the interventricular septum. Despite an absence of symptoms, persons with hypertrophic cardiomyopathy are at risk of sudden death during vigorous exercise due to the obstruction of aortic outflow from the left ventricle. None of the other choices describe the histopathology of hypertrophic cardiomyopathy.

Keywords: Hypertrophic cardiomyopathy

23 The answer is E: There is excess collagen in the alveolar septa. The patient's lung shows patchy, dense, interstitial fibrosis (i.e., scar tissue within alveolar septa). These histopathologic findings are seen in patients with pulmonary storage disorders (pneumoconiosis) such as silicosis and asbestosis. Asbestosis refers to the diffuse interstitial fibrosis that results from inhalation of asbestos fibers. Patients with hypersensitivity pneumonitis may have air spaces filled with eosinophils (choice A). Type II pneumocytes (choice D) produce surfactant lipids and proteins and also serve as pulmonary stem cells. None of the other choices describe histopathologic features of pulmonary asbestosis.

Keywords: Asbestosis, pulmonary fibrosis

24 The answer is A: The cell type of the surface epithelium has changed. This biopsy of the distal esophagus reveals a glandular surface epithelium with numerous goblet cells (cells with large, pale intracellular vacuoles). A reversible change in cell differentiation in response to injury is termed "metaplasia." Intestinal metaplasia with goblet cells in the distal esophagus is referred to as "Barrett esophagus." This pathologic condition is typically seen in patients with chronic gastroesophageal reflux. The lesion is characterized histologically by intestine-like epithelium, composed of goblet cells incompletely intestinalized gastric mucosa. Barrett esophagus is more resistant to peptic juices than normal squamous epithelium and appears to be an adaptive mechanism that serves to limit the harmful effects of gastroesophageal reflux. None of the other choices describe intestinal metaplasia.

Keywords: Barrett esophagus, metaplasia

25 The answer is B: Alteration of the submucosal vasculature. This autopsy specimen shows varices (varicose

veins) in the esophageal submucosa. These dilated veins are prone to rupture and hemorrhage. They arise in the lower third of the esophagus in patients with portal hypertension, secondary to hepatic cirrhosis (end-stage liver disease). Engorged collateral veins in the submucosa of the lower esophagus and upper stomach become dilated and protrude into the lumen. When esophageal varices become greater than 5 mm in diameter, they are likely to rupture causing life-threatening hemorrhage. The prognosis of patients with bleeding esophageal varices is poor, with a 40% mortality rate. The other choices are not associated with the histopathology of esophageal varices.
Keywords: Esophageal varices

26 **The answer is B: The gastric mucosa has been eroded.** Incidental findings are frequently encountered at autopsy. In this case, a peptic ulcer is identified in the distal stomach. Histologic examination of the lesion shows focal destruction of the mucosa and full-thickness replacement of the muscularis with collagen-rich connective tissue (shown in the image on the right). Gastric ulcers are usually single and less than 2 cm in diameter. Ulcers on the lesser curvature are commonly associated with chronic gastritis, whereas those on the greater curvature are often related to use of nonsteroidal anti-inflammatory drugs (NSAIDs). None of the other choices describe the histopathology of peptic ulcer disease.
Keywords: Gastric ulcer, peptic ulcer disease

27 **The answer is B: The hepatic architecture has been distorted by scar tissue.** This liver biopsy shows hepatic nodules of various sizes surrounded by irregular fibrous septa. Chronic liver injury (e.g., chronic viral hepatitis B or C) is associated with the development of collagenous scars within the hepatic parenchyma. The end stage of chronic injury to the liver is termed cirrhosis. Hepatocytes form regenerative nodules that lack central veins and expand to obstruct blood vessels and bile flow. Portal hypertension and jaundice ensue. Excess iron deposition in the liver (choice D) is seen in patients with familial hemochromatosis and can be visualized using Prussian blue stain. Cholestasis (choice A) is encountered in patients with intrahepatic or extrahepatic biliary obstruction. None of the other choices describe histopathologic features of hepatic cirrhosis.
Keywords: Hepatic cirrhosis, viral hepatitis

28 **The answer is A: The absorptive surface has been attenuated.** The child's biopsy reveals blunting and attenuation of intestinal villi. The mucosal surface shows loss of tall, slender intestinal villi and infiltration of the lamina propria by chronic inflammatory cells. These histopathologic findings are seen in patients with celiac sprue (also referred to as gluten-sensitive enteropathy). Celiac sprue is characterized by (1) generalized malabsorption, (2) small intestinal mucosal lesions, and (3) prompt clinical and histopathologic response to the withdrawal of gluten-containing foods from the diet. Critical factors in the development of celiac sprue include genetic predisposition and antigen exposure. The hallmark of celiac disease is a flat mucosa, with blunting of intestinal villi, damaged epithelial cells, intraepithelial T cells, and increased plasma cells in the lamina propria. None of the other choices describe these histopathologic findings.
Keywords: Celiac sprue, gluten-sensitive enteropathy

29 **The answer is D: Fat accumulation within hepatocytes.** This biopsy reveals hepatocytes that are distended by large, intracellular fat vacuoles that push nuclei to the periphery. Excessive alcohol consumption induces fat accumulation within hepatocytes, enlarging the liver to as much as three times the normal weight. The amount of fat deposited varies with the amount of alcohol consumed, as well as with the patient's hormonal status and diet. Triglyceride accumulation by itself is not ordinarily damaging, and the condition is fully reversible upon discontinuation of alcohol abuse (abstinence). None of the other choices describe histopathologic features of alcoholic fatty liver.
Keywords: Alcoholic fatty liver, alcoholism

30 **The answer is C: Defect in the wall of the colon.** Examination of the patient's colon reveals segments of mucosa (including muscularis mucosae) that have herniated through defects in the bowel wall, producing diverticula (shown in the image on right). Diverticular disease refers to two entities: a condition termed diverticulosis and an inflammatory complication termed diverticulitis. Diverticulosis is generally asymptomatic. Diverticulitis results from the irritation caused by retained fecal material that obstructs the lumen of a diverticulum. Diverticula are most common in the sigmoid colon, which is affected in 95% of cases. Rupture, followed by peritonitis and sepsis are serious complications. None of the other choices describe histopathologic features of diverticulosis.
Keywords: Diverticulosis

31 **The answer is B: The glomerulus is hypercellular.** The patient's glomerulus appears hypercellular, because it contains numerous neutrophils and increased numbers of mesangial cells. This case is illustrative of nephritic syndrome in the setting of poststreptococcal glomerulonephritis. Nephritic syndrome is characterized by hematuria, variable degrees of proteinuria, and decreased glomerular filtration. It results in elevations of blood urea nitrogen (BUN) and serum creatinine, as well as oliguria, salt and water retention, edema, and hypertension. None of the other choices describe histopathologic features of nephritic syndrome.
Keywords: Glomerulonephritis, nephritic syndrome

32 **The answer is B: There has been a neoplastic change in the epithelium.** The patient's colon biopsy reveals a neoplasm that is referred to as an adenomatous polyp.

Villous and tubular elements are observed in this polyp. Microscopic examination of the stalk further reveals a focus of mucus-producing adenocarcinoma (malignant neoplasm capable of invasion and metastasis). As long as dysplastic foci remain confined to the polyp mucosa, these lesions are almost always cured by surgical resection. None of the other choices describe the histopathology of an adenomatous polyp of the colon.

Keywords: Adenocarcinoma of the colon, adenomatous polyp of the colon

33 **The answer is C: There is expansion of the mesangium-forming nodular lesions.** The patient's renal biopsy reveals a prominent increase in the mesangial matrix, forming several nodular lesions. These microscopic findings are seen in patients with diabetic glomerulosclerosis. PAS reagent stains complex carbohydrates that are conjugated extracellular matrix proteins via nonenzymatic glycosylation—a reaction that occurs at an accelerated rate in diabetics with hyperglycemia. Diabetes mellitus, a complex metabolic disease associated with glucosuria and polyuria, is the leading cause of end-stage renal disease in the United States, accounting for a third of all patients with chronic renal failure. In patients with diabetic glomerulosclerosis, the renal glomeruli show diffuse mesangial matrix expansion with focal, segmental, and nodular lesions. Diabetic glomerulosclerosis eventually results in progressive renal failure. None of the other choices describe histopathologic findings evident in this biopsy specimen.

Keywords: Diabetic nephropathy, diabetes mellitus

34 **The answer is A: The cell type of the epithelium has been changed.** The patient's bladder biopsy shows squamous metaplasia of the urothelium. In this patient, parasitic infestation of the bladder caused the normal transitional cell epithelium to be replaced by a protective, stratified squamous epithelium. Squamous cell carcinoma of the bladder can develop in foci of squamous metaplasia, and a high incidence of bladder cancer is found in countries with endemic schistosomiasis. The other choices do not reflect squamous metaplasia of the bladder mucosa.

Keywords: Squamous cell carcinoma of the bladder

35 **The answer is C: There is a proliferation of abnormal germ cells.** The patient's testis shows no signs of spermatogenesis (i.e., no signs of haploid male germ cells) but does show large, atypical cells within the seminiferous epithelium. Recent studies indicate that these large cells are triploid. These atypical cells are confined within the tubular basement membrane and represent an example of carcinoma in situ. Half of men with intratubular germ cell neoplasia will develop invasive cancer (e.g., seminoma or embryonal carcinoma) within 5 years. Nuclear transcription factors OCT3 and OCT4 are reliable markers for these atypical germ cells. None of the other choices

describe the histopathologic findings evident in this patient's testicular biopsy.

Keywords: Seminoma, testicular cancer

36 **The answer is E: Proliferation of epithelial cells.** The prostate needle biopsy shows new uncontrolled proliferation of the glandular epithelium (adenocarcinoma). In 1990, prostatic adenocarcinoma became the cancer most frequently diagnosed in American men, surpassing the incidence of lung cancer for the first time. It is generally accepted that prostatic intraepithelial neoplasia lesions progress to invasive prostatic adenocarcinoma. There is no evidence that prostatic adenocarcinoma originates from hyperplastic nodules seen in patients with nodular prostatic hyperplasia. Prostatic adenocarcinomas are commonly multicentric and located in peripheral zones of the prostate gland. None of the other choices describe the histopathology of prostate cancer.

Keywords: Prostate cancer, adenocarcinoma of the prostate

37 **The answer is D: Perinuclear halos.** Compared to normal cervical epithelial cells (image on left), the patient's Pap smear (image on right) reveals atypical cells with enlarged nuclei and prominent perinuclear clear spaces. These atypical cells are referred to as koilocytes. For this Pap smear, the cytology report will note cervical squamous cells with "koilocytotic atypia." Human papillomavirus (HPV) is a DNA virus that infects a variety of skin and mucosal surfaces to produce wart-like lesions (verrucae and condylomata). In the female reproductive tract, HPV infections are linked to the pathogenesis of cervical cancer. The morphologic hallmark of HPV infection is koilocytotic atypia, a term that denotes the presence of sharply demarcated, large perinuclear halos, combined with alterations in the chromatin pattern of squamous epithelial cells. These perinuclear halos are filled with replicating virus HPV particles. Lewy bodies (choice A) are intracellular aggregates of synuclein protein found in dopaminergic neurons of patient's with Parkinson disease. Nuclear pyknosis (choice B) is hallmark of cell death, in which nuclear chromatin undergoes irreversible clumping and condensation. The normal Pap smear shows two cells with pyknotic nuclei (arrows). The patient's Pap smear does not show cellular aggregates with papillary morphology (choice C). Endocervical cells may undergo squamous metaplasia (choice E), but Pap smears taken from the ectocervix of the adult typically show squamous cell morphology.

Keywords: Cervix, Pap smear, human papillomavirus

38 **The answer is C: There is enlargement and growth of follicular cells.** This thyroid biopsy reveals active follicles lined by hyperplastic, tall columnar epithelial cells. The colloid appears scalloped at the periphery of the follicle. Scalloping represents active uptake of thyroglobulin for processing and transport to the systemic circulation. Inactive thyroid follicles are typically lined by a low cuboidal epithelium (image on left). These clinicopathologic findings are consistent with hyperthyroidism. Graves disease is the most frequent cause of hyperthyroidism in young adults. It is an autoimmune disorder characterized by diffuse goiter, hyperthyroidism, and exophthalmos. Patients with Graves disease are hyperthyroid due to the presence of stimulating IgG antibodies that bind to the TSH receptor expressed on the plasma membrane of follicular cells. Patients note the gradual onset of nonspecific symptoms, such as nervousness, emotional lability, tremor, weakness, and weight loss. They are intolerant of heat, seek cooler environments, tend to sweat profusely, and may report heart palpitations. None of the other choices describe histopathologic features of hyperthyroidism.

Keywords: Graves disease, hyperthyroidism

39 **The answer is B: Carcinoma in situ.** The patient's breast biopsy reveals intraductal carcinoma in situ (DCIS), which arises in the terminal duct lobular unit, greatly distorting the ducts by its growth (image on right). DCIS carries a 20% to 30% risk of developing invasive carcinoma in the same breast over the ensuing 20 years. Atypical ductal hyperplasia (choice A) is a component of benign, fibrocystic change of the breast. Intraductal papilloma (choice C) is a benign tumor that usually arises in a terminal lactiferous duct and causes nipple discharge. Examination of this patient's breast biopsy at low magnification does not reveal evidence of tumor cells within either blood or lymphatic vessels (choice D) nor does it reveal tumor cells leaving ducts and invading the adjacent stromal connective tissue (choice E).

Keywords: Breast cancer, intraductal carcinoma in situ

40 **The answer is E: There is increased cellularity of the gland.** This thyroid biopsy reveals increased cellularity, with monomorphic cells forming small follicular structures filled with colloid. A single, well-circumscribed, thyroid nodule in a young patient most likely represents a follicular adenoma—a benign neoplasm that exhibits follicular differentiation. It is the most common tumor of the thyroid and typically presents in euthyroid persons as a solitary "cold" nodule (i.e., a tumor that does not take up radiolabeled iodine). Follicular adenoma is an encapsulated neoplasm in which the cells are arranged in follicles that resemble normal thyroid tissue. None of the other choices describe histopathologic features of thyroid neoplasia.

Keywords: Follicular adenoma of the thyroid

Appendix A
Normal Reference Range*

Laboratory Test	Reference Range
Clinical Chemistry Tests (Serum)	
Alanine aminotransferase (ALT)	
Male	1–45 IU/L @ 37°C
Female	1–30 IU/L @ 37°C
Albumin	3.0–5.0 g/dL
Alkaline phosphatase	
0–17 yr	40–400 IU/L @ 37°C
18–99 yr	30–160 IU/L @ 37°C
Alpha-1-antitrypsin, total	96–199 mg/dL
Ammonia	11–35 µmol/L
Amylase	<132 U/L
Aspartate aminotransferase (AST)	
Male	7–42 IU/L @ 37°C
Female	7–35 IU/L @ 37°C
Bilirubin, direct	0.0–0.4 mg/dL
Bilirubin, total	0.2–1.2 mg/dL
Calcium	8.5–10.5 mg/dL
Cardio C-reactive protein (low-risk)	<1.2 mg/dL
Chloride	98–109 mmol/L
Cholesterol, HDL (desirable)	>60 mg/dL
Cholesterol, LDL (desirable)	<100 mg/dL
Cholesterol, total	<200 mg/dL
CO_2	24–32 mmol/L
Complement C-3	88–201 mg/dL
Complement C-4	16–47 mg/dL
Creatine kinase (CK)	
Male	25–215 IU/L @ 37°C
Female	25–185 IU/L @ 37°C
Creatinine	0.5–1.4 mg/dL
Ferritin	
Male	15–300 ng/mL
Female	10–160 ng/mL
Folate (folic acid)	3–18 ng/mL
Folate, red cell	145–540 ng/mL
Glucose, fasting	50–100 mg/dL
Hemoglobin A2	1.7%–3.4%
Hemoglobin, plasma, free	0–10 mg/dL
Immunoglobulins	
IgA	69–382 mg/dL
IgG	723–1,685 mg/dL
IgM	63–277 mg/dL
Insulin	10–26 mIU/mL
Iron	
Male	55–160 µg/dL
Female	40–155 µg/dL
Iron-binding capacity	250–400 µg/dL
Lactate dehydrogenase (LD)	100–200 U/L
Lead	
Child	0–9.9 µg/dL
Adult	0–25 µg/dL
Lipase	<52 U/L
Magnesium	1.3–2.1 mEq/L
Mercury	0–13 µg/L
Phosphate	2.5–4.5 mg/dL
Potassium	3.5–5.0 mmol/L
Protein, total	6.0–8.5 g/dL
Sodium	135–146 mmol/L
Triglycerides (desirable)	<150 mg/dL
Troponin I	<0.5 ng/mL
Urate (uric acid)	
Male	3.5–8.0 mg/dL
Female	2.2–7.0 mg/dL
Urea-*N* (blood urea nitrogen)	10–30 mg/dL
Vitamin B$_{12}$ (cobalamin)	200–1,100 pg/dL
Arterial Blood Gases (Heparinized Whole Blood)	
pH	7.35–7.45
pO_2	83–108 mm Hg
pCO_2	31–45 mm Hg

*Normal Reference Range data provided by Clinical Laboratories, Department of Pathology, Thomas Jefferson University Hospital, Philadelphia. Normal reference range data vary considerably between institutions.

Hematology Tests
Complete Blood Count Adult Male

Leukocytes	$4–11 \times 10^9$/L
Erythrocytes	$4.5–6.0 \times 10^{12}$/L
Hemoglobin	14–17 g/dL
Hematocrit	42%–52%
MCV	80–99 fL
MCH	26–34 pg
MCHC	32–36.5 g/dL
RDW	11.0%–15.8%
Platelets	$140–400 \times 10^9$/L
MPV	9–13 fL
Erythrocyte sedimentation rate	0–10 mm/h

Complete Blood Count Adult Female

Leukocytes	$4–11 \times 10^9$/L
Erythrocytes	$3.7–5.2 \times 10^{12}$/L
Hemoglobin	12.5–15 g/dL
Hematocrit	36%–46%
MCV	80–99 fL
MCH	26–34 pg
MCHC	32–36.5 g/dL
RDW	11.0%–15.8%
Platelets	$140–400 \times 10^9$/L
MPV	9–13 fL
Erythrocyte sedimentation rate	0–20 mm/h

Automated Differential (Adult)

	Relative %	Absolute ($\times 10^9$/L)
Neutrophils	40–73	1.7–7.0
Lymphocytes	20–44	1–4.0
Monocytes	3–13	0.2–0.9
Eosinophils	0–6	0.1–0.5
Basophils	0–3	0.0–0.2
Reticulocytes	0.5–1.5	20–76

Coagulation Tests (Citrated Plasma)

D-Dimer	<0.45 µg/mL
Partial thromboplastin time (PTT), activated	22–38 s
Prothrombin time (PT)	12.0–15.4 s
Fibrinogen	226–454 mg/dL

Endocrine Tests And Tumor Markers (Serum)

Alpha-fetoprotein (AFP), nonmaternal	<7.7 ng/mL
Angiotensin converting enzyme (ACE)	35–140 nmol/mL/min
Carcinoembryonic antigen (CEA)	
Non-smoker	3.5 ng/mL
Smoker	0–5.0 ng/mL
Corticotropin (ACTH)	9–52 pg/mL
Cortisol, serum	
8–10 AM	4–24 µg/dL
4–6 PM	2–12 µg/dL
Growth hormone	
0–1 yr	15–40 ng/mL (fasting)
1 yr to adult	0–5 ng/mL (fasting)
Human chorionic gonadotropin (hCG)	
Time after conception:	
1st week	0–50 mIU/mL
1 month	1,000–20,000 mIU/mL
3 months	20,000–200,000 mIU/mL
Insulin	10–26 mIU/mL
17-Ketosteroids, total	5–20 mg/24 h
Parathyroid hormone, intact	
Child	1–43 pg/mL
Adult	10–55 pg/mL
Prolactin	0–19 ng/mL
Prostate-specific antigen (PSA), male >40 yr	0–4 ng/mL
Triiodothyronine (T-3), total	90–200 ng/dL
Thyroxine (T-4), free	0.7–1.6 ng/dL
Testosterone, total	
Male	270–1,070 ng/dL
Female	10–70 ng/dL
Thyroid-stimulating hormone (TSH)	0.4–4.8 µIU/mL

Urine Tests

Calcium, quantitative	0–150 mg/24 h
Cortisol, free	<50 µg/24 h
Creatinine	
Male	1,000–2,000 mg/24 h
Female	800–1,800 mg/24 h
Electrolytes (24-h collection or 10 mL)	
Potassium	25–120 mmol/24 h
Sodium	40–220 mmol/24 h
Chloride	110–250 mmol/24 h
Glucose, quantitative	<500 mg/24 h

17-Hydroxycorticosteroids	3–11 mg/24 h
Magnesium	1.0–24.0 mEq/24 h
Mercury	0–20 µg/L
Osmolality (10 mL random specimen)	300–900 mOsmol/kg
Oxalate	3.6–38 mg/24 h
pH	5.0–8.0
Phosphate	400–1,400 mg/24 h
Protein, total	<150 mg/24 h
Urate (uric acid)	250–750 mg/24 h

Cerebrospinal Fluid

Glucose	40–70 mg/dL
Protein	
Neonate	15–130 mg/dL
Adult	15–55 mg/dL

Body Mass Index

BMI (adult)	19–25 kg/m^2

Appendix B
Common Abbreviations

Abbreviation	Expanded Form
ACTH	Corticotropin
ADH	Antidiuretic hormone
AFP	Alpha-fetoprotein
AIDS	Acquired immunodeficiency syndrome
ALL	Acute lymphoblastic leukemia
ALT	Alanine aminotransferase
AML	Acute myeloblastic leukemia
ANA	Antinuclear antibody
ANCA	Antineutrophil cytoplasmic antibody
AST	Aspartate aminotransferase
ATP	Adenosine triphosphate
ATPase	Adenosine triphosphatase
BMI	Body mass index
BPH	Benign prostatic hyperplasia
BUN	Blood urea nitrogen
C	Complement
cAMP	Cyclic adenosine monophosphate
CBC	Complete blood cell count
CD	Clusters of differentiation
CEA	Carcinoembryonic antigen
CFU	Colony-forming unit
cGMP	Cyclic guanosine monophosphate
CIN	Cervical intraepithelial neoplasia
CK	Creatine kinase
CMV	Cytomegalovirus
CNS	Central nervous system
CT	Computed tomography
Da	Dalton
DIC	Disseminated intravascular coagulation
DNA	Deoxyribonucleic acid
DNase	Deoxyribonuclease
EBV	Epstein–Barr virus
ECG	Electrocardiogram
EM	Electron microscope
FISH	Fluorescence in situ hybridization
FSH	Follicle-stimulating hormone
GBM	Glomerular basement membrane
GI	Gastrointestinal
H&E	Hematoxylin and eosin
Hb	Hemoglobin
HbS	Sickle cell hemoglobin
HBsAg	Hepatitis B surface antigen
HBV	Hepatitis B virus
hCG	Human chorionic gonadotropin
HCV	Hepatitis C virus
HDL	High-density lipoprotein
hGH	Human growth hormone
HIV	Human immunodeficiency virus
HLA	Human leukocyte antigen
HMG-CoA	3-hydroxy-3-methylglutaryl coenzyme A
HPF	High-power field
HPV	Human papillomavirus
HSV	Herpes simplex virus
HTLV	Human T-lymphotrophic virus
Ig	Immunoglobulin (IgM, IgG, IgA, IgE)
IL	Interleukin
ITP	Idiopathic thrombocytopenic purpura
IV	Intravenous
Kb	Kilobase (DNA)
LDH	Lactate dehydrogenase
LDL	Low-density lipoprotein
LH	Luteinizing hormone
MCH	Mean corpuscular hemoglobin
MCHC	Mean corpuscular hemoglobin concentration
MCV	Mean corpuscular volume
MEN	Multiple endocrine neoplasia
MRI	Magnetic resonance imaging
mRNA	Messenger RNA
NK	Natural killer
NSAID	Nonsteroidal anti-inflammatory drug
$PaCO_2$	Partial pressure of carbon dioxide, arterial
PaO_2	Partial pressure of oxygen, arterial
PAS	Periodic acid-Schiff
PCR	Polymerase chain reaction
pH	Hydrogen ion concentration
PID	Pelvic inflammatory disease
PSA	Prostate-specific antigen
PT	Prothrombin time
PTH	Parathyroid hormone
PTT	Partial thromboplastin time
PRL	Prolactin
RBC	Red blood cell
RNA	Ribonucleic acid
RSV	Respiratory syncytial virus
SIDS	Sudden infant death syndrome
STD	Sexually transmitted disease
SLE	Systemic lupus erythematosus
T3	Triiodothyronine
T4	Thyroxine
TB	Tuberculosis
TNF-α	Tumor necrosis factor-α
TSH	Thyrotropin
TTP	Thrombotic thrombocytopenic purpura
UV	Ultraviolet
WBC	White blood cell

Appendix C
Figure Credits

Images generated from virtual microscopic slides contributed by the University of Iowa Virtual Slide Box

Chapter 2
Questions 2, 3, 9, 12, and 14.

Chapter 3
Questions 1, 3, 5, 28, and 31.

Chapter 4
Questions 4, 13, 18, 27, 32, and 45.

Chapter 6
Questions 1, 2, and 18.

Chapter 7
Questions 1, 21, and 41.

Chapter 8
Questions 21, 22, 23, 27, 34, and 37.

Chapter 9
Question 19.

Chapter 10
Questions 2, 3, 4, 8, 20, and 28.

Chapter 11
Questions 20, 21, 30, 38, 40, 54, and 56.

Chapter 12
Questions 5, 6, 7, 10, and 11.

Chapter 13
Question 51.

Chapter 14
Questions 2, 3, 6, 11, and 14.

Chapter 15
Questions 7, 8, 9, 11, 15, 40, 42, 48, 49, and 50.

Chapter 16
Questions 31, 32, 42, and 44.

Chapter 17
Questions 27, 30, 33, 35, 39, 41, 54, 55, and 57.

Chapter 18
Questions 14, 28, 31, 32, 34, 39, and 43.

Chapter 19
Questions 3, 11, 13, 15, 17, 18, 19, 21, 23, 27, 33, 41, 42, 43, 45, 46, 48, 49, and 50.

Chapter 20
Questions 1, 2, 3, 5 11, 14, 15, 16, 24, 29, 30, 32, 33, 46, 49, 50, 52, 53, 54, 57, 58, 59, 60, 63, and 69.

Chapter 21
Questions 11L, 14L, 27L, 29L, and 39L.

Images generated from virtual microscopic slides contributed by the Thomas Jefferson University Virtual Slide Box

Chapter 1
Questions 5, 6, 7, 11, 12, 13, and 15.

Chapter 2
Questions 5, 6, 10, 15, 18, 20, 22, 23, and 25.

Chapter 3
Questions 23, 25, 26, and 29.

Chapter 4
Questions 9, 11, 14, 28, 29, 33, and 35.

Chapter 5
Questions 4, 15, 27, and 31.

Chapter 6
Questions 3, 12, 17, 19, and 22.

Chapter 7
Questions 9, 20, 22, 32, 33, 35, 36, 40, 46, 48, and 49.

Chapter 8
Questions 1, 2, 4, 5, 8, 28, 31, 35, and 36.

Chapter 9
Questions 3, 5, 6, 9, 10, 13, 15, 21, 22, 24, 27, 32, 34, 37, and 39.

Chapter 10
Questions 13, 14, 16, 17, 18, 22, 26, 27, 30, 33, 34, 39, 42, 43, 44, 45, 48, and 49.

Chapter 11
Questions 6, 22, 25, 28, 29, 33, 34, 35, 43, and 49.

Chapter 12
Questions 2, 8, 12, 14, 15, 17, 18, and 19.

Chapter 13
Questions 3, 7, 9, 10, 16, 17, 21, 26, 27, 29, 31, 32, 33, 36, 37, 40, 42, 46, 48, 49, and 50.

Chapter 14
Questions 19, 20, 22, 23, 25, and 27.

Chapter 15
Questions 12, 13, 16, 17, 30, 33, 35, 37, and 47.

Chapter 16
Questions 9, 13, 15, 19, 28, 34, 35, 36, 39, 40, 46, 47, and 49.

Chapter 17
Questions 5, 6, 7, 8, 9, 11, 14, 21, 22, 23, 25, 26, 36, 37, 48, and 59.

Chapter 18
Questions 1, 7, 9, 16, 22, 26, 36, 40, and 44.

Chapter 20
Questions 4, 6, 7, 8, 9, 10, 12, 13, 17, 18, 19, 20, 21, 22, 23, 25, 26, 27, 28, 31, 36, 40, 51, 56, 61, 62, 64, 65, 67, 68, 70,71, 72, 73, and 74.

Chapter 21
Questions 1, 2, 4, 6, 10L, 10R, 11R, 12L, 13L, 15L, 15R, 16L, 16R, 17L, 18L, 18R, 19L, 20L, 22L, 23L, 24L, 24R, 25L, 26L, 28L, 30L, 32L, 32R, 33L, 35L, 36L, 38L, 39R, 40L, and 40R.

Images from Rubin R, Strayer D, eds. *Rubin's Pathology: Clinicopathologic Foundations of Medicine.* 6th ed. Philadelphia, PA: Lippincott Williams & Wilkins, 2012.

Chapter 1
Questions 10, 23, 24, 25, 26, 28, and 31.

Chapter 2
Questions 27 and 28.

Chapter 3
Question 9.

Chapter 4
Questions 38 and 39.

Chapter 5
Questions 9, 13, 33, 41, and 44.

Chapter 6
Question 8.

Chapter 7
Questions 15, 25, 27, 30, and 31.

Chapter 8
Questions 10, 11, 17, 19, 25, and 26.

Chapter 9
Questions 14 and 31.

Chapter 10
Questions 19, 23, 41, and 50.

Chapter 12
Questions 3 and 16.

Chapter 13
Questions 5 and 52.

Chapter 15
Questions 20, 21, 24, and 27.

Chapter 18
Questions 19 and 47.

Chapter 19
Questions 1 and 16.

Chapter 21
Questions 3, 5, 7, 8, 9, 12R, 13R, 14R, 19R, 20R, 21L, 21R, 22R, 23R, 25R, 26R, 27R, 29R, 30R, 31L, 31R, 33R, 34L, 34R, 35R, 36R, and 38R.

Images from Fenderson BA, Strayer DS, Rubin R, et al. *Lippincott's Illustrated Q&A Review of Rubin's Pathology.* 2nd ed. Philadelphia, PA: Lippincott Williams & Wilkins, 2011.

Chapter 1
Question 9.

Chapter 5
Question 17.

Chapter 21
Questions 37L and 37R.

Images provided by David Weaver and Gyorgy Hajnoczky, Department of Pathology, Anatomy & Cell Biology, Thomas Jefferson University.

Chapter 1
Questions 16, 18, 20, and 22.

Images from Gartner L, Hiatt J. *Color Atlas of Histology.* 5th ed. Philadelphia, PA: Lippincott Williams & Wilkins, 2009.

Chapter 6
Question 5.

Chapter 7
Question 5.

Chapter 11
Question 11.

Image from Cui D. *Atlas of Histology with Functional and Clinical Correlations.* Philadelphia, PA: Lippincott Williams & Wilkins, 2011.

Chapter 11
Question 15.

Image from Bullough PG, Vigorita VJ. *Atlas of Orthopaedic Pathology.* New York: Gower Medical Publishing, 1984.

Chapter 4
Question 23.

Image from Mitros FA. *Atlas of Gastrointestinal Pathology.* New York: Gower Medical Publishing, 1988.

Chapter 13
Question 24.

Image courtesy of UBC Pulmonary Registry, St. Paul's Hospital.

Chapter 21
Question 17R.

Index